LARGE ANIMAL DERMATOLOGY

with 48 full color illustrations

Danny W. Scott, D.V.M.

Diplomate, American College of Veterinary Dermatology
Associate, American Society of Dermatopathology
Affiliate, American Academy of Dermatology
Associate Professor of Medicine
Department of Clinical Sciences
New York State College of Veterinary Medicine
Cornell University
Ithaca, New York

W. B. SAUNDERS COMPANY □ **1988**
Harcourt Brace Jovanovich, Inc.
Philadelphia London Toronto Montreal Sydney Tokyo

W. B. SAUNDERS COMPANY
Harcourt Brace Jovanovich, Inc.

West Washington Square
Philadelphia, PA 19105

Library of Congress Cataloging-in-Publication Data

Scott, Danny W.

Large animal dermatology.

Includes index.

1. Veterinary dermatology.   I. Title.

SF901.S38 1988   636.089′65   87–4936

ISBN 0–7216–8553–6

Editor: Darlene Pedersen
Designer: Karen Giacomucci
Production Manager: Bill Preston
Manuscript Editor: Gina Scala
Illustration Coordinator: Walt Verbitski
Indexer: Julie Schwager

LARGE ANIMAL DERMATOLOGY   ISBN   0–7216–8553–6

Last digit is the print number: 9   8   7   6   5   4   3   2   1

To Kris, Travis, and Tracy . . .
the real *side of life . . .*
without whom I'd be
incomplete, ineffective,
and probably intolerable

PREFACE

A few words of explanation are in order, because this book is a bit unusual. First, to my knowledge, it is the only textbook devoted exclusively to the skin and skin disorders of large (farm) animals: horses, cattle, sheep, goats, and swine. It is written from the perspective of a veterinary dermatologist and may, therefore, be less than keenly insightful in some areas of extracutaneous disease manifestations and animal husbandry.

Second, this book is, perhaps, uncommonly detailed and overly replete with references for the average textbook. Large animal dermatology has, in general, lagged behind human and small animal (dogs and cats) dermatology as concerns clinical and research interest and activities. Course time devoted to the teaching of large animal dermatology in veterinary schools has traditionally been . . . shall we say . . . "skeletal" (how about "lacking"!). Still, there is a plethora of articles scattered throughout the veterinary literature on various aspects of large animal dermatology. In addition to being widely scattered, this information is often confusing, contradictory, and anecdotal.

Thus, my burning desire was to get all the available information and references in one place, attempt to organize and summarize them, and encourage other investigators to take up the quest of discovery, clarification, repudiation, and ultimate *progress*. We are only beginning, and *much* remains to be done. My prayer is that many of you will be encouraged to critically investigate, publish, and inform veterinary medicine of your findings, so that the next edition of this book will be ever-so-much more scientific and factual.

For the present, I have tried to keep the references "out of the way," as much as possible, at the end of each chapter. In future editions of this book, we should be able to get by with reference back to this original literary depot, and a selection of current discovery and review articles.

Another area I have struggled with is terminology. The literature in large animal dermatology is adorned with a wealth of colorful and imaginative words and phrases for everything from primary and secondary skin lesions (bumps, sores, galls, sitfasts) to actual disease entities ("summer sores," "sweet itch," "mud fever," "rain scald," "strawberry foot-rot"). In addition, there are terms used to denote certain diseases (pityriasis rosea, acne, "sweating sickness") that draw upon erroneous analogies to human conditions, or inaccurate assessments of what is happening in a certain diseasse. Thus, I have attempted to name most diseases on an etiologic basis, or according to major clinical and/or pathologic features of the conditions. In some instances, I had no satisfactory nomenclature substitutes, and the diseases (and their name tags) were steeped in such history that I did not want the diseases to get lost in the science (at least not for *this* edition!). Reconsiderations and name changes will be necessary as progress in the understanding of these diseases increases.

Large animal dermatology is important! *Animal suffering*—through annoyance, irritability, pruritus, disfigurement, secondary infections, myiasis, and increased susceptibilty to other diseases—is often great. *Economic losses*—through decreased food intake, decreased weight gains or weight loss, decreased feed efficiency, decreased milk production, hide damage, wool loss, difficulties in estrus detection, death, and the financial burdens of diagnostic, therapeutic, or preventive programs—can be astronomic. *Zoonotic dermatoses*—dermatophytosis, dermatophilosis, sarcoptic mange, pseudocowpox, contagious viral pustular dermatitis—are potential sources of *human* suffering.

Well, it is now time to let this book speak for itself. I truly hope that this book can speak to everyone in veterinary medicine: academicians, practitioners, researchers, and students. Let me know what you think!

DANNY W. SCOTT

ACKNOWLEDGMENTS

Acknowledgments are difficult . . . almost as difficult as the writing of the book, itself. So many contribute to an effort like this—rendering any attempt at brevity only slightly shy of ingratitude. Having drawn attention to these inherent inadequacies, let me attempt to prioritize some ever-so-important driving forces behind this book.

1. My Lord and Savior, Jesus Christ, in whom all things are possible.
2. My wife, Kris. There were times when the task seemed just too big, when my desire was waning, when my spirit seemed close to broken, when I wanted to quit. But, Kris was always there with just the right words, just the right look, just the right encouragement to remotivate me. As much as myself, *Kris* finished this book.
3. My "employer," the New York State College of Veterinary Medicine at Cornell University. I have been blessed with a very enthusiastic, supportive clinical and academic environment, not to mention the natural beauty and peace of Ithaca, New York, where I can also *forget* about veterinary medicine and try to ponder and live the more important things in life.
4. My colleagues in the Large Animal and Ambulatory Clinics—especially Bill Rebhun, Mary Smith, Steve Dill, and Chuck Guard—who have humored me in my dermatologic dabblings over the years, and so facilitated and encouraged my participation in our large animal practice. Thanks, gang! I couldn't have done it without you!
5. My favorite veterinary pathologist, John King, who has always encouraged, supported, and challenged me and who supplied me with several lovely pictures and specimens.
6. Three outstanding investigators and teachers in large animal dermatology— Tony Stannard, Bill McMullan, Reg Pascoe—who have been not only informative but also inspirational to me.
7. Two lovely ladies—Sue Hubert and Joyce Reyna—who worked extremely hard in typing the manuscript.

Thanks, gang. This book belongs to *all* of us.

CONTENTS

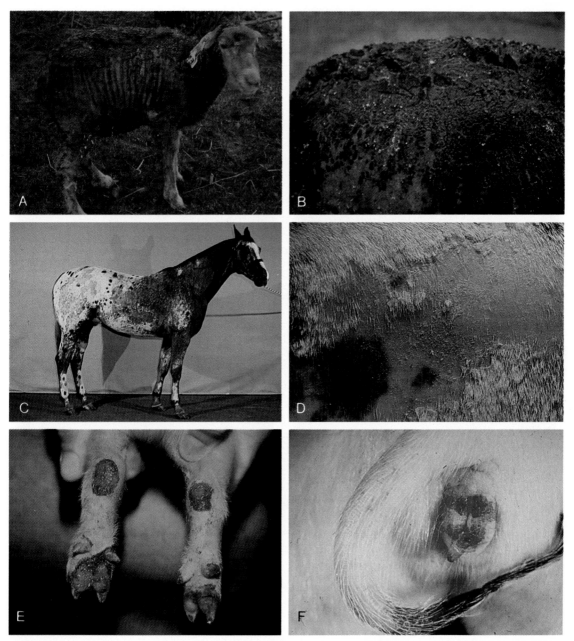

PLATE I. A, *Third-degree burns in a sheep caught in a barn fire (Courtesy M. C. Smith).* B, *Same sheep as in A. Note alopecia and "charcoaling" of skin (Courtesy M. C. Smith).* C, *Severe contact dermatitis in a horse after application of motor oil.* D, *Same horse as in C. Note alopecia, erythema, scaling, and erosions.* E, *Porcine skin necrosis. Note ulcers on hocks and feet (Courtesy R. D. Cameron).* F, *Porcine skin necrosis. Note ulcers on vulva and necrosis of distal tail (Courtesy R. D. Cameron).*

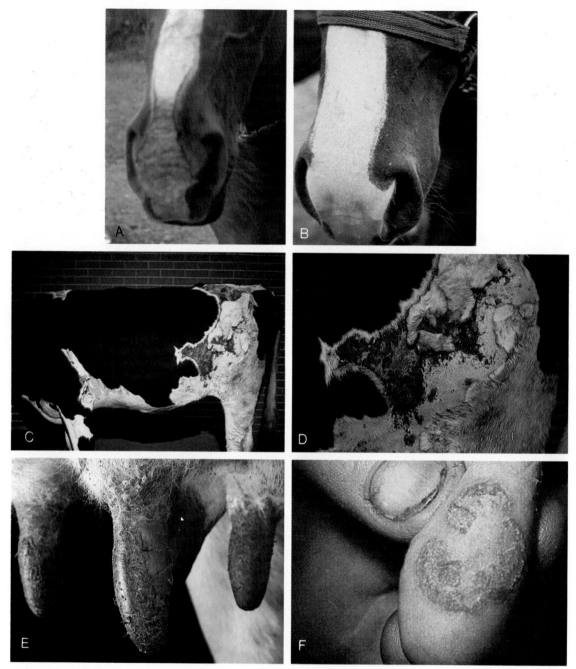

PLATE II. A, Hepatic photosensitization in a horse. Note erythema of muzzle. B, Photosensitization in association with dermatophilosis. Note erythema and crusting of muzzle. C, Hepatic photosensitization in a cow. Skin lesions are limited to white areas. D, Same cow as in C. Note sloughing, ulceration, alopecia, and erythema. E, Hepatic photosensitization in a cow. Note necrosis, sloughing, and ulceration of teats. F, Pseudocowpox in a cow. Note characteristic "horseshoe" crust (Courtesy P. Eyre).

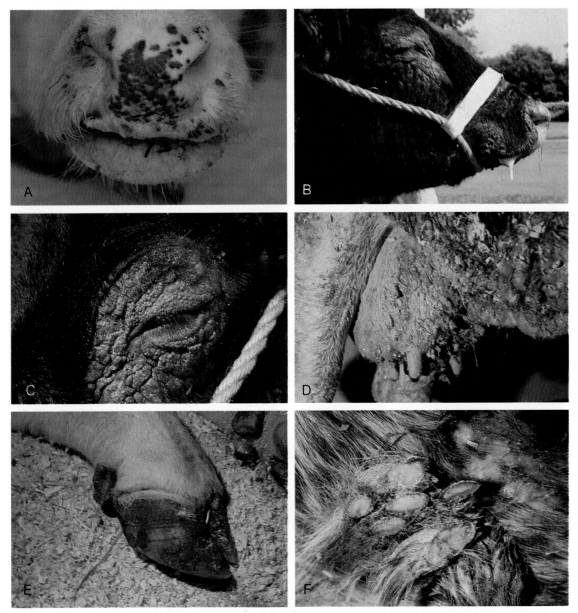

PLATE III. A, Bovine papular stomatitis. Note papules on lips. B, Malignant catarrhal fever. Note erythema and crusting around eye and on nose. C, Malignant catarrhal fever. Erythema and crusting around eye. D, Malignant catarrhal fever. Severe erythema and crusting of udder and ventrum. E, Malignant catarrhal fever. Note coronitis. F, Dermatophilosis in a horse. Note typical "paintbrush" crusts with adherent greenish pus.

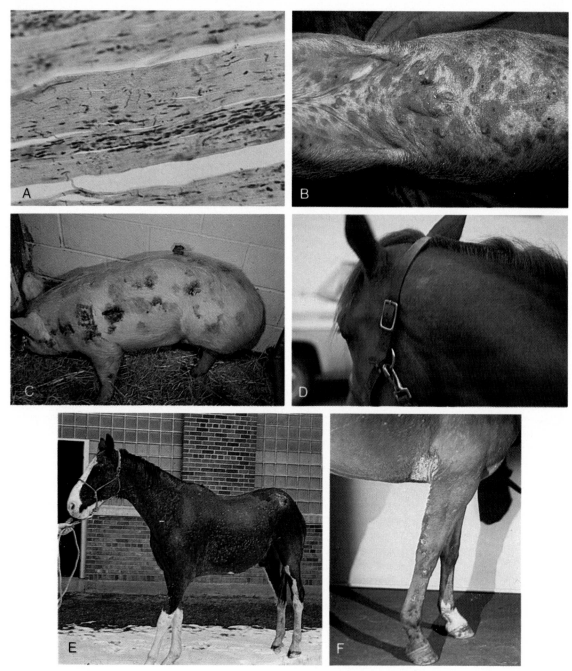

PLATE IV. A, Dermatophilus congolensis *in an AOG-stained crust.* B, Erysipelas in a pig. Erythematous papules and plaques, some of which show central necrosis (Courtesy R. D. Cameron). C, Chronic erysipelas in a pig. Rectangular and diamond-shaped areas of necrosis over entire body. D, Dermatophytosis due to Microsporum canis *in a horse.* Note patchy alopecia caudal to halter. E, Generalized alopecia due to Tricophyton equinum *in a horse.* F, Dermatophytosis in a horse due to T. equinum. Note annular areas of alopecia and crusting on chest and leg.

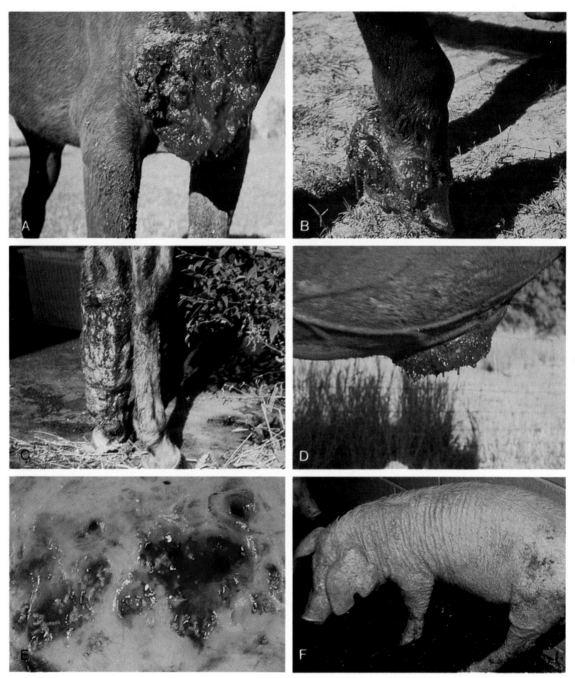

PLATE V. A, Basidiobolomycosis in a horse. Note large ulcerative granuloma on chest *(Courtesy R. Miller)*. B, Pythiosis in a horse. Ulcerative granuloma on the pastern *(Courtesy R. Miller)*. C, Pythiosis in a horse. Ulcerative granuloma involving entire metatarsal area *(Courtesy R. Miller)*. D, Pythiosis in a horse. Ulcerative granuloma on ventral abdomen *(Courtesy R. Miller)*. E, Pythiosis. Numerous coral-like "leeches" in necrotic sinuses *(Courtesy R. Miller)*. F, Generalized erythema and lichenification in a pig with chronic sarcoptic mange *(Courtesy R. D. Cameron)*.

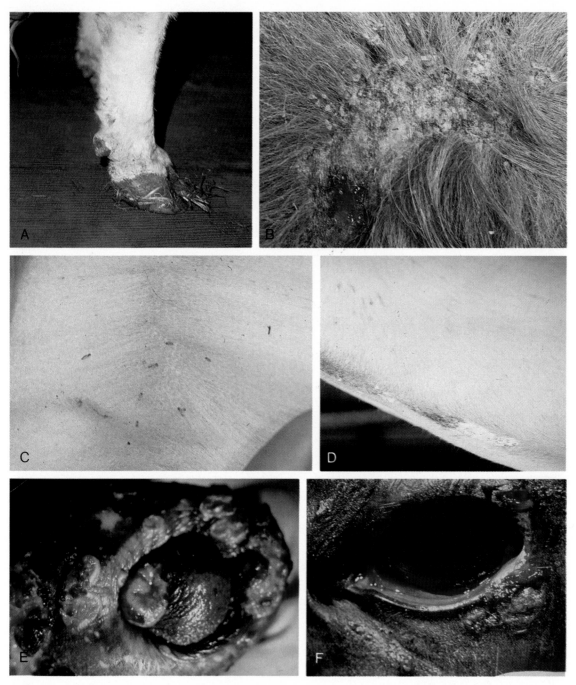

PLATE VI. A, *Chorioptic mange in a cow. Erythema and alopecia on the pastern of a hind foot.* B, *Pediculosis in a horse. Note lice, crusts, and focal excoriation.* C, *Pediculosis in a sheep. Note lice and scaling.* D, *Ventral midline dermatitis in a horse. Note linear alopecia, crusting, and hyperpigmentation.* E, *Habronemiasis in a horse. Multiple ulcerated papules with granular surface on prepuce.* F, *Habronemiasis in a horse. Multiple ulcerated, crusted papules on eyelid and conjunctiva (Courtesy T. J. Kern).*

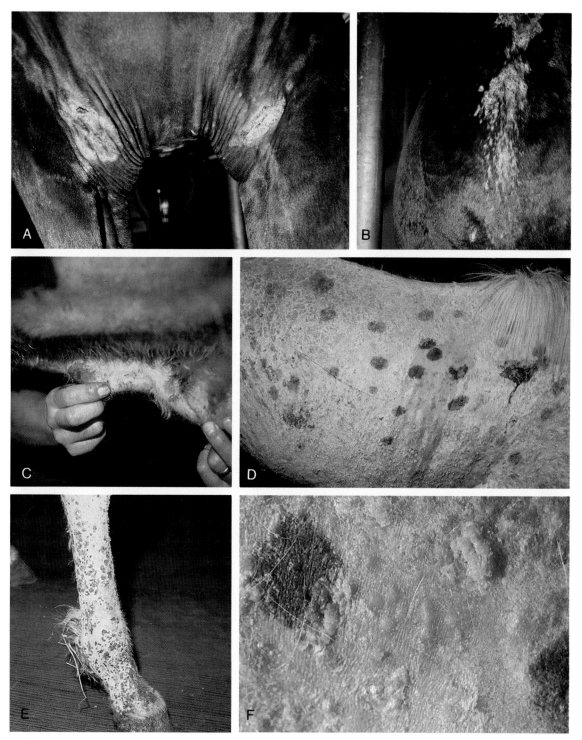

PLATE VII. A, *Onchocerciasis in a horse. Alopecic, crusted, hypopigmented plaques in the axillary regions.* B, *Onchocerciasis in a horse. Widespread alopecia and inflammation on the ventrum.* C, *Stephanofilariasis in a cow. Alopecia, erythema, and crusting of the ventrum.* D, *Pemphigus foliaceus in a horse. Generalized alopecia, crusting, and erythema.* E, *Same horse as in D. Alopecia, crusting, and erythema of the legs.* F, *Same horse as in D and E. Intact vesicles on the thorax.*

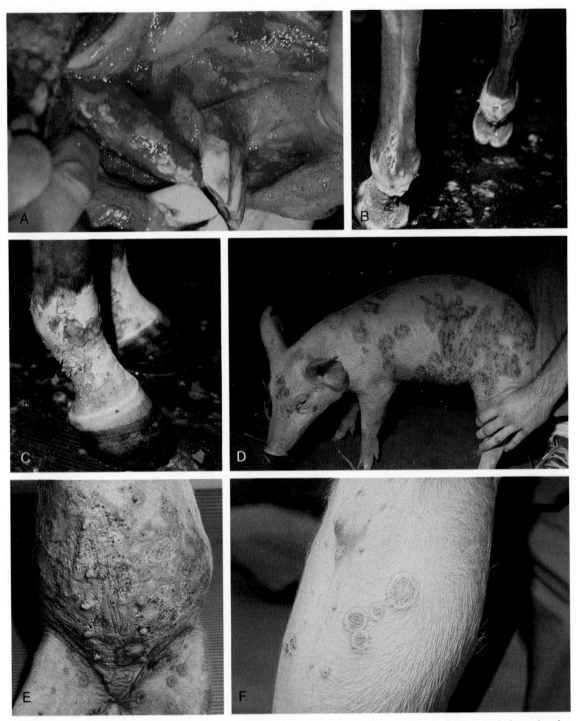

PLATE VIII. A, *Bullous pemphigoid in a horse. Ulcerative stomatitis.* B, *Vasculitis in a horse. Erythema and alopecia of the pasterns.* C, *Same horse as in B. Erythema, necrosis, and alopecia.* D, *Porcine juvenile pustular and psoriasiform dermatitis. Annular areas of erythema and crusting.* E, *Porcine juvenile pustular and psoriasiform dermatitis. Erythematous plaques with central "branlike" scales and crusts.* F, *Porcine juvenile pustular and psoriasiform dermatitis. Annular plaques with central "branlike" scales and crusts.*

CHAPTER 1

STRUCTURE AND FUNCTION OF THE SKIN

What a glorious organ it is! The skin, the largest organ in the body, is the anatomic and physiologic barrier between animal and environment. It provides protection from physical, chemical, and microbiologic injury, and its sensory components perceive heat, cold, pain, pruritus, touch, and pressure. In addition, the skin is synergistic with internal organ systems and, thus, reflects pathologic processes that either are primary elsewhere or are shared with other tissues. Not only is the skin an organ with its own reaction patterns, but also it is a mirror, reflecting the *milieu interieur* and, at the same time, the capricious world to which it is exposed.

Common parlance reflects the unique significance of the skin in the life of contemporary man:

> Skin is synonymous with "life" in the phrase "to save my skin"; human sensibilities are measured by "thin-skinned" or "thick-skinned"; a shallow person is "skin deep," and a miser is a "skin-flint"; a friendly greeting is "give me a little skin," and an unfriendly feeling is "skin him alive"; relief is expressed by "the skin of my teeth," unconcern by "no skin off my back," and annoyance by "getting under my skin," and nude swimming is "skinny dipping."[320]

Considerable histologic and histochemical information on the skin of large animals, especially swine,* has shown that significant species differences exist. In addition, these data, along with percutaneous absorption studies,† have shown that the skin of the domestic pig has morphologic and functional characteristics comparable with those of humans. Thus, porcine skin is commonly used as an experimental model for investigations of human skin.[152, 171–179, 181, 182]

*References 11, 75, 193–196, 222, 223, 285, 290–300, 309–311, 328, 349, 451–453, 454, 486, 494
†References 31, 62, 77, 161, 162, 188, 285, 298, 361, 470

GENERAL FUNCTIONS OF THE SKIN

The general functions of the skin have been modified to apply to animal skin as follows:*

Enclosing Barrier. The most important function of the skin is to make possible an internal environment for all other organs by maintaining an effective barrier to the loss of water, electrolytes, and macromolecules.

Environmental Protection. A corollary function is the exclusion of external injurious agents—chemical, physical, and microbiologic—from entrance into the internal environment.

Sensory Perception. The skin is the prime sense organ for touch, pressure, pain, itch, heat, and cold.

Temperature Regulation. The skin plays a role in the regulation of body temperature through its support of hair coat, regulation of cutaneous blood supply, and sweat gland function.

Motion and Shape. The flexibility, elasticity, and toughness of the skin allow motion and provide shape and form.

Adnexa Production. The skin produces keratinized structures such as hair, hooves, horn, and the horny layer of the epidermis.

Storage. The skin is an important reservoir of water, electrolytes, vitamins, fat, carbohydrates, protein, and other materials.

Secretion. The skin is a secretory organ by virtue of its apocrine and sebaceous glands.

Excretion. The skin functions in a limited way as an excretory organ.

Blood Pressure Control. Changes in the peripheral vascular bed affect blood pressure.

Pigmentation. Processes in the skin (melanin formation, vascularity, and keratinization) help determine the coat and skin color. Pigmentation of the skin helps prevent damage from solar radiation.

*References 57, 122, 184–188, 311, 322, 369, 425, 433

Antimicrobial Action. The skin surface has antibacterial and antifungal properties.

Immunoregulation. Keratinocytes, Langerhans's cells, and lymphocytes together provide the skin with an immunosurveillance capability that effectively prejudices against the development of cutaneous neoplasms and persistent infections.[433]

Indicator. The skin may be an important indicator of general health and the effects of medicine taken internally.

ONTOGENY

The embryology of the skin has been studied in sheep,* cattle,[191, 260, 261] goats,[27, 472] and swine.[127, 163, 302, 399] Initially, the embryonic skin consists of a single layer of ectodermal cells and a dermis containing loosely arranged mesenchymal cells embedded in ground (interstitial) substance. The ectodermal covering progressively develops into two layers (the basal cell layer, or stratum germinativum, and the outer periderm), three layers (the stratum intermedium forms between the other two layers), and then into an adult-like structure. Melanocytes and Langerhans's cells become identifiable during this period of ectodermal maturation.

Dermal development is characterized by increasing thickness and numbers of fibers, decreasing ground substance, and the transition of mesenchymal cells into fibroblasts. Elastin fibers appear later than collagen fibers. Histiocytes, Schwann's cells, and dermal melanocytes also become recognizable. In humans, fetal skin contains a large percentage of Type III collagen, in contrast with the skin of the adult, which contains a large proportion of Type I collagen.[240, 303] Fat cells (adipocytes, lipocytes) begin to develop in the subcutis from spindle-shaped mesenchymal precursor cells in the second half of gestation.

The embryonal stratum germinativum differentiates into hair germs (primary epithelial germs), which give rise to hair follicles, sebaceous glands, and apocrine sweat glands. Hair germs initially consist of an area of crowding of deeply basophilic cells in the basal layer of the epidermis. Subsequently, the areas of crowding become buds that protrude into the dermis. Beneath each bud lies a group of mesenchymal cells, from which the dermal hair papilla is later formed.

As the hair germ lengthens and develops into hair follicle and hair, three bulges appear. The lowest of the bulges develops into the attachment for the arrector pili muscle; the middle bulge differentiates into the sebaceous gland; the uppermost bulge evolves into the apocrine sweat gland. These appendages develop on the ental side of primary hair follicles, while secondary hair follicles develop on the opposite or ectal side.

Eccrine gland germs also begin as areas of crowding of deeply basophilic cells in the basal layer of the epidermis. They initially differ from hair germs only slightly, by being narrower and by showing fewer mesenchymal cells at their base.

GROSS ANATOMY AND PHYSIOLOGY

At each body orifice, skin is continuous with the mucous membrane located there (digestive, respiratory, ocular, or urogenital). The skin and hair coat vary in quantity and quality between species, breeds within a species, and individuals within a breed; from one area to another on the body; and according to age and sex.

In general, skin thickness decreases dorsally to ventrally on the trunk and proximally to distally on the limbs.* The skin is thickest on the forehead, dorsal neck, dorsal thorax, and base of the tail. It is thinnest on the pinnae and the axillary, inguinal, and perianal areas. The reported average thickness of the general body skin of adult large animals is as follows: horse, 3.8 mm;[444, 450] cow, 6.0 mm;[2, 7, 133, 136, 450] sheep, 2.6 mm;[70, 232, 263, 450] goat, 2.9 mm;[385, 450] and pig, 2.2 mm.[271, 450]

Hair is characteristic of mammals and is important in thermal insulation and sensory perception and as a barrier against chemical and physical injury to the skin.[41, 95, 158, 311, 425] The ability of the hair coat to regulate body temperature correlates closely with length, thickness, and medullation of individual hair fibers.† In general, hair coats composed of short, thick, medullated fibers are most efficient at high environmental temperatures. Conversely, hair coats composed of long, fine, poorly medullated fibers, with coat depth in-

---

*References 27, 128, 131, 151, 168, 178, 259, 266, 279, 372, 380, 428, 429, 479

*References 136, 191, 232, 263, 271, 309, 311, 404, 444
†References 81–83, 85, 95, 158, 392, 426, 455, 456, 482, 483, 489, 490

creased by piloerection, are most efficient for thermal insulation at low environmental temperatures.[42, 365, 366, 393, 456] In addition, coat color is of some importance in thermal regulation, with light-colored coats being more efficient in hot, sunny weather.[43, 158, 232, 363] Primary (guard, outercoat, kemp) and larger secondary (undercoat) hairs are medullated.* Smaller secondary hairs in goats are nonmedullated (lanugo hairs). Secondary hairs are more numerous than primary hairs in the goat and sheep (3:1 to 25:1).[126, 191, 380–382, 401]

In sheep and Angora goats, there are three main kinds of hair fibers.[47, 147, 346, 380] *True* wool fibers are fine, tightly crimped, and usually nonmedullated. *Kemp* fibers are very coarse, poorly crimped, fairly short in length, and heavily medullated. *Hair* fibers are intermediate between wool and kemp fibers. Kemp fibers are undesirable in good wool because the large medulla causes brittleness and leaves little solid substance to take up dye. In general, sheep have wool on the trunk and hair on the extremities.

Hair Cycle

Hairs do not grow continuously, but in cycles. Each cycle consists of a growing period (anagen), during which the follicle is actively producing the hair, and a resting period (telogen), when the hair is retained in the follicle as a dead, or "club," hair that is subsequently lost. There is also a transitional period (catagen) between these two stages.

The hair cycle, and thus the hair coat, are controlled by photoperiod, ambient temperature, nutrition, hormones, general state of health, genetics, and poorly understood "intrinsic factors."† Hair replacement in the goat, sheep, cow, and horse is mosaic in pattern, is unaffected by castration, and responds predominantly to photoperiod and, possibly, ambient temperature.‡ Two exceptions to this are (1) the wool follicles of most sheep, in which virtually no cyclic activity occurs, and (2) the coarse permanent hairs of the equine mane, tail, and fetlock ("horsehairs"). Normal goats, cattle, and horses in temperate latitudes such as the northern United States may shed noticeably in the spring and fall.[95, 96, 242, 382, 383, 401]

Hair follicle activity is maximal in summer and minimal in winter. In winter, up to 100 percent of the primary hair follicles and 50 percent of the secondary hair follicles are in telogen.

Because hair is predominantly protein, nutrition has a profound effect on its quality and quantity (see Chapter 12, discussion on protein deficiency).* Poor nutrition may produce a dull, dry, brittle, or thin hair coat and may result in retention of the winter coat in cattle and horses.

Under conditions of ill health or generalized disease, anagen may be considerably shortened. Accordingly, a large percentage of body hairs may be in telogen at one time. Telogen hairs tend to be more easily lost, so the animal may shed excessively. Disease states may also lead to faulty formation of hair cuticle, resulting in a dull, lusterless hair coat. Severe illness (e.g., septicemia and marked pyrexia) or systemic stress (e.g., pregnancy and parturition) may cause many hair follicles to enter into telogen synchronously and precipitously. Thus, shedding of these hairs (telogen defluxion) occurs simultaneously, often resulting in visible thinning of the hair coat or actual alopecia. In sheep, excessive amounts of glucocorticoids, exogenous or endogenous (e.g., stresses associated with injury or disease), are associated with a "tender" fleece and "wool-break."[115]

The hair cycle and hair coat are also affected by hormonal changes.[87, 115, 154, 322, 371, 380, 466] Anagen is initiated and advanced and hair growth rate is accelerated by thyroid hormones (see Chapter 13, discussion on hypothyroidism).† Conversely, excessive amounts of glucocorticoids inhibit anagen, suppress hair growth rate, and produce a tender fleece in sheep (wool-break) (see Chapter 13, discussion on hyperadrenocorticism).[87, 115, 246]

The skin surfaces of haired mammals are, in general, acidic.[92, 198, 206] In cattle, skin surface pH varies between different body regions and tends to be lower on the ventrum (5.40) compared with the rump (5.75). Physiologic changes have a greater influence on skin surface pH than do changes in ambient temperature. The skin surface pH of cattle is not significantly different at different times of the day or on different days of the week.[198] The skin surface pH of the horse was reported to range between 4.8 and 6.8 and to increase to as much as 7.9 with sweating.[233]

---

*References 41, 47, 105, 126, 136, 147, 191, 232, 263, 271, 309, 311, 380, 381, 385, 444
†References 34, 35, 48, 66, 68, 72, 87, 95, 96, 114, 115, 169, 212, 237, 326, 342, 371, 380, 384, 407–411, 457
‡References 33, 37, 41, 84, 95, 96, 154–158, 169, 170, 190, 230, 319, 379–383, 410, 435, 480–483, 489, 490

---

*References 48, 72, 86, 115, 158, 168, 237, 347, 362, 368, 373–375, 380, 384, 388, 412, 484, 491
†References 36, 87, 96, 135, 227, 270, 281, 371

MICROSCOPIC ANATOMY AND PHYSIOLOGY

The microanatomy of the skin has been the subject of several studies in horses,[105, 413, 436, 444, 450] cattle,[76, 105, 136, 326, 450] sheep,* goats,[105, 272, 273, 385, 401, 450] and swine.†

Epidermis

The outer layer of the skin, or epidermis, is composed of multiple layers of cells ranging from columnar to flat. These are of four distinct types: keratinocytes, melanocytes, Langerhans's cells, and Merkel's cells. For purposes of identification, certain areas of the epidermis are classified as layers and are named, from within outward, as follows: basal layer (stratum basale), spinous layer (stratum spinosum, "prickle cell" layer), granular layer (stratum granulosum), clear layer (stratum lucidum), and horny layer (stratum corneum). The thickness of the epidermis in hairy skin ranges from 30 to 95 µm in horses, 16 to 145 µm in cattle, 27 to 42 µm in sheep, and 20 to 40 µm in goats. The epidermis is thickest where hair covering is sparsest.

Basal Layer

The basal layer is a single row of columnar to cuboidal cells resting on the basement membrane that separates the epidermis from the dermis.‡ Most of these cells are keratinocytes, but a few are melanocytes (about one melanocyte per every 10 to 20 keratinocytes). The keratinocytes are constantly reproducing and pushing upward to replenish the epidermal cells above. The daughter cells move into the outer layers of the epidermis and are ultimately shed as dead horny cells. Mitotic figures are occasionally seen in the basal layer, especially in areas of skin with thicker epidermis (e.g., muzzle, mucocutaneous areas, and coronet).

Melanocytes and Melanogenesis. Melanocytes, the second type of cell found in the basal layer of the epidermis,§ are also found in the outer root sheath and the hair matrix of hair follicles, the ducts of sebaceous and sweat glands, and perivascularly in the superficial

---

*References 51, 76, 105, 232, 262, 263, 272, 450
†References 105, 217, 241, 242, 271, 309, 321, 415, 450
‡References 105, 136, 232, 241, 263, 271–273, 385, 415, 444
§References 8, 123, 124, 186, 217, 228, 232, 263, 264, 271, 309, 385, 394, 395, 415, 444, 488.

dermis. Since melanocytes do not stain readily with hematoxylin and eosin (H & E) and because they undergo artifactual cytoplasmic shrinkage during tissue processing, they appear as "clear cells." They are derived from the neural crest and migrate into the epidermis in early fetal life. Although melanocytes are of nondescript appearance, with special stains (dopa reaction; Fontana's ammoniacal silver nitrate) they can be shown to have long cytoplasmic extensions (dendrites) that weave among the keratinocytes. Ultrastructurally, melanocytes are characterized by typical intracytoplasmic melanosomes and premelanosomes and a cell membrane–associated basal lamina. Most of the melanin pigment in skin is located in the basal layer of the epidermis, but in dark-skinned animals, melanin may be found throughout the entire epidermis as well as within superficial dermal melanocytes.

Melanin pigments are chiefly responsible for the coloration of skin and hair. Melanins embrace a wide range of pigments, including the brown-black eumelanins, yellow or red-brown phaeomelanins, and other pigments whose physiochemical natures are intermediate between the two. Despite the different properties of the various melanins, they all arise from a common metabolic pathway in which dopaquinone is the key intermediate.[231, 239, 351] Tyrosine is converted to dopa, which is then oxidized to dopaquinone. Both reactions are catalyzed by the same copper-containing enzyme, tyrosinase. Melanin formation is under the control of genetics and melanocyte-stimulating hormone (MSH) from the pituitary gland. In addition, ultraviolet light and inflammation increase the production of melanin locally in affected skin.

Melanogenesis takes place in membrane-bound organelles called melanosomes,[123, 186, 240, 353] designated Types I through IV according to maturation. Melanosomes originate from the Golgi apparatus, where the tyrosinase enzyme is formed. Type I melanosomes contain no melanin and are electron-lucent. As melanin is progressively laid down on protein matrices, melanosomes become increasingly electron-dense. At the same time, they migrate to the periphery of the dendrites, where transfer of melanin to adjacent epidermal cells takes place. Transfer involves the endocytosis of the tips of the dendrites, and incorporated Type IV melanosomes, by the adjacent keratinocytes. Dermal melanocytes are often referred to as "continent" melanocytes, because they do not transfer melanosomes like the epidermal, or "secretory," melanocytes. Skin color is determined mainly by the number, size, type, and distribution of melanosomes. Melanins not only are responsible for coloration but also play important roles in photoprotection and free-radical scavenging.[122, 123, 186, 240] Studies have indicated that white Merino sheep fail to tan in response to ultraviolet light exposure, making them potentially vulnerable to the many damaging effects of ultraviolet light.[125]

Langerhans's Cells. Langerhans's cells are mononuclear dendritic cells located in the epidermis, from the stratum basale to the stratum spinosum.* These cells are epidermal clear cells that resemble melanocytes but do not stain for melanin with dopa. The cells have characteristic intracytoplasmic organelles on electron microscopic examination. These organelles, called Langerhans's or Birbeck's granules, often have a tennis racquet–like appearance. Langerhans's cells are aureophilic, have Fc-IgG and C3 receptors, and serve antigen-processing and alloantigen-stimulating functions. They are of bone marrow origin.

Merkel's Cells. Merkel's cells are epidermal clear cells confined to the stratum basale of the tylotrich pads.† These cells function as slow-adapting mechanoreceptors. They possess desmosomes and characteristic dense-core cytoplasmic granules on electron microscopic examination and may be of neural crest or keratinocyte origin. Merkel's cells have been shown to possess neuron-specific enolase, suggesting that they may belong to the diffuse neuroendrocrine amine precursor uptake and carboxylation (APUD) system.[146]

Basement Membrane Zone. The basement membrane zone is the physiochemical interface between the epidermis and the dermis. This zone is often poorly differentiated in hematoxylin and eosin preparations but stains nicely with periodic acid–Schiff (PAS).‡ The basement membrane zone is most prominent in the horse. By light microscopy, the basement membrane zone comprises only the fibrous zone of the sub-basal lamina and is about 20 times thicker than the actual basal lamina. Ultrastructurally, the basement membrane zone is composed of four components: (1) the basal cell plasma membrane, (2) the lamina lucida, (3) the basal lamina, and (4) the sub-basal lamina fibrous components.[50]

In all large animals except the pig, the undersurface of the epidermis is smoothly undulating and roughly parallel to the skin surface. In pigs and humans, this dermoepidermal junction is thrown into distinct folds called rete ridges. In horses, cattle, sheep, and goats, rete ridges are usually found only in glabrous (nonhaired) areas of normal skin; they are found in haired skin areas as a result of pathologic processes.

Spinous Layer

The stratum spinosum is composed of the daughter cells of the basal layer. In haired skin, this layer is two to four cells thick and is composed of lightly basophilic to eosinophilic, nucleated, polyhedral to flattened cuboidal cells.* It is much thicker where the hair coat is thinner or absent. The keratinocytes of the stratum spinosum appear to be connected by fine intercellular bridges (prickles). Ultrastructurally, keratinocytes are characterized by tonofilaments and desmosomes.[93, 140, 405, 406]

Granular Layer

The stratum granulosum is variably present in haired skin, ranging from one to three cells thick in most areas where it occurs.† In nonhaired skin or at the infundibulum of hair follicles, the granular layer may be several cells thick. Cells in this layer are flattened (parallel to the surface) and basophilic and contain shrunken nuclei and large, deeply basophilic keratohyalin granules. The function of keratohyalin granules is incompletely understood but is thought to be concerned with keratinization and barrier function.[184, 286, 311] Bovine keratohyalin granules have been extensively studied by biochemical, histochemical, ultrastructural, and immunologic techniques.[103, 104, 148, 458–462] Studies indicate that keratohyalin (1) is synthesized rapidly in cytoplasm, (2) concentrates histidine, arginine, serine, and glycine, and (3) is synthesized as a monomer, with orderly polymerization to higher molecular weight species.

Clear Layer

The stratum lucidum is a fully keratinized, compact thin layer of dead cells.‡ This layer is

---

*References 164, 186, 220, 240, 312, 313, 448
†References 49, 111, 186, 240, 247, 265, 269, 430, 432
‡References 136, 191, 232, 263, 271, 385, 401, 437, 444, 445

---

*References 136, 217, 232, 240, 241, 263, 271, 385, 401, 444
†References 136, 217, 232, 242, 263, 271, 385, 401, 444
‡References 136, 191, 232, 263, 271, 309, 354, 385, 401, 444

anuclear, homogeneous, and hyalin-like and contains refractile droplets (eleidin). The stratum lucidum is rarely, if ever, seen in haired skin. It has been described in sheep (muzzle, lip, and coronet), cattle (coronet and perianal area), goats (muzzle and coronet), and swine (snout).

Horny Layer

The stratum corneum is the outer layer of completely keratinized tissue that is constantly being shed. This layer, consisting of flattened anuclear, eosinophilic cells, is thicker in lightly haired or glabrous skin.* Its gradual desquamation normally is balanced by proliferation of the basal cells, which maintains a constant epidermal thickness.

The living epidermis and stratum corneum of haired skin from cattle and sheep were studied in frozen sections.[250, 251] In cattle, both the living epidermis and stratum corneum were found to be about 30 μm thick, with the stratum corneum containing about 30 cell layers and the living epidermis containing only 4. In sheep, the stratum corneum was found to be about 31 μm thick, and the living epidermis about 17 μm thick. Clipping and histologic processing involving fixation, dehydration, and paraffin embedding resulted in the loss of half of the stratum corneum and proved unsuitable for study of this layer.[250, 251, 253]

The structure of the stratum corneum was found to be very different in cattle and sheep.[250, 251] Only the densely packed columnar structure of the proximal half of the ovine stratum corneum is similar to that of the bovine. The distal layers in the sheep are found separating from the basal region in an apparently disorganized and haphazard manner.

Epidermal lipid was restricted to the stratum corneum, the surfaces of the hairs, and the sebaceous glands in cattle and sheep.[200, 250, 251] In the stratum corneum of cattle, the lipid was found in layers between the cornified cells. Lipid was present on the epidermal surface in an apparently irregular distribution, often in the form of globules and leaving much of the cornified layer exposed. No lipid was found in the basal layers of the stratum corneum or in the living epidermis or the sweat glands. The distribution and histochemistry of the lipid indicated that the sebaceous gland is the major source and that it represents an emulsion of sebum and sweat.

The distribution of lipid within the stratum corneum of sheep was quite different from that in cattle. In sheep, the lipid permeated the entire stratum corneum and apparently formed a film over the skin surface approximately 9 μm thick.

Epidermopoiesis and Keratogenesis. The most important product of the epidermis is the highly stable, disulfide bond–containing fibrous protein, keratin. This substance is the major barrier between animal and environment, the literal "Miracle Wrap" of the body. Prekeratin, the fibrous protein synthesized in the keratinocytes of the stratum basale and stratum spinosum, appears to be the precursor of the fully differentiated stratum corneum proteins.[30, 238]

The epidermis is ectodermal in origin and normally undergoes an orderly pattern of differentiation and keratinization. The factors controlling epidermal differentiation and keratinization are incompletely understood.* Among the intrinsic factors known to play a modulating role in these processes are the dermis, epidermal growth factor, epidermal chalone, calmodulin, and various hormones, particularly epinephrine and cortisol.† Recent work suggests that adrenergic agents and prostaglandins operate through their second messenger, cyclic adenosine monophosphate (cAMP), to regulate epidermal metabolic activity and proliferation.[20, 171–179, 229, 340] In addition, there appears to be a host of hormones and enzymes that can either or both induce and increase the activity of the enzyme ornithine decarboxylase. This enzyme is essential for the biosynthesis of polyamines (putrescine, spermidine, and spermine), which encourage epidermal cell proliferation. Numerous nutritional factors are also known to be important for normal keratinization, including protein, fatty acids, zinc, copper, vitamin A, and B vitamins.

As keratinocytes leave the stratum basale and move upwards within the epidermis they undergo changes not only in shape and orientation but also in their cytoplasmic structure and composition, which eventually lead to the transformation of viable, actively synthesizing cells into the dead, cornified cells of the stratum corneum. Basal keratinocytes are cuboidal to columnar in shape, whereas those of the stratum spinosum are polyhedral, those of the

---

*References 6, 136, 232, 242, 263, 271, 309, 385, 401, 444

*References 122, 153, 184, 223–225, 311, 364, 369, 425
†References 21–25, 134, 150, 165, 176, 288, 314–317, 344, 345

stratum granulosum are elliptic, and those of the stratum corneum are flattened, anuclear, cornified lamellae.

Modern research in epidermal cellular and molecular biology recognizes four distinct cellular events in the process of cornification: (1) keratinization (synthesis of the principal fibrous proteins of the keratinocyte), (2) keratohyalin synthesis (also referred to as histidine-rich protein, stratum corneum basic protein, or filaggrin), (3) formation of the highly cross-linked, insoluble stratum corneum peripheral envelope (involucrin is a protein precursor of this structure), and (4) generation of neutral lipid-enriched intercellular domains, resulting from the secretion of distinctive structures called keratinosomes (lamellar bodies, membrane-coating granules, Odland's bodies, or cementosomes).[101, 102, 130, 217, 240] The keratinosomes are synthesized primarily within the keratinocytes of the stratum spinosum and are then displaced to the apex and periphery of the cell as it reaches the stratum granulosum. They fuse with the plasma membrane and secrete their contents (neutral sugars linked to either or both lipids and proteins; hydrolytic enzymes; and free sterols). Intercellular lipids then undergo substantial alterations and assume an integral role in the regulation of stratum corneum barrier function and desquamation.

Cutaneous Ecology. The skin forms a protective barrier without which life would be impossible. This defense has three components: physical, chemical, and microbial.[335, 336] Hair forms the first physical line of defense to prevent contact of pathogens with the skin and to minimize external physical or chemical insult to the skin. Hair may also harbor microorganisms.

The stratum corneum forms the basic physical defense barrier. Its thick, tightly packed keratinized cells are permeated by an emulsion of sebum and sweat. This emulsion, concentrated in the outer layers of keratin, also functions as a physical barrier. In addition to its physical properties, the emulsion provides a chemical barrier to potential pathogens.* Fatty acids, especially linoleic acid, have antibacterial and antifungal properties. Water-soluble substances in the emulsion include inorganic salts and proteins that inhibit microorganisms. Sodium chloride and the antiviral glycoprotein interferon, albumin, transferrin, complement, glucocorticoid, and immunoglob-

ulins are present in the emulsion. Immunoglobulins A, G, and M have been demonstrated on the skin surface of cattle and sheep.[201, 249] In addition, studies on the distribution of immunoglobulins in the normal skin of cattle and sheep have shown the following: (1) IgA is present in the intercellular substance of epidermis and in sweat gland ducts, (2) IgG is present in the intercellular substance of epidermis, in the dermis, and in the endothelial cells of blood vessels, and (3) IgM is present in the basement membrane zone, in hair papillae, and in the walls of dermal blood vessels.[254]

The single factor with the greatest influence on the flora is the degree of hydration of the stratum corneum.[335, 336] Increasing the quantity of water at the skin surface (increased ambient temperature, increased relative humidity, or occlusion) enormously increases the number of microorganisms. In general, the moist or greasy areas of the skin support the greatest populations of microorganisms.

The normal skin microflora also contributes to skin defense.[335, 336] Bacteria and, occasionally, yeasts and filamentous fungi are located in the superficial epidermis (especially the intercellular spaces) and the infundibulum of hair follicles.[250–252, 335, 336] The normal flora is a mixture of bacteria that live in symbiosis. The flora may change with different cutaneous environments, which include such factors as pH, salinity, moisture, albumin level, and fatty acid level. The close relationship between the host and the microorganisms enables bacteria to occupy microbial niches and inhibit colonization by invading organisms.

Some organisms are believed to live and multiply on the skin, forming a permanent population; these are known as residents, and they may be reduced in number by degerming methods but not eliminated.[335, 336] The resident skin flora is not spread out evenly over the surface but is aggregated in microcolonies of various sizes. Other microorganisms are merely contaminants acquired from the environment, can be removed by simple hygienic measures, and are called transients.

In humans, evidence points to a number of sites for microbial growth.[252, 335, 336] Hair follicles have populations of *Propionibacterium* deep in the follicle and *Staphylococcus* and *Malassezia* (*Pityrosporon*) nearer the surface. Coagulase-negative staphylococci, coryneforms (diphtheroids, *Brevibacterium*, and *Corynebacterium*), *Micrococcus* spp., *Peptococcus* spp., and *Acinetobacter* spp. (*Mima-*

---

*References 198, 200–202, 249–252, 332–336

Herellea) inhabit the skin surface. Dermatophytes can also be recovered from clinically normal individuals who do not ultimately develop clinical disease.

Studies on the normal microbial flora of large animal skin have been strictly qualitative.* It is clear from studies in humans and dogs that the skin is an exceedingly effective environmental sampler, providing a temporary haven and way station for all sorts of organisms.[322, 335, 336] Thus, only repetitive quantitative studies allow reliable distinction between resident and transient bacteria.

While quantitative studies of microbial flora are not available for large animal skin, qualitative studies show that large animal skin and hair are a veritable "cesspool" of bacteria and fungi (Table 1–1). Thus, skin and hair must be adequately prepared prior to culturing for bacteria and fungi, if meaningful results are to be obtained on a patient.

Dermis

The dermis (corium) is an integral part of the body's connective tissue system and is of mesodermal origin. In areas of thick haired skin, the dermis accounts for most of the depth, whereas the epidermis is thin. In very thin skin, the decreased thickness results from the thinness of the dermis. The dermis is composed of fibers, ground substance, and cells. It also contains the epidermal appendages, arrector pili muscles, blood and lymph vessels, and nerves. Because the normal haired skin of large animals, except the pig, does not have epidermal rete ridges, dermal papillae are not usually seen. Thus, a true papillary and recticular dermis, as described in humans, is not present in large animals (except swine). The terms superficial and deep dermis are preferred. The dermis accounts for the majority of the tensile strength and elasticity of skin.

Dermal Fibers

The dermal fibers are formed by fibroblasts and are collagenous, reticular, and elastic.† *Collagenous* fibers (collagen) have great tensile strength and are the largest and most numerous (approximately 90 percent of all dermal fibers are collagen). They are thick bands composed of multiple protein fibrils and are differentially stained by Masson's trichrome. *Reticular* fibers (reticulin) are fine-branching structures that become closely approximated to collagen with age. They can be detected best with special silver stains. *Elastic* fibers (elastin) are composed of single, fine branches that possess great elasticity. They are well visualized by Verhoeff's and van Gieson's elastin stains.

There are at least seven and possibly ten genetically and structurally different types of collagen molecules in the body.[303] Type I collagen predominates in the dermis, and Type IV collagen is present in the epidermal basement membrane zone. The biosynthesis of collagen is a complex process of gene transposition and translation, intracellular modifications, packaging and secretion, extracellular modifications, and fibril assembly and crosslinking.[303] Collagen abnormalities may result from genetic defects, deficiencies of vitamin C, iron, and copper, and β-aminoproprionitrite poisoning (lathyrism).

In general, the superficial dermis contains fine, loosely arranged collagen fibers that are irregularly distributed and a network of fine elastin fibers. The deep dermis contains thick, densely arranged collagen fibers that tend to parallel the skin surface and elastin fibers that are thicker and less numerous than those in the superficial dermis. Small amounts of mucin (a blue-staining, granular to stringy-appearing substance) may be seen in the interstitial areas of the dermis, especially around vessels and appendages.

A special layer composed of fine collagenous fibers interwoven with fine elastic and reticular fibers occurs in horses.[397, 413, 442, 444] Because of its shiny gross appearance this layer has been called the "horse mirror" or "Ross-Spiegel." This structure is divided into three parts—upper and lower connective tissue layers and its own reticular layer having a characteristic treelike morphology. The dorsal thorax, croup, and the entire dorsal surface of the back, from the base of the tail to the tuber coxae, contain this additional connective tissue layer.

Dermal Ground Substance

The ground (interstitial) substance, the main component of the dermis, is a mucoid gel-sol of fibroblast origin composed of proteoglycans,

---

*References 1, 3, 18, 29, 69, 73, 78, 79, 94, 106, 128, 166, 167, 183, 283, 323, 337, 360, 400, 402, 420, 440, 441, 468

†References 136, 186, 191, 232, 263, 271, 278, 309, 311, 385, 401, 444

TABLE 1–1. Bacteria and Fungi Isolated from Normal Skin and Hair

Species	Bacteria	Fungi
Horse		*Absidia* spp.
		Acremonium spp.
	Acinetobacter sp.	*Alternaria* spp.
	Aerococcus sp.	*Aspergillus* spp.
	Aeromonas sp.	*Aureobasidium* sp.
		Candida spp.
		Cephalosporium spp.
	Bacillus spp.	*Chaetomium* spp.
		Chrysosporium spp.
	Corynebacterium sp.	*Cladosporium* spp.
		Cryptococcus spp.
		Diplosporium sp.
	Flavobacterium sp.	*Doratomyces* sp.
	Micrococcus spp.	*Fusarium* sp.
		Geomyces sp.
		Helminthosporium spp.
		Hormodendrum spp.
		Monotospora sp.
	Nocardia sp.	*Mucor* spp.
	Staphylococcus aureus	*Nigrospora* sp.
	Staphylococcus spp., coagulase-negative	*Paecilomyces* sp.
		Penicillium spp.
		Phoma spp.
		Rhodotorula spp.
	Staphylococcus spp., coagulase-positive	*Rhizopus* spp.
		Sordaria sp.
		Stemphylium spp.
		Thamnidium sp.
	Streptococcus spp., nonhemolytic	*Trichoderma* sp.
		Trichothecium sp.
		Ulocladium spp.
Cow		*Acremonium* spp.
	Bacillus spp.	*Arthrinium* spp.
	Corynebacterium bovis	*Arthroderma* spp.
	Escherichia coli	*Aspergillus* spp.
	Klebsiella pneumoniae	*Aureobasidium* sp.
		Botrytis spp.
		Candida spp.
	Proteus sp.	*Chaetomium* spp.
	Pseudomonas sp.	*Cladosporium* spp.
	Staphylococcus aureus	*Epicoccum* spp.
	Staphylococcus hyicus	*Fusarium* sp.
	Staphylococcus saprophyticus	*Mucor* spp.
		Penicillium spp.
		Phoma spp.
		Rhodotorula spp.
	Streptococcus agalactiae	*Scopulariopsis* spp.
	Streptococcus faecalis	*Trichothecium* sp.
	Streptococcus uberis	
	Streptococcus sp., hemolytic	
	Streptococcus sp., nonhemolytic	
Goat	*Staphylococcus aureus*	*Aspergillus* spp.
	Staphylococcus spp., coagulase-negative	*Mucor* spp.
Sheep	*Bacillus* spp.	
	E. coli	
	Micrococcus spp.	
	Staphylococcus aureus	
	Staphylococcus epidermidis	
	Streptococcus spp.	
Pig	*E. coli*	*Alternaria* spp.
	Klebsiella pneumoniae	*Aspergillus* spp.
	Proteus sp.	*Candida* spp.
	Pseudomonas sp.	*Cephalosporium* spp.
	Staphylococcus aureus	*Chaetomium* spp.
	Staphylococcus epidermidis	*Mortierella* spp.
	Staphylococcus hyicus	*Mucor* spp.
	Staphylococcus spp., coagulase-negative	*Oospora* spp.
	Streptococcus bov is	*Penicillium* spp.
	Streptococcus faecalis	*Rhizopus* spp.
		Scopulariopsis spp.
		Trichothecium spp.

principally hyaluronic acid, dermatan sulfate (chondroitin sulfate B), chondroitin-4-sulfate (chondroitin sulfate A), and chondroitin-6-sulfate (chondroitin sulfate C).[122, 186, 236] It fills the spaces and surrounds other structures of the dermis but allows electrolytes, nutrients, and cells to traverse it in passing from the dermal vessels to the avascular epidermis. The proteoglycans function in water storage and homeostasis; selective screening of substances (e.g., protein and electrolytes); and supporting dermal structure, lubrication, and collagen fibrillogenesis, orientation, growth, and differentiation. As animals age, the ground substance decreases in amount.

Cell surface fibronectin is an adhesive glycoprotein that mediates cell-to-cell interaction and cell adhesion to substratum and modulates microvascular integrity, vascular permeability, and wound healing.[113] Fibronectin is synthesized by fibroblasts, macrophages, and endothelial cells.

Dermal Cellular Elements

The dermis is usually sparsely populated with cells.* Fibroblasts are present throughout. Melanocytes may be seen near the superficial dermal blood vessels. Horses and ruminants tend to have a mild perivascular accumulation of small (lymphoid) and large (histiocytic) mononuclear cells in the superficial dermis.

Mast cells are most abundant around superficial dermal blood vessels and appendages, especially in the pinna, eyelid, face, ventral abdomen, scrotum, and interdigital areas.† They are best visualized with special stains such as toluidine blue or acid orcein–Giemsa. In goats, there are two morphologic forms of mast cells seen in skin: One is small and spindle-shaped resembling a fibroblast; the other is large and ovoid.[385] Healthy, parasite-free swine were shown to have an average of 32 mast cells/mm² of skin, and the numbers decreased markedly when the swine were stressed.[359]

Eosinophils are frequently seen in small numbers in the normal dermis of large animals.[91, 136, 359, 463] It has been reported that the number of eosinophils in the skin of normal cattle approximately doubles in the summer as compared with winter.[91] Presumably, this re-flects exposure to biting insects and arthropods and would be expected to happen in all large animals.

Hair Follicles

The hair shaft is divided into medulla, cortex, and cuticle.* The *medulla*, the innermost region of the hair, is composed of longitudinal rows of cuboidal cells, or cells flattened from top to bottom. The cells are solid near the hair root, but the rest of the hair shaft contains air and glycogen vacuoles. The *cortex*, the middle layer, consists of completely cornified, spindle-shaped cells, whose long axis is parallel to the hair shaft. These cells contain the pigment that gives the hair its color. Pigment may also be present in the medulla, but there it has little influence on the color of the hair. In general, the hairs of swine are mostly cortex. The *cuticle*, the outermost layer of the hair, is formed by flat, cornified, anuclear cells arranged like slate on a roof, the free edge of each cell facing the tip of the hair. In general, wool fibers from sheep have a relatively thin cuticle, with little overlapping of scales. Secondary hairs have a narrower medulla and a more prominent cuticle than do primary hairs. Lanugo hairs have no medulla.

Hair follicles are usually positioned at a 30 to 60 degree angle to the skin surface and occur in two basic arrangements: simple and compound.[191] In the simple hair follicle arrangement, characteristic of horses and cattle (Figs. 1–1 to 1–4), hair follicles occur singly and at random, displaying no obvious pattern of distribution.[41, 105, 136, 191, 444, 450] Each hair follicle is accompanied by sebaceous and sweat glands and an arrector pili muscle. Each hair emerges from a separate follicular opening. There are no secondary hair follicles.

In the compound hair follicle arrangement, characteristic of sheep and goats (Figs. 1–5 and 1–6), hair follicles occur in clusters of variable composition.† In general, a cluster consists of two to five large primary hairs surrounded by groups of smaller secondary hairs. One of the primary hairs is the largest (central primary hair), while the remaining primary hairs are smaller (lateral primary hairs). Each primary hair has sebaceous and

---

*References 136, 186, 191, 232, 263, 271, 278, 309, 311, 385, 401, 444
†References 186, 197, 232, 263, 271, 359, 385, 401, 444, 463

*References 41, 68, 136, 187, 191, 232, 234, 263, 277, 309, 311, 346, 385, 425, 444, 450
†References 28, 191, 232, 258, 263, 272–274, 376, 378, 385

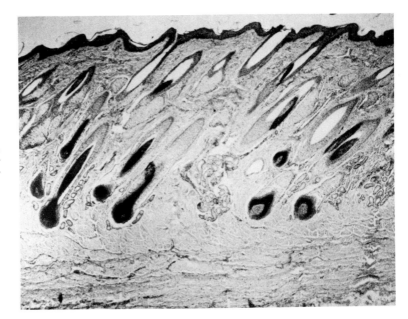

FIGURE 1–1. Normal horse skin. Note simple hair follicle arrangement and relatively thick epidermis.

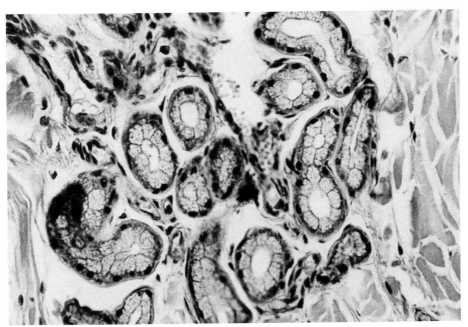

FIGURE 1–2. Normal horse skin. Note tightly coiled apocrine sweat glands exhibiting plump secretory epithelium and absence of visible secretion.

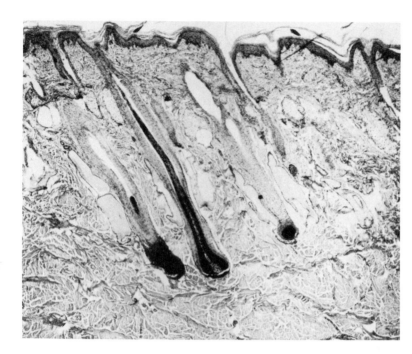

FIGURE 1–3. Normal cow skin. Note simple hair follicle arrangement and relatively thick epidermis.

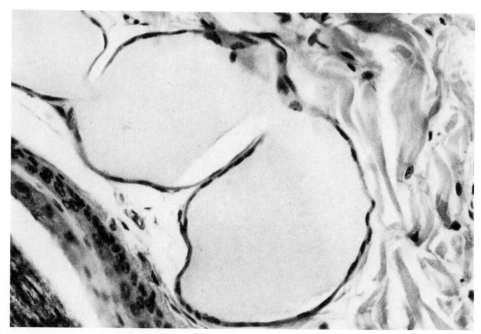

FIGURE 1–4. Normal cow skin. Note dilated apocrine sweat glands exhibiting flattened secretory epithelium and voluminous secretions.

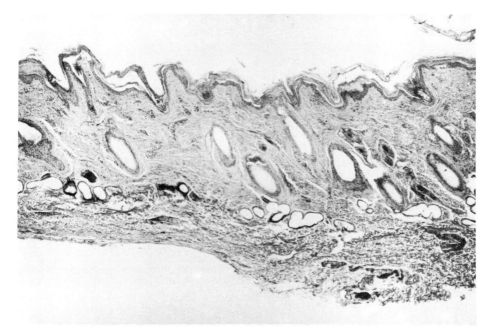

FIGURE 1–5. Normal goat skin. Note simple and compound hair follicle arrangements and relatively thin epidermis.

sweat glands and an arrector pili muscle. Secondary hairs may be accompanied by sebaceous glands, but that is all. The primary hairs generally emerge independently through separate pores, while the secondary hairs emerge through a common pore. From 5 to 25 secondary hairs may accompany each primary hair, depending on the breed of sheep or goat.* In sheep, wool follicles are characteristically spiral or twisted.

*References 59–61, 191, 232, 263, 272–274, 385

In sheep, the S/P ratio (ratio of the number of secondary follicles to each primary follicle) has received much study.[59–61, 112, 191, 372, 380] The greater the S/P ratio, the finer the fleece. Mountain breeds of sheep have mean S/P ratios of 3:1 to 4:1, long-wool breeds 4:1 to 5:1, down breeds 5:1 to 8:1, and Merinos 20:1. The S/P ratio can be a useful indication of fleece type in breeding experiments designed to improve the wool grown.

The hair follicle arrangement of the *pig* (Fig. 1–7) is intermediate between simple and com-

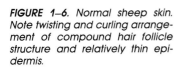

FIGURE 1–6. Normal sheep skin. Note twisting and curling arrangement of compound hair follicle structure and relatively thin epidermis.

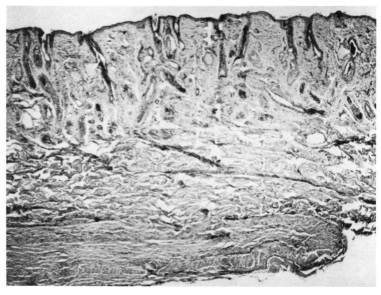

pound.[191, 281, 309, 415] Hair follicles may occur singly or in clusters of two or three.

The density of hair follicles (number of follicles per unit area of skin) varies between species, breeds, individuals, and regions of the body; for instance, the pig may average 30 hairs/cm^2 of skin, while the cow and sheep may average 900/cm^2 and 10,000/cm^2, respectively. In addition, follicle density is greater in the young, increases during drought conditions, and decreases with increased body weight.*

The hair follicle has five major components: the dermal hair papilla, the hair matrix, the hair, the inner root sheath, and the outer root sheath (Fig. 1–8).[41, 159, 187, 191, 240] The pluripotential cells of the hair matrix give rise to the hair and the inner root sheath. The outer root sheath represents a downward extension of the epidermis. Large hair follicles produce large hairs. For descriptive purposes, the hair follicle is divided into three anatomic segments: (1) the *infundibulum*, or pilosebaceous region (the upper portion, which consists of the segment from the entrance of the sebaceous duct to the skin surface), (2) the *isthmus* (the middle portion, which consists of the segment between the entrance of the sebaceous duct and the attachment of the arrector pili muscle), and (3) the *inferior segment* (the lower portion,

which extends from the attachment of the arrector pili muscle to the dermal hair papilla).

The inner root sheath is composed of three concentric layers, which from inside to outside include (1) the *inner root sheath cuticle* (a flattened, single layer of overlapping cells that point toward the hair bulb and interlock with the cells of the hair cuticle), (2) the *Huxley layer* (one to three nucleated cells thick), and (3) the *Henle layer* (a single layer of nonnucleated cells).* These layers contain eosinophilic cytoplasmic granules, called trichohyalin granules. The inner root sheath keratinizes and disintegrates when it reaches the level of the isthmus of the hair follicle.

The outer root sheath is thickest near the epidermis and gradually decreases in thickness toward the hair bulb.† In its lower portion (from the isthmus of the hair follicle downward), the outer root sheath is covered by the inner root sheath and does not undergo keratinization, and its cells have a clear, vacuolated cytoplasm (glycogen). In the middle portion of the hair follicle (isthmus), the outer root sheath is no longer covered by the inner root sheath and undergoes trichilemmal keratinization (keratohyalin granules are not formed). In the upper portion of the hair follicle (infundibulum), the outer root sheath undergoes keratinization in the same fashion as the sur-

---

*References 53, 54, 58–61, 65, 191, 376, 457

*References 41, 67, 71, 187, 191, 240, 431
†References 41, 71, 187, 191, 240, 341, 376, 380

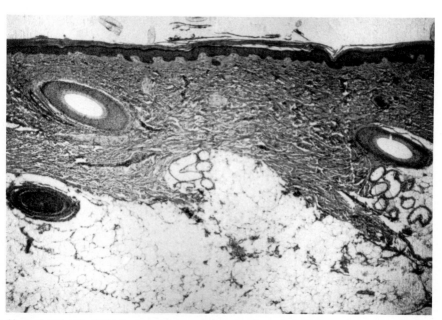

FIGURE 1–7. Normal pig skin. Note large, widely spaced simple hair follicle arrangement and relatively thick epidermis with rete ridge formation.

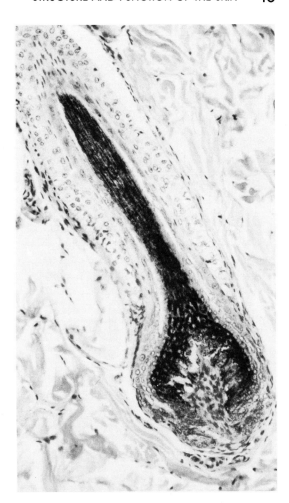

FIGURE 1-8. *Normal anagen hair follicle from a horse. Note relationships between outer and inner root sheaths, hair bulb, and dermal papilla.*

face epidermis. The outer root sheath is surrounded by two other prominent structures: a basement membrane zone, or "glassy" membrane (a downward reflection of the epidermal basement membrane zone), and a fibrous root sheath (a layer of dense connective tissue).

The dermal hair papilla is continuous with the dermal connective tissue and is covered by a thin continuation of the basement membrane zone.* The inner root sheath and hair grow from a layer of plump, nucleated epithelial cells that cover the papilla. These cells regularly show mitosis and are called the hair matrix.

The hair follicles of animals with straight hair are straight.† Conversely, the wool follicles of sheep are curved spirally, and the hair bulbs have a bend. This spiral configuration is associated with the waviness, or crimp, of wool fibers. In addition, hyperplastic epithelial bulbs, or cysts, arising from the suprabulbar outer root sheath of some wool follicles are seen in about half of the sheep examined carefully.[28, 64, 160, 263, 374]

Follicular folds have been described in the hair follicles of large animals.[136, 232, 271, 385, 444] These structures represent multiple (1 to 23) corrugations of the inner root sheath, which project into the pilary canal immediately below the sebaceous duct opening. These folds are believed to be artifacts of fixation and processing, as they are not seen in unprocessed sections cut by hand.[322]

Two specialized types of tactile hairs are found in mammalian skin: sinus hairs and tylotrich hairs. *Sinus hairs* (vibrissae) are found on the muzzle, lip, eyelid, face, and throat.* These hairs are thick, stiff, and tapered distally. Sinus hairs are characterized by an endothelium-lined blood sinus interposed be-

*References 41, 71, 129, 187, 191, 240, 389, 403, 431
†References 112, 136, 271, 327, 380, 385, 425, 444

*References 105, 121, 136, 232, 263, 271, 280, 309, 385, 404, 415, 444, 450

tween the external root sheath of the follicle and an outer connective tissue capsule. The sinus is divided into a superior nontrabecular ring, or annular sinus, and an inferior cavernous, or trabecular, sinus. A cushion-like thickening of mesenchyme ("sinus pad," or "ringwulst") projects into the annular sinus. The cavernous sinuses are traversed by trabeculae containing many nerve fibers. Skeletal muscle fibers attach to the outer layer of the follicle. Pacinian corpuscles are situated close to the sinus hair follicles. Sinus hairs are thought to function as slow-adapting mechanoreceptors.

Tylotrich hairs are scattered among ordinary body hairs.[247, 269, 310, 311, 430, 432] Tylotrich hair follicles are larger than surrounding follicles and contain a single stout hair and an annular complex of neurovascular tissue that surrounds the follicle at the level of the sebaceous glands. Tylotrich hairs are thought to function as rapid-adapting mechanoreceptors.

Each tylotrich follicle is associated with a tylotrich pad (Haarscheibe, touch spot, or touch corpuscle).* Tylotrich pads are composed of a thickened and distinctive epidermis underlaid by a convex area of fine connective tissue that is highly vascularized and well innervated. Unmyelinated nerve fibers end as flat plaques in association with Merkel's cells, which serve as slow-adapting touch receptors.

Sebaceous Glands

Sebaceous (holocrine) glands are simple or branched alveolar glands distributed throughout all haired skin.† The glands usually open through a duct into the pilary canal in the infundibulum (pilosebaceous follicle). Sebaceous glands tend to be largest in areas where hair follicle density is lowest. They are largest and most numerous near mucocutaneous junctions, the coronet, and over the dorsal neck and rump. Sebaceous glands are largest in the horse and smallest in the pig. These glands increase in size in intact male goats at the beginning of the rut period.[195, 381]

Sebaceous lobules are bordered by a basement membrane zone, upon which sits a single layer of deeply basophilic basal cells (reserve cells). The cells become progressively more lipidized and eventually disintegrate to form sebum toward the center of the lobule. Seba-

ceous ducts are lined with squamous epithelium.

The oily secretion (sebum) produced by the sebaceous glands tends to keep the skin soft and pliable by forming a surface emulsion that spreads over the surface of the stratum corneum to retain moisture and thus maintain proper hydration. The oil film also spreads over the hair shafts and gives them a glossy sheen. During periods of illness or malnutrition, the hair coat may become dull and dry as a result of inadequate sebaceous gland function. In addition to its action as a physical barrier, the sebum-sweat surface emulsion forms a chemical barrier against potential pathogens. Many of sebum's fatty acid constituents (linoleic, myristic, oleic, and palmitic acids) are known to have antimicrobial actions.[418, 419] Both the number and the area of sebaceous glands per unit length of skin were shown to decrease with age in *sheep*.[464, 467]

Sebaceous glands have an abundant blood supply and appear to be innervated.[192–194, 196, 401, 417] Their secretion is thought to be under hormonal control, with androgens causing hypertrophy and hyperplasia and estrogens and glucocorticoids causing involution. In cattle, it has been reported that sebum output is greater in summer than in winter and that prolonged exposure to a warm environment results in a higher output of sebum, together with an increased percentage of linoleic acid in the secretion.[416–419] The lipid composition of the skin surface often varies significantly between species.* In large animals, the surface lipids are predominantly produced by the sebaceous glands, with minor contributions from the epidermis. In general, the composition of surface lipids consists of varying percentages of triglycerides, phospholipids, cholesterol, cholesteryl esters, and unesterified fatty acids. Conspicuously absent, except for small amounts in cattle, is a characteristic lipid constituent of humans, squalene.

Studies of mammalian epidermal lipids show that these are predominantly highly polar compounds, consisting of ceramides, glucosylceramides, and gangliosides, and do not vary significantly among species.[40, 142–145, 473–477] These polar lipids are extruded from epidermal cells to occupy the intercellular spaces of the stratum corneum, where they are at least partially responsible for the epidermal barrier to water diffusion.

---

*References 111, 247, 263, 269, 310, 311, 430, 432
†References 100, 105, 136, 232, 263, 271, 276, 309, 310, 385, 413, 415, 444, 450, 464, 467

---

*References 88–90, 245, 256, 329, 330, 332–334, 338, 339, 348, 352, 418, 419, 477

Sweat Glands

Apocrine sweat glands are generally coiled and saccular or tubular and are distributed throughout all haired skin.* The glands are localized below the sebaceous glands and usually open through a duct into the pilary canal in the infundibulum, above the sebaceous duct opening. Aprocrine sweat glands tend to be largest in areas where hair follicle density is lowest. They are largest and most numerous near mucocutaneous junctions, the coronet, and over the dorsal neck and rump. Apocrine sweat glands are distinctively saccular and non-coiled in cattle and are usually filled with secretory colloid.

The secretory portions of apocrine sweat glands consist of a single row of flattened to columnar epithelial (secretory) cells and a single layer of fusiform myoepithelial cells. The excretory duct generally consists of two layers of cuboidal epithelial cells. In general, apocrine sweat glands do not appear to be innervated, except in the horse.[192–194, 196, 310, 311, 439]

Specialized glandular structures have been described in the skin of large animals. Nasolabial glands occur in the muzzle and lip of cattle, sheep, and goats.† These multilobular, tubuloalveolar, seromucoid glands are thought to secrete almost constantly in cattle. Seromucoid glands are also found in the snout and lip and at the caudomedial aspect of the carpus (carpal gland) of swine.[243, 271, 310, 450] These glandular structures occur at the junction of the deep dermis and subcutis, consist of deeply (dark) and faintly (clear) basophilic cuboidal to columnar epithelial cells, and contain large myoepithelial cells. The *mental*, or mandibular, organ of swine, a round, raised structure located in the intermandibular space, consists of large sebaceous and apocrine glands and very coarse sinus hairs (vibrissae).[309, 310]

Sweating and Thermoregulation

Horses are known to sweat moderately to markedly in response to exercise, heat (high ambient temperature or fever), pain, and secretion of catecholamines (resulting from stress or pheochromocytoma) as well as when they have Cushing's syndrome (see Chapter 13,

discussion on hyperadrenocorticism).* In fact, horses and humans are unique in their ability to produce copious amounts of sweat as a major component of thermoregulation.[39, 188, 208] Sweating is also thought to be a significant channel for heat loss in cattle.† Sweating can be evoked in cattle by local heat, high ambient temperature, and catecholamines. It has been shown that Brahman and crossbreeds of Brahman cattle (1) have a higher density of sweat glands, (2) sweat less at various ambient temperatures, and (3) have greater heat tolerance than do British breeds of cattle.[19, 324, 325, 390, 396]

In goats and sheep, both the local application of heat and exposure to a hot environment result in increased sweat production.‡ Sweating in response to heat but not to epinephrine was absent in areas deprived of sympathetic nerve supply. Apocrine sweating in goats and sheep is stimulated by the local administration of epinephrine and norepinephrine but not of pilocarpine, acetylcholine, nicotine, or histamine. Sweating in these two species occurs in discrete intermittent discharges, which gradually decrease in amount as the rate of expulsion exceeds the rate of production (fatigue).

In summary, only in horses and cattle is sweating thought to be important in thermoregulation. In all large animals, other factors in thermoregulation include peripheral vasculature and arteriovenous anastomoses, all of which modify the effects of radiation, convection, and conduction in heat loss.

In all large animals, other proposed functions of apocrine sweat include (1) excretion of waste products, (2) supplying moisture to assist the flow of sebum (protective role), and (3) scent signaling.[188, 191, 290, 311, 425, 427]

Because of the interest in racing, endurance riding, anhidrosis (see Chapter 14, discussion on anhidrosis), and comparative physiology and pathophysiology, sweat and sweating have been extensively studied in the horse. In primates, the neural control of eccrine sweating is primarily via cholinergic receptors, but adrenergic receptors also play a role in control.[39, 188] In the horse, even though a rich supply of acetylcholine esterase has been reported in equine apocrine sweat glands,[196] investigations have concluded that these glands are insensitive to cholinergic agonists and are predomi-

---

*References 10, 58, 80, 105, 108, 120, 136, 149, 188, 191, 199, 203, 210, 232, 243, 263, 271, 275, 309, 310, 324, 325, 327, 349, 385, 391, 413, 438, 447, 450, 465, 486, 487
†References 136, 232, 243, 263, 267, 310, 385, 450, 485, 493

*References 19, 32, 39, 56, 110, 191, 218, 219, 289, 310, 312, 370, 427, 447
†References 4, 5, 9, 13, 17, 46, 99, 118–120, 191, 198, 205, 207, 208, 216, 268, 290, 324, 325, 343, 427, 449
‡References 5, 45, 46, 52, 99, 132, 188, 191, 204, 205, 208, 213, 215, 221, 284, 318, 356–358, 367, 465

nantly under β-adrenergic control.* Decreased sweating rates seen during epinephrine infusion in horses suggest that the apocrine sweat glands of the horse can become refractory (fatigue) upon continuous exposure to adrenergic agonists. The average loss of body weight per hour during heat exposure and endurance exercise in horses was reported to be 0.8 and 1.5 percent, respectively.[370]

Sweat produced by all stimuli (prolonged epinephrine exposure, heat exposure, and exercise) in horses was found to be hypertonic (relative to plasma) for sodium, potassium, and chloride (in humans, eccrine sweat is hypotonic for sodium and chloride and isotonic for potassium).† Equine sweat protein (initially hypotonic), calcium (isotonic), and magnesium (initially hypertonic) concentrations decreased with time; urea levels (hypertonic) remained constant; and glucose was only detectable when plasma glucose levels increased. Equine sweat is alkaline during sweating (eccrine sweat in humans is acidic). Horses have an extremely high concentration of protein in sweat compared with other species.‡

Arrector Pili Muscles

Arrector pili muscles are of mesenchymal origin and consist of smooth muscle with intra- and extracellular vacuoles.§ Smooth muscle cells are characterized ultrastructurally by central nuclei, peripheral basement membrane, and intracytoplasmic myofilaments.[240] They are present in all haired skin and are largest in the dorsal neck and rump. Arrector pili muscles originate in the superficial dermis and insert approximately perpendicularly on a bulge of the primary hair follicles. Branching of these muscles is often seen in the superficial dermis.

Little has been written concerning the function of arrector pili muscles in large animals. In horses, cattle, and sheep, these muscles are known to contract in response to epinephrine or norepinephrine, producing piloerection, which may be helpful for thermoregulation.[63, 107, 109, 355, 367]

In sheep, the arrector pili muscles were shown not to be simple isolated strands of smooth muscle.[63] They are branched and interconnected by numerous strands of connective tissue, particularly just below the epidermis and near the level of their junctions with primary hair follicles. Arrector pili muscles in sheep skin were shown to have the ability to produce skin contraction in two directions at right angles and were theorized to be important in producing the crimp in wool fibers.

It has also been theorized that arrector pili muscles play a role in the emptying of sebaceous glands.[232]

An interfollicular smooth muscle that spans hair follicle triads has been studied in swine.[434] This muscle (1) lies opposite the arrector pili muscle on the follicle, (2) has its fiber orientation perpendicular to that of the arrector pili muscle, and (3) is not continuous with the arrector pili muscle. Its function is unknown.

Blood Vessels

Cutaneous blood vessels are generally arranged in three intercommunicating plexuses of arteries and veins.* The deep plexus is found at the interface of the dermis and subcutis. Branches from this plexus descend into the subcutis and ascend to supply the lower portions of the hair follicles and the apocrine sweat glands. These ascending vessels continue upward to feed the middle plexus, which lies at the level of the sebaceous glands. The middle plexus gives off branches to the arrector pili muscles, ascending and descending branches that supply the middle portions of the hair follicles and the sebaceous glands, and ascending branches to feed the superficial plexus. Capillary loops immediately below the epidermis emanate from the superficial plexus and supply the epidermis and upper portion of the hair follicles. Blood vessel endothelial cells are characterized ultrastructurally by a peripheral basement membrane and intracytoplasmic Weibel-Palade bodies (rod-shaped tubular structures enveloped in a continuous single membrane).[185, 235, 240, 471]

Arteriovenous anastomoses are normal connections between arteries and veins that allow arterial blood to enter the venous circulation without passing through capillary beds. Because of the size and position of these anastomoses, they can alter circulation dynamics and the blood supply to tissues. Arteriovenous

---

*References 38, 39, 56, 107, 109, 214, 218, 219, 244, 370, 421–423
†References 56, 188, 211, 218, 289, 312, 370, 423, 424
‡References 97, 207, 209, 282, 370, 414, 486
§References 63, 105, 136, 191, 232, 263, 271, 309–311, 355, 385, 401, 444, 450

---

*References 14, 15, 98, 116, 138, 185, 191, 255, 311, 373, 401, 425

anastomoses have been described in the skin of all large animals.* They occur in all areas of the skin but are commonest over the extremities (especially the legs and ears). They occur at all levels of the dermis, but especially in the deep dermis.

Arteriovenous anastomoses show considerable variation in structure, ranging from simple slightly coiled vessels to such complex structures as the glomus. The glomus is a special arteriovenous shunt located within the deep dermis. Each glomus consists of an arterial and a venous segment. The arterial segment (Sucquet-Hoyer canal) branches from an arteriole. The wall shows a single layer of endothelium, surrounded by a basement membrane zone, and a medium that is densely packed with four to six layers of glomus cells. These cells are large and plump, have a clear cytoplasm, and resemble epithelioid cells. Glomus cells are generally regarded as being modified smooth muscle cells. The venous segment of the glomus is thin-walled and has a wide lumen.

Arteriovenous anastomoses are concerned with thermoregulation. Constriction or dilatation of the shunt restricts or enhances, respectively, the blood flow to an area.[42, 185, 240, 306, 469, 478] Acetylcholine and histamine cause dilatation, while epinephrine and norepinephrine cause constriction.

Lymph Vessels

Lymphatics arise from capillary networks that lie in the superficial dermis and surround the adnexa.[188, 240, 401] The vessels arising from these networks drain into a subcutaneous lymphatic plexus. Lymph vessels are not usually seen above the middle dermis in routine histologic preparations of normal skin.

The lymphatics are essential for nutrition because they control the true microcirculation of the skin, which is the movement of interstitial tissue fluid. The supply, permeation, and removal of tissue fluid is important for proper function. The lymphatics are the drains that take away the debris and excess matter resulting from daily wear and tear in the skin. They are essential channels for the return of protein and cells from the tissues into the blood stream and for linking the skin and regional lymph nodes in an immunoregulatory capacity.

In general, lymph vessels are distinguished from blood capillaries by (1) possessing a wider and more angular lumen, (2) having flatter and more attenuated endothelial cells, (3) having no pericytes, and (4) containing no blood. However, even the slightest injury disrupts the wall of a lymphatic or blood vessel or the intervening connective tissue. Consequently, traumatic fistulae are commonplace. These account for the frequent observation of "blood flow" in lymphatics in inflamed skin.

Nerves

In general, cutaneous nerve fibers are associated with blood vessels (dual autonomic innervation of arteries), various cutaneous endorgans (tylotrich pad, pacinian corpuscle, Meissner's corpuscle, and mammalian end-organ), sebaceous glands, hair follicles, and arrector pili muscles and occur as a subepidermal plexus.* Only in the horse do the apocrine sweat glands appear to be innervated.[192-194, 196] Some free nerve endings even penetrate the epidermis. Under the light microscope, small cutaneous nerves and free nerve endings can be demonstrated satisfactorily only by methylene blue, metallic impregnation, or histochemical techniques.

In addition to the all-important function of sensory perception (touch, heat, cold, pressure, pain, and itch), the dermal nerves promote the survival and proper functioning of the epidermis (so-called trophic influences).

The area of skin supplied by the branches of one spinal nerve is known as its dermatome.[122, 185, 369] Dermatomes have been mapped out for sheep,[226, 248] cattle,[26, 386, 398] and goats.[248]

Subcutis

The subcutis (hypodermis) is the deepest and usually thickest layer of the skin.[189, 311, 425] It is a fibrofatty structure, consisting of lobules of fat cells (lipocytes, adipocytes) interwoven with connective tissue. The subcutis functions (1) as an energy reserve, (2) in heat insulation, (3) as a protective padding, and (4) in maintaining surface contours.

---

*References 16, 74, 117, 139, 185, 240, 263, 304–307, 331, 350, 443

*References 12, 111, 185, 192–194, 196, 232, 247, 263, 269, 301, 309, 354, 385, 413, 430, 432, 444, 446

REFERENCES

1. Adegoke, G. O., and Ojo, M. O.: Biochemical characterization of staphylococci isolated from goats. Vet. Microbiol. 7:463, 1982.
2. Agasti, M. K., et al.: Studies on the skin fold thickness in cross-bred cattle of first calving. Indian J. Anim. Health 12:183, 1973.
3. Aho, R.: Saprophytic fungi isolated from the hair of domestic and laboratory animals with suspected dermatophytosis. Mycopathologia 83:65, 1983.
4. Allen, T. E.: Responses of Zebu, Jersey, and Zebu and Jersey cross-bred heifers to rising temperature with particular reference to sweating. Aust. J. Agric. Sci. 13:165, 1962.
5. Allen, T. E., and Bligh, J.: A comparative study of the temporal patterns of cutaneous water vapour loss from some domesticated animals with epitrichial sweat glands. Comp. Biochem. Physiol. 31:347, 1969.
6. Amakiri, S. F.: A comparative study of the thickness of the stratum corneum in Nigerian breeds of cattle. Br. Vet. J. 129:227, 1973.
7. Amakiri, S. F.: Seasonal changes in bovine skin thickness in relation to the incidence of *Dermatophilus* infection in Nigeria. Res. Vet. Sci. 17:351, 1974.
8. Amakiri, S. F.: Melanin and dopa-positive cells in the skin of tropical cattle. Acta Anat. 103:434, 1979.
9. Amakiri, S. F., and Mordi, R.: The rate of cutaneous evaporation in some tropical and temperate breeds of cattle. Anim. Prod. 20:63, 1975.
10. Amakiri, S. F.: Sweat gland measurements in some tropical and temperate breeds of cattle in Nigeria. Anim. Prod. 18:285, 1974.
11. Amakiri, S. F.: Alkaline phosphatase activity in normal and *Dermatophilus congolensis* infected bovine skin. Nigerian Vet. J. 1:46, 1972.
12. Amakiri, S. F., et al.: Nerves and nerve endings in the skin of tropical cattle. Acta Anat. 100:391, 1978.
13. Amakiri, S. F., and Adepoju, J. J.: Changes in sweat gland morphology in cattle before and during heat stimulation. Acta Anat. 105:140, 1979.
14. Amakiri, S. F., and Nwufoh, K. J.: Changes in cutaneous blood vessels in bovine dermatophilosis. J. Comp. Pathol. 91:439, 1981.
15. Amakiri, S. F.: Vascular arrangement in the skin of tropical cattle. Acta Anat. 94:585, 1976.
16. Amakiri, S. F.: Arteriovenous anastomoses in the skin of tropical cattle. Acta Anat. 96:285, 1976.
17. Amakiri, S. F., and Onwuka, S. K.: Quantitative studies of sweating rate in some cattle breeds in a humid tropical environment. Anim. Prod. 30:383, 1980.
18. Amtsberg, G.: Untersuchungen zum Vorkommen von *Staphylococcus hyicus* beim Schwein bzw von *Staphylococcus epidermidis* Biotyp 2 bei anderen Tierarten. Dtsch. Tierärztl. Wschr. 85:385, 1978.
19. Aoki, T., et al.: On the responsiveness of the sweat glands in the horse. J. Invest. Dermatol. 33:441, 1959.
20. Aoyagi, T., et al.: Effect of hydrocortisone on the adenylate cyclase system. Br. J. Dermatol. 105:257, 1981.
21. Aoyagi, T., et al.: The effects of epidermal growth factor on the cyclic nucleotide system in pig epidermis. J. Invest. Dermatol. 74:238, 1980.
22. Aoyagi, T., et al.: Stimulation of protein phosphorylation by epidermal growth factor in pig skin. J. Invest. Dermatol. 74:421, 1980.
23. Aoyagi, T., et al.: Epidermal growth factor stimulates phosphorylation of pig epidermal keratin protein. J. Invest. Dermatol. 81:49, 1983.
24. Aoyagi, T., et al.: Epidermal growth factor stimulates tyrosine phosphorylation of pig epidermal fibrous keratin. J. Invest. Dermatol. 84:118, 1985.
25. Aoyagi, T., et al.: Epidermal growth factor stimulates release of arachidonic acid in pig epidermis. J. Invest. Dermatol. 84:168, 1985.
26. Arnold, J. P., and Kitchell, R. L.: Experimental studies of the innervation of the abdominal wall of cattle. Am. J. Vet. Res. 18:229, 1957.
27. Arvas, H.: Macroscopic and microscopic investigations on the skin of sheep (Akkaraman) and goat (Kil) in Elazig (District). Anat. Histol. Embryol. 11:356, 1982.
28. Auber, L.: The anatomy of follicles producing wool fibers with special reference to keratinization. Trans. R. Soc. Edinb. 62:191, 1952.
29. Ayers, J. L.: Corynebacterial infections. *In*: Howard, J. L. (ed.): *Current Veterinary Therapy, Food Animal Practice.* Philadelphia, W. B. Saunders Co., 1981, p. 658.
30. Baden, H. P., et al.: The fibrous proteins of stratum corneum. J. Invest. Dermatol. 67:573, 1976.
31. Bartek, M. J., et al.: Skin permeability *in vitro*: Rat, rabbit, pig, and man. J. Invest. Dermatol. 56:409, 1971.
32. Bell, F. R., and Evans, C. L.: The relation between sweating and the innervation of sweat glands in the horse. J. Physiol. 134:421, 1957.
33. Bennett, J. W., et al.: Annual rhythm of wool growth. Nature 194:651, 1962.
34. Berg, R.: Anatomische und physiologische Grundlagen der Woll produktion 1. Monat. Vet. Med. 32:259, 1977.
35. Berg, R.: Anatomische und physiologische Grundlagen der Woll produktion 2. Monat. Vet. Med. 32:265, 1977.
36. Berman, A.: Peripheral effects of L-thyroxine on hair growth and coloration in cattle. J. Endocrinol. 20:288, 1960.
37. Berman, A., and Volcani, R.: Seasonal and regional variations in coat characteristics of dairy cattle. Aust. J. Agric. Res. 12:528, 1961.
38. Bijman, J., and Quinton, P. M.: *In vitro* pharmacological stimulation of equine sweat glands shows equine sweating is predominantly under beta-adrenergic control. Physiologist 25:279, 1982.
39. Bijman, J., and Quinton, P. M.: Predominantly beta-adrenergic control of equine sweating. Am. J. Physiol. 246:R349, 1984.
40. Birkley, C. S., et al.: The polar lipids from keratinized tissues of some vertebrates. Comp. Biochem. Physiol. 73B:239, 1982.
41. Blackburn, P. S.: The hair of cattle, horse, dog, and cat. *In*: Rook, A. J., and Walton, G. S.: *Comparative Physiology and Pathology of the Skin.* Oxford, Blackwell Scientific Publications, 1965, p. 201.
42. Blaxter, K. L., et al.: Environmental temperature, energy metabolism and heat regulation in sheep. J. Agric. Sci. 52:25, 1959.
43. Blaxter, K. L., and Wainman, F. W.: Environmental temperature and the energy metabolism and heat emission of steers. J. Agric. Sci. 56:81, 1961.
44. Blaxter, K. L., and Wainman, F. W.: The effect of increased air movement on the heat production and emission of steers. J. Agric. Sci. 62:207, 1964.
45. Bligh, J.: Synchronous discharge of apocrine sweat glands of Welsh Mountain sheep. Nature 189:582, 1961.
46. Bligh, J.: A thesis concerning the process of secretion and discharge of sweat. Environ. Res. 1:28, 1967.
47. Bonadonna, T.: Observations histologiques et mensurations sur le poil des chevres d'Angora. Rec. Med. Vet. 134:611, 1958.
48. Bowstead, J. E., and Larose, P.: Wool growth and quality as affected by certain nutritional and climatic factors. III. Results and conclusions. Can. J. Res. D 16:361, 1938.
49. Breathnach, A. S.: Branched cells in the epidermis: An overview. J. Invest. Dermatol. 75:6, 1980.
50. Briggman, R. A., and Wheeler, C. E.: The epidermal-dermal junction. J. Invest. Dermatol. 65:71, 1975.
51. Britt, A. G., et al.: Structure of the epidermis of Australian Merino sheep over a 12-month period. Aust. J. Biol. Sci. 38:165, 1985.
52. Brook, A. H., and Short, B. F.: Sweating in sheep. Aust. J. Agric. Res. 11:557, 1960.
53. Burns, M., and Clarkson, H.: Some observations of the dimensions of follicles and of other structures in the skin of sheep. J. Agric. Sci. 39:315, 1949.
54. Burns, M.: The development of the fleece and follicle population in Herdwick sheep. J. Agric. Sci. 44:443, 1954.
55. Camek, J.: Investigations of the hair of different breeds of cattle. J. Agric. Sci. 10:12, 1920.
56. Carlson, G. P., and Ocen, P. O.: Composition of equine sweat following exercise in high environmental tempera-

tures and in response to intravenous epinephrine administration. J. Equine Med. Surg. 3:27, 1979.

57. Carruthers, C.: *Biochemistry of Skin in Health and Disease.* Springfield, IL: Charles C Thomas Pub., 1962.

58. Carter, H. B., and Dowling, D. F.: The hair follicle and apocrine gland population of cattle skin. Aust. J. Agric. Res. 5:745, 1954.

59. Carter, H. B.: The hair follicle group in sheep. Anim. Breed. Abstr. 23:101, 1955.

60. Carter, H. B., and Clarke, W. H.: The hair follicle group and skin follicle population of Australian Merino sheep. Aust. J. Agric. Res. 8:91, 1957.

61. Carter, H. B.: Variation in the hair follicle population of the mammalian skin. *In*: Lyne, A. G., and Short, B. F. (eds.): *Biology of the Skin and Hair Growth.* New York, American Elsevier Publishing Co., 1965, p. 25.

62. Chan, C. C., and Ford-Hutchinson, A.: Effects of synthetic leukotrienes on local blood flow and vascular permeability in porcine skin. J. Invest. Dermatol. 84:154, 1985.

63. Chapman, R. E.: The ovine arrector pili musculature and crimp formation in wool. *In*: Lyne, A. G., and Short, B. F. (eds.): *Biology of the Skin and Hair Growth.* New York, American Elsevier Publishing Co., 1965, p. 201.

64. Chapman, R. E., et al.: Abnormal crimping in Merino and Polwarth wools. Nature 187:960, 1960.

65. Chapman, R. E., and Young, S. S. Y.: A study of wool production per unit area of skin in Australian Merino sheep. Aust. J. Agric. Res. 8:723, 1957.

66. Chapman, R. E.: Cell migration in wool follicles of sheep. J. Cell Sci. 9:791, 1971.

67. Chapman, R. E., and Gemmell, R. T.: Formation and breakdown of the inner sheath and features of the pilary canal epithelium in the wool follicle. J. Ultrastruct. Res. 36:355, 1971.

68. Chapman, R. E., and Gemmell, R. T.: The origin of cortical segmentation in wool follicles. J. Invest. Dermatol. 57:377, 1971.

69. Chengappa, M. M., et al.: Isolation and identification of yeasts and yeast-like organisms from clinical veterinary sources. J. Clin. Microbiol. 19:427, 1984.

70. Choudhury, G., et al.: Studies on skin fold thickness in Sahawadi and Nellore sheep and their crosses in relation to live weight gain at different ages. Indian J. Anim. Health 13:121, 1974.

71. Cohen, J.: The dermal papilla. *In*: Lyne, A. G., and Short, B. F. (eds.): *Biology of the Skin and Hair Growth.* New York, American Elsevier Publishing Co., 1965, p. 183.

72. Coop, I. E.: Wool growth as affected by nutrition and by climatic factors. J. Agric. Sci. 43:456, 1953.

73. Cullen, G. A., and Harbert, C. N.: Some ecological observations on micro-organisms inhabiting bovine skin, teat canals, and milk. Br. Vet. J. 123:14, 1967.

74. Daniel, P. M., and Pritchard, M. M. L.: Arteriovenous anastomoses in the external ear. Q. J. Exp. Physiol. 41:107, 1956.

75. Davies, H. W., and Trotter, M. D.: Synthesis and turnover of membrane glycoconjugates in monolayer culture of pig and human epidermal cells. Br. J. Dermatol. 104:649, 1981.

76. Dempsey, M.: The structure of the skin and leather manufacture. J. R. Microsc. Soc. 67:21, 1948.

77. DesGrossilliers, J. P., et al.: Distribution of ^{3}H-betamethasone-17-valerate after topical application in the domestic pig. J. Invest. Dermatol. 53:270, 1969.

78. Devriese, L. A.: Isolation and identification of *Staphylococcus hyicus.* Am. J. Vet. Res. 38:787, 1977.

79. Devriese, L. A., and Derycke, J.: *Staphylococcus hyicus* in cattle. Res. Vet. Sci. 26:346, 1979.

80. Dowling, D. F.: The hair follicle and apocrine gland populations of Zebu and Shorthorn cattle skin. Aust. J. Agric. Res. 6:645, 1955.

81. Dowling, D. F.: An experimental study of heat tolerance in cattle. Aust. J. Agric. Res. 7:469, 1956.

82. Dowling, D. F.: The medullation characteristic of the hair coat as a factor in the heat tolerance of cattle. Aust. J. Agric. Res. 10:736, 1959.

83. Dowling, D. F.: The significance of the coat in heat tolerance of cattle. Aust. J. Agric. Res. 10:744, 1959.

84. Dowling, D. F., and Nay, T.: Cyclic changes in the follicles and hair coat in cattle. Aust. J. Agric. Res. 11:1064, 1960.

85. Dowling, D. F.: The significance of the coat in heat tolerance of cattle. II. Effect of solar radiation on body temperatures. Aust. J. Agric. Res. 11:871, 1960.

86. Downes, A. M.: A study of the incorporation of labelled cystine into growing wool fibres. *In*: Lyne, A. G., and Short, B. F. (eds.): *Biology of the Skin and Hair Growth.* New York, American Elsevier Publishing Co., 1965, p. 345.

87. Downes, A. M., and Wallace, A. L. C.: Local effects on wool growth of intradermal injections of hormones. *In*: Lyne, A. G., and Short, B. F. (eds.): *Biology of the Skin and Hair Growth.* New York, American Elsevier Publishing Co., 1965, p. 679.

88. Downing, D. T., et al.: Measurement of the time between synthesis and surface excretion of sebaceous lipids in sheep and man. J. Invest. Dermatol. 64:215, 1975.

89. Downing, D. T., and Colton, S. W.: Skin surface lipids of the horse. Lipids 15:323, 1980.

90. Downing, D. T., and Lindholm, J. S.: Skin surface lipids of the cow. Comp. Biochem. Physiol. 73B:327, 1982.

91. Dragnev, H.: Seasonal changes in the number of mast cells and eosinophil leucocytes in the skin of cattle. Vet. Med. Nauki 7:73, 1970.

92. Draize, H. H.: The determinations of the pH of the skin of man and common laboratory animals. J. Invest. Dermatol. 5:77, 1942.

93. Drochmans, P., et al.: Structure and biochemical composition of desmosomes and tonofilaments isolated from calf muzzle epidermis. J. Cell Biol. 79:427, 1978.

94. Dunne, H. W., and Leman, A. D.: *Diseases of Swine IV.* Ames, Iowa State University Press, 1975.

95. Ebling, F. J.: Comparative and evolutionary aspects of hair replacement. *In*: Rook, A. J., and Walton, G. S.: *Comparative Physiology and Pathology of the Skin.* Oxford, Blackwell Scientific Publications, 1965, p. 87.

96. Ebling, F. J.: Systemic factors affecting the periodicity of hair follicles. *In*: Lyne, A. G., and Short, B. F. (eds.): *Biology of the Skin and Hair Growth.* New York, American Elsevier Publishing Co., 1965, p. 507.

97. Eckersall, D., et al.: An investigation into the proteins of equine sweat. Comp. Biochem. Physiol. 73B:375, 1982.

98. El-Bab, M. R. F., et al.: The morphogenesis of the vasculature in bovine fetal skin. J. Anat. 136:561, 1983.

99. Elder, H. Y., et al.: Structural changes in the glands during sweating in ungulates. J. Physiol. 273:39P, 1977.

100. Elder, H. Y., et al.: The use of computer-linked planimetry in the image analysis of serial sections from horse sebaceous glands. J. Physiol. 343:21P, 1983.

101. Elias, P. M.: Epidermal lipids, barrier function, and desquamation. J. Invest. Dermatol. 80(Suppl. 6):44S, 1983.

102. Elias, P. M.: Epidermal lipids, membranes, and keratinization. Int. J. Dermatol. 20:1, 1981.

103. Elias, P. M., et al.: Kinetics of *in vitro* bovine keratohyalin synthesis. Br. J. Dermatol. 95:115, 1976.

104. Elias, P. M., et al.: *In vitro* studies on the kinetics, composition, and homology of bovine keratohyalin. Exp. Cell Res. 73:95, 1972.

105. Ellenberger, W.: *Handbuch der Vergleichenden Mikroskopischen Anatomie der Haustiere.* Berlin, Paul Parey, 1906.

106. Euzeby, J., et al.: Investigations mycologiques. I. Recherches sur quelques pseudodermatophytes. Bull. Soc. Sci. Vet. Med. Comp. Lyon 75:355, 1973.

107. Evans, C. L., and Smith, D. F. G.: Sweating response in the horse. Proc. R. Soc. Lond. B 145:61, 1956.

108. Evans, C. L., et al.: A histological study of the sweat glands of normal and dry-coated horses. J. Comp. Pathol. 67:397, 1957.

109. Evans, C. L., et al.: Physiological factors in the condition of "dry-coat" in horses. Vet. Rec. 69:1, 1957.

110. Evans, L. H., et al.: Clinico-pathologic conference. J. Am. Vet. Med. Assoc. 159:209, 1971.

111. Evans, M. H.: Sensory receptors in the sheep's foot. J. Physiol. 235:355, 1973.

112. Fayez, I., et al.: Wool follicle characteristics in the Awassi fat-tailed sheep. Acta Anat. 96:55, 1976.

113. Feldman, B. F., and Thomson, D. B.: Fibronectin: Its

diagnostic and therapeutic implications. J. Am. Anim. Hosp. Assoc. 19:1027, 1983.

114. Ferguson, K. A., et al.: Studies of comparative fleece growth in sheep. I. The quantitative nature of inherent differences in wool-growth rate. Aust. J. Sci. Res. B 2:42, 1949.

115. Ferguson, K. A., et al.: Hormonal regulation of wool growth. In: Lyne, A. G., and Short, B. F. (eds.): *Biology of the Skin and Hair Growth*. New York, American Elsevier Publishing Co., 1965, p. 655.

116. Findlay, J. D., and Yang, S. H.: Capillary distribution in cow skin. Nature 161:1012, 1948.

117. Findlay, J. D., and Goodall, A. M.: Arteriovenous anastomoses in the perichondrium and skin of the ear of the Ayrshire calf. J. Physiol. 121:46P, 1953.

118. Findlay, J. D., and Robertshaw, D.: The role of the sympatho-adrenal system in the control of sweating in the ox (*Bos taurus*). J. Physiol. 179:285, 1965.

119. Findlay, J. D., and Jenkinson, D. M.: Sweat gland function in the Ayrshire calf. Res. Vet. Sci. 5:109, 1965.

120. Findlay, J. D., and Jenkinson, D. M.: The morphology of bovine sweat glands and the effect of heat on the sweat glands of the Ayrshire calf. J. Agric. Sci. 55:247, 1960.

121. Fitzgerald, M. J. T.: Postnatal growth of the nerves of vibrissae. J. Anat. 96:521, 1962.

122. Fitzpatrick, T. B., et al.: *Dermatology in General Medicine II*. New York, McGraw-Hill Book Co., 1979.

123. Fitzpatrick, T. B., et al.: *Biology and Diseases of Dermal Pigmentation*. Tokyo, University of Tokyo Press, 1981.

124. Forrest, J. W., et al.: Characterization of melanocytes in wool-bearing skin of Merino sheep. Aust. J. Biol. Sci. 38:245, 1985.

125. Forrest, J. W., and Fleet, M. R.: Lack of tanning in white Merino sheep following exposure to ultraviolet light. Aust. Vet. J. 62:244, 1985.

126. Fotedar, H. L., and Chopra, S. L.: A note on skin follicular array in Beetal and its crosses with Alpine and Anglo-Nubian. Indian J. Anim. Sci. 45:51, 1976.

127. Fowler, E. H., and Calhoun, M. L.: The microscopic anatomy of developing fetal pig skin. Am. J. Vet. Res. 25:156, 1964.

128. Fraser, A. S.: Development of the skin follicle population in Merino sheep. Aust. J. Agric. Res. 5:737, 1954.

129. Fraser, I. E. B.: Cellular proliferation in the wool follicle bulb. In: Lyne, A. G., and Short, B. F. (eds.): *Biology of the Skin and Hair Growth*. New York, American Elsevier Publishing Co., 1965, p. 427.

130. Freinkel, R. K., and Traczyk, T. N.: Acid hydrolases of epidermis: Subcellular localization and relationship to cornification. J. Invest. Dermatol. 80:441, 1983.

131. Galpin, N.: The prenatal development of the coat of the New Zealand Romney lamb. J. Agric. Sci. 25:344, 1935.

132. Ghosal, A. K., et al.: A note on some aspects of sweat composition and their effect on canary colouration on Nali sheep. Indian J. Anim. Sci. 47:501, 1977.

133. Ghosal, A. K., and Guha, S.: Study on skin thickness in relation to its growth rate in Hariana calf. Indian J. Anim. Health 9:69, 1970.

134. Gillespie, J. M., et al.: Changes in the proteins of wool following treatment of sheep with epidermal growth factor. J. Invest. Dermatol. 79:197, 1982.

135. Godfrey, N. W., and Tribe, D. E.: The effect of thyroxine implantation on wool growth. J. Agric. Sci. 53:369, 1959.

136. Goldsberry, S., and Calhoun, M. L.: The comparative histology of the skin of Hereford and Aberdeen Angus cattle. Am. J. Vet. Res. 20:61, 1959.

137. Gonzalez-Jiminez, E., and Blaxter, K. L.: The metabolism and thermal regulation of calves in the first month of life. Br. J. Nutr. 16:199, 1962.

138. Goodall, A. M., and Yang, S. H.: The vascular supply of Ayrshire calves and embryos. J. Agric. Sci. 44:1, 1954.

139. Goodall, A. M.: Arterio-venous anastomoses in the skin of the head and ears of the calf. J. Anat. 89:100, 1955.

140. Gorbsky, G., and Steinberg, M. S.: Isolation of the intercellular glycoproteins of desmosomes. J. Cell Biol. 90:243, 1981.

141. Gravesen, S., et al.: Demonstration, isolation, and identification of culturable microfungi and bacteria in horse hair and dandruff. Allergy 33:89, 1978.

142. Gray, G. M., and Yardley, H. J.: Lipid composition of cells isolated from pig, human, and rat epidermis. J. Lipid Res. 16:434, 1975.

143. Gray, G. M., and Yardley, H. J.: Different populations of pig epidermal cells: Isolation and lipid composition. J. Lipid Res. 16:441, 1975.

144. Gray, G. M., et al.: 1-(3'-O-acyl)-β-glucosyl-N-dihydroxypentatriacontadienoylsphingosine, a major component of the glucosylceramides of pig and human epidermis. Biochem. Biophys. Acta 528:127, 1978.

145. Gray, G. M., and White, R. J.: Glycosphingolipids and ceramides in human and pig epidermis. J. Invest. Dermatol. 70:336, 1978.

146. Gu, J., et al.: Neuron-specific enolase in the Merkel cells of mammalian skin. Am. J. Pathol. 104:63, 1981.

147. Guillermo, L.: The hair of the Angora goat. Rev. Elv. Med. Vet. Pays Trop. 3:161, 1979.

148. Guss, S. B., and Ugel, A. R.: Immunofluorescent antibodies to bovine keratohyalin and immunologic confirmation of homology. J. Histochem. Cytochem. 20:97, 1972.

149. Hafez, E. S. E., et al.: Skin structure of Egyptian buffaloes and cattle with particular reference to sweat glands. J. Agric. Sci. 46:19, 1955.

150. Halprin, K. M., et al.: Control of epidermal cell proliferation in vitro. Br. J. Dermatol. 111:13, 1984.

151. Hardy, M. H., and Lyne, A. G.: The prenatal development of wool follicles in Merino sheep. Aust. J. Biol. Sci. 9:423, 1956.

152. Harmon, C. S., et al.: Effect of ischemia and reperfusion of pig skin flaps on epidermal glycogen metabolism. J. Invest. Dermatol. 86:69, 1986.

153. Harris, R. R., and MacKenzie, I. C.: The effects of alpha and beta adrenergic agonists and cyclic adenosine 3':5'-monophosphate on epidermal metabolism. J. Invest. Dermatol. 77:337, 1981.

154. Hart, D. S.: Photoperiodic and hormone response of wool growth in sheep. Proc. N. Z. Soc. Anim. Prod. 15:57, 1955.

155. Hart, D. S.: The effect of light-dark sequences on wool growth. J. Agric. Sci. 56:235, 1961.

156. Hart, D. S., et al.: Reversed periodic seasons and wool growth. Nature 198:310, 1963.

157. Hayman, R. H., and Nay, T.: Observations on hair growth and sheddiing in cattle. Aust. J. Agric. Res. 12:513, 1961.

158. Hayman, R. H.: Hair growth in cattle. In: Lyne, A. G., and Short, B. F. (eds.): *Biology of the Skin and Hair Growth*. New York, American Elsevier Publishing Co., 1965, p. 575.

159. Henderson, A. E.: Relationship of wool follicle and wool fibre dimensions. In: Lyne, A. G., and Short, B. F. (eds.): *Biology of the Skin and Hair Growth*. New York, American Elsevier Publishing Co., 1965, p. 447.

160. Henrikson, R. C., and Chapman, R. E.: Cysts of the outer root sheath of wool follicles: A study of abnormal keratinization. J. Ultrastruct. Res. 31:116, 1970.

161. Hensby, C. N., et al.: Mini-pig skin as a potential alternative for predicting human skin pharmacological reactions. Int. J. Immunopharmacol. 4:352, 1982.

162. Hensby, C. N., et al.: Superfused mini-pig skin. A new method for studying the interaction of drugs with prostaglandin biosynthesis. Br. J. Dermatol. 111:136, 1984.

163. Hickl, A.: Die Gruppierung der Haaranlagen ("Wild Zeichnung") in der Entwickelung des Hausschweines. Anat. Anz. 44:393, 1913.

164. Hollis, D. E., and Lyne, A. G.: Acetylcholinesterase-positive Langerhans' cells in the epidermis and wool follicles of the sheep. J. Invest. Dermatol. 58:211, 1972.

165. Hollis, D. E., et al.: Morphological changes in the skin and wool fibres of Merino sheep infused with mouse epidermal growth factor. Aust. J. Biol. Sci. 36:419, 1983.

166. Horter, R.: Zur Pilzflora hautkranker und-gesunder Schweine. Deut. Tierarztl. Wschr. 69:217, 1962.

167. Hunter, D., et al.: Exudative epidermitis of pigs. The serological identification and distribution of the associated *Staphylococcus*. Br. Vet. J. 126:225, 1970.

168. Hutchinson, G., and Mellor, D. J.: Effects of maternal nutrition on the initiation of secondary wool follicles in foetal sheep. J. Comp. Pathol. 93:577, 1983.

169. Hutchinson, J. C. D.: Photoperiodic control of the annual rhythm of wool growth. *In*: Lyne, A. G., and Short, B. F. (eds.): *Biology of the Skin and Hair Growth*. New York, American Elsevier Publishing Co., 1965, p. 565.

170. Hutchinson, K. J.: Climate corrections to the seasonal wool growth rhythm of sheep grazing in a southern Australian environment. Proc. Aust. Soc. Anim. Prod. 4:34, 1962.

171. Iizuka, H., et al.: Histamine H_2 receptor–adenylate cyclase system in pig skin. Biochem. Biophys. Acta 437:150, 1976.

172. Iizuka, H., et al.: The epinephrine activation of pig skin adenylate cyclase *in vivo* and subsequent refractoriness to the activation. J. Invest. Dermatol. 70:111, 1978.

173. Iizuka, H., et al.: Effects of hydrocortisone on the adrenaline–adenylate cyclase system of the skin. Br. J. Dermatol. 102:703, 1980.

174. Iizuka, H., et al.: Effects of trypsin on the cyclic AMP system of pig skin. J. Invest. Dermatol. 76:511, 1981.

175. Iizuka, H., and Ohkawara, A.: Effects of glucocorticoids on the beta-adrenergic adenylate cyclase system of pig skin. J. Invest. Dermatol. 80:524, 1983.

176. Iizuka, H., et al.: Pig-skin epidermal calmodulin: Effects of antagonists of calmodulin on DNA synthesis of pig-skin epidermis. Arch. Dermatol. Res. 278:133, 1985.

177. Iizuka, H., et al.: Adenosine and adenine nucleotides stimulation of skin (epidermal) adenylate cyclase. Biochem. Biophys. Acta 444:685, 1976.

178. Iizuka, H., et al.: Regulation of beta-adrenergic adenylate cyclase responsiveness of pig skin epidermis by suboptimal concentrations of epinephrine. J. Invest. Dermatol. 81:549, 1983.

178a. Ikai, K., and McGuire, J. S.: Phosphorylation of keratin polypeptides. Biochim. Biophys. Acta 760:371, 1983.

178b. Ikai, K., and McGuire, J. S.: Dephosphorylating activity of phosphorylated keratin polypeptides in calf snout epidermis. Arch. Dermatol. Res. 278:423, 1986.

178c. Ikai, K., and McGuire, J. S.: Cyclic AMP–dependent protein kinase in calf snout epidermis. Arch. Dermatol. Res. 278:367, 1986.

179. Ishizawa, H., et al.: Effects of betamethasone-17-valerate on the cyclic AMP system of the pig skin epidermis. J. Dermatol. 10:321, 1983.

180. Jacobs, R., et al.: Effect of hypoxia in the initiation of secondary wool follicles in the fetus. Aust. J. Biol. Sci. 39:79, 1986.

181. Iizuka, H., et al.: Effects of retinoids on the cyclic AMP system of pig skin epidermis. J. Invest. Dermatol. 85:324, 1985.

182. Iizuka, H., et al.: Colchicine-induced alteration of hormone-stimulated cyclic AMP synthesis in pig skin (epidermis). J. Invest. Dermatol. 82:357, 1984.

183. Jaksch, W.: Dermatomykosen der Equiden, Karnivoren und einiger Beitrag zur normalien Pilzflora der Haut. Wien. Tierarztl. Monat. 50:645, 1963.

184. Jarrett, A.: *The Physiology and Pathophysiology of the Skin I.* New York, Academic Press, 1973.

185. Jarrett, A.: *The Physiology and Pathophysiology of the Skin II.* New York, Academic Press, 1973.

186. Jarrett, A.: *The Physiology and Pathophysiology of the Skin III.* New York, Academic Press, 1974.

187. Jarrett, A.: *The Physiology and Pathophysiology of the Skin IV.* New York, Academic Press, 1977.

188. Jarrett, A.: *The Physiology and Pathophysiology of the Skin V.* New York, Academic Press, 1978.

189. Jarrett, A.: *The Physiology and Pathophysiology of the Skin VII.* New York, Academic Press, 1982.

190. Jeffries, B. C.: Changes in face cover of Merino and Corriedale sheep throughout the year. Aust. J. Exp. Agric. Anim. Husb. 4:118, 1964.

191. Jenkinson, D. M.: The skin of domestic animals. *In*: Rook, A. J., and Walton, G. S.: *Comparative Physiology and Pathology of the Skin*. Oxford, Blackwell Scientific Publications, 1965, p. 591.

192. Jenkinson, D. M., et al.: The distribution of nerves, monoamine oxidase, and cholinesterase in the skin of cattle. J. Anat. 100:593, 1966.

193. Jenkinson, D. M., and Blackburn, P. S.: The distribution of nerves, monoamine oxidase, and cholinesterase in the skin of the sheep and goat. J. Anat. 101:333, 1967.

194. Jenkinson, D. M., et al.: The distribution of nerves, monoamine oxidase, and cholinesterase in the skin of the pig. Res. Vet. Sci. 8:306, 1967.

195. Jenkinson, D. M., et al.: Seasonal changes in the skin glands of the goat. Br. Vet. J. 123:541, 1968.

196. Jenkinson, D. M., and Blackburn, P. S.: The distribution of nerves, monoamine oxidase, and cholinesterase in the skin of the horse. Res. Vet. Sci. 9:165, 1968.

197. Jenkinson, D. M., et al.: Histochemical studies on mast cells in cattle skin. Histochem. J. 2:419, 1970.

198. Jenkinson, D. M., and Mabon, R. M.: The effect of temperature and humidity on skin surface pH and the ionic composition of skin secretions in Ayrshire cattle. Br. Vet. J. 129:282, 1973.

199. Jenkinson, D. M., and Nay, T.: The sweat glands and hair follicles of different species of bovidae. Aust. J. Biol. Sci. 28:55, 1975.

200. Jenkinson, D. M., and Lloyd, D.H.: The topography of the skin surface of cattle and sheep. Br. Vet. J. 135:376, 1979.

201. Jenkinson, D. M., et al.: The antigenic composition and source of soluble proteins on the surface of the skin of sheep. J. Comp. Pathol. 89:43, 1979.

202. Jenkinson, D. M., and Mabon, R. M.: The corticosteroid content of cattle skin washings. Res. Vet. Sci. 19:94, 1975.

203. Jenkinson, D. M., and Nay, T.: The sweat glands and hair follicles of European cattle. Aust. J. Biol. Sci. 25:585, 1972.

204. Jenkinson, D. M., and Robertshaw, D.: Studies of the nature of sweat gland "fatigue" in the goat. J. Physiol. 212:455, 1971.

205. Jenkinson, D. M., et al.: The ultrastructure of the sweat glands of the ox, sheep, and goat during sweating and recovery. J. Anat. 129:117, 1979.

206. Jenkinson, D. M.: The skin surface: An environment of *Dermatophilus congolensis*. *In*: Lloyd, D. H., and Sellers, K. C. (eds.): *Dermatophilus Infection in Animals and Man*. New York, Academic Press, 1976, p. 146.

207. Jenkinson, D. M., et al.: The effect of temperature and humidity on the losses of nitrogenous substances from the skin of Ayrshire cattle. Res. Vet. Sci. 17:75, 1974.

208. Jenkinson, D. M.: Comparative physiology of sweating. Br. J. Dermatol. 88:397, 1973.

209. Jenkinson, D. M., et al.: Sweat protein. Br. J. Dermatol. 90:175, 1974.

210. Jenkinson, D. M., and Nay, T.: The sweat glands and hair follicles of Asian, African, and South American cattle. Aust. J. Biol. Sci. 26:259, 1973.

211. Jirka, M., and Kotas, J.: Some observations on the chemical composition of horse sweat. J. Physiol. 147:74, 1959.

212. Johnson, E.: Inherent rhythms of activity in the hair follicle and their control. *In*: Lyne, A. G., and Short, B. F. (eds.): *Biology of the Skin and Hair Growth*. New York, American Elsevier Publishing Co., 1965, p. 491.

213. Johnson, K. G.: Sweat glands as a factor influencing sweat discharge in sheep. J. Physiol. 235:523, 1973.

214. Johnson, K. G., and Creed, K. E.: Sweating in the intact horse and isolation perfused horse skin. Comp. Biochem. Physiol. 73C:259, 1982.

215. Johnson, K. G., and Linzell, J. L.: Sweat gland function in isolated perfused sheep and goat skin. J. Physiol. 226:25P, 1972.

216. Johnson, K. G.: Sweating rate and the electrolyte content of skin secretions of *Bos taurus* and *Bos indicus* cross-bred cows. J. Agric. Sci. 75:397, 1970.

217. Kapp, P., and Kovacs, A. B.: Ultrastructural details of the coronary band of swine foot. Acta Vet. Acad. Sci. Hung. 23:343, 1973.

218. Kerr, M. G., and Snow, D. H.: Composition of sweat of the horse during prolonged epinephrine (adrenaline) infusion, heat exposure, and exercise. Am. J. Vet. Res. 44:1571, 1983.

219. Kerr, M. G., et al.: Equine sweat composition during prolonged heat exposure. J. Physiol. 307:52P, 1980.

220. Khalil, H. M., et al.: Alkaline phosphatase–positive Langerhans' cells in the epidermis of cattle. J. Invest. Dermatol. 79:47, 1982.

221. Kimura, S., and Aoki, T.: Functional activity of the apocrine sweat gland in the goat. Tohoku J. Exp. Med. 76:8, 1962.

222. King, I. A., and Gray, G. M.: Incorporation of L-(^{3}H) fucose and D-(^{3}H) glucosamine into pig epidermal cell surface glycoproteins. Biochem. Soc. Trans. 6:1354, 1978.

223. King, I. A., and Tabiowo, A.: The dermis is required for the synthesis of extracellular glycosaminoglycans in cultured pig epidermis. Biochem. Biophys. Acta 632:234, 1980.

224. King, I. A., and Tabiowo, A.: Isolation and characterization of plasma membrane glycoproteins from pig epidermis. Biochem. J. 201:287, 1984.

225. King, I. A., et al.: Electrophoretic and immunoelectrophoretic analysis of pig epidermal plasma membrane glycoproteins. J. Invest. Dermatol. 83:42, 1984.

226. Kirk, E. J.: The dermatomes of the sheep. J. Comp. Neurol. 134:553, 1968.

227. Kirton, A. H., et al.: Some effects of thyroxine on live weight, metabolism, and wool growth of Romney ewes. N. Z. J. Agric. Res. 2:1143, 1959.

228. Klein, L. E., and Norlund, J. J.: Genetic basis of pigmentation and its disorders. Int. J. Dermatol. 20:621, 1981.

229. Koizumi, H., et al.: Calcium-activated, phospholipid-dependent protein kinase in pig epidermis. J. Invest. Dermatol. 83:261, 1984.

230. Kooistra, L. H., and Ginther, O. J.: Effect of photoperiod on reproductive activity and hair in mares. Am. J. Vet. Res. 36:1413, 1975.

231. Korner, A., and Pawelek, J.: Mammalian tyrosinase catalyzes three reactions in the biosynthesis of melanin. Science 217:1163, 1982.

232. Kozlowski, G. P., and Calhoun, M. L.: Microscopic anatomy of the integument of sheep. Am. J. Vet. Res. 30:1267, 1969.

233. Kral, F., and Schwartzman, R. M.: *Veterinary and Comparative Dermatology.* Philadelphia, J. B. Lippincott Co., 1964.

234. Kratochvil, Z.: Microscopic evaluation of hairs of the mane and tail of the wild horse *(Equus prezewalskii)* in comparison with the modern and historical domesticated horse *(Equus prezewalskii f. caballus).* Acta Vet. Brno 40:23, 1971.

235. Lamar, C. H., et al.: Equine endothelial cells *in vitro.* Am. J. Vet. Res. 47:956, 1986.

236. Lamberg, S. I., and Stoolmiller, A. C.: Glycosaminoglycans: A biochemical and clinical review. J. Invest. Dermatol. 63:433, 1974.

237. Larose, P., and Tweedle, A. S.: The influence of nutritional and climatic factors on wool growth and quality. II. Laboratory methods used in measurement of wool characters. Can. J. Res. D 16:166, 1938.

238. Lee, L. D., et al.: Immunology of epidermal fibrous proteins. J. Invest. Dermatol. 67:521, 1976.

239. Lerner, A. B.: Behavior of pigment cells. J. Invest. Dermatol. 75:121, 1980.

240. Lever, W. F., and Schumburg-Lever, G.: *Histopathology of the Skin VI.* Philadelphia, J. B. Lippincott Co., 1983.

241. Karasek, J., and Oehlert, W.: Ultrastructure of the pig epidermis. I. Stratum basale and stratum spinosum. Z. Mikrosk. Anat. Forsch. 78:133, 1968.

242. Karasek, J., and Oehlert, W.: Ultrastructure of the pig epidermis. II. Stratum granulosum and stratum corneum. Z. Mikrosk. Anat. Forsch. 79:157, 1968.

243. Kurosumi, K., and Kitamura, T.: Occurrence of foldings of plasma membrane (beta-membrane) in cells of pig's carpal organ as revealed by electron microscopy. Nature 181:489, 1958.

244. Langley, J. N., and Bennett, S.: Action of pilocarpine, arecoline and adrenaline on sweating in the horse. J. Physiol. 57:lxxxi, 1923.

245. Lindholm, J. S., et al.: Variation of skin surface lipid composition among mammals. Comp. Biochem. Biophys. 69B:75, 1981.

246. Lindner, H. R., and Ferguson, K. A.: Influence of the adrenal cortex on wool growth and its relation to break and tenderness of the fleece. Nature 177:188, 1956.

247. Link, L.: Uber das Vorkommen von "Haarscheiben" in der Haut von Saugetieren. Berl. Munch. Tierarztl. Wochenschr. 87:127, 1974.

248. Linzell, J. L.: The innervation of the mammary glands in the sheep and goat with some observations on the lumbosacral autonomic nerves. Q. J. Exp. Physiol. 44:160, 1959.

249. Lloyd, D. H., et al.: The antigenic constituents of cattle skin washings. J. Comp. Pathol. 87:75, 1977.

250. Lloyd, D. H., et al.: Structure of the epidermis in Ayrshire bullocks. Res. Vet. Sci. 26:172, 1979.

251. Lloyd, D. H., et al.: Structure of the sheep epidermis. Res. Vet. Sci. 26:180, 1979.

252. Lloyd, D. H., et al.: Location of the microflora in the skin of cattle. Br. Vet. J. 135:519, 1979.

253. Lloyd, D. H., et al.: The effects of some surface sampling procedures on the stratum corneum of bovine skin. Res. Vet. Sci. 26:250, 1979.

254. Lloyd, D. H., et al.: Location of immunoglobulins in the skin of cattle and sheep. Res. Vet. Sci. 26:47, 1979.

255. Loeffler, K.: Die Blutgefassversorgung der Haut des Rindes. Berl. Munch. Tierarztl. Wochenschr. 79:365, 1966.

256. Long, V. J. W.: Variations in lipid composition at different depths in the cow snout epidermis. J. Invest. Dermatol. 55:269, 1970.

257. Lowery, O. H., et al.: The demonstration of collagen and elastin in tissues, with results obtained in various normal tissues from different species. J. Biol. Chem. 139:795, 1941.

258. Lyne, A. G.: Bundles of primary follicles in sheep. Nature 179:825, 1957.

259. Lyne, A. G.: The development of the epidermis and hair canals in the Merino sheep foetus. Aust. J. Biol. Sci. 10:10, 1957.

260. Lyne, A. G., and Heideman, M. J.: The prenatal development of skin and hair in cattle *(Bos taurus L.).* Aust. J. Biol. Sci. 12:72, 1959.

261. Lyne, A. G., and Heideman, M. J.: The prenatal development of skin and hair in cattle. II. *Bos indicus* cross *Bos taurus L.* Aust. J. Biol. Sci. 13:584, 1960.

262. Lyne, A. G.: The postnatal development of wool follicles, shedding, and skin thickness in inbred Merino and Southdown-Merino crossbred sheep. Aust. J. Biol. Sci. 14:141, 1961.

263. Lyne, A. G., and Hollis, D. E.: The skin of the sheep: A comparison of body regions. Aust. J. Biol. Sci. 21:499, 1968.

264. Lyne, A. G., and Hollis, D. E.: Effects of freezing the skin and plucking the fibres in sheep with special reference to pigmentation. Aust. J. Biol. Sci. 21:981, 1968.

265. Lyne, A. G., and Hollis, D. E.: Merkel cells in sheep epidermis during fetal development. J. Ultrastruct. Res. 34:464, 1971.

266. Lyne, A. G., and Hollis, D. E.: The structure and development of the epidermis in sheep fetuses. J. Ultrastruct. Res. 38:444, 1972.

267. Mackie, A. G., and Nisbet, A. G.: The histology of the bovine muzzle. J. Agric. Sci. 52:376, 1959.

268. MacLean, J. A.: The regional distribution of cutaneous moisture vaporization in the Ayrshire calf. J. Agric. Sci. 61:275, 1963.

269. Mann, S. J.: Haarscheiben in the skin of sheep. Nature 205:1228, 1965.

270. Maqusood, M.: Effects of the thyroid gland on fleece growth in sheep. Br. Vet. J. 111:163, 1955.

271. Marcarian, N. Q., and Calhoun, M. L.: Microscopic anatomy of the integument of adult swine. Am. J. Vet. Res. 27:765, 1966.

272. Margolena, L. A.: Influence of the season on the anatomy of the skin and follicles of wooled sheep and dairy goats. Va. J. Sci. 9:393, 1958.

273. Margolena, L. A.: Skin and hair follicle development in dairy goats. Va. J. Sci. 10:33, 1959.

274. Margolena, L. A.: Season and comparative activity of wool follicles. Anat. Rec. 138:368, 1960.

275. Margolena, L. A.: Sudoriferous glands of sheep and goats. Z. Mikrosk. Anat. Forsch. 69:217, 1962.

276. Margolena, L. A.: Sebaceous glands of sheep and goats. Va. J. Sci. 14:170, 1963.

277. Margolena, L. A.: Ziehl-Neelsen's stain for skin sections to show wool and hair follicles. Stain Technol. 38:145, 1963.

278. Margolena, L. A., and Dolnick, E. H.: Differential staining method for elastic fibers, collagen fibers, and keratin. Stain Technol. 26:119, 1951.

279. Margolena, L. A., and Dolnick, E. H.: Cell division in the epidermis of foetuses and young lambs of Karakul sheep. Va. J. Sci. 4:71, 1953.

280. Marshall, F. H. A.: On hair in the equidae. Vet. J. 54:34, 1902.

281. Marston, H. R., and Peirce, A. W.: The effects following thyroidectomy in Merino sheep. Aust. J. Exp. Biol. Med. Sci. 10:203, 1932.

282. Martin, A. K.: Some errors in the determination of nitrogen retention of sheep by nitrogen balance studies. Br. J. Nutr. 20:325, 1966.

283. Marzouk, M. A., et al.: Studies on commensal micro-organisms inhabiting bovine skin in Sharkia Governorate. J. Egypt. Vet. Med. Assoc. 40:61, 1980.

284. Marzulli, F. N., and Callahan, J. F.: The capacity of certain laboratory animals to sweat. J. Am. Vet. Med. Assoc. 131:80, 1957.

285. Marzulli, F. N., and Maibach, H. I.: *Dermatotoxicology and Pharmacology*. New York, John Wiley & Sons, 1977.

286. Matoltsy, A. G.: Desmosomes, filaments, and keratohyaline granules: Their role in the stabilization and keratinization of the epidermis. J. Invest. Dermatol. 65:127, 1975.

287. McMaster, J. D., et al.: The lipid composition of bovine sebum and dermis. Br. Vet. J. 141:34, 1985.

288. McDonald, B. J., et al.: Effect of epidermal growth factor on wool fibre morphology and skin histology. Res. Vet. Sci. 35:91, 1983.

289. Meyer, H., et al.: Untersuchungen uber Schweiffmenge und Schweiffzusammensetzung beim Pferd. Tierarztl. Umsch. 33:330, 1978.

290. Meyer, W., et al.: Zur Bedeutung der apokrinen Hautdrusen der allgemeinen Korperdecke bei verschiedenen Haussaugetierarten. Dtsch. Tierarztl. Wochenschr. 85:194, 1978.

291. Meyer, W., et al.: Aspects of fibre arrangements in the skin of the pig. Anat. Histol. Embryol. 9:367, 1980.

292. Meyer, W., and Neurand, K.: Distribution and activities of the oxidative enzymes in the apocrine skin glands of the pig. Anat. Histol. Embryol. 5:189, 1976.

293. Meyer, W., and Neurand, K.: Distribution and activities of hydrolytic enzymes in the apocrine skin glands of the domestic pig. Acta Anat. 97:103, 1977.

294. Meyer, W., and Neurand, K.: The distribution of enzymes in the skin of the domestic pig. Lab. Anim. 10:237, 1976.

295. Meyer, W., and Neurand, K.: Verteilung und Aktivaten hydrolytischer Enzyme in den apokrinen Hautdrusen des Schweines. Zbl. Vet. Med. C 51:189, 1976.

296. Meyer, W., and Neurand, K.: Enzymhistochemische Untersuchungen an der Epidermis des Hausschweines. Z. Mikrosk. Anat. Forsch. 89:961, 1975.

297. Meyer, W., and Neurand, K.: Verteilung und Aktivaten hydrolytischer Enzyme in den apokrinen Hautdrusen des Hausschweines. Acta Anat. 97:103, 1977.

298. Meyer, W., et al.: The skin of domestic mammals as a model for the human skin, with specific reference to the domestic pig. Curr. Probl. Dermatol. 7:39, 1978.

299. Meyer, W., et al.: Elastic fibre arrangement in the skin of the pig. Arch. Dermatol. Res. 270:391, 1981.

300. Meyer, W., et al.: Collagen fibre arrangement in the skin of the pig. J. Anat. 134:139, 1982.

301. Meyer, W., and Neurand, K.: The demonstration of Krause end bulbs (Pacinian corpuscles) in the hairy skin of the pig. Anat. Histol. Embryol. 11:283, 1982.

302. Meyer, W., and Gorgen, S.: Development of hair coat and skin glands in fetal porcine integument. J. Anat. 144:201, 1986.

303. Minor, R. R.: Collagen metabolism. Am. J. Pathol. 98:227, 1980.

304. Molyneux, G. S., and Griffin, C. J.: Arteriovenous anastomoses in body skin of Merino sheep. J. Dent. Res. 42:6, 1963.

305. Molyneux, G. S.: Observations on the distribution of arteriovenous anastomoses in sheep skin. J. Anat. 98:483, 1964.

306. Molyneux, G. S.: Observations on the structure, distribution, and significance of arteriovenous anastomoses in sheep skin. *In*: Lyne, A. G., and Short, B. F. (eds.): *Biology of the Skin and Hair Growth*. New York, American Elsevier Publishing Co., 1965, p. 591.

307. Molyneux, G. S.: The interrelationship of smooth muscle cells in arteriovenous anastomoses in sheep skin. J. Anat. 106:202, 1970.

308. Molyneux, G. S.: Occurrence of non-adrenergic axons containing large granular vesicles in arteriovenous anastomoses in the skin of sheep. J. Anat. 121:420, 1976.

309. Montagna, W., and Yung, J. S.: The skin of the domestic pig. J. Invest. Dermatol. 42:11, 1964.

310. Montagna, W.: Comparative anatomy and physiology of the skin. Arch. Dermatol. 96:357, 1967.

311. Montagna, W., and Parakkal, P. F.: *The Structure and Function of Skin III*. New York, Academic Press, 1974.

312. Montgomery, I., et al.: The effects of thermal stimulation of the ultrastructure of the fundus and duct of the equine sweat gland. J. Anat. 135:13, 1982.

313. Montgomery, I., et al.: The ultrastructure of the sweat gland duct of the ox, sheep, and goat before and during sweating. J. Anat. 134:741, 1982.

314. Moore, G. P. M., et al.: Epidermal growth factor causes shedding of the fleece of Merino sheep. Search 12:128, 1981.

315. Moore, G. P. M., et al.: Inhibition of wool growth in Merino sheep following administration of mouse epidermal growth factor and a derivative. Aust. J. Biol. Sci. 35:163, 1982.

316. Moore, G. P. M., et al.: Treatment of ewes at different stages of pregnancy with epidermal growth factor. Acta Endocrinol. 105:558, 1984.

317. Moore, G. P. M., et al.: Epidermal hyperplasia and wool follicle regression in sheep infused with epidermal growth factor. J. Invest. Dermatol. 84:172, 1985.

318. Moore, T., et al.: Observations on excretory patterns of sodium, potassium, and water in different genetic groups of sheep under high ambient temperature. Indian J. Anim. Sci. 50:182, 1980.

319. Morris, L. R.: Photoperiodicity of seasonal rhythm of wool growth in sheep. Nature 190:102, 1961.

320. Moschella, S. L., et al.: *Dermatology*. Philadelphia, W. B. Saunders Co., 1975.

321. Mowafy, M., and Cassens, R. G.: A histological study of skin from the pig. J. Anim. Sci. 35:205, 1972.

322. Muller, G. H., et al.: *Small Animal Dermatology III*. Philadelphia, W. B. Saunders Co., 1983.

323. Nasser, M., et al.: Carrier-states of staphylococci in domestic animals and in contact persons. J. Egypt. Vet. Med. Assoc. 40:23, 1980.

324. Nay, T., and Hayman, R. H.: Sweat glands in Zebu and European cattle. Aust. J. Agric. Res. 7:482, 1956.

325. Nay, T.: Sweat glands in cattle: Histology, morphology, and evolutionary trends. Aust. J. Agric. Res. 10:121, 1959.

326. Nay, T., and Hayman, R. H.: Some skin characters in five breeds on European (*B. taurus L.*) dairy cattle. Aust. J. Agric. Res. 14:294, 1963.

327. Nay, T., and Dowling, D. T.: Size of sweat glands in Shorthorn strains and Zebu cross Shorthorn cattle. Aust. J. Agric. Res. 8:385, 1957.

328. Neurand, K., and Meyer, W.: Enzyme histochemical studies on the sebaceous glands of the pig. Anat. Anz. 140:286, 1976.

329. Nicolaides, N., et al.: The skin surface lipids of man compared with those of eighteen species of animals. J. Invest. Dermatol. 51:83, 1968.

330. Nicolaides, N., et al.: Diester waxes in surface lipids of animal skin. Lipids 5:299, 1970.

331. Nisbet, A. M.: Arteriovenous anastomoses in the teat of a cow. Nature 178:1477, 1956.

332. Noble, R. C., et al.: Presence of linoleic acid in the skin surface lipids of the ox. Res. Vet. Sci. 17:372, 1974.

333. Noble, R. C., et al.: Relationships between lipids in plasma and skin secretions of neonatal calf with particular reference to linoleic acid. Lipids 10:128, 1975.

334. Noble, R. C., et al.: Lipid composition of the bovine epidermis. Res. Vet. Sci. 37:120, 1984.

335. Noble, W. C.: *Microbiology of Human Skin II*. London, Lloyd-Luke, 1981.

336. Noble, W. C.: *Microbial Skin Disease: Its Epidemiology*. London, Butler and Tanner, Ltd., 1983.

337. Nwufoh, K. J., and Amakiri, S. F.: The normal skin bacterial flora of some cattle breeds in Nigeria. Bull. Anim. Health Prod. Afr. 29:103, 1981.

338. O'Kelly, J. C., et al.: Sebum composition of tropical and temperate breeds of cattle. Comp. Biochem. Physiol. 67B:217, 1980.

339. O'Kelly, J. C., and Reich, H. P.: The effect of environmental temperature on sebum composition of tropical and temperate breeds of cattle. Lipids 17:19, 1982.

340. Ohkawara, A., and Iizuka, H.: Glucocorticoid-induced alteration of beta-adrenergic adenylate cyclase response of epidermis. Arch. Dermatol. Res. 277:88, 1985.

341. Orwin, D. F. G., and Thomson, R. W.: The distribution of coated vesicles in keratinizing cells of the wool follicle. Aust. J. Biol. Sci. 24:573, 1972.

342. Pan, Y. S.: Variation in hair characters over the body in Sahiwal Zebu and Jersey cattle. Aust. J. Agric. Res. 15:346, 1964.

343. Pan, Y. S., et al.: Sweating rate at different body regions on cattle and its correlation with some quantitative components of sweat gland volume for a given area of skin. Aust. J. Agric. Res. 20:396, 1969.

344. Panaretto, B. A., et al.: Plasma concentrations and urinary excretion of mouse epidermal growth factor associated with the inhibition of food consumption and of wool growth in Merino wethers. J. Endocrinol. 94:191, 1982.

345. Panaretto, B. A., et al.: Inhibition of DNA synthesis in dermal tissue of Merino sheep treated with depilatory doses of mouse epidermal growth factor. J. Endocrinol. 100:25, 1984.

346. Pant, K. P.: Medullated Mohair fibres of Angora, Gaddi, and their crossbred goats. Indian Vet. J. 46:125, 1969.

347. Platt, B. S.: Nutritional influences on the skin: Experimental evidence. In: Rook, A. J., and Walton, G. S.: Comparative Physiology and Pathology of the Skin. Oxford, Blackwell Scientific Publications, 1965, p. 245.

348. Poon, W. Y., et al.: In vivo changes in the composition of cattle skin surface lipid with time. Res. Vet. Sci. 25:234, 1978.

349. Prasad, G.: Observations on the fine structure of bovine sweat glands. Nord. Vet. Med. 25:163, 1973.

350. Pritchard, M. M. L., and Daniel, P. M.: Arteriovenous anastomoses in the tongue of the sheep and the goat. Am. J. Anat. 95:203, 1954.

351. Prota, G.: Recent advances in the chemistry of melanogenesis in mammals. J. Invest. Dermatol. 75:122, 1980.

352. Purohit, S. K., et al.: A note on agar-gel electrophoretogram of skin secretions and serum of Nali sheep. Indian J. Anim. Sci. 48:321, 1978.

353. Quevedo, W. C., and Fleischmann, R. D.: Developmental biology of mammalian melanocytes. J. Invest. Dermatol. 75:116, 1980.

354. Qualliam, T. A., et al.: Epidermal innervation in the pig's snout. J. Anat. 115:156, 1973.

355. Rackow, J.: Beitrag zur Histologie und Physiologie des glatten Hautmuskels des Pferdes. Arch. Tierheilk. 24:273, 1898.

356. Rai, A. K., et al.: Sweating in sheep and goats. Indian J. Anim. Sci. 49:546, 1979.

357. Rai, A. K., et al.: Cutaneous water loss and respiration rates of various breeds of sheep at high ambient temperatures. Trop. Anim. Health Prod. 11:51, 1979.

358. Rai, A. K., et al.: Composition of sweat in sheep exposed to high ambient temperatures. Indian J. Anim. Sci. 52:1056, 1982.

359. Rang, H.: Quantitative und Qualitative Untersuchungen an Mastzellen des Schweines. Zbl. Vet. Med. A 20:546, 1973.

360. Razavi-Rohani, M., and Bramley, A. J.: A study of the frequency and distribution of Streptococcus uberis contamination on the body of lactating and nonlactating cows. Indian Vet. J. 58:804, 1981.

361. Reifenrath, W. G., et al.: Percutaneous penetration in the hairless dog, weanling pig, and grafted athymic nude mouse: Evaluation of models for predicting skin penetration in man. Br. J. Dermatol. 111:123, 1984.

362. Reis, P. J.: Variations in the sulphur content of wool. In: Lyne, A. G., and Short, B. F. (eds.): Biology of the Skin and Hair Growth. New York, American Elsevier Publishing Co., 1965, p. 365.

363. Rhoad, A. O.: Absorption and reflection of solar radiation in relation to coat colour in cattle. Proc. Am. Soc. Anim. Prod. 33:291, 1940.

364. Rieger, M. M.: Epidermal ornithine decarboxylase. Int. J. Dermatol. 21:455, 1982.

365. Riemerschmid, G.: The amount of solar radiation and its absorption on the hairy coat of cattle under South African and European conditions. J. S. Afr. Vet. Med. Assoc. 14:121, 1943.

366. Riemerschmid, G., and Elder, J. S.: The absorptivity for solar radiation of different coloured hairy coats of cattle. Onderstepoort J. Vet. Sci. 20:223, 1945.

367. Robertshaw, D.: The pattern and control of sweating in the sheep and the goat. J. Physiol. 198:531, 1968.

368. Rogers, G. E., and Clarke, R. M.: An approach to the investigation of protein biosynthesis in hair follicles. In: Lyne, A. G., and Short, B. F. (eds.): Biology of the Skin and Hair Growth. New York, American Elsevier Publishing Co., 1965, p. 329.

369. Rook, A., et al.: Textbook of Dermatology III. Oxford, Blackwell Scientific Publications, 1979.

370. Rose, R. J., et al.: Plasma and sweat electrolyte concentrations in the horse during long distance exercise. Equine Vet. J. 12:19, 1980.

371. Rougeot, J.: The effect of thyroid hormones on the morphology of the wool cuticle. In: Lyne, A. G., and Short, B. F. (eds.): Biology of the Skin and Hair Growth. New York, American Elsevier Publishing Co., 1965, p. 625.

372. Ryder, M. L.: The prenatal development of follicle population in the Romney lamb. J. Agric. Sci. 47:6, 1956.

373. Ryder, M. L.: Studies on the nutrition of wool follicles in sheep: The anatomy of the general blood supply to the skin. J. Agric. Sci. 45:311, 1955.

374. Ryder, M. L.: Observations of nutritional and seasonal changes in the fleece of some Masham sheep. J. Agric. Sci. 47:129, 1956.

375. Ryder, M. L.: Nutritional factors influencing hair and wool growth. In: Montagna, W., and Ellis, R. A. (eds.): The Biology of Hair Growth. New York, Academic Press, 1958, p. 359.

376. Ryder, M. L.: A survey of the follicle populations in a range of British breeds of sheep. J. Agric. Sci. 49:275, 1957.

377. Ryder, M. L.: Some observations on the glycogen of the wool follicle. Q. J. Micro. Sci. 99:221, 1958.

378. Ryder, M. L.: Some unusual outgrowths from secondary follicles in Soay sheep. Nature 183:1831, 1959.

379. Ryder, M. L.: Preliminary observations on seasonal changes in the fleeces of unshorn Merino sheep. Proc. Aust. Soc. Anim. Prod. 4:46, 1962.

380. Ryder, M. L.: Wool growth in sheep. In: Rook, A. J., and Walton, G. S.: Comparative Physiology and Pathology of the Skin. Oxford, Blackwell Scientific Publications, 1965, p. 161.

381. Ryder, M. L.: Coat structure and seasonal shedding in goats. Anim. Prod. 8:289, 1966.

382. Ryder, M. L.: Structure and seasonal change of the coat in Scottish wild goats. J. Zool. 161:355, 1970.

383. Ryder, M. L.: Growth cycles in the coat of ruminants. Int. J. Chronobiol. 5:369, 1978.

384. Sackville, J. P., and Bowstead, J. E.: The influence of nutritional and climatic factors on wool growth and quality. I. Statement of problem and experimental procedure. Can. J. Res. D 16:153, 1938.

385. Sar, M., and Calhoun, M. L.: Microscopic anatomy of the integument of the common American goat. Am. J. Vet. Res. 27:444, 1966.

386. Schaller, O.: Die periphere sensible Innervation der Haut am Rumpfe des Rhindes. Wien. Tierarztl. Monatsschr. 43:346, 1956.

387. Schinckel, P. G.: The relationship between follicle numbers and wool production. Aust. J. Agric. Res. 8:512, 1957.

388. Schinckel, P. G., and Short, B. F.: The influence of nutritional level during prenatal and early post-natal life on adult fleece and body characters. Aust. J. Agric. Res. 12:176, 1961.

389. Schinckel, P. G.: Mitotic activity in wool follicle bulbs. Aust. J. Biol. Sci. 14:659, 1961.

390. Schleger, A. V., and Turner, H. G.: Sweating rates of cattle in the field and their reaction to diurnal and seasonal changes. Aust. J. Agric. Res. 16:92, 1965.

391. Schleger, A. V.: Relationship between cyclic changes in the hair follicle and sweat gland size in cattle. Aust. J. Biol. Sci. 19:607, 1966.

392. Schleger, A. V., and Turner, H. G.: Analysis of coat characters of cattle. Aust. J. Agric. Res. 11:875, 1960.

393. Schleger, A. V.: Physiological attributes of coat colour in beef cattle. Aust. J. Agric. Res. 13:943, 1962.

394. Schleger, A. V., and Bean, K. G.: The melanocyte system of cattle skin. I. Amelanotic dendritic cells of epidermis. Aust. J. Biol. Sci. 26:973, 1973.

395. Schleger, A. V., and Bean, K. G.: The melanocyte system of cattle skin. II. Melanotic melanocytes of epidermis and dermis. Aust. J. Biol. Sci. 26:985, 1973.

396. Schleger, A. V., and O'Kelly, J. C.: Esterase activity in the bovine sweat gland: Genetic differences and the effect of temperature. Acta Anat. 125:229, 1986.

397. Schonberg, F.: Der Ross-Spiegel. Eine Eigentumlichkeit des integumentum pelvis beim Pferde. Berl. Munch. Tierarztl. Wochenschr. 42:777, 1926.

398. Schreiber, J.: Die anatomischen Grundlagen der Leitungsanasthesis beim Rhind. Wien. Tierarztl. Monatsschr. 42:129, 1955.

399. Schwarz, R., et al.: The prenatal development of the cutaneous vascular architecture of the pig. Anat. Histol. Embryol. 11:377, 1982.

400. Scott, D. W.: Folliculitis and furunculosis. *In*: Robinson, N. (ed.): *Current Therapy in Equine Medicine*. Philadelphia, W. B. Saunders Co., 1985, p. 542.

401. Scott, D. W., et al.: Caprine dermatology. Part I. Normal skin and bacterial and fungal disorders. Compend. Cont. Ed. 6:S190, 1984.

402. Scott, F. M. M., et al.: Staphylococcal dermatitis of sheep. Vet. Rec. 107:572, 1980.

403. Short, B. F., et al.: Proliferation of follicle matrix cells in relation to wool growth. *In*: Lyne, A. G., and Short, B. F. (eds.): *Biology of the Skin and Hair Growth*. New York, American Elsevier Publishing Co., 1965, p. 409.

404. Sisson, S., and Grossman, J. D.: *Anatomy of Domestic Animals*. Philadelphia, W. B. Saunders Co., 1956.

405. Skerrow, C. J., and Matoltsy, A. G.: Isolation of epidermal desmosomes. J. Cell Biol. 63:513, 1974.

406. Skerrow, C. H., and Matoltsy, A. G.: Chemical characterization of isolated epidermal desmosomes. J. Cell Biol. 63:524, 1974.

407. Slee, J., and Carter, H. B.: A comparative study of fleece growth in Tasmanian Fine Merino and Wiltshire Horn ewes. J. Agric. Sci. 47:11, 1961.

408. Slee, J., and Carter, H. B.: Fibre shedding and fibre-follicle relationships in the fleeces of Wiltshire Horn cross Scottish Blackface sheep crosses. J. Agric. Sci. 58:309, 1962.

409. Slee, J.: Birthcoat shedding in Wiltshire Horn lambs. Anim. Prod. 5:301, 1963.

410. Slee, J.: Seasonal patterns of moulting in Wiltshire Horn sheep. *In*: Lyne, A. G., and Short, B. F. (eds.): *Biology of the Skin and Hair Growth*. New York, American Elsevier Publishing Co., 1965, p. 545.

411. Slee, J.: The genetics of hair growth. *In*: Rook, A. J., and Walton, G. S.: *Comparative Physiology and Pathology of the Skin*. Oxford, Blackwell Scientific Publications, 1965, p. 103.

412. Slen, S. B., and Whiting, F.: Wool production as affected by the level of protein in the ration of mature ewes. J. Anim. Sci. 11:156, 1952.

413. Smith, F.: The histology of the skin of the horse. Vet. J. 26:333, 1888.

414. Smith, F.: Note on the composition of the sweat of the horse. J. Physiol. 11:497, 1890.

415. Smith, J. L., and Calhoun, M. L.: The microscopic anatomy of the integument of newborn swine. Am. J. Vet. Res. 25:165, 1964.

416. Smith, M. E., and Jenkinson, D. M.: Effect of age, sex, and season on sebum output of Ayrshire calves. J. Agric. Sci. 84:57, 1975.

417. Smith, M. E., and Jenkinson, D. M.: The mode of secretion of the sebaceous glands of cattle. Br. Vet. J. 131:610, 1975.

418. Smith, M. E., et al.: The effect of environment on sebum output and composition in cattle. Res. Vet. Sci. 19:253, 1975.

419. Smith, M. E., and Ahmed, S. U.: The lipid composition of cattle sebaceous glands: A comparison with skin surface lipid. Res. Vet. Sci. 21:250, 1976.

420. Smith, R. F., and Evans, B. L.: Bacteria of porcine skin, xenografts, and treatment with neomycin sulfate. Appl. Microbiol. 23:293, 1972.

421. Snow, D. H.: Identification of the receptor involved in adrenaline-mediated sweating in the horse. Res. Vet. Sci. 23:247, 1977.

422. Snow, D. H.: Metabolic and physiological effects of adrenoreceptor agonists and antagonists in the horse. Res. Vet. Sci. 27:372, 1979.

423. Snow, D. H., et al.: Alterations in blood, sweat, urine, and muscle composition during prolonged exercise in the horse. Vet. Rec. 110:377, 1982.

424. Soliman, M. K., and Nadim, M. A.: Calcium, sodium, and potassium levels in the serum and sweat of horses after strenuous exercise. Zbl. Vet. Med. A 14:53, 1967.

425. Spearman, R. I. C.: *The Integument*. London, Cambridge University Press, 1973.

426. Speed, J. G.: The importance of the coat in Exmoor and other mountain and moorland ponies living out of doors. Br. Vet. J. 116:91, 1960.

427. Stephen, E., and Redecker, R.: Die Rolle der Haut bei der Thermoregulation von Haustieren. Dtsch. Tierarztl. Wochenschr. 77:628, 1970.

428. Stephenson, S. K.: Wool follicle development in the New Zealand Romney and N-type sheep. Aust. J. Agric. Res. 8:371, 1957.

429. Stephenson, S. K.: Wool follicle development in the New Zealand Romney and N-type sheep. V. The prenatal relationships between growth, skin expansion, and primary follicle number. Aust. J. Agric. Res. 10:453, 1959.

430. Straile, W. E.: Sensory hair follicles in mammalian skin: The tylotrich follicle. Am. J. Anat. 106:133, 1960.

431. Straile, W. E.: Root sheath–dermal papilla relationships and the control of hair growth. *In*: Lyne, A. G., and Short, B. F. (eds.): *Biology of the Skin and Hair Growth*. New York, American Elsevier Publishing Co., 1965, p. 35.

432. Straile, W. E.: Encapsulated nerve end-organs in the rabbit, mouse, sheep, and man. J. Comp. Neurol. 136:317, 1969.

433. Streilein, J. W.: Skin-associated lymphoid tissues (SALT): Origins and functions. J. Invest. Dermatol. 80:12S, 1983.

434. Stromberg, M. W., et al.: Interfollicular smooth muscle in the skin of the domesticated pig (*Susscrofa*). Anat. Rec. 201:455, 1981.

435. Symington, R. B.: Light regulation of coat shedding in a tropical breed of hair sheep. Nature 184:1076, 1959.

436. Szeligowski, E.: Contribution to the histology of the skin of the horse. Folia Morphol. 13:531, 1954.

437. Szodoray, L.: The structure of the junction of the dermis and epidermis. Arch. Dermatol. Syph. 23:920, 1931.

438. Takagi, S., and Tagawa, M.: A cytological and cytochemical study of the sweat gland of the horse. Jap. J. Physiol. 9:153, 1959.

439. Takagi, S., and Tagawa, M.: Nerve fibers supplying the horse sweat gland. Jap. J. Physiol. 11:158, 1961.

440. Takatori, K., et al.: Occurrence of equine dermatophytosis in Hokkaido. Jap. J. Vet. Sci. 43:307, 1981.

441. Takatori, K., et al.: Fungal flora of equine skin with or without dermatophytosis. Jap. J. Vet. Med. Assoc. 34:580, 1981.

442. Talukdar, A. H., and Calhoun, M. L.: A modified dermal part in the skin of the croup region of the horse. Pak. J. Vet. Sci. 1:84, 1967.

443. Talukdar, A. H., et al.: Specialized vascular structures in the skin of the horse. Am. J. Vet. Res. 33:335, 1972.

444. Talukdar, A. H., et al.: Microscopic anatomy of the skin of the horse. Am. J. Vet. Res. 33:2365, 1972.

445. Talukdar, A. H.: A histological study of the dermoepidermal junction in the skin of horse. Res. Vet. Sci. 15:328, 1973.

446. Talukdar, A. H., et al.: Sensory end organs in the upper lip of the horse. Am. J. Vet. Res. 31:1751, 1970.
447. Talukdar, A. H., et al.: Sweat glands of the horse: A histologic study. Am. J. Vet. Res. 31:2179, 1970.
448. Tamakijk, K., and Katz, S. I.: Ontogeny of Langerhans' cells. J. Invest. Dermatol. 75:12, 1980.
449. Taneja, G. C.: Sweating in cattle. IV. Control of sweat glands secretion. J. Agric. Sci. 52:66, 1959.
450. Trautman, A., and Fiebiger, J.: Fundamentals of Histology of Domestic Animals. Ithaca, Comstock Publishing Associates, 1957.
451. Tsukise, A., and Yamada, K.: The histochemistry of complex carbohydrates in the scrotum of the boar. Histochemistry 72:511, 1981.
452. Tsukise, A., et al.: Histochemistry of complex carbohydrates in the skin of the pig snout, with special reference to eccrine glands. Acta Anat. 115:141, 1983.
453. Tsukise, A., and Meyer, W.: Histochemistry of complex carbohydrates in the hairy skin of the domestic pig. Histochem. J. 15:845, 1983.
454. Tsukise, A., et al.: Histochemistry of complex carbohydrates in the skin of the pig. Anat. Histol. Embryol. 11:377, 1982.
455. Turner, H. G.: Effect of clipping the coat on performance of calves in the field. Aust. J. Agric. Res. 13:180, 1962.
456. Turner, H. G., and Schleger, A. V.: The significance of coat type in cattle. Aust. J. Agric. Res. 11:645, 1960.
457. Turner, H. G., et al.: The hair follicle population of cattle in relation to breed and body weight. Aust. J. Agric. Res. 13:960, 1962.
458. Ugel, A. R.: Keratohyalin: Extraction and in vitro aggregation. Science 166:250, 1969.
459. Ugel, A. R., and Idler, W.: Stratum granulosum: Dissection from cattle hoof epidermis. J. Invest. Dermatol. 55:350, 1970.
460. Ugel, A. R.: Studies on isolated aggregating oligoribonucleo-proteins of the epidermis with histochemical and morphological characteristics of keratohyalin. J. Cell Biol. 49:405, 1971.
461. Ugel, A. R., et al.: Fractionation and characterization of an oligomeric series of bovine keratohyalin by polyacrylamide gel electrophoresis. Anal. Biochem. 43:410, 1971.
462. Ugel, A. R., and Idler, W.: Further characterization of bovine keratohyalin. J. Cell Biol. 52:453, 1972.
463. Vegad, J. L.: Staining of mast cells and eosinophils in the sheep skin. N. Z. Vet. J. 18:31, 1970.
464. Vulov, T.: Age changes in microstructure of the skin in fine-fleeced sheep. Vet. Med. Nauki 11:35, 1974.
465. Waites, G. M. H., and Voglmayr, J. K.: Apocrine sweat glands of the scrotum of the ram. Nature 196:965, 1962.
466. Walton, G. S.: Abnormal hair growth in domestic animals. In: Rook, A. J., and Walton, G. S.: Comparative Physiology and Pathology of the Skin. Oxford, Blackwell Scientific Publications, 1965, p. 211.
467. Warren, G. H., et al.: A morphometric analysis of the changes with age in the skin surface wax and the sebaceous gland area of Merino sheep. Aust. Vet. J. 60:238, 1983.
468. Watson, W. A.: The carriage of pathogenic staphylococci by sheep. Vet. Rec. 77:477, 1965.
469. Webster, M. E. D., and Johnson, K. G.: Distribution of temperature in the skin of sheep exposed to moderate environments. Nature 201:208, 1965.
470. Webster, R. C., and Maibach, H. I.: Percutaneous absorption in man and animal: A perspective. In: Drill, V. A., and Lazar, P. (eds.): Cutaneous Toxicity. New York, Academic Press, 1977, p. 111.
471. Weibel, E. R., and Palade, G. E.: New cytoplasmic components in arterial endothelia. J. Cell Biol. 23:101, 1964.
472. Wentzel, D., and Vosloo, L. P.: Prenatal development of hair follicle groups in Angora goats. Agroanimalia 6:13, 1974.
473. Wertz, P. W., and Downing, D. T.: Glycolipids in mammalian epidermis: Structure and function in the water barrier. Science 217:1261, 1982.
474. Wertz, P. W., and Downing, D. T.: Acylglycosylceramides from pig epidermis: Structure determination. J. Lipid Res. 24:753, 1983.
475. Wertz, P. W., and Downing, D. T.: Ceramides of pig epidermis: Structure determination. J. Lipid Res. 24:759, 1983.
476. Wertz, P. W., and Downing, D. T.: Glucosylceramides of pig epidermis: Structure determination. J. Lipid Res. 24:1135, 1983.
477. Wertz, P. W., et al.: Comparison of the hydroxyacids from the epidermis and from the sebaceous glands of the horse. Comp. Biochem. Physiol. 75B:217, 1983.
478. Whittow, G. C.: The significance of the extremities of the ox (Bos taurus) in thermoregulation. J. Agric. Sci. 58:109, 1962.
479. Wildman, A. B.: Coat and fibre development in some British sheep. Proc. Zool. Soc. Lond. 1932:257, 1932.
480. Wildman, A. B.: Photoperiodicity and wool growth in Romney rams and wethers. Nature 180:296, 1957.
481. Williams, A. J.: The effect of daily photoperiod on the wool growth of Merino rams subjected to unrestricted and restricted feeding regimens. Aust. J. Exp. Agric. Anim. Husb. 4:124, 1964.
482. Wodzicka, M.: Seasonal variations in wool growth and heat tolerance of sheep. I. Wool growth. Aust. J. Agric. Res. 11:75, 1960.
483. Wodzicka, M.: Seasonal variations in wool growth and heat tolerance of sheep. II. Heat tolerance. Aust. J. Agric. Res. 11:85, 1960.
484. Worden, A. N.: Nutritional influences on the skin in domestic animals. In: Rook, A. J., and Walton, G. S.: Comparative Physiology and Pathology of the Skin. Oxford, Blackwell Scientific Publications, 1965, p. 261.
485. Wrobel, K. H., and Lindner, E.: Die Histopochemie und ultrastruktur der Glandulae nasolabiales des Rindes. Berl. Munch. Tierarztl. Wochenschr. 85:480, 1972.
486. Yang, S. H.: Histochemical studies of bovine sweat glands. J. Agric. Sci. 42:155, 1952.
487. Yang, S. H., and Goodall, A. M.: Myoepithelial cells in bovine sweat glands. J. Agric. Sci. 42:159, 1952.
488. Yang, S. H.: A method of assessing cutaneous pigmentation in bovine skin. J. Agric. Sci. 42:465, 1952.
489. Yeates, N. T. M.: Photoperiodicity in cattle. I. Seasonal changes in coat character and their importance in heat regulation. Aust. J. Agric. Res. 6:891, 1955.
490. Yeates, N. T. M.: Photoperiodicity in cattle. II. The equatorial light environment and its effects on the coat of European cattle. Aust. J. Agric. Res. 8:733, 1957.
491. Yeates, N. T. M.: Observations on the role of nutrition in coat shedding in cattle. J. Agric. Sci. 50:110, 1958.
492. Yeates, N. T. M., and Southcott, W. H.: Coat type in relation to cold adaptation of cattle. Proc. Aust. Soc. Anim. Prod. 2:102, 1958.
493. Zimmerman, A.: Zur Histologie des Nasenlippen-Spiegels des Rindes. Morphol. Jahrb. 74:105, 1934.
494. Zvara, J., and Hradil, I.: Histochemistry of lipids and carbohydrates in the hair follicle and accessory glands in the pig. Folia Morphol. 22:241, 1974.

CHAPTER 2

DERMATOHISTOPATHOLOGY*

Dermatohistopathology has only recently received significant attention from researchers in veterinary dermatology. This has been due largely to the interest of clinical veterinary dermatologists in studying all aspects of animal skin disease. As a result of this increasing interest in dermatohistopathology, we have witnessed an explosion in the number of "new" skin diseases described in large animals since 1975 (e.g., pemphigus foliaceus, bullous pemphigoid, discoid lupus erythematosus, leukocytoclastic vasculitis, staphylococcal folliculitis and furunculosis, zinc-responsive dermatosis, vitamin C–responsive dermatosis, equine eosinophilic granuloma, axillary nodular necrosis, unilateral papular dermatosis, linear keratosis, and sarcoidosis).

The clinical veterinary dermatologist is in the perfect position to examine the historical, physical, laboratory, therapeutic, and prognostic features of animal skin disease and to establish meaningful histopathologic correlates. As more veterinary dermatologists are trained and certified, we can expect an increasing recognition of new skin diseases and a more thorough appreciation of the therapeutic and prognostic as well as the diagnostic value of dermatohistopathology in veterinary medicine.

THE BIOPSY

Skin biopsy is not performed as often as it should be, and when it is, it is often performed too late, with poor specimen selection or poor technique, or both. Skin biopsy should not be regarded as merely a diagnostic aid in the difficult case. It provides a permanent record of the pathology present at a particular moment in time, and knowledge of this pathology acts as a stimulus for the clinician to think more deeply about the basic cellular changes underlying the disease.

When to Biopsy

Hard and fast rules on when to perform a skin biopsy cannot be made. The following suggestions are offered as general guidelines. Biopsy should be performed on (1) all obviously neoplastic or suspected neoplastic lesions, (2) all persistent ulcerations, (3) a dermatosis that is not responding to apparently rational therapy, (4) any dermatosis that in the experience of the clinician is unusual or appears serious, and (5) any suspected diagnosis for which the therapy is expensive, dangerous, or time-consuming enough to necessitate a definitive diagnosis before beginning treatment. In general, skin biopsy should be performed within *three weeks* in any dermatosis that is not responding to what appears to be appropriate therapy. This early intervention (1) helps obviate the nonspecific, masking, and misleading changes of chronicity, topical and systemic medicaments, excoriation, and secondary infection and (2) allows more rapid institution of specific therapy, thus reducing permanent disease sequelae (scarring and alopecia), patient suffering, and needless financial involvement of the owner.

What to Biopsy

In most instances, histologic examination of a fully developed primary lesion provides more information than does examination of early or late lesions. Exceptions to this rule are vesicular, bullous, and pustular lesions, in which very early lesions are selected in order to eliminate secondary changes that can obscure the diagnosis (degeneration, regeneration, or secondary infection). Because these fluid-filled

---

*Portions of this material first appeared in Muller, G. H., Kirk, R. W., and Scott, D. W.: *Small Animal Dermatology*, 3rd ed. Philadelphia, W. B. Saunders Co., 1983.

lesions are often quite fragile and transient in large animal skin (often lasting only two to six hours), it may be necessary to examine patients every two to four hours in order to find early intact lesions for biopsy. Vesicles, bullae, and pustules that have been present for over 12 hours should not be biopsied.

Often, the histologic diagnosis is facilitated by taking multiple biopsy specimens. By using this technique, lesions in different stages of development are sampled, and it is probable that one sample will establish the diagnosis. Together, the samples document a pathologic continuum. Whenever possible, biopsy spontaneous, primary lesions (macules, papules, pustules, vesicles, bullae, nodules, and tumors) and avoid lesions that are marred by excoriation, chronicity, or medication.

How to Biopsy

In general, a 6- to 9-mm biopsy punch provides an adequate specimen. It is imperative not to include any significant amount of normal skin margin with punch biopsies. Unless the person taking the biopsy personally supervises the processing of the specimen, rotation in the wrong direction may result in failure to section the lesion portion of the specimen.

Excisional biopsy with a scalpel is often indicated (1) for larger lesions, (2) for vesicles, bullae, and pustules (the rotary and shearing action of a punch may damage the lesion), and (3) when disease of the subcutaneous fat is suspected (punches often fail to deliver diseased fat).

Skin biopsy is usually easily and rapidly accomplished using physical restraint and local anesthesia. Desired lesion sites are gently clipped (if needed), and the surface is gently cleansed by daubing or soaking with 70 percent alcohol. *Under no circumstances* should biopsy sites be scrubbed or prepared with other antiseptics (e.g., iodophors). Such endeavors remove important surface pathology and create iatrogenic lesions, all of which render the specimen useless or misleading. After the surface has air-dried, the desired lesion is undermined with an appropriate amount (usually 1 to 2 ml) of local anesthetic (2 percent lidocaine), injected subcutaneously. An exception to this would be when disease of the fat is suspected, in which case regional or ring blocks or general anesthesia should be used. The desired lesion is then punched or excised, including the underlying fat. Great care should be exercised

when manipulating the biopsy specimen, avoiding the use of large forceps and using instead tiny mosquito hemostats or the syringe needle through which the local anesthetic was injected. The biopsy site is then sutured closed. Postbiopsy complications (infection and dehiscence) are extremely rare.

What to Do with the Biopsy

Skin biopsy specimens should be gently blotted to remove artifactual blood and placed, with the subcutaneous side down, on pieces of wooden tongue depressor or cardboard. They should be gently pressed flat for 30 to 60 seconds to facilitate adherence. Placing the specimens on a flat surface allows proper anatomic orientation and obviates potentially drastic anatomic artifacts associated with curling and folding. The specimen and its adherent splint are then immersed in fixative within one to two minutes, since artifactual changes develop rapidly in room air.

In most instances, the fixative of choice is 10 percent neutral phosphate-buffered formalin (100 ml of 40 percent formaldehyde, 900 ml of tap water, 4 gm of acid sodium phosphate monohydrate, and 6.5 gm of anhydrous disodium phosphate). The volume of the fixative should be 10 to 20 times that of the specimen, and the specimen should be fixed for at least 24 hours. This formalin fixative freezes at about −11°C, and specimens exposed to cold prior to fixation will develop freezing artifacts. This situation can be avoided by keeping fixed specimens at room temperature for at least six hours prior to cold exposure or by using an alcoholic formalin solution (formol). This is composed of 100 ml of 40 percent formaldehyde and 900 ml of 95 percent ethyl alcohol. Alternatively, one can use 70 percent ethyl or isopropyl alcohol. The latter two alternatives are less desirable, as alcohol solutions produce tissue hardening and shrinkage, resulting in significant artifacts.

The last critical consideration in what to do with a skin biopsy sample is whom to send it to. Obviously, the clinician wants to send it to the person who can provide the most information. The choices should be prioritized as follows: (1) a veterinary dermatologist or pathologist with a special interest and expertise in dermatohistopathology, (2) a general veterinary pathologist, or (3) a physician pathologist. A word of caution is in order here: Physician pathologists are often singularly unhelpful or misleading in the interpretation of animal skin pathology.

Tissue Stains

Hematoxylin and eosin (H & E) is the most widely used routine stain for skin biopsies. In the author's laboratory, acid orcein–Giemsa (AOG) is also used as a routine stain for skin biopsies. The routine use of AOG markedly reduces the need for ordering special stains (Table 2–1). Table 2–2 contains guidelines for the use of various special stains.

ARTIFACTS IN DERMATOHISTOPATHOLOGY

Numerous artifacts can be produced by the improper selection, preparation, taking, handling, fixation, and processing of skin biopsies. It is very important that the clinician and the pathologist be cognizant of these potentially disastrous distortions of the truth.

1. Artifacts resulting from *improper selection* include excoriations and other physicochemical effects (e.g., maceration, inflammation, necrosis, and staining abnormalities caused by topical medicaments).

2. Artifacts produced by *improper preparation* include inflammation; staining abnormalities; removal of surface pathology (from surgical scrubbing and antiseptics); collagen separation (pseudoedema); and pseudosinus formation (intradermal injection of local anesthetic).

3. Artifacts due to *improper taking and handling* include pseudovesicles, pseudoclefts, and shearing (dull punch or poor technique); pseudopapilloma or pseudonodule, pseudosclerosis, pseudosinus, pseudocyst, and lobules of sebaceous glands within hair follicles or on the skin surface or both (squeeze artifacts due to use of forceps); marked dehydration, elongation, and polarization of cells and cell nuclei (electrodesiccation); and intercellular edema, clefts, and vesicles (friction).

4. Artifacts resulting from *improper fixation and processing* include dermoepidermal separation, intracellular edema, and fractures (autolysis); curling and folding (failure to use wooden or cardboard splints); intracellular edema, vacuolar alteration, and multinucleated epidermal giant cells (freezing); "formalin pigment" in blood vessels and extravascular phagocytes (use of nonbuffered formalin); hardening, shrinkage, and loss of cellular detail (alcohol in fixative); poor staining and soft, easily displaced and distorted tissue (Bouin's solution); thick, fragmented sections (inadequate dehydration during tissue processing); pseudoacanthosis (tangential sections associated with poor orientation of specimen); and dermoepidermal separation and displacement of dermal tissues into epidermis (cutting sections from dermis to epidermis).

TABLE 2–1. Staining Characteristics of Various Cutaneous Components with Acid Orcein–Giemsa (AOG)

Test Component	Color
Nuclei	Dark blue
Cytoplasm of keratinocytes	Blue-purple
Cytoplasm of smooth muscle cells	Light blue
Keratin	Blue
Collagen	Pink
Elastin	Dark brown to black
Mast cell granules	Purple
Some acid mucopolysaccharides	Purple
Melanin	Dark green to black
Hemosiderin	Yellow-brown to green
Erythrocytes	Green-orange
Eosinophil granules	Red
Cytoplasm of plasma cells	Dark blue to gray-blue
Cytoplasm of histiocytes, lymphocytes, and fibrocytes	Light blue
Cytoplasm of neutrophils	Clear to light blue
Amyloid	Sky blue to gray-blue
Hyalin	Pink
Fibrin and fibrinoid	Green-blue
Keratohyalin	Dark blue
Trichohyalin	Red
Bacteria, fungal spores, and hyphae	Dark blue
Serum	Light blue

THE VOCABULARY OF DERMATOHISTOPATHOLOGY

Dermatohistopathology has a specialized vocabulary, as many of the histopathologic changes that occur are unique to the skin. Unfortunately, as is true of most sciences, the dermatologic and general medical literature abounds with confusing and sometimes inappropriate dermatohistopathologic terms. The following is a definition of terms, based on an amalgamation of such considerations as precision of definition, descriptive value, popular usage, and historical precedent, and a discussion of their diagnostic significance in dermatohistopathology.

TABLE 2–2. Staining Characteristics of Various Substances with Special Stains

Stain	Tissue and Color
van Gieson's	Mature collagen, red; immature collagen, keratin, muscle, and nerves, yellow
Masson's trichrome	Mature collagen, blue; immature collagen, keratin, muscle, and nerves, red
Verhoeff's	Elastin and nuclei, black
Gomori's aldehyde fuchsin	Elastin, sulfated acid mucopolysaccharides, and certain epithelial mucins, purple
Oil red O ⎫ Requires frozen sections of	Lipids, dark red
Sudan black B ⎬ formalin-fixed tissue	Lipids, green-black
Scarlet red ⎭	Lipids, red
Gomori's or Wilder's reticulin stain	Reticulin, melanin, and nerves, dark brown to black
Periodic acid–Schiff (PAS)	Glycogen, neutral mucopolysaccharides, fungi, and tissue debris, red
Alcian blue	Acid mucopolysaccharides, blue
Hale's colloidal iron	Acid mucopolysaccharides, blue
Toluidine blue	Acid mucopolysaccharides and mast cell granules, purple
Grocott's methenamine silver	Fungi, black
Gram or Brown and Brenn	Gram-positive bacteria, blue; Gram-negative bacteria, red
Fite's modified acid-fast	Acid-fast bacteria, red
Fontana's ammoniacal silver nitrate	Premelanin and melanin, black (hemosiderin usually positive too, but less intense)
Prussian blue	Ferrous and ferric iron, dark blue
von Kossa's	Calcium salts, dark brown to black
Alizarin red	Calcium salts, red
Crystal violet ⎫ Can be done on routine	Amyloid, orange to red with green birefringence on polarized light
Congo red ⎬ sections, but best on frozen	
Thioflavine T ⎭ sections	Amyloid, blue to green with fluorescence microscopy
Foot's or Snook's silver nitrate	Nerves and reticulum, black
Giemsa	Mast cell granules, purple; eosinophil granules, red; Leishman-Donovan bodies, red
Dopa reaction—fresh frozen tissues	Peroxidase-containing cells (melanocytes, granulocytes, and mast cells), positive
Feulgen's reaction	Deoxyribonucleic acid (DNA), magenta
Methyl green–pyronine	Ribonucleic acid (RNA), pink; DNA, green

EPIDERMAL CHANGES

Hyperkeratosis

Hyperkeratosis is an increased thickness of the stratum corneum and may be absolute (an actual increase in thickness—the most common situation) or relative (an apparent increase resulting from thinning of the underlying epidermis—rare). The type of hyperkeratosis is further specified by the adjectives orthokeratotic (anuclear) (see Fig. 11–8, Chapter 11) and parakeratotic (nucleated) (see Fig. 12–10, Chapter 12). Orthokeratotic and parakeratotic hyperkeratoses are commonly, but less precisely, referred to as hyperkeratosis and parakeratosis, respectively. Other adjectives commonly used to further describe the nature of hyperkeratosis include basket-weave (e.g., dermatophytosis and endocrinopathies), compact (e.g., lichenoid dermatoses and cutaneous horns), and laminated (e.g., ichthyosis).

Orthokeratotic and parakeratotic hyperkeratoses may be seen as alternating layers in the stratum corneum. This implies episodic changes in epidermopoiesis. If the changes are generalized, the lesions present as horizontal layers. If the changes are focal, the resultant lesion is a vertical defect in the stratum corneum. Orthokeratotic and parakeratotic hyperkeratoses are common, nondiagnostic findings in virtually any chronic dermatosis. They simply imply altered epidermopoiesis, whether inflammatory, hormonal, neoplastic, or developmental. Diffuse parakeratotic hyperkeratosis is suggestive of ectoparasitism, seborrhea, zinc-responsive dermatosis, dermatophytosis, and dermatophilosis. Focal areas (caps) of parakeratotic hyperkeratosis with underlying edema (papillary squirting) are seen with seborrheic dermatitis.

Hypokeratosis

Hypokeratosis is a decreased thickness of the stratum corneum. It is much less common than hyperkeratosis and reflects an exceptionally rapid epidermal turnover time and/or decreased cohesion between cells of the stratum corneum. Hypokeratosis may be found in seborrheic and other exfoliative skin disorders and also may be produced by excessive surgical preparation of the biopsy site or by friction and maceration in intertriginous areas.

Dyskeratosis

Dyskeratosis is a premature and faulty keratinization of individual cells. Dyskeratosis is also used, though less commonly, to indicate a general fault in the keratinization process and, thus, in the state of the epidermis as a whole. Dyskeratotic cells are characterized by an eosinophilic, swollen cytoplasm and a condensed, dark-staining nucleus. Such cells are often difficult to distinguish from necrotic keratinocytes on light microscopic examination. The judgment usually rests on whether the rest of the epithelium is thought to be keratinizing or necrosing.

Dyskeratosis may be seen in a number of inflammatory dermatoses (especially the lichenoid dermatoses and the pemphigus and seborrheic complexes) and neoplastic dermatoses (especially papilloma and squamous cell carcinoma).

Hypergranulosis and Hypogranulosis

Hypergranulosis and hypogranulosis indicate, respectively, increased and decreased thicknesses of the stratum granulosum. Both entities are common and nondiagnostic. Hypergranulosis may be seen in any dermatosis in which there is epidermal hyperplasia and orthokeratotic hyperkeratosis. Hypogranulosis is often seen in dermatoses in which there is parakeratotic hyperkeratosis.

Hyperplasia

Hyperplasia is an increased thickness of the noncornified epidermis resulting from an increased number of epidermal cells (see Fig. 16–7, Chapter 16). The term acanthosis is often used interchangeably with hyperplasia. However, acanthosis specifically indicates an increased thickness of the stratum spinosum and may be due to hyperplasia (true acanthosis—most common) or hypertrophy (pseudoacanthosis—uncommon). Epidermal hyperplasia is often accompanied by rete ridge formation (irregular hyperplasia resulting in

"pegs" of epidermis that appear to project downward into the underlying dermis). Rete ridges are not found in normal haired skin of large animals, except for the pig.

Epidermal hyperplasia may be further specified by the following adjectives: (1) irregular (uneven, elongated, pointed rete ridges with an obliterated or preserved rete-papilla configuration), (2) regular, or psoriasiform (approximately evenly elongated rete ridges with preservation of the rete-papilla configuration), (3) papillated (digitate projections of the epidermis above the skin surface), and (4) pseudocarcinomatous, or pseudoepitheliomatous, (extreme, irregular hyperplasia, which may include increased mitoses, squamous eddies, and horn pearls, thus resembling squamous cell carcinoma; however, there is no cellular atypia, and the basement membrane zone is not breached). These four forms of epidermal hyperplasia may be seen in various combinations in the same specimen.

Epidermal hyperplasia is a common, nondiagnostic feature of virtually any chronic inflammatory process. Additionally, the four types of epidermal hyperplasia are, for the most part, useful descriptive terms, having little specific diagnostic significance. Pseudocarcinomatous hyperplasia is most commonly associated with underlying dermal suppurative, granulomatous, or neoplastic processes and with chronic ulcers. Papillated hyperplasia is most commonly seen with neoplasia and callosities.

Hypoplasia and Atrophy

Hypoplasia is a decreased thickness of the noncornified epidermis resulting from a decreased number of cells. Atrophy is a decreased thickness of the noncornified epidermis due to the decreased size of cells. An early sign of epidermal hypoplasia or atrophy is the loss of rete ridges in areas of skin where they are normally present (the nonhaired skin in large animals).

Epidermal hypoplasia and atrophy are uncommon in skin diseases of large animals but are occasionally seen with hormonal (hyperadrenocorticism and hypothyroidism), developmental (cutaneous asthenia), and inflammatory (discoid lupus erythematosus) dermatoses.

Necrosis

Necrosis is the death of cells or tissues in a living organism and is determined primarily on the basis of nuclear morphology. Necrolysis is often used synonymously with necrosis but actually implies a separation of tissue as a consequence of the death of cells (e.g., erythema multiforme). Nuclear changes indicative of necrosis include karyorrhexis (nuclear fragmentation), pyknosis (nuclear shrinkage and consequent hyperchromasia), and karyolysis (nuclear "ghosts"). With all three necrotic nuclear changes, individual keratinocytes are characterized by loss of intercellular bridges, with resultant rounding of the cell, and a normal-sized or swollen eosinophilic cytoplasm. Necrosis is further specified by the adjectives coagulation (cell outlines preserved but cell detail lost) or caseation (complete loss of all structural details, the tissue being replaced by a granular material containing nuclear debris).

Epidermal necrosis may be focal (see Fig. 5–14, Chapter 5) (drug eruptions, microbial infections, and lichenoid dermatoses) or generalized, as a result of physiochemical trauma (primary irritant contact dermatitis and burns), interference with blood supply (vasculitis, thromboembolism, subepidermal bullae, and dense subepidermal cellular infiltrates), or an immunologic mechanism (erythema multiforme). A unique type of epidermal necrosis has been described in graft-versus-host disease in humans and horses and in cattle with malignant catarrhal fever. This satellite cell necrosis (satellitosis) is characterized by individual keratinocyte necrosis in association with a contiguous (satellite) lymphoid cell.

Intercellular Edema

Intercellular edema (spongiosis) of the epidermis is characterized by a widening of the intercellular spaces, with accentuation of the intercellular bridges, giving the involved epidermis a spongy appearance (see Fig. 9–11, Chapter 9). Severe intercellular edema may lead to rupture of the intercellular bridges and the formation of spongiotic vesicles within the epidermis. Severe spongiotic vesicle formation may, in turn, blow out the basement membrane zone in some areas, giving the appearance of subepidermal vesicles. Intercellular edema is a common, nondiagnostic feature of any acute or subacute inflammatory dermatosis.

Intracellular Edema

Intracellular edema (hydropic degeneration, vacuolar degeneration, and ballooning degeneration) of the epidermis is characterized by increased size, cytoplasmic pallor, and displacement of the nucleus to the periphery of the affected cell (see Fig. 17–9, Chapter 17). Severe intracellular edema may result in reticular degeneration and intraepidermal vesicles.

Intracellular edema is a common, nondiagnostic feature of any acute or subacute inflammatory dermatosis. Caution must be exercised not to confuse intracellular edema and freezing artifact, delayed fixation artifact, or the intracellular accumulation of glycogen seen in the outer root sheath of normal hair follicles and secondary to epidermal injury.

Ballooning Degeneration

Ballooning degeneration is a specific type of degenerative change seen in epidermal cells and characterized by swollen eosinophilic cytoplasm without vacuolization, by enlarged or condensed and occasionally multiple nuclei, and by a loss of cohesion resulting in acantholysis. Ballooning degeneration is a specific feature of viral infections (see Fig. 5–1, Chapter 5).

Reticular Degeneration

Reticular degeneration is caused by severe intracellular edema of epidermal cells, in which the cells burst, resulting in multilocular intraepidermal vesicles whose septae are formed by resistant cell walls. It may be seen with any acute or subacute inflammatory dermatosis.

Hydropic Degeneration of Basal Cells

Hydropic degeneration (liquefaction degeneration and vacuolar alteration) of the basal epidermal cells is a term used to describe intracellular edema restricted to cells of the stratum basale (see Figs. 10–33 and 10–36, Chapter 10). This process may also affect the basal cells of the outer root sheath of hair follicles. Hydropic degeneration of basal cells is usually focal but, if severe and extensive, may result in subepidermal clefts or vesicles resulting from dermoepidermal separation. Hydropic degeneration of basal cells is an uncommon finding and is usually associated with lichenoid dermatoses, drug eruptions, lupus erythematosus, and erythema multiforme.

Acantholysis

Acantholysis (dyshesion, desmolysis, and desmorrhexis) is a loss of cohesion between epidermal cells, resulting in intraepidermal clefts, vesicles, and bullae (see Fig. 10–24, Chapter 10). Free epidermal cells in the vesicles are called acantholytic cells. This process may also involve the outer root sheath of hair follicles and glandular ductal epithelium. Acantholysis is further specified by reference to the level at which it occurs (i.e., subcorneal, intragranular, intraepidermal, or suprabasilar).

Acantholysis may be caused by severe spongiosis (any acute or subacute inflammatory dermatosis), ballooning degeneration (viral infection), proteolytic enzymes released by neutrophils (bacterial and fungal dermatoses), autoantibodies against intercellular cement substance (pemphigus complex), developmental defects (familial acantholysis), and neoplastic transformation (squamous cell carcinoma).

Exocytosis

Exocytosis is the migration of inflammatory cells or erythrocytes, or both, through the intercellular spaces of the epidermis (see Fig. 9–11, Chapter 9). Exocytosis of inflammatory cells is a common, nondiagnostic feature of any inflammatory dermatosis. Exocytosis of erythrocytes implies purpura (e.g., vasculitis and coagulation defect).

Clefts

Clefts (lacunae) are slitlike spaces, which do not contain fluid, within the epidermis or at the dermoepidermal junction. Clefts may be caused by acantholysis or hydropic degeneration of basal cells (Max Joseph spaces). However, clefts may also be caused by mechanical trauma and tissue retraction associated with the taking, fixation, and processing of biopsy specimens.

Microvesicles, Vesicles, and Bullae

Microvesicles, vesicles, and bullae are microscopic and macroscopic fluid-filled, relatively acellular spaces within or below the epidermis. Such lesions are often loosely referred to as blisters. These lesions may be caused by severe intercellular or intracellular edema, ballooning degeneration, acantholysis, hydropic degeneration of basal cells, subepidermal edema, or other factors resulting in dermoepidermal separation (e.g., the autoantibodies in bullous pemphigoid). Thus, microvesicles, vesicles, and bullae may be further

described as subcorneal, intragranular, intraepidermal, suprabasilar, intrabasal, or subepidermal (see Table 2–3, p. 45). When these lesions contain larger numbers of inflammatory cells, they may be referred to as vesicopustules.

Microabscesses and Pustules

Microabscesses and pustules are microscopic or macroscopic intraepidermal and subepidermal cavities filled with inflammatory cells. Microabscesses and pustules are further described on the basis of location and cell type: (1) spongiform pustules of Kogoj, a multilocular accumulation of neutrophils within and between keratinocytes, especially those of the stratum granulosum and stratum spinosum, whose cell boundaries form a spongelike network (seen in microbial infections), (2) Munro's microabscess, small, desiccated accumulations of neutrophils within or below the stratum corneum (seen in microbial infections), (3) Pautrier's microabscess, small, focal accumulations of abnormal lymphoid cells (seen in some lymphoproliferative malignancies), (4) eosinophilic microabscess, seen in ectoparasitism, eosinophilic granuloma, eosinophilic folliculitis, dermatosis vegetans, and the pemphigus complex, and (5) subcorneal microabscesses and pustules, subcorneal accumulations of predominantly neutrophils. The last are seen in microbial infections (see Fig. 6–2, Chapter 6) and pemphigus foliaceus (see Fig. 10–21, Chapter 10).

Hyperpigmentation

Hyperpigmentation (hypermelanosis) refers to excessive amounts of melanin deposited within the epidermis and, often, concurrently in dermal melanophages. Hyperpigmentation may be focal or diffuse and may be confined to the stratum basale or present throughout all epidermal layers. It is a common, nondiagnostic finding in chronic inflammatory and hormonal dermatoses as well as in some developmental and neoplastic disorders. Hyperpigmentation must always be cautiously assessed with regard to the patient's normal pigmentation.

Hypopigmentation

Hypopigmentation (hypomelanosis) refers to decreased amounts of melanin in the epidermis (see Fig. 17–10, Chapter 17). It may be associated with congenital or acquired idi-

opathic defects in melanization (e.g., leukoderma and vitiligo), toxic effects of certain
chemicals on melanocytes (e.g., monobenzyl
ether of dihydroquinone in rubbers and plas-
tics), inflammatory disorders that affect melanization or destroy melanocytes, hormonal disorders, and dermatoses featuring hydropic
degeneration of basal cells (e.g., lupus erythematosus). In those hypopigmented dermatoses
associated with hydropic degeneration of basal
cells, the underlying superficial dermis usually
reveals pigmentary incontinence.

Crust

A crust is a consolidated, desiccated surface
mass composed of varying combinations of
keratin, serum, cellular debris, and, often,
microorganisms (see Fig. 6–29, Chapter 6).
Crusts are further described on the basis of
their composition: (1) serous (mostly serum),
(2) hemorrhagic (mostly blood), (3) cellular
(mostly inflammatory cells), and (4) serocel-
lular, or exudative (a mixture of serum and
inflammatory cells).

Crusts merely indicate a prior exudative
process and are rarely of diagnostic significance. However, crusts should always be
closely scrutinized, since they may contain
important diagnostic clues: (1) dermatophyte
spores and hyphae, (2) the filaments and coccoid elements of *Dermatophilus congolensis*,
and (3) large numbers of acantholytic keratinocytes (pemphigus complex). Bacteria and
bacterial colonies are common inhabitants of
surface debris and are of no diagnostic significance. Palisading crusts (alternating horizontal
layers of keratin and exudate) are seen in
dermatophilosis and dermatophytosis.

Dells

Dells are small depressions, or hollows, in
the surface of the epidermis and are usually
associated with focal epidermal atrophy and
orthokeratotic hyperkeratosis. Dells may be
seen in lichenoid dermatoses, especially lupus
erythematosus.

Epidermal Collarette

The term epidermal collarette refers to the
formation of elongated, hyperplastic rete
ridges at the lateral margins of a pathologic
process that appears to curve inward toward
the center of the lesion. Epidermal collarettes

may be seen with neoplastic, granulomatous,
and suppurative dermatoses.

Horn Cysts, Pseudohorn Cysts, Horn Pearls, and Squamous Eddies

Horn cysts (keratin cysts) are circular cystic
structures surrounded by flattened epidermal
cells and containing concentrically arranged
lamellar keratin. Horn cysts are features of
trichoepitheliomas and basal cell tumors. Pseu-
dohorn cysts are illusory cystic structures
formed by the irregular invagination of a hyperplastic, hyperkeratotic epidermis. They are
seen in numerous hyperplastic or neoplastic
epidermal dermatoses. Horn pearls (squamous
pearls) are focal, circular, concentric layers of
squamous cells showing gradual keratinization
toward the center, often accompanied by cellular atypia and dyskeratosis. They are features
of squamous cell carcinoma and pseudocarcinomatous hyperplasia. Squamous eddies are
whorl-like patterns of squamoid cells with no
atypia, dyskeratosis, or central keratinization.
Squamous eddies are features of numerous
neoplastic and hyperplastic epidermal disorders.

DERMAL CHANGES

Collagen Changes

Dermal collagen is subject to a number of
pathologic changes: (1) hyalinization, a confluence and increased eosinophilic, glassy, refractile appearance (seen in chronic inflammation
and connective tissue diseases), (2) fibrinoid
degeneration, deposition of or replacement
with a brightly eosinophilic fibrillar or granular
substance resembling fibrin (seen in connective
tissue diseases), (3) lysis, a homogeneous, eosinophilic, complete loss of structural detail
(see Fig. 9–37, Chapter 9) (seen in microbial
infections, habronemiasis, and ischemia), (4)
degeneration, a structural and tinctorial
change characterized by slight basophilia,
granular appearance, and frayed edges of collagen fibrils (see Fig. 15–5, Chapter 15) (seen
in equine eosinophilic granuloma), (5) dystrophic mineralization, deposition of calcium
salts as basophilic, amorphous, granular material along collagen fibrils (see Fig. 15–6,
Chapter 15) (seen in equine eosinophilic granuloma and mastocytoma), (6) atrophy, thin
collagen fibrils and decreased fibroblasts, with
resultant decreased dermal thickness (seen in
hormonal dermatoses), (7) disorganization and

fragmentation (seen in cutaneous asthenia), and (8) alignment in vertical streaks, elongated, parallel strands of collagen in the superficial dermis, perpendicular to the epidermal surface (seen in chronic pruritus and rubbing).

Fibroplasia, Desmoplasia, Fibrosis, and Sclerosis

Fibroplasia, the formation and development of fibrous tissue in increased amounts, is often used synonymously with granulation tissue. Fibroplasia is characterized by a fibrovascular proliferation in which the blood vessels with prominent endothelial cells are oriented roughly perpendicular to the surface of the skin. The new collagen fibrils, with prominent fibroblasts, are oriented roughly parallel with the surface of the skin. Edema and inflammatory cells are constant features of fibroplasia. Desmoplasia is the term commonly used to refer to the fibroplasia induced by neoplastic processes.

Fibrosis (see Fig. 9–49, Chapter 9) is a later stage of fibroplasia in which increased numbers of fibroblasts and collagen fibrils are the characteristic findings. There is little or no inflammation present. Sclerosis (scar) may be the end point of fibrosis, wherein the increased numbers of collagen fibrils have a thick, eosinophilic, hyalinized appearance and the number of fibroblasts is greatly reduced.

Papillomatosis, Villi, and Festoons

Papillomatosis refers to the projection of dermal papillae above the surface of the skin, resulting in an irregular undulating configuration of the epidermis. Papillomatosis is often associated with epidermal hyperplasia and is seen with chronic inflammatory and neoplastic dermatoses. Villi are dermal papillae, covered by one to two layers of epidermal cells, that project into a vesicle or bulla. Villi are seen in pemphigus vulgaris. Festoons are dermal papillae, devoid of attached epidermal cells, that project into the base of a vesicle or bulla. Festoons are seen in porphyria, bullous pemphigoid, and epidermolysis bullosa (see Fig. 4–8, Chapter 4).

Pigmentary Incontinence

Pigmentary incontinence refers to the presence of free melanin granules within the subepidermal dermis and within dermal macrophages (melanophages). Pigmentary incon-

tinence may be seen with any process that damages the stratum basale and the basement membrane zone, especially hydropic degeneration of basal cells (lichenoid dermatoses, lupus erythematosus, and erythema multiforme).

Edema

Dermal edema is recognized by dilated lymphatics (not visible in normal skin), widened spaces between blood vessels and perivascular collagen (*perivascular edema*), or widened spaces between large areas of dermal collagen (*interstitial edema*). The dilated lymphatics and widened perivascular and interstitial spaces may or may not contain a lightly eosinophilic homogeneous, frothy-appearing substance (serum).

Dermal edema is a common, nondiagnostic feature of any inflammatory dermatosis. Severe edema of the superficial dermis may result in subepidermal vesicles and bullae, necrosis of the overlying epidermis, and predisposition to artifactual dermoepidermal separation during handling and processing of biopsy specimens.

Mucinous Degeneration

Mucinous degeneration (myxedema, mucoid degeneration, myxoid degeneration, and mucinosis) is characterized by increased amounts of an amorphous, stringy, granular, basophilic material that separates, thins, or replaces dermal collagen fibrils and surrounds blood vessels and appendages in sections stained with hematoxylin and eosin. Only small amounts of mucin are ever visible in normal skin, mostly around appendages and blood vessels. Mucin is more easily demonstrated with stains for acid mucopolysaccharides, such as Hale's and alcian blue. Mucinous degeneration may occasionally be seen in numerous inflammatory, neoplastic, and developmental dermatoses and in hypothyroidism.

Grenz Zone

A grenz zone is a marginal zone of relatively normal collagen that separates the epidermis from an underlying dermal alteration. It may be seen in neoplastic and granulomatous disorders.

Follicular Changes

Follicular epithelium is affected by most of the histopathologic changes described for the epidermis. Follicular (poral) keratosis, plugging, and dilatation are common features of such diverse conditions as inflammatory, hormonal, and developmental dermatoses. Perifolliculitis, folliculitis, and furunculosis (penetrating or perforating folliculitis) refer to varying degrees of follicular inflammation (Figs. 2–10, 2–11, and 2–12). Follicular atrophy refers to the gradual involution and disappearance characteristic of hormonal dermatoses. Hair follicles should be closely examined to determine what phase of the growth cycle they are in. A predominance of telogen hair follicles is characteristic of hormonal dermatoses and stages of telogen defluxion (stress, disease, or drugs).

Glandular Changes

Sebaceous and apocrine sweat glands may be involved in various dermatoses. Sebaceous glands may be involved in many suppurative and granulomatous inflammations (sebaceous adenitis). They may become atrophic (reduced in number and size, with pyknotic nuclei predominating) and cystic in hormonal and developmental dermatoses, in occasional chronic inflammatory processes, and as a senile change. Sebaceous glands may also become hyperplastic in chronic inflammatory dermatoses and in senile nodular sebaceous hyperplasia. Sebaceous gland atrophy and hyperplasia must always be cautiously assessed with regard to the area of the body from which the skin specimen was taken.

Apocrine sweat glands are commonly involved in suppurative and granulomatous dermatoses (hidradenitis). They may become dilated or cystic in many inflammatory, developmental, and hormonal dermatoses, in apocrine cystomatosis, and as a senile change. The recognition of apocrine gland atrophy by light microscopy is a moot point, since dilated apocrine secretory coils containing flattened epithelial cells are a feature of the normal postsecretory state.

Vascular Changes

Cutaneous blood vessels exhibit a number of histologic changes, including dilatation (ectasia), endothelial swelling, hyalinization, fibrinoid degeneration, vasculitis, thromboembolism, and extravasation (diapedesis) of erythrocytes (purpura) (see Fig. 10–41, Chapter 10).

SUBCUTANEOUS FAT CHANGES

The subcutaneous fat (panniculus adiposus and hypodermis) is subject to the connective tissue and vascular changes described earlier. It is frequently involved in suppurative and granulomatous dermatoses. In addition, subcutaneous fat may exhibit its own inflammatory changes (panniculitis and steatitis) without any significant involvement of the overlying dermis and epidermis (nutritional steatitis and bacterial and fungal panniculitis) and may atrophy in various hormonal, inflammatory (Wucher's atrophy), and idiopathic dermatoses.

MISCELLANEOUS CHANGES

Civatte Bodies

Civatte bodies (colloid bodies, hyaline bodies) are degenerate basal epidermal cells that appear as round, homogeneous, eosinophilic bodies in the stratum basale or just below. They are features of lichenoid dermatoses.

Thickened Basement Membrane Zone

By light microscopy, thickening of the basement membrane zone appears as focal, linear, homogeneous, eosinophilic bands below the stratum basale. The basement membrane zone is better demonstrated with periodic acid–Schiff (PAS) stain. Thickening of the basement membrane zone is a feature of lichenoid dermatoses, especially lupus erythematosus.

Dysplasia

Dysplasia is faulty or abnormal development of individual cells. The term is also commonly used to describe abnormal development of the epidermis as a whole. Dysplasia may be a feature of neoplastic, hyperplastic, and developmental dermatoses.

Anaplasia

Anaplasia (atypia) is a feature of neoplastic cells, in which there is a loss of normal differentiation and organization.

Metaplasia

Metaplasia is a change in the type of mature cells in a tissue into a form that is not normal for that tissue.

Nests

Nests (theques) are well-circumscribed clusters or groups of cells within the epidermis or the dermis. Nests are seen in some neoplastic and hamartomatous dermatoses, such as melanocytic nevi and melanomas.

Lymphoid Nodules

Lymphoid nodules are rounded, discrete masses of primarily mature lymphocytes. They are often found perivascularly in the deep dermis or subcutis, or both. They appear to be uncommon in large animals, being most frequently recognized in the eosinophilic granuloma complex, connective tissue diseases, and insect bite nodules (pseudolymphoma).

Multinucleated Epidermal Giant Cells

Multinucleated epidermal giant cells are found in viral infections and in a number of nonviral and non-neoplastic dermatoses characterized by epidermal hyperplasia, dyskeratosis, chronicity, or pruritus.

CONFUSING TERMS

Necrobiosis

Necrobiosis is the degeneration and death of cells or tissue, followed by replacement. Examples of necrobiosis would be the constant degeneration and replacement of epidermal and hematopoietic cells.

The term necrobiosis has been used in dermatohistopathology to describe various degenerative changes in collagen found in equine eosinophilic granuloma, and human granuloma annulare, necrobiosis lipoidica, and rheumatoid and pseudorheumatoid nodules. The use of the term necrobiosis to describe a pathologic change is inappropriate and confusing, both histologically and etymologically, and should be discouraged. It is better to use the more specific terms described previously under collagen changes.

Nevus and Hamartoma

Nevus literally means spot or birthmark. The term is often used clinically to describe any congenital skin lesion and histologically for cells (nevus cells, or nevocytes) that compose the common pigmented mole (nevus pigmentosus) of humans. The widest application of nevus is anything odd, abnormal, or faulty that is related to conception, gestation, and postnatal development and that stems from heritable or embryogenic fault, abnormality, or oddity. A more precise and preferable definition of nevus is a circumscribed stable malformation of the skin, congenital or tardive in onset and consisting of the local excess of one or several of the normal mature constituents of the skin. The term *nevus* should never be used alone but always with a modifier such as melanocytic, epidermal, vascular, connective tissue, or organoid.

Hamartoma literally means a tumor-like proliferation of normal or embryonal cells. In other words, a hamartoma is a macroscopic hyperplasia of normal tissue elements.

In common usage and medical literature, the terms nevus and hamartoma are used interchangeably, albeit with considerable unresolved confusion and disagreement. Whereas the term hamartoma is used to describe malformations in *any* organ system, the term nevus is used only for the skin.

CELLULAR INFILTRATES

Dermal cellular infiltrates are described in terms of (1) the types of cells present and (2) the pattern of cellular infiltration. In general, cellular infiltrates are either monomorphous (one cell type) or polymorphous (more than one cell type). Further clarification as to the predominant cells is accomplished by modifiers such as lymphocytic, histiocytic, neutrophilic, eosinophilic, and plasmacytic.

Cellular infiltration usually exhibits one or more of the following basic patterns: (1) perivascular (angiocentric—located around blood vessels), (2) perifollicular and periglandular (appendagocentric, periappendageal, and periadnexal—located around follicles and glands), (3) lichenoid (assuming a "band like" configuration that parallels and hugs the overlying epidermis), (4) nodular (occurring in basically well-defined groups or clusters at any site), and (5) diffuse (interstitial—scattered lightly or solidly throughout the dermis).

The types of cells and patterns of infiltration present are important clues to the diagnosis of many dermatoses.

THE DERMATITIS REACTION

The dermatitis reaction is a nondiagnostic cutaneous inflammatory response, with concomitant changes in the epidermis and dermis.

Acute dermatitis is characterized grossly by vesicles, papules, erythema, edema, and exudation and histologically by spongiotic vesicles, spongiosis, intracellular edema, leukocytic exocytosis, and superficial dermal edema, vascular dilatation, and perivascular inflammatory cells.

Subacute dermatitis is characterized grossly by erythema, edema, and exudation, with or without crusts and mild to moderate vesiculation, and histologically by epidermal and dermal changes similar to those described in acute dermatitis, with the addition of varying degrees of epidermal hyperplasia and orthokeratotic or parakeratotic hyperkeratosis.

Chronic dermatitis is characterized grossly by mild erythema, scaling, crusts, lichenification, and pigmentary disturbances and histologically by variable epidermal hyperplasia and orthokeratotic or parakeratotic hyperkeratosis and mild to moderate degrees of dermal edema, vascular dilatation, and perivascular inflammatory cells.

The dermatitis reaction is not a particularly useful concept from the standpoint of diagnostic or therapeutic specificity. However, it is a useful and frequently employed concept for histopathologic description and morphologic diagnosis. Although the dermatitis reaction may be the only abnormality the tissue shows, it is most frustrating to clinicians to receive a histopathologic diagnosis of chronic dermatitis, chronic nonsuppurative dermatitis, or chronic nonspecific dermatitis. Such histopathologic diagnoses should always be amended with "consistent or compatible with," and a differential diagnosis listed.

DERMATOLOGIC DIAGNOSIS BY HISTOPATHOLOGIC PATTERNS

Central reference works on the histopathology of neoplasms of large animal skin are readily accessible (see Chapter 17). However, information on the histopathologic features of non-neoplastic large animal dermatoses is fragmentary and scattered throughout the veterinary medical literature. A detailed description and discussion of the histopathology of these disorders is beyond the scope of this chapter, and pertinent aspects of each will be presented as the dermatoses themselves are discussed.

In 1978, Ackerman published a textbook on the histopathologic aspects of inflammatory dermatoses in humans. The essence of this book was histopathologic diagnosis by pattern analysis, that is, first categorizing inflammatory dermatoses by their appearance on the scanning objective of the light microscope and then homing in on a specific diagnosis, wherever possible, by the assimilation of fine details gathered on low- and high-power scrutiny. This approach has been very helpful in the examination of large animal inflammatory dermatoses.

The following scheme is an application of Ackerman's method, modified by the author, for the histologic evaluation of large animal inflammatory dermatoses. In addition, a discussion of hormonal dermatoses is included. This scheme is based on the author's experience and a review of the literature.

PERIVASCULAR DERMATITIS

In perivascular dermatitis, the predominant inflammatory reaction is centered around either or both the superficial and the deep dermal blood vessels (Fig. 2–1). Perivascular dermatitis is subdivided, on the basis of accompanying epidermal changes, into four types: (1) pure perivascular dermatitis (perivascular dermatitis without significant epidermal changes), (2) interface dermatitis (perivascular dermatitis with obscuring of the dermoepidermal interface), (3) spongiotic dermatitis (perivascular dermatitis with spongiosis), and (4) hyperplastic dermatitis (perivascular dermatitis with epidermal hyperplasia). Most perivascular dermatitides involve predominantly the superficial dermal blood vessels. Concurrent involvement of deep dermal blood vessels always suggests a systemic disease (e.g., infection and immune-mediated disease). In the horse, most perivascular dermatitides are both superficial and deep.

Pure Perivascular Dermatitis

The cellular infiltrate in perivascular dermatitis may be monomorphous or polymorphous. Most perivascular dermatitides are caused by ectoparasitism, hypersensitivity reactions, and contact dermatitis. Any perivascular dermatitis containing numerous eosinophils should be suspected first of representing ectoparasitism or hypersensitivity. Focal areas of epidermal edema, eosinophilic exocytosis, and necrosis are suggestive of ectoparasitism ("epidermal nibbles"). Other perivascular dermatitides that may contain numerous eosinophils include juvenile pustular and psoriasi-

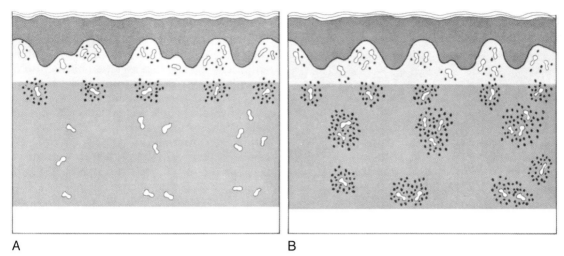

FIGURE 2–1. A, *Superficial perivascular dermatitis.* B, *Superficial and deep perivascular dermatitis. (With permission from Ackerman, A. B.:* Histologic Diagnosis of Inflammatory Skin Diseases. *Philadelphia, Lea & Febiger, 1978.)*

form dermatitis of swine, zinc-responsive dermatoses, and exfoliative eosinophilic dermatitis of horses. Diffuse parakeratotic hyperkeratosis is suggestive of ectoparasitism, zinc-responsive dermatoses, dermatophilosis, and dermatophytosis. Parakeratotic caps with underlying papillary squirting are seen with seborrheic dermatitis.

Interface Dermatitis

In interface dermatitis, the dermoepidermal junction is obscured by hydropic degeneration, lichenoid cellular infiltrate, or both (Fig. 2–2). The hydropic type of interface dermatitis is seen with drug eruptions, lupus erythematosus, erythema multiforme, rinderpest, bovine viral diarrhea, and graft-versus-host reactions. The lichenoid type is seen with drug eruptions, lupus erythematosus, pemphigus, pemphigoid, malignant catarrhal fever, and idiopathic lichenoid dermatoses.

Spongiotic Perivascular Dermatitis

Spongiotic perivascular dermatitis is characterized by varying degrees of spongiosis and spongiotic vesicle formation (Fig. 2–3). Severe spongiotic vesiculation may blow out the basement membrane zone, resulting in subepidermal vesicles. The epidermis frequently shows varying degrees of hyperplasia and hyperker-

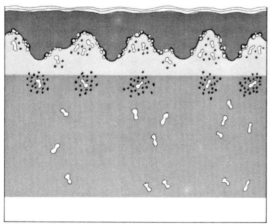

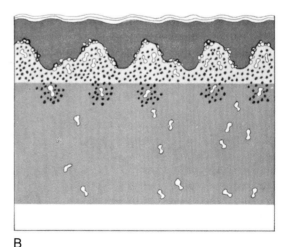

FIGURE 2–2. A, *Interface dermatitis with vacuolar alteration.* B, *Interface dermatitis with lichenoid infiltrate. (With permission from Ackerman, A. B.:* Histologic Diagnosis of Inflammatory Skin Diseases. *Philadelphia, Lea & Febiger, 1978.)*

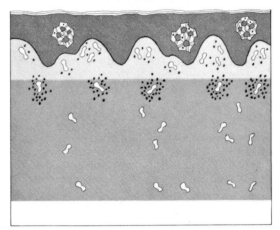

FIGURE 2–3. Spongiotic dermatitis. (With permission from Ackerman, A. B.: Histologic Diagnosis of Inflammatory Skin Diseases. *Philadelphia, Lea & Febiger, 1978.)*

atosis. Spongiotic dermatitis may be monomorphous or polymorphous. The differential considerations are as discussed earlier for pure perivascular dermatitis.

Hyperplastic Perivascular Dermatitis

Hyperplastic perivascular dermatitis is characterized by varying degrees of epidermal hyperplasia and hyperkeratosis, with little or no spongiosis (Fig. 2–4). This is a common, nondiagnostic, chronic dermatitis reaction and is commonly seen with hypersensitivity reactions, ectoparasitism, contact dermatoses, seborrheic dermatoses, and postinflammatory dermatoses.

VASCULITIS

Vasculitis is an inflammatory process in which inflammatory cells are present within and around blood vessel walls, and there are concomitant signs of damage to the blood vessels (e.g., degeneration and lysis of vascular and perivascular collagen, degeneration and swelling of endothelial cells, extravasation of erythrocytes, thrombosis, effacement of vascular architecture, and fibrinoid degeneration) (Fig. 2–5). Vasculitides are usually classified on the basis of the dominant inflammatory cell within vessel walls. There are neutrophilic, eosinophilic, and lymphocytic types.

Neutrophilic vasculitis may be leukocytoclastic (associated with karyorrhexis of neutrophils, resulting in "nuclear dust") or nonleukocytoclastic and is seen in connective tissue disorders, hypersensitivity reactions (drug eruptions, infections, and toxins), septicemia, thrombophlebitis (intravenous catheters and thromboembolism), and hog cholera and as an idiopathic disorder.

Lymphocytic vasculitis may be seen in malignant catarrhal fever, equine viral arteritis, drug eruptions, and ectoparasitism and as an idiopathic disorder.

Eosinophilic vasculitis has been reported as an idiopathic, presumably immune-mediated disorder in the horse.

Nodular and Diffuse Dermatitis and Granulomatous Inflammation

Nodular dermatitis denotes discrete clusters of cells (Fig. 2–6). Such dermal nodules are

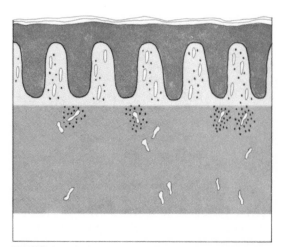

FIGURE 2–4. Hyperplastic dermatitis. (With permission from Ackerman, A. B.: Histologic Diagnosis of Inflammatory Skin Diseases. *Philadelphia, Lea & Febiger, 1978.)*

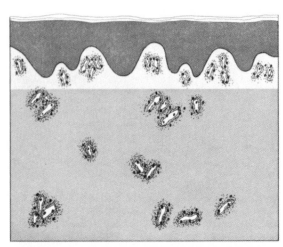

FIGURE 2–5. Vasculitis. (With permission from Ackerman, A. B.: Histologic Diagnosis of Inflammatory Skin Diseases. *Philadelphia, Lea & Febiger, 1978.)*

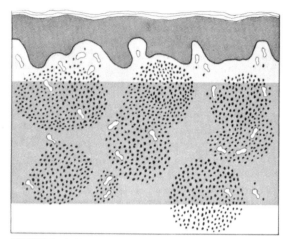

FIGURE 2–6. Nodular dermatitis. (With permission from Ackerman, A. B.: Histologic Diagnosis of Inflammatory Skin Diseases. Philadelphia, Lea & Febiger, 1978.)

usually multiple but occasionally may be large and solitary.

Diffuse dermatitis denotes a cellular infiltrate so dense that discrete cellular aggregates are no longer easily recognized (Fig. 2–7).

Granulomatous inflammation represents a heterogeneous pattern of tissue reactions in response to various stimuli. There is no simple, precise, universally accepted way of defining granulomatous inflammation. A commonly proposed definition of granulomatous inflammation is a circumscribed tissue reaction, subacute to chronic, located around one or more foci, wherein the histiocyte or macrophage is a predominant cell type. Thus, granulomatous dermatitis may be nodular or diffuse, but not all nodular and diffuse dermatoses are granulomatous. Granulomatous infiltrates that contain large numbers of neutrophils are frequently called pyogranulomatous.

Cell Types

Nodular dermatitis and diffuse dermatitis are often associated with certain unusual inflammatory cell types.

Foam cells are histiocytes with vacuolated cytoplasm due to their contents (lipids, debris, and microorganisms).

Epithelioid cells are histiocytes with elongated or oval vesicular nuclei and abundant finely granular, eosinophilic cytoplasm with ill-defined cell borders. They are called epithelioid because they appear to cluster and adjoin as epithelial cells.

Multinucleated giant cells are histiocytic variants that assume three morphologic forms: (1)

Langhans's (nuclei form a circle or semicircle at the periphery of the cell), (2) foreign body (nuclei are scattered throughout the cytoplasm), and (3) Touton's (nuclei form a wreath that surrounds a central, homogeneous, amphophilic core of cytoplasm, which is in turn surrounded by abundant foamy cytoplasm). In general, these three forms of giant cells have no diagnostic specificity, although the Touton variety is fairly specific for xanthomas.

Certain general principles apply to the examination of all nodular and diffuse dermatitides. Those processed should be (1) polarized (foreign material), (2) stained for bacteria and fungi, and (3) cultured. In general, microorganisms are most likely to be found near areas of suppuration and necrosis.

Nodular and diffuse dermatitis may be characterized by predominantly neutrophilic, histiocytic, eosinophilic, or mixed cellular infiltrates.

Neutrophils (dermal abscess) often predominate in dermatoses associated with bacteria, mycobacteria, actinomycetes, fungi, *Prototheca* species, and foreign bodies.

Histiocytes may predominate in the chronic stage of any of the entities just listed and in xanthomas. Granulomas that are composed chiefly of histiocytic elements are often referred to as tuberculoid (histiocytes and epithelioid cells surrounded by giant cells, then a layer of lymphocytes, and then an outer layer of fibroblasts), as in tuberculosis and caseous lymphadenitis, or sarcoidal (naked epithelioid cells), as in equine scarcoidosis. Palisading granulomas are characterized by the alignment of histiocytes as staves around a central focus

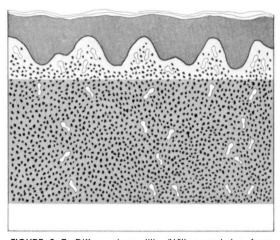

FIGURE 2–7. Diffuse dermatitis. (With permission from Ackerman, A. B.: Histologic Diagnosis of Inflammatory Skin Diseases. Philadelphia, Lea & Febiger, 1978.)

of collagen degeneration (equine eosinophilic granuloma and equine mastocytoma), lipids (xanthoma), other foreign material, and some infections (pythiosis and conidiobolomycosis).

Eosinophils may predominate in equine eosinophilic granuloma, in certain parasitic dermatoses, in certain fungal dermatoses (e.g., pythiosis), and where hair follicles have ruptured. Mixed cellular infiltrates contain most commonly neutrophils and histiocytes (pyogranuloma), eosinophils and histiocytes (eosinophilic granuloma), or some combination thereof.

Plasma cells are common components of nodular and diffuse dermatitides and are of no particular significance. Hyperactive plasma cells may contain eosinophilic intracytoplasmic inclusions (Russell's bodies). These accumulations of glycoprotein are largely globulin and may be large enough to push the cell nucleus eccentrically.

Reactions to ruptured hair follicles are a common cause of nodular and diffuse pyogranulomatous dermatitides, and any such dermal process should be carefully scrutinized for keratinous and epithelial debris, with a serial section being performed to rule out this possibility.

INTRAEPIDERMAL VESICULAR AND PUSTULAR DERMATITIS

Vesicular and pustular dermatitides show considerable microscopic and macroscopic overlap (Fig. 2–8). This is because vesicles

tend to accumulate leukocytes very early and rapidly. Thus, vesicular dermatitides in large animals frequently appear pustular or vesiculopustular, both macroscopically and microscopically.

Intraepidermal vesicles and pustules may be produced by intercellular or intracellular edema (any acute to subacute dermatitis reaction), ballooning degeneration (viral infections), acantholysis (the autoantibodies of pemphigus, the proteolytic enzymes from neutrophils in microbial infections, and familial acantholysis), and hydropic degeneration of basal cells (lupus erythematosus, erythema multiforme, and drug eruptions). It is very useful to classify intraepidermal vesicular and pustular dermatitides according to their anatomic level of occurrence within the epidermis (Table 2–3).

SUBEPIDERMAL VESICULAR AND PUSTULAR DERMATITIS

Subepidermal vesicles and pustules may be formed through hydropic degeneration of basal cells (lupus erythematosus, erythema multiforme, and drug eruptions), dermoepidermal separation (bullous pemphigoid, epidermolysis bullosa, porphyria, and drug eruptions), severe subepidermal edema or cellular infiltration (especially urticaria, cellulitis, vasculitis, and ectoparasitism), and severe intercellular edema, with blow out of the basement membrane zone (spongiotic perivascular dermatitis) (Fig. 2–9). Concurrent epidermal and dermal inflamma-

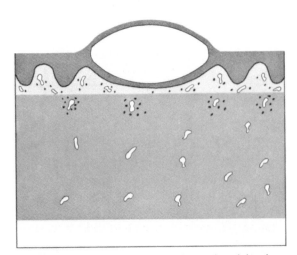

FIGURE 2–8. Intraepidermal vesicular and pustular dermatitis. (With permission from Ackerman, A. B.: Histologic Diagnosis of Inflammatory Skin Diseases. Philadelphia, Lea & Febiger, 1978.)

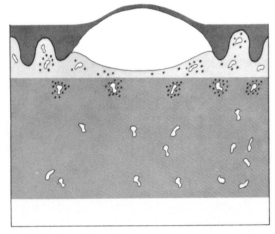

FIGURE 2–9. Subepidermal vesicular dermatitis. (With permission from Ackerman, A. B.: Histologic Diagnosis of Inflammatory Skin Diseases. Philadelphia, Lea & Febiger, 1978.)

TABLE 2–3. Histopathologic Classification of Intraepidermal and Subepidermal Vesicular and Pustular Dermatoses

Anatomic Location	Other Helpful Findings
INTRAEPIDERMAL	
Subcorneal	
Microbial infection	Microorganisms (bacteria and fungi), with or without acantholysis
Pemphigus foliaceus	Acantholysis (marked), granular "cling-ons," with or without follicular involvement
Drug eruption	
Bovine exfoliative dermatitis	Neutrophils
Intragranular	
Pemphigus foliaceus	Acantholysis (marked), granular cling-ons, with or without follicular involvement
Intraepidermal	
Spongiotic dermatitis	Eosinophilic exocytosis suggests ectoparasitism and pemphigus
Dermatosis vegetans	Eosinophils and neutrophils, papillomatosis
Viral dermatoses	Ballooning degeneration, with or without inclusion bodies
Intrabasal	
Lupus erythematosus	Hydropic degeneration of basal cells
Drug eruption	Hydropic degeneration of basal cells, with or without necrotic keratinocytes
Erythema multiforme	Hydropic degeneration of basal cells, epidermal coagulation necrosis
Graft-versus-host disease	Hydropic degeneration of basal cells, satellitosis
SUBEPIDERMAL	
Bullous pemphigoid	Subepidermal vacuolar alteration, with or without inflammation
Porphyria	Little or no inflammation; festooning; hyalinization of blood vessels
Epidermolysis bullosa	Little or no inflammation
Lupus erythematosus	Hydropic degeneration of basal cells
Drug eruption ⎫ Erythema multiforme ⎭	Hydropic degeneration of basal cells, with or without epidermal coagulation necrosis
Severe subepidermal edema or cellular infiltration	
Severe intercellular edema	Spongiotic vesicles

tory changes are important diagnostic clues (Table 2–3). Caution is warranted when examining older lesions, as re-epithelialization may result in subepidermal vesicles' and pustules' assuming an intraepidermal location. Such re-epithelialization is usually recognized as a single layer of flattened, elongated basal epidermal cells at the base of the vesicle or pustule.

PERIFOLLICULITIS, FOLLICULITIS, AND FURUNCULOSIS

Perifolliculitis denotes the accumulation of inflammatory cells around a hair follicle and the exocytosis of these cells through the follicular epithelium (Fig. 2–10). Folliculitis implies the accumulation of inflammatory cells within follicular lumina (Fig. 2–11). Furunculosis (penetrating or perforating folliculitis) signifies hair follicle rupture (Fig. 2–12). Obviously,

perifolliculitis, folliculitis, and furunculosis usually represent a pathologic continuum and may all be present in the same specimen. Follicular inflammation is a common gross and microscopic finding, and one must always be cautious in assessing its importance. It is a common secondary complication in pruritic dermatoses (e.g., hypersensitivities and ectoparasitism), seborrheic dermatoses, and hormonal dermatoses. Thus, a thorough search for underlying causes is mandatory.

Follicular inflammation may be caused by bacteria, fungi, and parasites (*Demodex* spp. and *Pelodera strongyloides*) and is seen in eosinophilic folliculitis and unilateral papular dermatosis. The folliculitides associated with bacteria, fungi, and parasites are usually suppurative initially. Any chronic folliculitis, particularly when there is furunculosis, can become pyogranulomatous or granulomatous. Furunculosis, regardless of the initiating cause, is frequently associated with moderate to

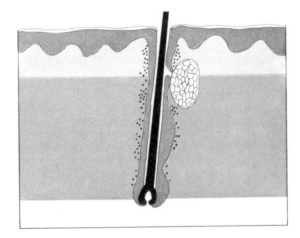

FIGURE 2–10. Perifolliculitis. (With permission from Ackerman, A. B.: Histologic Diagnosis of Inflammatory Skin Diseases. *Philadelphia, Lea & Febiger, 1978.*)

FIGURE 2–11. Folliculitis. (With permission from Ackerman, A. B.: Histologic Diagnosis of Inflammatory Skin Diseases. *Philadelphia, Lea & Febiger, 1978.*)

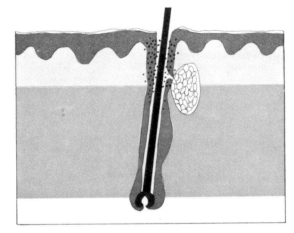

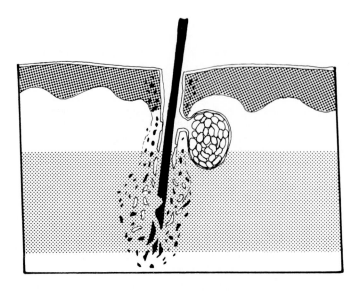

FIGURE 2–12. Furunculosis. (With permission from Muller, G. H., et al.: Small Animal Dermatology, 3rd ed. *Philadelphia, W. B. Saunders Co., 1983, p. 87.*)

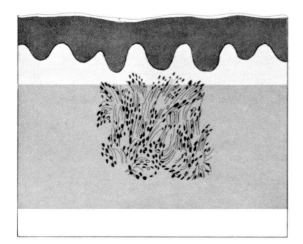

FIGURE 2–13. Fibrosing dermatitis. (With permission from Ackerman, A. B.: Histologic Diagnosis of Inflammatory Skin Diseases. Philadelphia, Lea & Febiger, 1978.)

marked tissue eosinophilia. The significance of this finding is unknown. The early lesions of alopecia areata are characterized by a lymphocytic perifolliculitis that is directed at anagen hair follicle bulbs.

It must be remembered that involvement of the hair follicle outer root sheath is a feature of pemphigus and that any significant degree of acantholysis mandates a consideration of this disorder. Likewise, the hair follicle outer root sheath may be involved in the hydropic degeneration and the lichenoid cellular infiltrates of lupus erythematosus.

FIBROSING DERMATITIS

Fibrosis, which presages the resolving stage of an intense or insidious inflammatory process, results mainly from collagen destruction. Fibrosis that is recognizable histologically does not necessarily produce a visible clinical scar. Scarring does not usually result from ulcers that cause damage to collagen in the upper portion of the superficial dermis only, whereas virtually all ulcers that extend into the deep dermis inexorably proceed to fibrosis and clinical scars.

Fibrosing dermatitis follows severe insults, of many types, to dermal collagen (Fig. 2–13). Thus, fibrosing dermatitis itself is of minimal diagnostic value, other than as testimony to severe antecedent injury. The pathologist will have to look carefully for telltale signs of the antecedent process, such as ruptured hair follicles, vascular disease, foreign material, lymphedema, and lupus erythematosus. The fibrosing dermatitis seen with caprine parelaphostrongylosis is associated with hydropic degeneration of epidermal basal cells.

PANNICULITIS

The panniculus is commonly involved as an extension of dermal inflammatory processes, especially suppurative and granulomatous dermatoses (Fig. 2–14). Likewise, there is usually some deep dermal involvement in virtually all panniculitides.

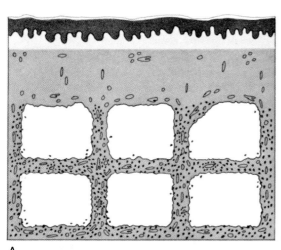

A

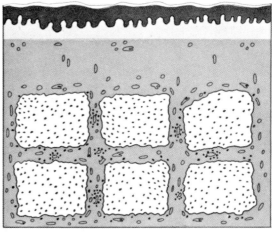

B

FIGURE 2–14. Panniculitis. A, Septal. B, Lobular. (With permission from Ackerman, A. B.: Histologic Diagnosis of Inflammatory Skin Diseases. Philadelphia, Lea & Febiger, 1978.)

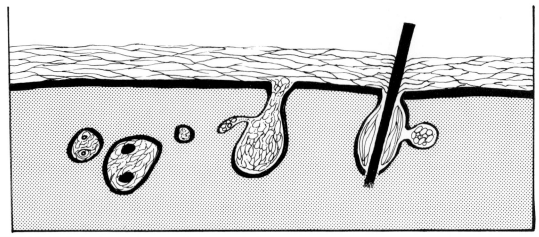

FIGURE 2–15. Endocrine dermogram. Nondiagnostic findings here suggest an endocrinopathy. Findings include orthokeratotic hyperkeratosis, follicular keratosis, follicular atrophy, follicular dilatation and plugging, mostly telogen hair follicles, epidermal hyperpigmentation, and sebaceous gland atrophy. (With permission from Muller, G. H., et al.: Small Animal Dermatology, 3rd ed. Philadelphia, W. B. Saunders Co., 1983, p. 89.)

Panniculitis is conveniently divided, on an anatomic basis, into a lobular type (primarily involving fat lobules), a septal type (primarily involving interlobular connective tissue septa), and combinations thereof. Lobular panniculitis is the most common type and is seen with microbial infections (bacteria and fungi), reactions to foreign bodies, and nutritional steatitis. Lobular panniculitis, depending on the stage of the reaction, may be primarily suppurative, pyogranulomatous, granulomatous, or fibrosing. Septal panniculitis is seen with vasculitides and erythema nodosum. Lobular inflammation and fat necrosis are not prominent features of septal panniculitis. Diffuse lobular and septal panniculitis suggests microbial infection.

ENDOCRINOPATHY

Endocrine dermatoses are those associated with various documented or presumed hormonal disturbances. These dermatoses have many histopathologic findings in common. The existence of an endocrinopathy is suggested by the following dermatohistopathologic findings: orthokeratotic hyperkeratosis, follicular keratosis, follicular atrophy, follicular dilatation and plugging, a predominance of telogen hair follicles, hair follicles devoid of hair, and sebaceous gland atrophy (Fig. 2–15). Although these findings are indicative of an endocrinopathy, they are nondiagnostic. Findings indicative of a specific endocrinopathy may or may not be present in any given specimen (see Chapter 13).

Inflammatory changes are a frequent and potentially misleading finding in the endocrine dermatoses and reflect the common occurrence of secondary seborrhea or pyoderma with these disorders (see Chapter 13). In such cases, it is essential that the clinician supply detailed data from the history and clinical examination and that the pathologist read between the lines and look beyond the distracting inflammatory changes.

CONCLUSION

A skin biopsy can be diagnostic, confirmatory, helpful, or inconclusive, depending on the dermatosis, the selection, handling, and processing of the specimen, and the skill of the histopathologist.

"The dermatopathologist has no right to make a diagnosis of nonspecific dermatitis or inflammation. Every biopsy specimen is a sample of some specific process, but the visible changes may be 'noncharacteristic' and may not permit a diagnosis."[12]

The clinician should always accept the terms nonspecific changes and nonspecific dermatitis with great reserve. The pathology of many entities that are now well recognized was once regarded as nonspecific! *Recourse to serial sections (the key pathologic changes may be very focal), special stains, second opinions, and further biopsies may be required.*

REFERENCES

1. Ackerman, A. B.: *Histopathologic Diagnosis of Inflammatory Skin Diseases*. Philadelphia, Lea & Febiger, 1978.
2. *Dorland's Illustrated Medical Dictionary*, 26th ed. Philadelphia, W. B. Saunders Co., 1981.
3. Fitzpatrick, T. B., et al.: *Dermatology in General Medicine*, 2nd ed. New York, McGraw-Hill Book Co., 1979.
4. Graham, J. H., et al.: *Dermal Pathology*. New York, Harper & Row, 1972.
5. Leider, M., and Rosenblum, M.: *A Dictionary of Dermatological Words, Terms, and Phrases*. New York, McGraw-Hill Book Co., 1968.
6. Lever, W. F., and Schaumburg-Lever, G.: *Histopathology of the Skin*, 5th ed. Philadelphia, J. B. Lippincott Co., 1975.
7. Milne, J. A.: *An Introduction to the Diagnostic Histopathology of the Skin*. Baltimore, Williams & Wilkins Co., 1972.
8. Montgomery, H.: *Dermatopathology*. New York, Harper & Row, 1967.
9. Moschella, S. L., et al.: *Dermatology*. 2nd ed. Philadelphia, W. B. Saunders Co., 1983.
10. Muller, G. H., et al.: *Small Animal Dermatology III*. Philadelphia, W. B. Saunders Co., 1983.
11. Okun, M. R., and Edelstein, L. M.: *Gross and Microscopic Pathology of the Skin*. Boston, Dermatopathology Foundation Press, 1976.
12. Pinkus, H., and Mehregan, A. H.: *A Guide to Dermatohistopathology*, 2nd ed. New York, Appleton-Century-Crofts, 1976.
13. Rook, A., et al.: *Textbook of Dermatology*, 3rd ed. Oxford, Blackwell Scientific Publications, 1979.
14. Yager, J. A., and Scott, D. W.: The skin and appendages. *In*: Jubb, K. V., et al.: *Pathology of Domestic Animals III*. New York, Academic Press, 1985, pp. 407–549.

CHAPTER 3

DIAGNOSTIC METHODS*

THE SYSTEMATIC APPROACH

If the veterinarian examines patients with skin disease in a cursory manner and attempts to make snap judgments, confusion and incorrect diagnoses will often result. In no other system of the body is a careful plan of examination and evaluation more important. Ideally, a thorough examination and appropriate diagnostic procedures should be accomplished the first time the patient is seen and before any masking treatments have been initiated. The following points should be systematically considered and correlated for a rational accurate dermatologic diagnosis.

STEPS TO A DERMATOLOGIC DIAGNOSIS

1. Clinical Examination.
   Record age, sex, breed, and general medical and dermatologic history. The inquiry should determine the chief complaint and data about the original lesion's location, appearance, onset, and rate of progression. Also determine the presence and degree of pruritus, contagion to other animals or people, and possible seasonal incidence. The relationship to diet and environmental factors as well as the response to previous medications is also important.
2. Physical Examination.
   a. Determine the distribution pattern and the regional location of affected areas.
   b. Closely examine the skin to identify primary and secondary lesions. Evaluate alopecias or hair abnormalities.
   c. Observe the configurations of specific skin lesions and their relationship to each other; certain patterns are diagnostically significant.

3. Diagnostic and Laboratory Aids.
   Diagnostic aids such as skin scrapings, impression smears, and fungal cultures should be done routinely. Biopsies, bacterial and viral cultures, hormonal assays, hemograms and chemistry panels, and other special tests are also performed when indicated by clinical findings.
4. Correlate the Data.
   Make a list of differential diagnoses.
5. Narrow the List of Differential Diagnoses.
   Plan additional tests, observations of therapeutic trials, and so on to narrow the list and provide a definitive diagnosis.

HISTORY

The medical history in a patient with skin disease should obviously be obtained with the same care as that exercised in a patient with any general medical or surgical illness. However, frequently such is not the case. Skin lesions are often too quickly assessed as trivial and unimportant. As a result, the history and physical examination may be totally inadequate, the precise extent of the skin lesions undetermined, and their possible general medical importance unsuspected.

Diseases, like criminals, are sometimes trapped by sudden flashes of intuitive diagnostic genius, but this is a hazardous substitute for painstaking collection of the essential medical evidence.[9]

With skin diseases, the necessity for being a heroic historian and dogged detective is paramount in accurate diagnosis and successful management. To this end, the use of a standard dermatologic history form or questionnaire is extremely helpful. Such a questionnaire will (1) involve the owners in the recording of historical data and save examination time, (2) provide a standard historical data base, allowing meaningful and valuable

---

*Portions of this material first appeared in Muller, G. H., Kirk, R. W., and Scott, D. W.: *Small Animal Dermatology*, 3rd ed. Philadelphia, W. B. Saunders Co., 1983.

data retrieval and disease surveillance and obviating failure to question the owner in one or more key areas, and (3) become an integral part of the patient's medical record, so that clinicians unfamiliar with the case can rapidly bring themselves up to date and not walk once-trodden ground again and again. An adequate dermatologic history, by questionnaire or interrogation, should include the following considerations.

Age. As with many other diseases, certain groups of skin conditions are seen much more frequently in various age groups. For instance, dermatophytosis, exudative epidermitis, and congenitohereditary dermatoses occur more commonly in young animals, whereas skin tumors and hyperadrenocorticism are more commonly seen in older animals. Nevertheless, great caution should be exerted not to allow age to become too much of a determining factor in arriving at a diagnosis.

Breed. Again, this may have some influence in the general considerations leading to a diagnosis, but it is rarely a crucial determining factor. Many skin disorders are known to occur with increased frequency in certain breeds, such as linear keratosis and unilateral papular dermatosis in quarter horses and dermatosis vegetans in Landrace pigs (Table 3–1).

Sex. The sex of the patient is rarely an

TABLE 3–1. Breed Predilections for Skin Diseases

Breed	Disease
Afrikander cattle	Hereditary goiter
Angus cattle	Familial acantholysis
Appaloosa horses	Pemphigus foliaceus
Arabian horses	Vitiligo; cutaneous asthenia
Ayrshire cattle	Curly coat; lymphedema
Bashkin horses	Curly coat
Belgian cattle	Cutaneous asthenia
Black Pied cattle	Hereditary zinc deficiency
Border Leicester-Southdown cross sheep	Cutaneous asthenia
Brangus cattle	Epidermolysis bullosa
Brown Swiss cattle	Ichthyosis; congenital porphyria
Charolais cattle	Cutaneous asthenia
Chianina cattle	Ichthyosis
Corriedale sheep	Congenitohereditary photosensitivity
Dorset sheep	Viable hypotrichosis
Finnish crossbred sheep	Cutaneous asthenia
Friesian cattle	Hereditary zinc deficiency, hypertrichosis
German Pinzgauer cattle	Ichthyosis
Guernsey cattle	Viable hypotrichosis
Hereford cattle	Viable hypotrichosis; semihairlessness; cutaneous asthenia; hereditary goiter; congenital porphyria; Chédiak-Higashi syndrome; curly coat
Holstein-Friesian cattle	Congenital porphyria; lethal hypotrichosis; streaked hypotrichosis; baldy calf syndrome; cutaneous asthenia; ichthyosis; vitiligo
Jersey cattle	Viable hypotrichosis
Landrace swine	Dermatosis vegetans
Limousin crossbred cattle	Protoporphyria
Merino sheep	Hereditary goiter; cutaneous asthenia
Mexican hairless swine	Viable hypotrichosis
Missouri Fox Trotting horses	Curly coat
Norwegian Dala sheep	Cutaneous asthenia
Norwegian Red Poll cattle	Ichthyosis
Percheron horses	Curly coat
Quarter horses	Cutaneous asthenia; linear keratosis; reticulated leukotrichia; unilateral papular dermatosis
Romney sheep	Cutaneous asthenia
Saanen-Dwarf cross goat	Hereditary goiter
Scottish Blackface sheep	Epidermolysis bullosa
Shorthorn cattle	Congenital porphyria
Simmental cattle	Cutaneous asthenia
Southdown sheep	Congenitohereditary photosensitivity; epidermolysis bullosa
Standardbred horses	Reticulated leukotrichia; equine viral arteritis
Suffolk sheep	Epidermolysis bullosa; scrapie
Swedish cattle	Curly coat
Thoroughbred horses	Reticulated leukotrichia; psychodermatoses

important diagnostic tool. For example, equine hyperadrenocorticism and bovine herpes mammillitis more commonly affect females, while equine mastocytoma and ovine *Clostridium novyi* infection are more common in males.

Familial Occurrence. Certain dermatoses have well-known hereditary predilections, such as cutaneous asthenia, dermatosis vegetans, hypotrichosis, and epidermolysis bullosa. Although data on familial occurrence of a dermatosis can be helpful in arriving at a diagnosis, frequently this information is unknown or unavailable.

Geographic Location. Some diseases are acquired under climatic and other circumstances that render these illnesses endemic in certain areas. Hence, blastomycosis, coccidioidomycosis, and pythiosis are confined to specific regions of the country. Remember, however, that geographic information must be gathered on both present and past environments.

Seasonal Influences. Some dermatoses have seasonal peaks, for known and unknown reasons. Thus, certain dermatoses may occur in summer (pollen-related atopy, foliage- and chemical-related contact dermatitis, insect hypersensitivity, and staphylococcal pyodermas), and others in winter (dermatophytosis, pediculosis, chorioptic mange, salt-related contact dermatitis, and frostbite). However, with repeated recurrences, the seasonal onset and end of many dermatoses may become less and less apparent.

Environmental Considerations. Crucial information that may be gathered includes (1) a detailed description of what the environment contains (bedding, flora, fauna, other contactants, and inhalants) and (2) what the animal is used for. This type of information is often critical in diagnosing and successfully managing contact dermatitis and contagious dermatoses.

Other Animals or People Affected. The history suggestive of contagion is often an important clue in ectoparasitisms and dermatophytosis. However, the presence or absence of evidence of contagion should never be the crucial diagnostic factor, since it is too unreliable.

Previous Skin Disease. Frequently, an accurate history regarding the previous occurrence of skin disease in a patient will be helpful in establishing a diagnosis and therapeutic plan. For example, a history of a similar or identical pruritic dermatosis occurring every year at the same time would be suggestive of allergic or ectoparasitic skin disease. A history of dry, flaky, greasy, or smelly skin (i.e., seborrhea) could give the clinician great insight into the reason for recurrent pyoderma and allow him or her to plan therapy more effectively. However, the clinician must be very sure to ascertain whether the previous skin disease was the same as the present one.

Previous Medical or Surgical Problems. Knowledge of previous medical or surgical problems of the patient may be helpful in arriving at a dermatologic diagnosis or in selecting appropriate therapy for a dermatosis.

Present Noncutaneous Symptoms. It is essential to question the owner concerning the presence of any noncutaneous symptoms. The presence of concurrent noncutaneous symptoms often helps to elucidate the etiology of a troublesome dermatosis. For instance, polydipsia, polyuria, and muscle wasting suggest hyperadrenocorticism. Lameness, fever, and lethargy could indicate systemic lupus erythematosus. Growth retardation, discolored teeth and urine, and anemia typify bovine erythropoietic porphyria. Of equal importance is the fact that the presence of other organ dysfunctions may significantly alter the clinician's approach to the dermatosis.

Previous and Current Therapy. Most animals presented for dermatologic disorders have been bathed, dipped, sprayed, powdered, and/or greased with one or more items procured by the owners, with or without the advice of a veterinarian, groomer, friend, or magazine article. Terribly important information can be gathered by the accurate determination of (1) what was used, (2) what dose was given, (3) how often it was given, (4) for how long it was given, and (5) what effect it had (good or bad).

An accurate knowledge of all drugs given to the patient may be the key to diagnosis of a problem dermatosis. Drug eruptions mimic virtually any dermatosis and can occur from the period of seven to ten days after drug therapy is begun, to weeks, months, or years later, to days after the drug is stopped. In addition, drugs being given to the patient at the time of evaluation may significantly interfere with any laboratory testing being considered.

Initial Skin Lesions. It is extremely important to determine, if possible, (1) the first skin lesions seen by the owner or others and (2) where the lesions were first seen. Many dermatoses have typical lesions and launch points.

Progression of the Skin Lesions. It is also important to determine how the initial skin lesions have changed (if at all) and how the dermatosis has spread (if at all). Is the dermatosis that the animal now has the same as what it had initially? Does the animal now have more than one skin problem? How might any previous therapy have influenced the clinical picture (drug-induced skin disease or drug-induced increased susceptibility to additional skin problems)?

Pruritus. Although the presence or absence of pruritus in association with a dermatosis is an important diagnostic consideration, it should seldom be the crucial diagnostic determinant. A commonly espoused but all too simplistic and frequently erroneous approach to skin diseases is to divide them into "them that itch" and "them that don't itch." Taken as a very general starting point, this type of categorization is useful. In general, allergic and parasitic dermatoses are pruritic, and endocrine dermatoses are not. Unfortunately, then we have all the dermatoses in between—including bacterial, fungal, and seborrheic—that are extremely variable and unpredictable with respect to pruritus. More important information is gained by these additional questions concerning pruritus: (1) Was pruritus the first thing noted, or did it develop later in the dermatosis? (2) How severe is the pruritus (occasional or constant)? and (3) How did the pruritus respond to known glucocorticoid regimens?

PHYSICAL EXAMINATION

Inasmuch as a visual appreciation of skin lesions is the essential factor in dermatologic diagnosis, the examiner's eye is undoubtedly the most important instrument at his or her disposal. Yet, the "standardization" of this instrument receives scant attention. Thus, Fitzpatrick writes, "Physicians are skilled in the physical examination of many organ systems, but not, usually, of the skin."[5]

The current prejudice in favor of laboratory tests that give numeric values as opposed to clinical observation is a theme that was challenged by Feinstein.[4] He wrote that clinicians try to be scientific in the use of inanimate objects but not in the use of their own sensory organs and brain and often believe that their own human equipment is a hindrance instead of an advantage, and is an apology, rather than an incentive, for science in clinical work. This argument is particularly apropos to dermatology, wherein the skin graciously lends itself to

the actual visualization of the gross pathology present. It has been estimated in pathology that 60 percent of diagnosis rests on gross and 40 percent on histopathologic examination. So why ignore or skim over the gross pathology and throw away 60 percent of the diagnosis?

Vital prerequisites for an adequate dermatologic examination are (1) good lighting (natural light or daylight-type lamps preferred), (2) clipping the animal's hair, when necessary, to adequately visualize lesions, (3) magnification, when critical to the accurate description of cutaneous lesions and debris, and (4) adequate restraint and positioning of the patient.

The crucial determinations to be made during the examination itself are (1) the type of lesions present, (2) the configuration of the lesions, and (3) the distribution of the lesions.

TYPES OF LESIONS

Dermatologic lesions are classified as primary or secondary. Primary lesions are the direct reflection or result of the underlying disease. These primary lesions, then, are the crucial ones to seek. Secondary lesions are evolutionary changes in the skin, dictated by the course of the primary lesions themselves and modified by factors such as secondary infections, self-trauma, and drug therapy. These secondary lesions are rarely helpful in making a specific diagnosis but, unfortunately, are usually the ones in greatest preponderance on the patient.

Primary Lesions

Macule. A macule (macula, spot) is a flat, circumscribed area of color change, equal to or less than 1 cm in diameter, that has no palpable mass. Macules may be produced by vasodilatation and inflammation (erythema), extravasation of blood (purpura), decreased melanin (hypopigmentation), and increased melanin (hyperpigmentation).

Patch. A patch is a macule that is greater than 1 cm in diameter.

Papule. A papule (papula, pimple) is a circumscribed, solid, usually rounded mass, equal to or less than 1 cm in diameter. Papules are usually elevated but may be intradermal or subcutaneous. Papules may be produced by hyperplasias (epidermal or dermal), cellular infiltrates (inflammatory or neoplastic), or metabolic products (lipid or amyloid) and, therefore, vary considerably in color, although most are erythematous. When papules are elevated and flat-topped, they are called lichenoid. It is imperative to establish whether papules are of follicular (hair projecting from center) or nonfollicular origin. Follicular papules usually indicate infection (bacterial, fungal, or parasitic) and are, thus, essential to distinguish from the nonfollicular papules of allergy and ectoparasitism. Lichenoid papules may be seen with drug eruptions and other poorly understood conditions.

Plaque. A plaque is a solid, elevated, flat-topped lesion, larger than 1 cm in diameter. Plaques often arise from a confluence of papules and, thus, have the color variations as well as the etiologic possibilities of papules. When a plaque is obviously made up of multiple, small, closely-packed, projected elevations, it is called a vegetation.

Nodule. A nodule (tubercle) is a circumscribed, solid, usually rounded mass, larger than 1 cm in diameter (a large papule). Nodules have the same positional and color variations and the same etiologic possibilities as papules. Gumma is an infrequently used term that implies a soft (gummy), deep (involving dermis and subcutis) nodule that has single or multiple punched-out ulcers over its surface.

Tumor. Tumor is a vague, general term for any mass, benign or malignant. Often, it is used to indicate a large nodule. Older, less frequently employed synonyms include tuber and phyma.

Vesicle. A vesicle (vesicula) is a circumscribed, elevated, dome-shaped, fluctuant lesion containing serum, equal to or less than 1 cm in diameter. Vesicles suggest an autoimmune, irritant, or viral etiology. It is essential to remember two things about vesicles in large animals: (1) the thin epidermis of these lesions makes them very fragile and transient (animals suspected of having a blistering disorder often require a "blister watch" every two to three hours) and (2) vesicles often fill rapidly with inflammatory cells, thus producing a vesicopustule or frank pustule, indistinguishable from the pustules of infection.

Bulla. A bulla (blister) is a vesicle larger than 1 cm in diameter. The etiologic considerations, transient nature, and precautionary statements mentioned for vesicles also apply to bullae. In addition, bullae may become hemorrhagic (red-purple in color).

Pustule. A pustule (pustula) is a vesicle filled with pus (inflammatory cells). It is essential to determine whether a pustule is follicular or nonfollicular, as follicular pustules indicate infection, whereas nonfollicular pustules may indicate infection but are also seen with other conditions. *Not all pustules are infected!* Pustules are also seen with autoimmune dermatoses. Pustules may be white (as in demodicosis), yellowish (staphylococcosis), yellowish-green (*Pseudomonas* infection), or reddish (hemorrhage), depending on the etiologic agent(s) involved and other factors.

Wheal. A wheal (urtica, hive) is a circumscribed, semisolid, raised, rounded, or flat-topped lesion that may produce blanching, slight erythema, or no color change in affected skin. The overlying epidermis and pelage are usually normal. Wheals are characteristically evanescent and vary in size from 3 to 4 mm (papular urticaria) to 10 to 12 cm (plaquelike) in diameter. Wheals may be immunologic or nonimmunologic in origin.

Other Primary Lesions. Other skin lesions occasionally classified as primary are the abscess, sinus, and cyst. An abscess is a well to poorly demarcated, fluctuant lesion involving the dermis and subcutis, the pus not being visible on the surface of the skin. A sinus is a draining tract from a suppurative cavity to the skin surface. A cyst is a well-demarcated, smooth, fluctuant sac that contains liquid or semisolid material (fluid, cells, and cell products).

Secondary Lesions

Scale. A scale (squame, or flake) is an accumulation of loose fragments of the stratum corneum. Scales may be white and nonadherent or, if mixed with sebaceous and apocrine secretion, yellowish to brown, greasy, and adherent. Scaling indicates altered epidermal maturation and turnover time, with or without glandular secretory abnormalities.

Hyperkeratosis. Hyperkeratosis is a localized, multifocal, or generalized accumulation of adherent keratinaceous material. It may be seen with such conditions as ichthyosis, linear keratosis, cannon keratosis, and cutaneous horns.

Crust. A crust (scab) is a dried, solid, adherent consolidation of varying combinations of serum, blood, pus, cutaneous debris, microorganisms, and medications. Crusts may be predominantly serous (yellowish), hemorrhagic (brown to red-black), purulent (greenish to yellow-green), or any combination thereof. An eschar is a crust resulting from a slough (for example, after a burn). A sphacelus is a densely adherent, dry, shiny, necrotic membrane, usually occurring on the floor of an ulcer.

Erosion. An erosion is a loss of epidermis to varying depths but not breaching the basement membrane. Erosions heal without scarring.

Ulcer. An ulcer is a loss of tissue that breaches the basement membrane. This is important prognostically, as ulcers may result in scarring. A *chancre* is a circumscribed indurated area of ulceration (most commonly used in human medicine to refer to the skin lesions of primary syphilis).

Excoriation. Excoriations are erosions and ulcers produced by self-trauma and are often linear. They are the hallmark of pruritus but can also be psychogenic in origin.

Lichenification. Lichenified skin is thickened, hardened, and its normal lines and markings are exaggerated. Lichenification is the hallmark of chronic inflammation and may be noted as early as 30 days into an inflammatory dermatosis.

Fissure. A fissure (crack, or rhagade) is a split in the skin, secondary to drying and loss of tone.

Pigmentary Disturbance. Hyperpigmentation (melanosis), an increase in either or both epidermal and dermal melanin, is associated with chronic inflammation, endocrinopathies, and many skin tumors and may be idiopathic. Hypopigmentation (hypomelanosis), a decrease in either or both epidermal and dermal melanin, may be seen in association with inflammatory disorders and as an idiopathic or congenital problem. Pigmentary disturbances may affect the skin (melanoderma and leukoderma, or achromoderma), hair (melanotrichia and leukotrichia, or achromotrichia), or both. In addition to disturbances in melanization, the skin color may reflect disturbances such as icterus (yellow), inflammatory or functional vasodilatation (red), purpura (red, purple, brown, or black), true or relative polycythemia (dull red to purplish), vascular collapse (pale and clammy), and cyanosis (blue).

Alopecia. Alopecia (atrichia, or atrichosis) is a complete absence of hair from where it is normally present. Hypotrichosis implies a less than normal amount of hair (partial alopecia). Alopecia and hypotrichosis may be inflammatory, hormonal, neoplastic, developmental, or idiopathic in nature. Hypertrichosis (hirsutism) is rare in large animals and may be hormonal (hyperadrenocorticism) or developmental (Border disease) in nature.

Comedo. A comedo is a plugged hair follicle. Comedones may be brown to black (open comedo, or blackhead) or white (closed comedo, or whitehead). Comedones are very commonly seen, especially in seborrheic, hormonal, and acneiform dermatoses. They frequently predispose to bacterial folliculitis.

Epidermal Collarette. An epidermal collarette is a circular rim of peeling epidermis surrounding a recent erosion or ulcer. Epidermal collarettes are the "footprints" of pustules, vesicles, and bullae. A pustule or blister watch may be in order to demonstrate the primary lesions.

Changes in Elasticity, Extensibility, and Thickness. The mechanical properties of skin are mainly dependent on the dermis. Skin tone is maintained by elastin, and skin toughness and tensile strength are maintained by collagen. Loss of elasticity (hypotonia) is manifested by skin that wrinkles excessively and fails to snap back into position when lifted away from the body and released; it may be seen with hyperadrenocorticism, catabolic states (malnutrition and diabetes mellitus), hereditary defects (cutaneous asthenia), and senility. Hyperelasticity and hyperextensibility are seen with cutaneous asthenia. Thin skin is usually generalized, is associated with cutaneous atrophy (and occasionally cutaneous asthenia), and is characterized by thinning, excessive fine wrinkling, and/or loss of normal skin markings and increased translucency (underlying vessels and fat more easily visualized). Thin skin may be seen with hyperadrenocorticism, catabolic states, and senility. Localized cutaneous atrophy (as occurs after dermatitis or panniculitis) may produce, in addition to the aforementioned, actual depressions in the skin. Thick skin may be generalized or localized (sclerosis) and usually indicates inflammation or infiltration (e.g., the myxedema of hypothyroidism).

Quality of Hair Coat. A hair coat (pelage) plagued by variable degrees of localized or generalized dryness, dullness, brittleness, and ease of epilation is common in most inflammatory and hormonal dermatoses and is a cutaneous expression of general systemic illness. It is important to determine (1) if easy epilation is occurring generally or only in areas of visible inflammation (hormonal versus inflammatory) and (2) in noninflammatory alopecias, if the easily epilated hairs are mostly undercoat and if the focal hair loss produced is incomplete (shedding, or telogen defluxion from disease, drugs, or stress), or if all hairs in focal areas are easily epilated, resulting in complete alopecia (hormonal).

Hyperhidrosis. Hyperhidrosis is excessive sweating. One sees multifocal or generalized accumulations of small, clear glistening beads of sweat in association with hair follicle openings. Fairly generalized hyperhidrosis may be seen with equine hyperadrenocorticism, equine pheochromocytoma, equine Japanese encephalitis, high ambient temperatures, vigorous exercise, severe pain (e.g., colic), and the administration of certain drugs (e.g., epinephrine, prostaglandin $F_{2\alpha}$). Localized hyperhidrosis may be seen with local injections of epinephrine, equine dourine, and Horner's syndrome.

Hematidrosis. Hematidrosis refers to blood in sweat and may be seen in equine infectious anemia, purpura hemorrhagica, and various bleeding diatheses.

Nikolsky's Sign. The Nikolsky sign is produced when the normal-appearing skin peripheral to vesicobullous and erosive or ulcerative lesions can be dislodged with sliding digital pressure. The Nikolsky sign may be present in pemphigus.

CONFIGURATION OF LESIONS

The configuration of skin lesions refers to their spatial relationship to each other (Fig. 3–1). These spatial relationships are occasionally helpful in arriving at a dermatologic diagnosis.

Linear. Linear skin lesions may suggest an exogenous cause (contact dermatitis or excoriation), developmental abnormalities (nevi), blood vessel (embolism or vasculitis) or lymphatic (lymphangitis) involvement, or miscellaneous idiopathic dermatoses (linear keratosis, cannon keratosis, or parelaphostrongylosis).

Annular or Arciform. Annular or arciform lesions suggest a point source of infection or inflammation that has spread peripherally and cleared centrally. Such lesions are often referred to as target, bull's eye, "iris," or ringworm-like. They usually indicate folliculitis (bacterial, fungal, or parasitic), impetiginous eruptions (bacterial), seborrheic eruptions, or blistering dermatoses. Annular lesions are also seen with bovine sterile eosinophilic folliculitis and alopecia areata.

Grouped. Grouping of lesions may be focal or multifocal and is most commonly seen with insect bites, ectoparasites, urticaria, and folliculitis. Terms occasionally employed for special groupings include (1) *corymbiform*, denoting a central large lesion, or cluster of lesions, surrounded by scattered, small satellite lesions (such as may be seen in papillomatosis, vegetative pyoderma, porcine juvenile pustular psoriasiform dermatitis, porcine dermatosis vegetans, and equine sarcoids), (2) *herpetiform*, indicating clusters of vesicles (herpes simplex in humans), and (3) *zosteriform*, signifying vesicles and bullae in a bandlike pattern, following a dermatome (herpes zoster in humans).

DISTRIBUTION OF LESIONS

Noting the distribution of skin lesions over the body is often helpful in arriving at a dermatologic diagnosis. A bilaterally symmetric dermatosis usually suggests an internal etiology (hormonal, allergic, or drug-related), whereas an asymmetric dermatosis usually suggests an external etiology (microorganisms or trauma). A ventrally distributed dermatosis would suggest contact origin, whereas a dorsally distributed dermatosis might suggest ectoparasitism. Charts for the regional diagnosis of large animal dermatoses have been devised (Table 3–2). In most instances, however, one distribution pattern may be most characteristic of, or most frequently seen with, a certain disease, but variations are common, and the differential diagnosis is lengthy. One must constantly remind oneself to (1) never say "never" and never say "always," (2) keep the mind open and the etiologic possibilities exhaustive, and (3) be meticulous in the case work-up. Patterns of distribution are best remembered in light of the following analogy: "To use a geographic metaphor, they are signs which point more or less accurately to large areas and well populated centers, but cannot include obscure but sometimes important diagnostic hamlets and byways."[9]

OTHER CONSIDERATIONS IN THE PHYSICAL EXAMINATION

It goes without saying that a cursory or complete (depending on the patient's medical history) general physical examination must be performed on all dermatologic patients. Never forget the skin is the window to the soul, the

Text continued on page 63

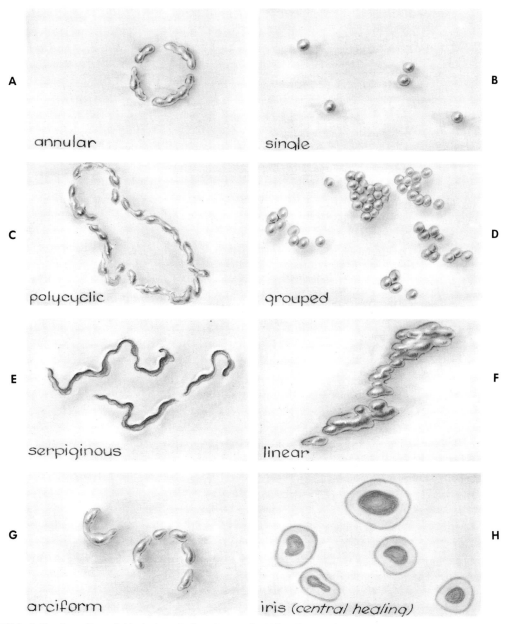

FIGURE 3–1. *Configuration of skin lesions. A, Annular configuration has a clear or less involved center and is found in folliculitides and other dermatoses. B, Single lesions are found in many dermatoses. C, Polycyclic configurations often result from the confluence of lesions or a spreading process. Examples are folliculitides and erythema multiforme. D, Grouped lesions are clusters, often the result of new foci developing around an old lesion. They are seen in folliculitis, ectoparasitisms, and other dermatoses. E, Serpiginous lesions develop as a result of spreading, such as in folliculitides and erythema multiforme. F, Linear configurations are best typified by lymphangitis, linear keratosis, or lesions resulting from contact with irritant materials streaked along the skin. G, Arciform lesions may result from spreading, as in folliculitides. H, Central-healing (target) configurations are produced when the skin heals behind an advancing front of a disease process. It is typical of folliculitides. (With permission from Muller, G.H., et al.: Small Animal Dermatology, 3rd ed. Philadelphia, W.B. Saunders Co., 1983.)*

TABLE 3–2. Regional Diagnosis of Skin Disease*

Area	Disease
Head and Neck	Dermatophytosis (papulocrustous)
	Dermatophilosis (pustulocrustous)
	Staphylococcal folliculitis (papulocrustous)
	Demodicosis (papulonodular)
	Exudative epidermitis (vesiculocrustous)
	Onchocerciasis (alopecia, scaling and crusts)
	Habronemiasis (papuloulcerative)
	Stephanofilariasis (alopecia, scaling and crusts)
	Elaeophoriasis (ulcerative)
	Fly bites (papulocrustous)
	Porcine spirochetosis (necroulcerative)
	Necrobacillosis (necroulcerative)
	Actinomycosis (nodular)
	Actinobacillosis (nodular)
	Bovine farcy (nodular)
	Clostridal infection (edematous)
	Sarcoptic mange (papulocrustous)
	Gasterophiliasis (papular, linear)
	Contagious viral pustular dermatosis (pustulocrustous)
	Ovine viral ulcerative dermatosis (ulcerative)
	Trombiculidiasis (papulocrustous)
	Porcine contagious streptococcal pustular dermatitis (pustulocrustous)
	Goatpox (pustulocrustous)
	Sheep-pox (pustulocrustous)
	Bovine malignant catarrhal fever (papulocrustous, necroulcerative)
	Bovine papular stomatitis (papular)
	Infectious bovine rhinotracheitis (erosion; crusting)
	Molluscum contagiosum (papular)
	Urticaria (papules, wheals)
	Anthrax (edematous)
	Edema disease (edematous)
	Alopecia areata (alopecia)
	Discoid lupus erythematosus (alopecia, scaling and crusts)
	Aplasia cutis (ulcerative)
	Atopy (pruritus, excoriations)
	Chlorinated naphthalene toxicosis (hyperkeratosis)
	Epidermolysis bullosa (vesiculoulcerative)
	Familial acantholysis (vesiculoulcerative)
	Bovine sterile eosinophilic folliculitis (papulocrustous)
	Pemphigus foliaceus (vesiculopustular, crusts)
	Zinc deficiency (crusts)
	Vitiligo (depigmentation)
	Contact dermatitis (variable)
	Viral papillomatosis (papulonodular)
	Equine sarcoid (alopecic or nodular)
	Equine mastocytoma (nodular)
	Melanoma (nodular)
	Squamous cell carcinoma (nodular or necroulcerative)
	Equine amyloidosis (nodular)
	Equine schwannoma (nodular)
Ear	Dermatophytosis (papulocrustous)
	Dermatophilosis (pustulocrustous)
	Sarcoptic mange (papulocrustous)
	Ear mites (otitis externa)
	Equine aural plaques (hyperkeratotic plaques)
	Fly bites (papulocrustous)
	Ticks (otitis externa)
	Porcine spirochetosis (necroulcerative)
	Porcine ear necrosis (necroulcerative)
	Vasculitis (necroulcerative)
	Pemphigus foliaceus (vesiculopustular, crusts)
	Ergotism (necrotizing)
	Fescue toxicosis (necrotizing)
	Frostbite (necrotizing)

TABLE 3–2. Regional Diagnosis of Skin Disease* *Continued*

Area	Disease
	Photodermatitis (edematous or necroulcerative)
	Equine sarcoid (nodular)
	Squamous cell carcinoma (nodular or necroulcerative)
	Temporal teratoma (cystic)
Mucocutaneous	Foot-and-mouth disease (vesiculoulcerative)
	Vesicular stomatitis (vesiculoulcerative)
	Vesicular exanthema (vesiculoulcerative)
	Swine parvovirus vesicular disease (vesiculoulcerative)
	Swine vesicular disease (vesiculoulcerative)
	Bovine virus diarrhea (erosion, crusts)
	Contagious viral pustular dermatitis (pustulocrustous)
	Goatpox (pustulocrustous)
	Blue tongue (erythema, edema)
	Sheep-pox (pustulocrustous)
	Exudative epidermitis (vesiculocrustous)
	Zinc deficiency (crusts)
	Bullous pemphigoid (vesiculoulcerative)
	Vasculitis (necroulcerative)
	Stachybotryotoxicosis (necroulcerative)
	Thallotoxicosis (necroulcerative)
	Epidermolysis bullosa (vesiculoulcerative)
	Familial acantholysis (vesiculoulcerative)
	Equine herpes coital exanthem (vesiculoulcerative)
	Horsepox (vesiculoulcerative)
	Pemphigus foliaceus (vesiculopustular, crusts)
	Candidiasis (pustular)
	Staphylococcal folliculitis (papulocrustous)
	Dermatophytosis (papulocrustous)
	Dermatophilosis (pustulocrustous)
	Drug eruption (vesiculoulcerative)
	Squamous cell carcinoma (nodular or necroulcerative)
Dorsum	Dermatophilosis (pustulocrustous)
	Pediculosis (scale)
	Fly bites (papulocrustous)
	Psoroptic mange (papulocrustous)
	Fleas (papulocrustous)
	Hypodermiasis (nodular)
	Porcine hyperkeratosis (keratosebaceous debris)
	Equine eosinophilic granuloma (nodular)
	Contact dermatitis (chemicals; variable)
	Bovine angiomatosis (nodular, bleeding)
Ventrum	Contact dermatitis (variable)
	Fly bites (papulocrustous)
	Dermatophilosis (pustulocrustous)
	Stephanofilariasis (alopecia, scaling and crusts)
	Impetigo (pustulocrustous)
	Trombiculidiasis (papulocrustous)
	Candidiasis (pustular)
	Tuberculosis (nodular)
	Sarcoptic mange (papulocrustous)
	Pelodera dermatitis (papulocrustous)
	Onchocerciasis (alopecia, scaling and crusts)
	Habronemiasis (nodular, ulcerative)
	Swinepox (pustulocrustous)
	Goatpox (pustulocrustous)
	Sheep-pox (pustulocrustous)
	Porcine spirochetosis (necroulcerative)
	Anthrax (edematous)
	Edema disease (edematous)
	Botryomycosis (nodular, ulcerative)
	Molluscum contagiosum (papular)
	Contagious viral pustular dermatitis (pustulocrustous)
	Porcine contagious streptococcal pustular dermatitis (pustulocrustous)

Table continued on following page

TABLE 3–2. Regional Diagnosis of Skin Disease* *Continued*

Area	Disease
	Bovine malignant catarrhal fever (papulocrustous)
	Infectious bovine rhinotracheitis (erosive, crusted)
	Zinc deficiency (crusts)
	Dracunculiasis (nodular, cystic)
	Porcine juvenile pustular psoriasiform dermatitis (pustulocrustous)
	Porcine dermatosis vegetans (pustulocrustous)
	C. pseudotuberculosis abscesses (abscess)
	Zygomycosis (nodular, ulcerative)
	Pythiosis (nodular, ulcerative)
	Lymphangioma (cystic)
Trunk	Dermatophytosis (papulocrustous)
	Dermatophilosis (pustulocrustous)
	Staphylococcal folliculitis (papulocrustous)
	Erysipelas (papular, urticarial, necrotizing)
	Psoroptic mange (papulocrustous)
	Psorergatic mange (pruritus, alopecia)
	Keds (pruritus, alopecia)
	Pediculosis (scaling, with or without pruritus)
	Parafilariasis (nodules, cysts, hemorrhage)
	Ovine fleece rot (moist dermatitis)
	Pemphigus foliaceus (vesiculopustular, crusts)
	Parelaphostrongylosis (vertical, linear, excoriation)
	Food hypersensitivity (pruritus, excoriation)
	Demodicosis (papulonodular)
	Bovine sterile eosinophilic folliculitis (papulocrustous)
	Exudative epidermitis (vesiculocrustous)
	Equine viral papular dermatitis (papulocrustous)
	Equine unilateral papular dermatosis (papular, unilateral)
	Caprine viral dermatitis (papulonodular)
	Equine axillary nodular necrosis (nodular)
	Scrapie (pruritus, excoriations)
	Seborrhea (scaling and crusts)
	Equine exfoliative eosinophilic dermatitis and stomatitis (scaling, crusts, ulcers)
	Equine sarcoidosis (scaling and crusts)
	Hypotrichoses (hair loss)
	Anagen defluxion (alopecia)
	Abnormal shedding (alopecia)
	Alopecia areata (alopecia)
	Hypertrichosis (excessive hair)
	Aplasia cutis (ulcers)
	Arsenic toxicosis (alopecia, scaling)
	Mercurialism (alopecia)
	Hairy vetch toxicosis (papulocrustous)
	Chlorinated naphthalene toxicosis (hyperkeratosis)
	Polybrominated biphenyl toxicosis (alopecia, scaling)
	Bovine lumpy skin disease (papulonodular)
	Bovine pseudolumpy skin disease (papulonodular)
	Besnoitiosis (papulonodular)
	Trypanosomiasis (wheals)
	Urticaria (papules, wheals)
	Erythema multiforme (papules, wheals)
	Hyalomma toxicosis (moist dermatitis)
	High-fat milk replacer dermatosis (scaling, alopecia)
	Iodine deficiency (scaling, alopecia)
	Hereditary goiter (scaling, alopecia)
	Protein deficiency (scaling, alopecia)
	Essential fatty acid deficiency (scaling, alopecia)
	Biotin deficiency (pustulocrustous, alopecia)
	Niacin deficiency (alopecia, scaling, crusts)
	Pantothenic acid deficiency (alopecia, scaling, crusts)
	Riboflavin deficiency (alopecia, scaling, crusts)
	Vitamin C–responsive dermatosis (alopecia, scales, purpura)
	Vitamin A deficiency (hyperkeratosis)
	Dermatosis responsive to vitamin E and selenium (scale)

TABLE 3–2. Regional Diagnosis of Skin Disease* Continued

Area	Disease
	Ichthyosis (hyperkeratosis)
	Bovine exfoliative erythroderma
	Systemic lupus erythematosus (alopecia, scaling, crusts)
	Panniculitis (nodular, cystic)
	Bovine dermatitis, pyrexia, and hemorrhage (papulocrustous)
	Reticulated leukotrichia
	Spotted leukotrichia
	Copper deficiency (depigmentation)
	Equine amyloidosis (nodular)
	Lymphosarcoma (nodular)
	Equine mastocytoma (nodular)
Hindquarters	Dermatophilosis (pustulocrustous)
	Staphylococcal folliculitis (papulocrustous)
	Chorioptic mange (papulocrustous)
	Louseflies
	Porcine tail necrosis
	Rinderpest (papulocrustous)
	Sorghum toxicosis (moist dermatitis)
	Melanoma (nodular)
Legs and Feet	Dermatophilosis (pustulocrustous)
	Dermatophytosis (papulocrustous)
	Staphylococcal folliculitis (papulocrustous)
	Chorioptic mange (papulocrustous)
	Ulcerative lymphangitis (nodular, ulcerative)
	Sporotrichosis (nodular, ulcerative)
	Equine histoplasmosis (nodular, ulcerative)
	Bovine farcy (nodular)
	Atypical mycobacteriosis (nodular)
	Actinomycosis (nodular, ulcerative)
	Nocardiosis (nodular, ulcerative)
	Pythiosis (nodular, ulcerative)
	Mycetoma (nodular, ulcerative)
	Glanders (nodular, ulcerative)
	Habronemiasis (nodular, ulcerative)
	Fly bites (papulocrustous)
	Contact dermatitis (variable)
	Hookworm dermatitis (papulocrustous)
	Strongyloidiasis (papulocrustous)
	Stephanofilariasis (alopecia, scaling, crusts)
	Trombiculidiasis (papulocrustous)
	Dracunculiasis (nodular, cystic)
	Elaeophoriasis (necroulcerative)
	Clostridial infection (edematous)
	Sarcoptic mange (papulocrustous)
	Zinc deficiency (crusts)
	Vitamin C–responsive dermatosis (erythema, alopecia, purpura)
	Atopy (pruritus, excoriation)
	Food hypersensitivity (pruritus, excoriation)
	Ovine viral ulcerative dermatosis (ulcerative)
	Snake bite (edematous)
	Spider bite (edematous)
	Equine viral arteritis (edematous)
	Equine purpura hemorrhagica (edematous)
	Systemic lupus erythematosus (edematous)
	Lymphedema
	Vasculitis (edematous, necroulcerative)
	Bovine lumpy skin disease (papulonodular)
	Botryomycosis (nodular, ulcerative)
	Pemphigus foliaceus (vesiculopustular, crusts)
	Aplasia cutis (ulcerative)
	Equine cannon keratosis (hyperkeratosis)
	Equine linear keratosis (hyperkeratosis)
	Epidermolysis bullosa (vesiculoulcerative)

Table continued on following page

TABLE 3–2. Regional Diagnosis of Skin Disease* *Continued*

Area	Disease
	Familial acantholysis (vesiculoulcerative)
	Dermatosis vegetans (pustulocrustous)
	Equine sarcoid (nodular, ulcerative)
	Equine mastocytoma (nodular)
	Angiomatosis (hyperkeratosis, hemorrhage)
	Polychlorinated biphenyl toxicosis (erythema)
Mane and Tail	Pediculosis (pruritus, scales)
	Psoroptic mange (pruritus, scales)
	Insect hypersensitivity (pruritus)
	Oxyuriasis (pruritus)
	Food hypersensitivity (pruritus)
	Mane and tail seborrhea (scales)
	Piedra (broken hairs)
	Mane and tail dystrophy (abnormal hairs)
	Trichorrhexis nodosa (broken hairs)
	Bovine papular stomatitis (hair loss)
	Sarcocystosis (hair loss)
	Selenosis (hair loss)
	Leucaenosis (hair loss)
	Mercurialism (hair loss)
Coronary Band	Pemphigus foliaceus (vesiculopustular, crust)
	Vasculitis (necroulcerative)
	Equine sarcoidosis (scaling, crusts)
	Equine exfoliative eosinophilic dermatitis and stomatitis (scaling, crusts, ulcers)
	Blue tongue (erythema)
	Contagious viral pustular dermatitis (pustulocrustous)
	Foot-and-mouth disease (vesiculoulcerative)
	Vesicular stomatitis (vesiculoulcerative)
	Vesicular exanthema (vesiculoulcerative)
	Swine vesicular disease (vesiculoulcerative)
	Porcine parvovirus vesicular disease (vesiculoulcerative)
	Ergotism (edematous)
	Fescue toxicosis (edematous)
	Zinc deficiency (crusts)
	Dermatosis vegetans (pustulocrustous)
	Exudative epidermitis (vesiculocrustous)
	Photodermatitis (erythema, edema)
	Dermatophilosis (pustulocrustous)
	Epidermolysis bullosa (vesiculoulcerative)
	Familial acantholysis (vesiculoulcerative)
Hoof	Zinc deficiency
	Biotin deficiency
	Exudative epidermitis
	Epidermolysis bullosa
	Familial acantholysis
	Pemphigus foliaceus
	Dermatosis vegetans
	Vasculitis
	Erysipelas
	Salmonellosis
	Streptococcosis
	Photodermatitis
	Selenosis
	Ergotism
	Fescue toxicosis
	Leucaenosis
	Foot-and-mouth disease
	Vesicular stomatitis
	Vesicular exanthema
	Swine vesicular disease
	Porcine parvovirus vesicular disease
	Chlorinated naphthalene toxicosis

TABLE 3–2. Regional Diagnosis of Skin Disease* *Continued*

Area	Disease
	Hog cholera
	Equine sarcoidosis
	Equine exfoliative eosinophilic dermatitis and dermatitis
	Polybrominated biphenyl toxicosis
	Blue tongue
Pressure Points	Pressure sore (ulcerative)
	Callus (hyperkeratosis)
	Epidermolysis bullosa (vesiculoulcerative)
	Familial acantholysis (vesiculoulcerative)
	Cutaneous asthenia (lacerations)
	Porcine skin necrosis (necroulcerative)
Pigment-Related	Photodermatitis
	Black and white hair follicle dystrophies
	Albinism
	Lethal white foal
	Chédiak-Higashi syndrome
	Vitiligo
	Leukoderma
	Reticulated leukotrichia
	Spotted leukotrichia
	Photo-activated vasculitis

*See also equine pastern dermatitis (Chapter 15, Table 15–3), gangrene (Chapter 4, discussion on gangrene), nodular skin disease (Chapter 15, Table 15–1), bovine udder and teat (Chapter 5, Table 5–1), and porcine erythema and cyanosis (Chapter 14, discussion on porcine erythema and cyanosis).

mirror reflecting the *milieu interieur*, and can be diseased in association with other organ systems as well as by itself.

Specialized cutaneous structures such as the hooves and horns may provide helpful hints to underlying etiologic agents. These may be dystrophic, brittle, cracked, discolored, or sloughed in various congenitohereditary disorders (familial acantholysis, epidermolysis bullosa, and hypotrichosis), disorders resulting from environmental factors (ergotism, fescue toxicosis, selenosis, and frostbite), autoimmune disorders, and vascular disorders.

In addition, the mucous membranes and mucocutaneous junctions should be carefully inspected. These areas may be involved in viral, autoimmune, vascular, toxic, and drug-induced disorders.

SUMMARY

"Dermatologists are physicians who can diagnose a rash!"[5] The most common error in dermatologic diagnosis is to regard skin lesions as nonspecific rashes, eczemas, or dermatitides rather than as aggregates or specific, individual lesions. Let's face it: (1) rash is defined as a temporary eruption on the skin, (2) eczema is defined as an inflammatory skin disease char-

acterized by lesions varying greatly in character, with vesiculation, infiltration, watery discharge, and the development of scales and crusts, and (3) dermatitis is defined as inflammation of the skin. What have we really said, and what heady diagnostic coups have we really accomplished when we use these rather meaningless terms?

Too often, clinicians adopt a speedy, superficial approach to the historical and physical aspects of skin disease, which they would not apply to any other organ system. A careful history and physical examination, particularly noting and recording the morphology, configuration, and distribution of the primary and secondary skin lesions, are the starting point for a comprehensive differential diagnosis, which, in turn, becomes the starting point for unraveling the diagnostic puzzle. In some instances, an accurate history and physical examination are the only aids to dermatologic diagnosis. In other cases, they allow the clinician's impressions to be substantiated by appropriate laboratory tests.

What is the most difficult of all? It is what appears the simplest: to see with your eyes what lies in front of your eyes.

GOETHE

TABLE 3–3. Dermatologic Tests

Test	References
Examinations for Parasites	
Acetate tape preparation	Chapter 9, ref. 10
Skin scraping	Chapter 9, refs. 6, 10
Fecal flotation	Chapter 9, refs. 6, 11
Examinations for Fungi	
Potassium hydroxide or mineral oil preparations	Chapter 7, refs. 7, 10
Wood's light examination	Chapter 7, refs. 7, 10
Fungal culture	Chapter 7, refs. 7, 10
Fungal slide cultures	Chapter 7, ref. 10
Stained slide preparations	Chapter 7, ref. 10
Examinations for Bacteria	
Direct or impression smears	Chapter 6, ref. 10
Bacterial cultures	Chapter 6, ref. 10
Antibacterial sensitivity tests	Chapter 6, ref. 10
Examinations for Viruses and Protozoa	
Viral culture	Chapter 5, refs. 2, 8
Serology	Chapter 5, refs. 2, 8, 11
Electron microscopy	Chapter 5, ref. 8
Histopathologic Examinations	
Skin biospy	Chapter 2
Fixing and staining	Chapter 2
Allergy Testing	
Patch tests	Chapter 10, ref. 10
Intradermal tests	Chapter 10, ref. 10
Immunologic Tests	
Immunofluorescent tests	Chapter 10, ref. 10
Antinuclear antibody tests	Chapter 10, ref. 10
Lupus erythematosus cell preparation	Chapter 10, ref. 10
Endocrine Tests	
Thyroid function	Chapter 13
Adrenal function	Chapter 13

DIAGNOSTIC AND LABORATORY PROCEDURES

Diagnostic tests and laboratory procedures are valuable aids in almost every dermatologic case. Most tests are simple, quick, and inexpensive to perform. Some tests should be done routinely, since many dermatoses are, in fact, complex problems with more than one cause. It would be embarrassing to miss a case of demodectic mange or dermatophytosis because a simple test was not run to check for a secondary problem in what superficially looked like a single primary disease.

Detailed discussions of dermatologic tests are best presented in the most appropriate disease section as well as in other in-depth textbooks. Table 3–3 provides cross-references to detailed directions for specific tests.

REFERENCES

1. Beutner, E., et al.: *Immunopathology of the Skin II.* New York, John Wiley & Sons, 1979.
2. Blood, D. C., et al.: *Veterinary Medicine VI.* Oxford, Baillière Tindall, 1983.
3. Fadok, V. A.: Equine dermatology. Mod. Vet. Pract. 64:A7, 1985.
4. Feinstein, A. R.: *Clinical Judgment.* Baltimore, Williams & Wilkins Co., 1967.
5. Fitzpatrick, T. B., et al.: *Dermatology in General Medicine.* New York, McGraw-Hill Book Co., 1979.
6. Georgi, J. R.: *Parasitology for Veterinarians IV.* Philadelphia, W. B. Saunders Co., 1985.
7. Jungerman, P. F., and Schwartzman, R. M.: *Veterinary Medical Mycology.* Philadelphia, Lea & Febiger, 1972.
8. Mohanty, S. B., and Dutta, S. K.: *Veterinary Virology.* Philadelphia, Lea & Febiger, 1981.
9. Moschella, S. L., et al.: *Dermatology.* Philadelphia, W. B. Saunders Co., 1975.
10. Muller, G. H., et al.: *Small Animal Dermatology III.* Philadelphia, W. B. Saunders Co., 1983.
11. Soulsby, E. J. L.: *Helminths, Arthropods, and Protozoa of Domesticated Animals VII.* London, Baillière Tindall, 1982.
12. Evans, A. G., and Stannard, A. A.: *Diagnostic approach to equine skin disease.* Compend. Cont. Ed. 8:652, 1986.

CHAPTER 4

ENVIRONMENTAL DISEASES

Environmental disorders are common and often a cause of substantial economic loss in livestock production. In many instances—chemical toxicoses, mycotoxicoses, and hepatotoxic plant toxicoses—the dermatologic abnormalities are clinically spectacular and of important diagnostic significance but are of rather trivial overall importance prognostically, therapeutically, and financially compared with abnormalities in other organ systems. An in-depth discussion of these disorders is beyond the scope of this chapter. The author has emphasized the dermatologic features of each condition. For detailed clinicopathologic information on these environmental disorders, the reader is referred to numerous excellent textbooks.*

MECHANICAL INJURIES

Intertrigo

Intertrigo is a superficial inflammatory dermatosis that occurs in places where skin is in apposition and is thus subject to the friction of movement, increased local heat, maceration from retained moisture, and irritation from accumulation of debris.[112] When these factors are present to a sufficient degree, dissolution of stratum corneum, exudation, and secondary bacterial infection are inevitable.

Intertrigo (udder dermatitis, flexural seborrhea) is most commonly seen in dairy cattle and occasionally in dairy goats and mares.[35, 319, 365a] Congestion of the udder at parturition is physiologic but may be sufficiently severe to cause edema of the belly, udder, and teats.[402, 402a] In most cases, the edema disappears within two to three days after parturition but, if extensive and persistent, it can lead to intertrigo where the skin of the udder contacts the skin of the medial thighs. Erythema is followed by oozing, crusting, secondary bacterial infec-

tion, and, in severe cases, necrosis and a foul odor. The frequency of the condition in German dairy cattle was reported to be about 2 percent in first-calf heifers and 0.06 percent in older animals.[365a]

Udder-thigh intertrigo is generally treated with gentle antiseptic soaps, astringent rinses, frequent massage, and diuretics (acetazolamide, 1–2 gm b.i.d. orally or parenterally; chlorothiazide, 2 gm b.i.d. orally or 0.5 gm b.i.d. intravenously or intramuscularly; furosemide, 0.5 gm b.i.d. intravenously) to reduce udder edema, and, when dry, dusting with powders to reduce friction. Healing is virtually always complete within 4 to 12 weeks.

Callus

A callus is a localized area of hyperkeratosis and epidermal hyperplasia caused by intermittent pressure and friction, resulting in recurring cutaneous ischemia and hyperplasia. Callosities are common over joints and bony prominences, especially the knee, fetlock, elbow, hock, and tuber ischii and are most commonly seen in swine housed on concrete floors with insufficient bedding.[229] The lesions are characterized by annular, well-circumscribed plaques of lichenification and hyperkeratosis. Secondary bacterial infection can intervene, producing callus pyoderma.

In most instances, callosities require no therapy and should *not* be removed unless the environmental circumstances that created them can be remedied. They are, after all, the body's attempt to protect itself! When environmental insults can be corrected, callosities may be softened with emollient ointments or creams or with lactic acid–containing sprays (Humilac, Hy Lyt EFA). Surgical excision is usually unsuccessful.

Hematoma

A hematoma is a circumscribed area of hemorrhage into the tissues. It arises from

---

*References 6, 18, 35, 46, 58, 60, 70, 95, 191, 194, 199, 214, 218, 226, 229, 241, 245, 299, 349a, 421

vascular damage associated with sudden, severe, blunt external trauma (e.g., a fall) or with more prolonged physical trauma (e.g., head shaking because of irritation from ear mites). The lesions are usually acute in onset, subcutaneous, and fluctuant and may or may not be painful.

Hematomas, most commonly seen in swine,[229, 330, 386] are usually located over the shoulders, flanks, and hindquarters and may develop rapidly after severe nonpenetrating trauma. Aural hematomas, most frequently found in lop-eared breeds of swine, are associated with head-shaking (from sarcoptic mange, pediculosis, or meal in ears from overhead feeders) or ear biting. Vulvar hematomas are seen in the post partum gilt and sow, associated with trauma from faulty farrowing crate doors or large piglets at farrowing.

Diagnosis is based on history and physical examinations. Needle aspiration and cytologic examination reveal blood. Most hematomas are simply allowed to organize and partially resolve. If surgical incision, evacuation, and repair are indicated, the hematoma should be allowed to organize first. Occasional herd outbreaks of hematomas, in which 10 percent of the sows died from massive hemorrhage, have been reported.[229] Increasing the level of vitamin K in the feed corrected the problem.

Pressure Sore

Pressure sores (decubitus ulcers) usually occur as a result of prolonged application of pressure concentrated in a relatively small area of the body and sufficient to compress the capillary circulation, causing tissue damage or frank necrosis.[112] Tissue anoxia and full-thickness skin loss rapidly progress from a small localized area to produce ulceration, which almost invariably becomes infected with a variety of pathogenic bacteria. Within a matter of 24 to 48 hours, the edges of the ulcerated area become undermined. The ulceration may later extend to underlying bone. Because of the area of capillary and venous congestion in the base of the ulcer and at the tissue margins, systemic antibiotic therapy is virtually useless, except in the case of bacteremia.

Pressure sores (bedsores, saddle sores, saddle galls, girth galls, "sit fasts," decubital ulcers) are caused by prolonged, continuous pressure—often relatively mild—leading to ischemic necrosis.* They are most commonly

*References 35, 53, 179, 229, 323, 383, 394

seen in horses and swine: Ill-fitting tack and hard floors (cement, wooden slats, and wire mesh), respectively, are major causes. Lesions are seen over pressure points such as bony prominences, joints, and other areas subject to sustained external pressure. Animals that are emaciated (decreased fat and muscle layers) or recumbent are at an increased risk.

Lesions are initially characterized by an erythematous to reddish-purple discoloration. This progresses to oozing, necrosis, and ulceration (Fig. 4–1). The resultant ulcers tend to be deep, undermined at the edges, secondarily infected, and very slow to heal. Scarring and leukotrichia after healing are not uncommon. Diagnosis is based on history and physical examination.

The most important aspect of therapy is to identify and correct the cause. Routine wound care includes daily cleansing and drying agents, and topical antiseptics or systemic antibiotics if indicated. Surgical débridement, surgical excision, or skin grafting may be necessary in certain instances. Prevention is vastly superior to any kind of therapy.

Foreign Body

Foreign bodies occasionally cause skin lesions in large animals.[35, 298, 394] Most commonly, the foreign material is of plant origin (e.g.,

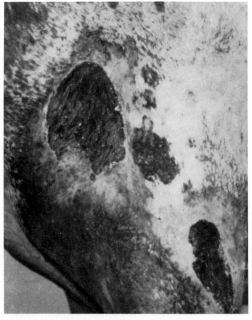

FIGURE 4–1. Pressure sores over the shoulder of a horse after anesthesia and surgery.

wood splinters and the seeds and awns of cheatgrass, needlegrass, poverty grass, crimson clover, and foxtail). Resultant skin lesions include papules or nodules (granulomas) or draining tracts (fistulae). Lesions are usually seen over the limbs and ventrolateral aspects of the body.

Diagnosis is based on history, physical examination, and skin biopsy. Therapy may entail surgical removal of the foreign body or excision of the entire lesion.

Gangrene

Gangrene is a clinical term used to describe severe tissue necrosis and sloughing.[33, 35, 240] The necrosis may be moist or dry. The pathologic mechanism of gangrene is an occlusion of either arterial or venous blood supply. Moist gangrene is produced by impairment of lymphatic and venous drainage plus infection (putrefaction) and is a complication of decubital ulcers associated with bony prominences and pressure points in recumbent animals. Moist gangrene presents as swollen, discolored areas with a foul odor and progressive tissue decomposition. Dry gangrene occurs when arterial blood supply is occluded, but venous and lymphatic drainage remain intact and infection is absent (mummification). Dry gangrene assumes a dry, discolored, leathery appearance.

The causes of gangrene include (1) external pressure (pressure sores, rope galls, constricting bands, ill-fitting tack, and porcine skin necrosis), (2) internal pressure (severe edema), (3) burns (thermal, chemical, friction, radiation, or electrical), (4) frostbite, (5) envenomation (snake bite), (6) vasculitis, (7) ergotism, (8) fescue toxicosis, and (9) various infections (salmonellosis, streptococcosis, spirochetosis, necrobacillosis, erysipelas, malignant catarrhal fever, bovine herpes mammillitis, bovine lumpy skin disease, and staphylococcal and clostridial infections). For diagnosis and management of these conditions, the reader is referred to appropriate sections of this book.

Subcutaneous Emphysema

Subcutaneous emphysema is characterized by free gas in the subcutis.[35, 227, 359, 390] Possible causes include (1) air entering through a cutaneous wound (from an accident or surgery), (2) lung punctured by the end of a fractured rib, (3) internal penetrating wounds (e.g., traumatic reticuloperitonitis), (4) rumen gases migrating from a rumenotomy or rumenal trocarization, (5) extension from pulmonary emphysema, (6) extension from tracheal rupture, (7) gas gangrene infections, and (8) bovine ephemeral fever.

Subcutaneous emphysema is characterized by soft, fluctuant, crepitant subcutaneous swellings. The lesions are usually nonpainful, and the animals are not acutely ill, except in the case of gas gangrene (e.g., clostridial infections; see Chapter 6, discussion on clostridial infections).

Diagnosis is based on history and physical examination. Treatment is directed at the underlying cause. Sterile subcutaneous emphysema requires no treatment unless extensive and incapacitating, in which case multiple skin incisions may be necessary.[35]

Black Pox

Black pox, a sporadic condition seen in dairy cattle,[35] is thought to be a traumatically induced teat disorder caused by poor milking machine techniques. *Staphylococcus aureus* is consistently cultured from the lesions but is presumed to be secondary.

Lesions occur most commonly on the tip of the teat and are characterized by crateriform ulcers with raised edges and a black spot in the pitted center. The affected area may spread to involve the teat sphincter, whereupon mastitis is a possible sequela.

Black pox is usually quite intractable to topical and systemic medicaments. The milking machinery should be carefully analyzed as concerns pressure and technique.

THERMAL INJURIES

Burns

Burns are occasionally seen in large animals and may be thermal (barn, forest, and bush fires or accidental spillage of hot solutions), electrical (electrocution or lightning strike), frictional (rope burns or abrasions from falling), chemical (blisters, improperly used topical medicaments, or maliciously utilized caustic agents), and radiational (x-ray therapy).* The reader is referred to two excellent articles[134, 356] for in-depth discussions of the pathophysiology of burns and the management of severely burned patients with extracutaneous compli-

---

*References 35, 126a, 134, 227, 323, 341, 356, 394

cations (cardiopulmonary, ocular, hematologic, or renal).

Burns are most commonly seen over the dorsum and the face (see Plate 1, A and B). Animals with burns over more than 50 percent of their body usually die. Burns have been classified according to severity.[134, 323] First-degree burns involve the superficial epidermis, are characterized by erythema, edema, and pain, and generally heal without complication. Second-degree burns affect the entire epidermis, are characterized by erythema, edema, pain, and vesicles, and usually re-epithelialize with proper wound care. Third-degree burns include the entire epidermis, dermis, and appendages and are characterized by necrosis, ulceration, anesthesia, and scarring. Diligent therapy and possibly skin grafting are indicated. Fourth-degree burns involve the entire skin, subcutis, and underlying fascia, muscle, and tendon.

Care of burn wounds usually includes one or more of the following: (1) thorough cleansing (povidone-iodine or chlorhexidine), (2) surgical débridement, (3) daily hydrotherapy, and (4) topical antibiotics.[126a, 134, 356] Occlusive dressings are avoided because of their tendency to produce a closed wound with bacterial proliferation and to delay healing. The wound should be cleaned two or three times daily, and the topical antibiotic reapplied. The most useful topical antibiotic is silver sulfadiazine, a painless, nonstaining, broad-spectrum antibacterial agent with the ability to penetrate eschar. Systemic antibiotics are *not* effective in preventing local burn wound infections and may permit the growth of resistant organisms. Burns heal slowly, and many weeks may be required to allow the wound to close by granulation.

Frostbite

Frostbite, an injury to the skin resulting from excessive exposure to cold,[112] is more common in neonates; animals that are sick, debilitated, or dehydrated; animals with heavily pigmented skin; and animals having preexisting vascular insufficiency (from ergotism, fescue toxicosis, or vasculitis). Also at risk are dairy cattle and goats turned out into cold weather after udders and teats have been washed but inadequately dried off.

Frostbite most commonly affects ears, tails, teats, scrotum, and feet (Fig. 4–2).* Mild cases

_____
*References 6, 33, 95, 109, 227, 280–284, 326, 359, 378, 379, 394

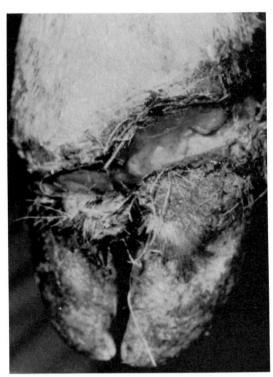

FIGURE 4–2. Frostbite in a cow. Necrosis and sloughing at the coronet.

present with erythema, scaling, and alopecia. Severe cases present with necrosis, dry gangrene, and sloughing. The affected skin is usually anesthetic.

Therapy varies with the severity of the frostbite. In mild cases, treatment is usually not needed. In more severe cases, rapid thawing in warm water (41 to 44°C) is indicated as soon as possible after it is known that refreezing can be prevented. Rewarming may be followed by the application of bland, protective ointments or creams. In very severe cases with necrosis and sloughing, symptomatic therapy with topical wet soaks and systemic antibiotics is indicated, and surgical excision is postponed until an obvious boundary between viable and nonviable tissue is present. Once-frozen tissue may be increasingly susceptible to cold injury.

PRIMARY IRRITANT CONTACT DERMATITIS

Primary irritant contact dermatitis is common in large animals and has numerous causes, and its dermatologic findings reflect the mode of encounter with the contactant.

Cause and Pathogenesis

Primary irritants have one thing in common: They invariably produce dermatitis if they come into direct contact with skin in sufficient concentration for a long enough period.[186, 382, 383] No sensitization is required. Moisture is an important predisposing factor, as it decreases the effectiveness of normal skin barriers and increases the intimacy of contact between the contactant and the skin surface. In this regard, the sweating horse is an ideal candidate for contact dermatitis over any area of the body.

Commonly incriminated causes of primary irritant contact dermatitis include body excretions (feces and urine), wound secretions, caustic substances (acids and alkalis), crude oil, diesel fuel, turpentine, leather preservatives, mercurials, various blisters, leg sweats, improperly utilized topical parasiticides (sprays, dips, and wipes), irritating plants (*Helenium microcephalum* [smallhead sneezeweed], *Cleome gynandra* [prickly spider flower], *Urtica ureus* and *U. dioica* [stinging nettle], and *Euphorbia* spp. [spurge]), wood preservatives, bedding, and a filthy environment.*

Clinical Features

Primary irritant contact dermatitis is far more common than contact hypersensitivity.[186, 278, 279] Age, breed, and sex are not factors in the incidence of the disease, except as they relate to frequency of encounter with the offending contactant. Because direct contact is required, the face, distal extremities, ventrum, and areas under tack are most commonly affected (see Plate 1, *C* and *D*). The dermatitis varies in severity (depending on the nature of the contactant) from erythema, papules, edema, and scaling to vesicles, erosions, ulcers, necrosis, and crusts. Pruritus and pain are variable. Severe irritants or self-trauma in response to pruritus can result in alopecia, lichenification, and scarring. Leukotrichia and leukoderma can be transient or permanent sequelae.

In most instances, the nature of the contactant can be inferred from the distribution of the dermatitis: muzzle and distal extremities (plants and environmental substances such as sprays and fertilizers); a single limb (blisters and sweats); face and dorsum (sprays, dips,

*References 35, 59, 95, 101, 102, 186, 227, 229, 256, 283, 284, 323, 342, 354, 382, 383

and wipes); perineum and rear legs (urine and feces); tack-associated areas (preservatives, dyes, and polishes); and ventrum (bedding and a filthy environment). Leukoderma or dermatitis around the mouth of horses has been attributed to contact with rubber bits and feed buckets (see Chapter 14, discussion on leukoderma).[256, 284]

Salt produces large, irregularly shaped erythematous plaques in contact areas of swine skin.[8] Pentachlorophenol (a component of waste motor oil, fungicides, wood preservatives, and moth-proofers) was reported to produce severe contact dermatitis in horses and swine and loss of the mane and tail in horses.[59, 95] During breeding season, the buck goat urinates on his own face, beard, and forelimbs when sexually excited, producing urine scald.[359, 378, 379] A dermatitis may be seen on the muzzle, lips, and ear tips of kids and calves fed milk or milk replacer from pans and buckets.[282, 359, 379, 387] Transit erythema is a contact dermatitis in swine, associated with exposure to lime.[229]

A condition analogous to immersion foot in humans has been reported in cattle and horses.[38a] All animals had been standing in cool water for over three days. Clinical signs included early pain, reluctance to move, and edema and erythema of the submerged areas of skin. Dermatitis progressed to necrosis and slough. Therapy included warming, symptomatic topical medicaments, and surgical intervention as required.

Diagnosis

Diagnosis is based on history, physical examination, and recovery when the offending contactant is removed. The cause is usually obvious but, occasionally, may require considerable detective work, especially when owners are unwilling to admit to using home remedies that have produced the dermatitis. Skin biopsy usually reveals varying degrees of superficial perivascular dermatitis (hyperplastic or spongiotic) wherein neutrophils or mononuclears are the predominant inflammatory cell types. Spongiotic vesicles or epidermal necrosis and ulceration may be seen. Biopsies from swine with salt-induced contact dermatitis revealed superficial and deep perivascular dermatitis with eosinophilia.[8]

Clinical Management

The contact irritant must be identified and eliminated. Residual contactant and other surface debris can be removed with copious amounts of water and gentle cleansing soaps. Moist, oozing dermatoses will benefit from the application of astringent soaks (aluminum acetate or magnesium sulfate in water) applied for five to ten minutes t.i.d. Other measures for treatment of symptoms, depending on the presence and severity of secondary bacterial infection or pruritus, may include topical antiseptic or antibiotic preparations or topical or systemic glucocorticoids. In most instances, if the irritant is removed, the dermatitis will improve markedly within three to seven days.

PORCINE SKIN NECROSIS

Porcine skin necrosis is trauma related and most commonly affects the knees, fetlocks, hocks, elbows, ears, and teats.

Cause and Pathogenesis

Porcine skin necrosis is becoming increasingly common as more and more swine are kept under intensive husbandry systems with only minimal bedding.[229] Necrotic lesions usually occur bilaterally over bony prominences and other areas that are easily damaged by environmental contact or fighting.[228, 326, 331] The occurrence of most forms of porcine skin necrosis has been associated with rough concrete flooring, alkaline pH (alkalis and lime-washed pens), and contact dermatitis (formalin and calcium hypochlorite disinfectants and other caustic agents).[229, 326, 331] Strips of adhesive plaster or gauze pads covered with adhesive tape placed over susceptible anatomic sites (knees, fetlocks, hocks, teats, and so forth) as soon as possible after birth will significantly reduce the incidence of skin necrosis in piglets.[326, 331]

Porcine ear necrosis is thought to be precipitated by fighting and bite wounds, which may become secondarily infected with *Staphylococcus hyicus* and β-hemolytic streptococci.[263, 345] Severe bacterial infection leads to vasculitis, thrombosis, and severe necrosis.

Clinical Features

Although most forms of porcine skin necrosis are epidemic, mortality is negligible with most forms.[229, 326, 331] At birth the piglet's skin is soft and moist, and at this stage, it could be particularly sensitive to irritants and trauma. In most instances, the initial skin lesion is a reddish-brown macule or patch over a joint or other prominent cutaneous site where contact is made with the ground. These lesions are always bilateral and may be seen within a few hours after birth. The lesions progress through necrosis, erosion, and ulceration, reaching maximum severity in about seven days (see Plate 1, *E*). A blackish-brown crust forms over the lesions, which begin to heal after about three weeks and are usually healed within five weeks of their onset. Lameness and local infections may or may not be seen. The knees are most commonly affected, followed in descending order of frequency by the fetlocks, hocks, elbows, coronets, chin, sternum, vulva, stifles, and rump.*

Teat necrosis is also a herd problem, being bilateral and most common in females and affecting the cranial pair of teats most frequently.[326, 327, 331] Tail biting and tail necrosis (see Plate 1, F) are often seen.[34, 296, 326, 328, 330, 331] A small abraded area appears on the dorsal or ventral surface of the tail root soon after birth and proceeds to necrose, ulcerate, and encircle the tail root, resulting in sloughing of the entire tail.

Ear necrosis begins as ear biting at the margins of the pinnae.[150, 195, 239, 263, 329, 345] Early lesions may resolve completely or evolve through a vesicular, exudative, and crusted phase (*S. hyicus* infection) and terminate as a scalloping of the ear margins. This mild form is of no concern to pig or pig producers. Sporadically, severe cellulitis develops (β-hemolytic streptococci) and progresses through vasculitis, thrombosis, and severe necrosis and ulceration. The severe form may be accompanied by sloughing of the entire ear, bacteremia, polyarthritis, and pneumonia.

Diagnosis is based on history and physical examination. Skin biopsy in porcine ear necrosis reveals an early intraepidermal pustular dermatitis phase (*S. hyicus*) and a later diffuse suppurative dermatitis and necrotizing vasculitis phase (β-hemolytic streptococci).[345]

Clinical Management

In most instances, therapy is of no benefit.[229, 326] Severe porcine ear necrosis has been reported to respond to tylosin (100 gm/T food),[345] ampicillin (10 to 20 mg/kg/day orally),[239] or sodium selenite (0.3 ppm in feed).[150]

Prevention is the key.[229, 326, 331] Ensuring proper bedding and freedom from exposure to irritating chemicals is critical. As mentioned

---

*References 22, 72, 169, 267, 325, 326, 331, 335

previously, gauze pads applied under adhesive tape over susceptible areas will reduce the incidence of porcine skin necrosis significantly.

OVINE FLEECE ROT

Ovine fleece rot is a superficial dermatitis resulting from bacterial proliferation induced by wetness at skin level and manifested by seropurulent exudation and matting of the wool fibers.

Cause and Pathogenesis

Under natural and experimental conditions, continued wetting of sheep, such that saturation of the skin surface persists, will produce fleece rot.[35, 151, 167, 168, 253, 353] Approximately a week of continual skin wetting is sufficient to produce the disease (eight or more wet days and a total of 100 mm or more of rain). Temperature itself is not an important factor. The seasonal incidence of fleece rot will thus coincide with the months of maximum rainfall.

Certain sheep show a predisposition to fleece rot, which may be attributed to variations in physical characteristics of the fleece and skin that exist among sheep of different breeds and strains and even among individual sheep.* Increasing staple length reduces penetration of rain to skin level, but once wet, a long fleece will dry out far more slowly. Conversely, fleeces of short staple length are rapidly penetrated but dry out more quickly. Character (staple conformation) and fleece architecture are important in that in compact fleeces, water tends to penetrate by diffusion only, while in less dense fleeces, direct wetting of the skin is permitted. Microanatomically, fleeces with a larger secondary:primary hair follicle ratio are more resistant to fleece rot.[234, 253, 353] Fleeces with a high wax (sebum) content are less susceptible to fleece rot, presumably because of the water-proofing effect of wax.[35, 146, 164, 192, 353] Last, a yellowish fleece color (high suint content) is indicative of susceptibility to fleece rot.[125, 253, 353]

Subsequent to wetting of the skin, a marked proliferation of bacteria, almost exclusively *Pseudomonas* spp., occurs on the skin and in the fleece.† This is followed by an exudation of serum and inflammatory cells, which mats

the fleece and attracts blowflies. Fleece discoloration is produced by chromogenic bacteria such as *Pseudomonas aeruginosa* (green) and *P. indigofera* (blue).

Clinical Features

Fleece rot (wool rot, yolk rot, water rot, canary stain) is common in most parts of Australia during wet years and causes considerable economic losses due to depreciation of the value of damaged fleeces.[35, 245, 353, 377, 398, 410] It is also of concern in South Africa and the United Kingdom. The incidence of fleece rot within a flock varies from 14 to 92 percent. Lesions are most common over the withers and along the back. Initially, the skin in affected areas assumes a deep purple hue. This is followed by the exudation and accumulation of seropurulent material, which causes the characteristic band of matted fleece. The wool in affected areas is always saturated and may be easily epilated. Discoloration of the wool by green, blue, brown, orange, or pink bands may occur at any level of the staple. The area of fleece rot emanates putrid odors, which attract gravid blowflies. Affected sheep are usually otherwise healthy.

Diagnosis

Diagnosis is based on history and physical examination.[35, 245, 353] The main differential diagnosis is dermatophilosis, which occurs under similar conditions. However, the characteristic crusting and ulceration of dermatophilosis is not present in fleece rot. Skin biopsy reveals suppurative intraepidermal pustular dermatitis and superficial folliculitis.[50, 353] Affected sheep may have leukocytosis and neutrophilia.[165]

Clinical Management

Therapy is not usually undertaken and is usually of no benefit.[35, 245] Chemical drying of the fleece decreases wetness and the incidence of fleece rot. A mixture of zinc and aluminum oxides with sterols and fatty acids applied to sheep as a mist was shown to offer protection for 10 to 12 weeks.[152] Immunization of sheep with a cell-free vaccine containing high concentrations of soluble antigens from *P. aeruginosa* was reported to reduce the severity of fleece rot.[51]

Prevention, through selecting sheep for inherent resistance to fleece rot, would appear to be the most logical approach to dealing with

---

*References 35, 74, 125, 167, 234, 245, 253, 322, 353, 409, 412
†References 50, 51, 167, 259, 260, 289, 353, 410

the problem.[35, 235, 253, 322, 353] A technique for measuring fleece wettability has been developed.[235, 322] A sample of staple is placed in a plastic cylinder with one end in water, and the mass of water that is taken up in a given time is measured. The technique has been shown to be consistent and capable of distinguishing resistant from susceptible sheep.

CHEMICAL TOXICOSES

Selenosis

Chronic selenium poisoning causes lameness, hoof changes, emaciation, and loss of the long hairs of the mane, tail, and distal limbs in horses and cattle.

CAUSE AND PATHOGENESIS

Selenosis is seen in the Great Plains and Rocky Mountain belt areas of the United States and in certain regions of Australia, Canada, Columbia, Israel, Mexico, and the United Kingdom.* The condition is associated with high levels of selenium in the soil (generally greater than 5 ppm) or the presence of selenium-concentrating plants. Selenium levels are highest in low-rainfall areas with alkaline soils. On seleniferous soils, "converter" or "indicator" plants such as *Astragalus bisulcatus, A. pattersonii, A. praelongus, A. pectinatus, A. racemosus, Acacia cana, Morinda reticulata, Neptunia amplexicaulis, Xylorrhiza* spp., *Oxytropis* sp., *Gutierrezia* spp., *Penstemon* spp., *Sideranthus* spp., *Grindelia* spp., *Greyia* spp., *Castilleja* spp., *Aster* spp., *Atriplex* spp., *Camandra pallida, Machaeranthera* spp., *Oonopsis* spp., *Haplopappus* spp., *Mentzelia* spp., and *Stanleya* spp. accumulate selenium to a much higher level (up to several thousand ppm) than do other plants on the same soil. In addition, these plants grow preferentially in seleniferous soil and have some value as indicators of possible toxicosis. Chronic selenosis can also be seen when drinking water contains as little as 0.1 to 2 ppm selenium. Selenium concentrations in feed should *not* exceed 5 ppm.

The pathologic mechanism of chronic selenosis is unclear.[35, 46, 58, 70, 213, 399a] Selenium probably interferes with oxidative enzyme systems that possess sulfur-containing amino acids. The defective hoof and hair keratinization characteristic of chronic selenosis probably results from the substitution of sulfur with selenium in the sulfur-containing amino acids.

CLINICAL FEATURES

Chronic selenosis (alkali disease, bob-tailed disease) is most commonly reported in horses and cattle but may be seen in sheep and swine.* Chronic selenosis has also been suspected to be the cause of alopecia in the flanks and beard of goats in the western United States.[280] Chronic selenosis generally occurs in livestock that consume grasses and cereal grains containing 5 to 40 ppm selenium. There are no apparent age, breed, or sex predilections. Typically, animals develop sore feet and lameness, which begins in the hind feet and progresses to involve all four feet. The coronary band area becomes tender, and transverse cracks and separations appear in the hoof. In severe cases, the hooves may become necrotic and slough. The hair coat is rough, and there is progressive depilation of the long hairs of the mane, tail, and fetlock region. Generalized alopecia may be seen in horses and swine.

DIAGNOSIS

The differential diagnosis includes chronic arsenic toxicosis, chronic mercurialism, leucaenosis, and malnutrition. The definitive diagnosis is based on history (exposure), physical examination, selenium levels in tissues, and selenium levels in soil, water, and feed.[35, 78, 241, 302, 302c, 323] Chronic selenosis is characterized by the following tissue levels of selenium: 1 to 4 ppm (blood), 11 to 45 ppm (hair), and 8 to 20 ppm (hoof).

CLINICAL MANAGEMENT

Fatalities are rare in chronic selenosis, but affected animals are often destroyed or sold because owners become impatient or discouraged with the chronic, prolonged recovery period, which usually takes several months.[35, 302, 302c, 323, 399a] The source of selenium intake must be identified and eliminated. Addition of inorganic arsenic, such as sodium arsenate, to drinking water (5 ppm) or salt supplements

---

*References 6, 35, 78, 189, 190, 222, 284, 287, 302, 323, 365, 399a

*References 6, 35, 78, 128, 141, 142, 222, 241, 287, 302c, 336, 399a

(30 to 40 ppm) is reported to be beneficial.* Naphthalene, given orally at a dosage of 4 to 5 gm for an adult horse once daily for five days, is reported to be effective.[35, 284, 302, 302c, 399a] The naphthalene is stopped for five days then readministered daily for a second five-day course. Other measures reported to be of some benefit include a high-protein diet (especially those high in sulfur-containing amino acids) and the daily oral administration of 2 to 3 gm of DL-methionine.[35, 70, 111, 182, 284, 399a] Pretreatment with copper is reported to be an effective preventive.[35, 284, 385, 399a]

Molybdenosis

Molybdenum poisoning causes a secondary copper deficiency in ruminants, characterized clinically by diarrhea and depigmentation of hair.† Cattle are more susceptible than sheep, and young growing animals are particularly susceptible. Forage molybdenum levels higher than 10 ppm are dangerous, although toxicity is also dependent on the intake of copper and sulfur. Excessive molybdenum intake interferes with hepatic storage of copper, which is exacerbated by a high intake of sulfur or a low intake of copper.

Molybdenosis has been recognized in the United States, the United Kingdom, Australia, and New Zealand. Clinical signs are those of hypocuprosis (see Chapter 12, discussion on copper deficiency). Diagnosis is based on history, physical examination, blood copper levels of less than 0.7 µg/ml, and blood molybdenum levels higher than 0.1 ppm. Treatment and prevention are as discussed under copper deficiency (see Chapter 12).

Arsenic Toxicosis

Chronic arsenic poisoning causes gastroenteritis, emaciation, and an exfoliative dermatitis in large animals.

CAUSE AND PATHOGENESIS

Sources of arsenic include parasiticide dips and sprays, weed and orchard sprays, insect baits, and arsenical medicaments.‡ Arsenic is a general tissue poison and combines with and inactivates sulfhydryl groups in tissue enzymes.

CLINICAL FEATURES

Arsenic toxicosis has been reported in all large animals,* with no apparent age, breed, or sex predilections. Clinical signs include gastroenteritis, emaciation, variable appetite, and a dry, dull, rough, easily epilated hair coat, progressing to alopecia and severe seborrheic skin disease. Occasionally, focal areas of skin necrosis and slow-healing ulcers may be seen. Horses may develop a long hair coat along with severe seborrhea.[323]

DIAGNOSIS

Differential diagnosis includes selenosis, mercurialism, leucaenosis, malnutrition, and equine hyperadrenocorticism. Definitive diagnosis is based on history, physical examination, and arsenic levels in the liver or kidneys higher than 10 ppm.[6, 35, 46, 58, 70, 127, 241]

CLINICAL MANAGEMENT

The source of arsenic intake must be identified and eliminated. Treatment recommendations have included (1) D-penicillamine at 11 mg/kg orally q.i.d. for 7 to 10 days,[298] or (2) for adult horses and cattle, 10 to 30 gm of sodium thiosulfate (10 to 20 percent aqueous solution) intravenously, followed by 20 to 60 gm orally q.i.d. for three to four days (sheep, goats, and swine receive ¼ of these doses),[35, 70, 127, 241, 298, 302b] or (3) dimercaprol (BAL) at 3 to 5 mg/kg q.i.d. intramuscularly for two days, then b.i.d. for eight more days,[35, 70, 127, 241, 298, 302b] or (4) thioctic acid (with or without BAL) at 50 mg/kg t.i.d. intramuscularly.[127, 162, 241, 302b]

Mercurialism

Chronic mercury poisoning causes gastroenteritis, lameness, emaciation, and progressive generalized alopecia in horses.

CAUSE AND PATHOGENESIS

Mercurialism is usually caused by the accidental feeding of grain that has been treated with organic mercurials used as antifungals.† It may also occur from the accidental overdosing of mercury-containing medicaments, the licking-off of mercury-containing skin dressings, or from the percutaneous absorption of

*References 35, 70, 241, 284, 302, 323, 404
†References 6, 35, 45, 70, 131, 153, 336, 401
‡References 35, 44, 58, 70, 127, 227, 258, 302b, 323, 414

*References 6, 35, 46, 70, 227, 229, 241, 298, 302b
†References 35, 46, 58, 70, 242, 313, 323, 349a

mercury-containing skin dressings. Mercury-containing topical medicaments (e.g., mercurial blisters) may produce severe primary irritant contact dermatitis.[227, 256, 323] The pathologic mechanism of mercurialism is not known.

CLINICAL FEATURES

Mercurialism has been reported in horses and cattle.* There are no apparent age, breed, or sex predilections. Clinical signs include gastroenteritis, depression, anorexia, emaciation, a generalized loss of body hair, and then the loss of the long hairs of the mane, tail, and fetlock regions.

DIAGNOSIS

Differential diagnosis includes selenosis, leucaenosis, arsenic toxicosis, and malnutrition. Definitive diagnosis is based on history, physical examination, and mercury levels in tissues.[35, 46, 70] Mercury is concentrated in the kidneys, and chronic mercurialism may be associated with levels of 100 ppm.

CLINICAL Management

The source of mercury intake must be identified and eliminated. Sodium thiosulfate as well as dimercaprol has been recommended for treatment (see discussion on arsenic toxicosis).[35, 70, 170, 313, 349a] In addition, 4 gm of potassium iodide given orally s.i.d. for 10 to 14 days has been reported to be beneficial in horses.[323]

Chlorinated Naphthalene Toxicosis

Chlorinated naphthalene toxicosis (CNT) causes severe hyperkeratos, emaciation, and increased susceptibility to many infections in cattle.

CAUSE AND PATHOGENESIS

Chlorinated naphthalenes were once widely used as industrial lubricant and wood preservative additives.[35, 70, 185, 307, 380] The ingestion or percutaneous absorption of these compounds interferes with the conversion of carotene to vitamin A. The clinical signs of CNT are believed to be caused by a combination of vitamin A deficiency and the direct toxic effects of chlorinated naphthalenes. CNT is essentially a man-made disease, with the principal source of contamination being a chlorinated naphthalene–containing lubricant used in machines for pelleting feed.

CLINICAL FEATURES

CNT (bovine hyperkeratosis, x disease, and Wendener's disease) was widespread in the United States and Germany during the 1940's and 1950's.* The disease was also reported in Australia[416] and New Zealand.[163] In the United States, annual economic losses resulting from CNT were estimated at $20 million. CNT is basically a historical disease today.

The cutaneous changes of CNT usually begin over the withers and sides of the neck and extend cranially, caudally, and ventrally. The skin becomes progressively more hyperkeratotic, scaly, thickened, alopecic, and fissured. Pruritus is absent. Horns may become loose and develop asymmetric growth. Other clinical signs include lacrimation, proliferative stomatitis, salivation, variable appetite, decreased milk production, emaciation, and increased susceptibility to many infections (metritis, mastitis, dermatophytosis, and viral papillomatosis).

DIAGNOSIS

Diagnosis is based on history, physical examination, and low vitamin A level in tissues (less than 10 μg/dl in plasma, less than 5 μg/gm dry matter in liver).[35, 244, 307] Skin biopsy reveals marked orthokeratotic hyperkeratosis, follicular keratosis, and variable epidermal hyperplasia (Fig. 4–3).[223, 224, 307] Dermal collagen was reported to be decreased.[244]

CLINICAL MANAGEMENT

Therapy, including vitamin A, is of no benefit.[175–177, 240, 307, 380, 413] The source of chlorinated naphthalene intake must be identified and eliminated. If cattle are not too severely poisoned and if secondary infections are controlled, recovery does occur.[307–310]

Thallotoxicosis

Thallium salts have been used in many parts of the world as rodenticides.[35, 46, 58, 70] Ingestion

---

*References 6, 35, 46, 70, 126, 161, 227, 256, 313, 323, 384, 394

*References 143, 144, 223, 224, 307, 380, 403

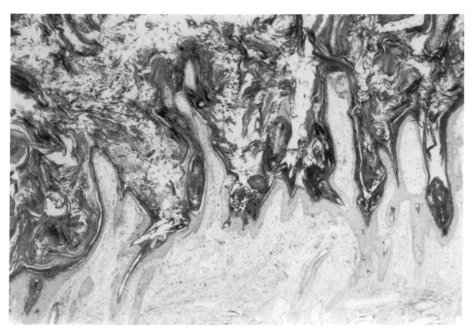

FIGURE 4–3. Chlorinated naphthalene toxicosis (CNT) in a cow. Marked orthokeratotic hyperkeratosis, papillated epidermal hyperplasia, and papillomatosis. (Courtesy J. M. King.)

of rodent poisons or poisoned rodents can produce severe toxicosis. The pathologic mechanism of thallotoxicosis is unknown.

In swine, chronic thallotoxicosis is reported to cause generalized alopecia and erythema, and necrosis and oozing of the skin around the eyes and mouth.[95] In addition, affected swine may manifest salivation, colic, diarrhea, dyspnea, weakness, impaired vision, hyperesthesia, and emaciation.

Diagnosis is based on history, physical examination, and urine thallium levels. Successful therapy has not been described. The source of thallium should be identified and eliminated.

Polybrominated and Polychlorinated Biphenyl Toxicoses

Polybrominated biphenyls (PBB) and polychlorinated biphenyls (PCB) are compounds with numerous industrial uses and with serious environmental contamination potentials.[35, 46, 70, 187, 391, 417] Because these compounds are lipophilic, they accumulate in animal body fat. The compounds also have a very low rate of biotransformation and excretion and persist in body fat for a very long time.

PBB toxicosis in cattle is characterized by anorexia and decreased milk production, followed in one month by hematomas and abscesses over the back, along the abdominal veins, and in the muscles of the rear legs.[96, 187, 268, 269, 391, 417] After two months, affected cattle develop abnormal hoof growth (long and curling upward and inward), matting of the coat, and alopecia with lichenification over the lateral thorax, neck, and shoulders. PCB toxicosis in swine is characterized by erythema of the snout and anus, diarrhea, reduced growth, and coma.[35, 261, 334]

Diagnosis is based on history, physical examination, and PBB or PCB levels in body fat or feed.[187] In the United States, the maximal limit of these compounds (as determined by gas-liquid chromatography) in fat is less than 1 ppm. Affected animals should be destroyed and removed from the environment, as it is highly unlikely that their body fat would ever test less than 1 ppm in their lifetimes.

Iodism

Excessive intake of iodine is usually due to therapeutic overdose or oversupplemented feeds.* Clinical signs include seromucoid nasal discharge, lacrimation, cough, variable appetite, and joint pain. Cutaneous changes are characterized by severe seborrhea sicca, with

---

*References 6, 46, 47, 70, 107, 174, 227, 229, 256, 265, 271, 284

or without partial alopecia, which is most commonly seen over the dorsum, neck, head, and shoulders. Because iodine is rapidly metabolized and excreted by the body, removal of the source results in rapid recovery.

DERMATOTOXIC PLANTS

Photodermatitis

Electromagnetic radiation comprises a continuous spectrum of wavelengths varying from fractions of angstroms (Å) to thousands of meters (m). A useful wavelength unit is the nanometer (nm) (1 nm equals 10^{-9} m, or 10 Å). The ultraviolet (UV) spectrum is of particular importance in dermatology.[112] UV-B (290 to 320 nm) is often referred to as the sunburn, or erythema, spectrum and is about 1000 times more erythemogenic than UV-A. UV-A (320 to 400 nm) is the spectrum associated with photosensitivity reactions.

Photodermatitis is defined as ultraviolet light (UVL)–induced inflammation of the skin. Phototoxicity is a dose-related response of all animals to light exposure (e.g., sunburn). Photosensitivity implies that the skin has been rendered increasingly susceptible to the damaging effects of UVL. Photoallergy is a reaction to a chemical (systemic or contact) and UVL in which an immune mechanism can be demonstrated. Photocontact dermatitis occurs when contactants cause photosensitivity or photoallergy. Phytophotodermatitis is caused by contact with certain plants.

The pathogenesis of UVL-induced dermatitis is complex and incompletely understood.[11, 112] Two main mechanisms have been proposed to account for the dermal vascular changes that follow UVL exposure. The diffusion mechanism theory postulates the diffusion of mediators released by UVL-damaged keratinocytes into the dermis. The direct-hit mechanism theory suggests a direct action of UVL on dermal blood vessels. Numerous mediator substances have been studied, including histamine, serotonin, free radicals, and especially prostaglandins.

Sunburn

Sunburn is a phototoxic reaction caused by excessive exposure to UV-B in animals that have lightly pigmented, thinly haired skin.[35, 194, 227, 229, 241, 359] Dairy goats that are light-skinned may develop sunburn, especially on the lateral aspects of the udder and teats, when turned outside in the summer.[359, 378, 379] The skin becomes erythematous and scaly and if severely burned, may exude, necrose, crust, and be painful. White udders often develop darkly pigmented skin after a summer in the sun. Prevention of sunburn involves moderation of exposure to sunlight for the first few weeks of summer and application of PABA-containing sunscreens (e.g., Sundown, Eclipse).

White pigs may develop sunburn, especially along the back and behind the ears.[52, 53, 95, 229, 281] Young pigs and pigs not previously exposed to sustained UV-B are most susceptible. Clinical signs and management are as previously described for dairy goats. Severely affected pigs may slough their ears and tails.

Dermatohistopathologic findings in sunburned skin include superficial perivascular dermatitis, dyskeratotic keratinocytes in the superficial epidermis, and, in chronic cases, solar elastosis (basophilic degeneration of elastin).[171, 172, 230]

Photosensitization

Photosensitization of domestic livestock, particularly sheep, goats, and cattle under range conditions, can be a major obstacle to livestock production.* Light-skinned animals of various livestock species, breeds, crosses, and sexes are susceptible to photodermatitis. Although photosensitized animals seldom die, resultant weight loss, damaged udders, refusal to allow the young to nurse, and the occurrence of secondary infections and fly strike may lead to appreciable economic losses.

There are three features basic to all types of photosensitization: (1) the presence of a photodynamic agent within the skin, (2) the concomitant exposure to a sufficient amount of certain wavelengths of UVL, and (3) the cutaneous absorption of this UVL, which is greatly facilitated by lack of pigment and hair coat.[382, 383]

Regardless of the type of photodynamic agent involved or how it reaches the skin, all instances involve the same basic pathogenesis.[112, 358, 374, 382, 383] Molecules of the photodynamic agent absorb light energy at a specific wavelength, entering a high-energy state. These "excited" molecules, usually in the pres-

---

*References 6, 35, 37, 66, 129, 194, 213, 220, 245, 295, 317, 318, 374, 415a ence of oxygen, are believed to enter a series of reactions with substrate molecules in the skin. Free radicals produced by such reactions cause structural changes in cell membranes, especially those of lysosomes, resulting in the release of hydrolytic enzymes and other chemical mediators of inflammation.

Photosensitization is classified according to the source of the photodynamic agent:[35, 66, 374, 382, 383] (1) primary photosensitization (a preformed or metabolically derived photodynamic agent reaches the skin by ingestion, injection, or contact), (2) hepatogenous photosensitization (blood phylloerythrin levels are elevated in association with liver abnormalities), (3) photosensitization due to aberrant pigment synthesis (porphyria), and (4) photosensitization of uncertain etiology.

The dermatologic findings in photosensitization are essentially identical, regardless of the cause.* Cutaneous lesions are often restricted to light-skinned, sparsely haired areas but, in severe cases, may extend into the surrounding dark-skinned areas as well (see Plate 2). The eyelids, lips, face, ears, perineum, and coronary band region are commonly involved. There is usually an acute onset of erythema, edema, and variable degrees of pruritus and/or pain. Vesicles and bullae may be seen, often progressing to oozing, necrosis, slough, and ulceration. In severe cases, the pinnae, eyelids, tail, teats, and feet may slough. Photodermatitis confined to the distal

extremities, muzzle, and ventrum is strongly suggestive of photocontact reactions (pasture plants, environmental sprays, or topical medicaments).[240, 284, 323, 382, 383]

Diagnosis of photosensitization is based on history, physical examination, and laboratory evaluation. Liver function tests should be performed on all animals with photosensitization, whether they are showing clinical signs of liver disease or not. *The number of animals at risk compared with the number of animals affected* helps to determine whether the photodermatitis is photosensitive (many animals affected) or photoallergic (one animal affected). *The distribution of the photodermatitis* aids in determining whether the photodynamic agent is systemic or a contactant. A thorough examination of the diet, pasture, and drug history is critical.

In general, the prognosis is favorable for primary photosensitization but poor for hepatogenous photosensitization and porphyria. The general principles of therapy include (1) identification and elimination of the source of the photodynamic agent, (2) avoidance of sunlight, and (3) symptomatic therapy for hepatic disease and other extracutaneous disorders.* The photodermatitis may be ameliorated with systemic glucocorticoids, for example, 1.1 mg/kg prednisone or prednisolone per day and nonsteroidal anti-inflammatory agents (e.g., aspirin and phenylbutazone). Systemic antibiotics may be required if secondary pyoderma

---

*References 35, 95, 194, 229, 236, 240, 245, 382, 383, 415a

*References 6, 32, 35, 46, 70, 213, 241, 245, 282–284, 323, 382, 383, 394, 415a

TABLE 4–1. Primary Photosensitization in Large Animals

Source	Photodynamic Agent	Species Affected
Plants		
St.-John's-wort (*Hypericum perforatum*)	Hypericin	All
Buckwheat (*Fagopyrum esculentum, Polygonum fagopyrum*)	Fagopyrin, photofagopyrin	All
Bishop's-weed (*Ammi majus*)	Furocoumarins (xanthotoxin, bergapten)	Ruminants
Dutchman's breeches (*Thamnosma texana*)	Furocoumarins	Ruminants
Wild carrot (*Daucus carota*), spring parsley (*Cymopterus watsonii*)	Furocoumarins	Ruminants
Perennial rye grass (*Lolium perenne*)	Perloline	All
Burr trefoil (*Medicago denticulata*)	Aphids	All
Chemicals		
Phenothiazine	Phenothiazine sulfoxide	All
Thiazides	?	All
Acriflavines	?	All
Rose bengal	?	All
Methylene blue	?	All
Sulfonamides	?	All
Tetracyclines	?	All

is present, and surgical débridement may be indicated if necrosis and sloughing are severe.

PRIMARY PHOTOSENSITIZATION

In primary photosensitization, the photodynamic agent is either preformed or produced metabolically within the body.[35, 66, 129, 240, 374] The photodynamic agent may be acquired by ingestion, injection, or contact. Table 4–1 contains information relative to primary photosensitization.

HEPATOGENOUS PHOTOSENSITIZATION

Phylloerythrin, a porphyrin compound formed by microbial degradation of chlorophyll in the gut, is normally conjugated in the liver and excreted in the bile. Liver dysfunction or biliary stasis, or both, result in the accu-

TABLE 4–2. Hepatogenous Photosensitization in Large Animals

Source	Hematotoxin	Species Affected
Plants		
Burning bush, fireweed (*Kochia scoparia*)	?	Ruminants, horse
Kleingrass (*Panicum coloratum*)	?	Sheep
Ngaio tree (*Myoporum* spp.)	Ngaione	All
Lechuguilla (*Agave lecheguilla*)	Saponins	Ruminants
Caltrops (*Tribulus terrestris*)	Saponins	Sheep
Rape, kale (*Brassica* spp.)	?	All
Coal-oil brush, spineless horsebush (*Tetradymia* spp.)	?	Ruminants
Sacahuiste (*Nolina texana*)	?	Ruminants
Salvation Jane (*Echium lycopsis*)	Pyrrolizidine alkaloids (echiumidine, echimidine)	Ruminants
Lantana (*Lantana camara*)	Triterpene (lantadene A)	Ruminants
Heliotrope (*Heliotropium europaeum*)	Pyrrolizidine alkaloids (lasiocarpine, heliotrine)	Ruminants, horse
Ragworts (*Senecio* spp.)	Pyrrolizidine alkaloids (retrorsine) jacobine	Horses, cattle
Tarweed, fiddle-neck (*Amsinckia* spp.)	Pyrrolizidine alkaloids	All
Crotalaria, rattleweed (*Crotalaria* spp.)	Pyrrolizidine alkaloids (monocrotaline, fulvine, crispatine)	All
Millet, panic grass (*Panicum* spp.)	?	Ruminants
Ganskweed (*Lasiopermum bipinnatum*)	?	Ruminants
Vervain (*Lippia rehmanni*)	Triterpenes (icterogenin, rehmannic acid)	Ruminants
Bog asphodel (*Narthecium ossifragum*)	Saponins	Ruminants
Alecrim (*Holocalyx glaziovii*)	?	Ruminants
Mycotoxicoses		
Pithomyces chartarum (on pasture, especially rye)	Sporidesmin	Cattle, sheep
Anacystis (*Microcystis*) spp. (blue-green algae in water)	Alkaloid	All
Periconia spp. (on Bermuda grass)	?	Ruminants
Phomopsis leptostromiformis (on lupins)	Acid-phenolic compound	All
Fusarium spp. (on moldy corn)	T-2 toxin (diacetoxyscirpenol)	Cattle, swine
Aspergillus spp. (on stored feeds)	Aflatoxin	Cattle, swine
Infection		
Leptospirosis	Leptospires	Cattle
Liver abscess	Bacteria/toxins	All
Parasitic liver cyst (flukes, hydatids)	Parasites	Cattle
Rift Valley fever	Virus	Cattle, sheep
Neoplasia		
Lymphosarcoma	Malignant lymphocytes	All
Hepatic carcinoma	Malignant hepatocytes	All
Chemicals		
Copper		All
Phosphorus		All
Carbon tetrachloride		All
Phenanthridium		All
Serum, antiserum	?(Viral? immunologic?)	Horse

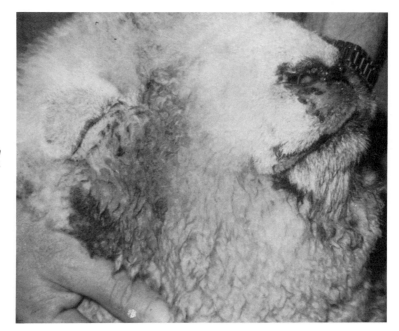

FIGURE 4–4. Pithomycotoxicosis in a sheep. Marked facial swelling. (Courtesy B. R. Jones.)

mulation of phylloerythrin in the blood and body tissues, with resultant photosensitization. It has been reported that a serum or plasma concentration of phylloerythrin in excess of 10 μg/dl is diagnostic.[245] Hepatogenous photosensitization is the most common form of photosensitization in large animals, and liver function tests should be run on any animal with photosensitization whether it is showing clinical signs of liver disease or not.[*] Table 4–2 contains information relative to hepatogenous photosensitization.

Pithomycotoxicosis (facial eczema) is a mycotoxicosis of sheep and cattle of all breeds,

ages, and sexes in Australia, New Zealand, and South Africa (Figs. 4–4 and 4–5).[*] The fungus *Pithomyces chartarum (Sporidesmium bakeri)* produces a hepatotoxin, sporidesmin, when growing on pasture, especially rye grass. The toxin causes an obstructive cholangiohepatitis and hepatogenous photosensitization.[†] Extensive fungal growth and high spore counts are produced when ambient temperature and humidity are high.[35, 56, 86, 262] Outbreaks usually occur in summer and fall, during warm sunny weather and a week or two after summer rains that follow a dry period. Good control has

---

[*]References 6, 35, 124, 194, 241, 245, 283, 284, 374, 382

[*]References 56, 67, 79, 99, 100, 180, 194, 236, 282
[†]References 55, 62, 66, 94, 251, 272–276, 332, 388, 389, 396

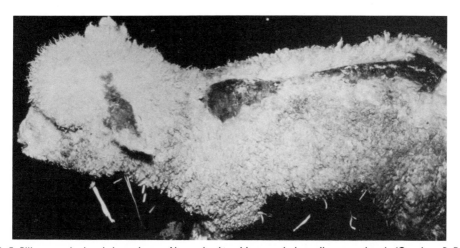

FIGURE 4–5. Pithomycotoxicosis in a sheep. Necrosis, sloughing, and ulceration over back. (Courtesy B. R. Jones.)

been achieved with applications of the fungicide thiabendazole to pasture (1 kg/acre).[54, 56, 194, 369, 370] The oral administration of $ZnSO_4$ (30 mg/kg/day for cattle; 0.5 to 2 gm/day for sheep) has been shown to have a protective effect in naturally occurring and experimentally produced pithomycotoxicosis.* However, because of the narrow safety range between protective and toxic doses of zinc, this mode of prophylaxis has been discouraged.[373]

Congenital hyperbilirubinemia and photosensitization have been reported in Southdown lambs.[63, 76, 154, 252] The condition, inherited as an autosomal recessive trait, represents a defect in hepatic uptake of certain organic ions. There is a marked delay in plasma clearance of bilirubin, sulfobromophthalein (BSP), rose bengal, sodium cholate, and indocyanine green. The liver is structurally normal.

---

*References 35, 56, 282, 346, 372, 375, 399

A hepatogenous photosensitization has been reported in Corriedale lambs with a brownish-black pigment in their livers.[75] The condition represents a presumably inherited defect in transfer of phylloerythrin, conjugated bilirubin, BSP, and iodopanoic acid from the liver into the bile. The condition appeared functionally identical to the Dubin-Johnson syndrome in humans.

PORPHYRIA

This condition is characterized by the abnormal accumulation of various photodynamic porphyrins in the blood and body tissues as a result of aberrant porphyrin synthesis (Fig. 4–6).[35, 112, 358] Porphyrins absorb UVL in the UV-A spectrum, resulting in photosensitization. Porphyrin molecules become excited in the presence of UV-A and oxygen, resulting in the

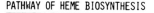

PATHWAY OF HEME BIOSYNTHESIS

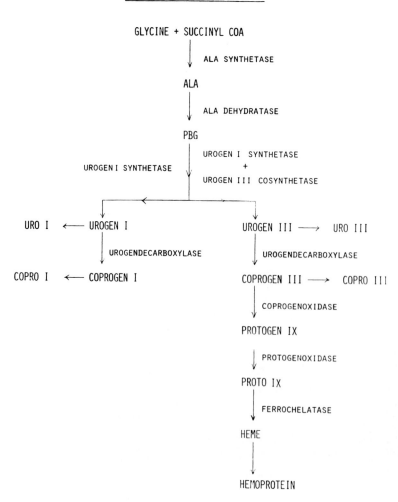

FIGURE 4–6. Outline of heme biosynthesis. ALA, δ-aminolevulinic acid; CoA, coenzyme A; PBG, porphobilinogen; URO and UROGEN, uroporphyrin and uroporphyrinogen; COPRO and COPROGEN, coproporphyrin and coproporphyrinogen; PROTO and PROTOGEN, protoporphyrin and protoporphyrinogen. (With permission from Fitzpatrick, T. B., et al.: The porphyrias. In: Dermatology in General Medicine. New York, McGraw-Hill, 1979.)

formation of free radicals and peroxide and subsequent tissue damage.

Bovine Protoporphyria. This condition has been reported in crossbred Limousin cattle in the United States.[39, 351, 352, 357] The condition, inherited as an autosomal recessive trait, is associated with decreased heme synthetase (ferrochelatase) levels.[39] Increased levels of protoporphyrin accumulate in the blood and deposit in tissues.

Clinical signs include photodermatitis and photophobia. Teeth and urine are normal in color. Mature cows may become tolerant to sunlight but, when maintained on pasture, have continual epidermal sloughing, crusting, partial healing, and reactivation of lesions.

Diagnosis is based on history, physical examination, and levels of protoporphyrin in blood and feces.[351, 357] Teeth and urine do not fluoresce under Wood's light.

Livestock should be permanently sheltered from sunlight. Affected animals and carriers should not be used for breeding. It has been reported that heterozygous (carrier) animals have about 50 percent of the activity of heme synthetase as compared with normal animals.[355] Homozygous (clinically diseased) animals have about 10 percent of the activity of heme synthetase as compared with normal animals.[355]

Bovine Erythropoietic Porphyria. Bovine erythropoietic porphyria (bovine congenital porphyria, pink tooth, ochronosis, osteohemochromatosis, porphyrinuria, hematoporphyrinuria) has been reported in many breeds of cattle from all over the world.* The condition, inherited as an autosomal recessive trait, is associated with decreased uroporphyrinogen III cosynthetase levels.[119, 120, 203, 231, 406] Increased levels of uroporphyrin I and coproporphyrin I accumulate in the blood and deposit in body tissues, resulting in a reddish-brown discoloration of teeth, bones, and nearly all soft tissues.

Clinical signs include retarded growth, discolored teeth and urine, pale mucous membranes, and photodermatitis (Fig. 4–7). Teeth vary in color from light pink, pinkish-red, purplish-red, red-brown, to mahogany. Urine is usually reddish-brown or turns red on exposure to sunlight; however, it may be normal in color but still contain excessive porphyrins.

The anemia of bovine erythropoietic porphyria, usually macrocytic and normochromic,

*References 5, 31, 35, 103, 115–117, 121, 202, 204, 205, 238, 294, 339, 344, 348, 349, 408

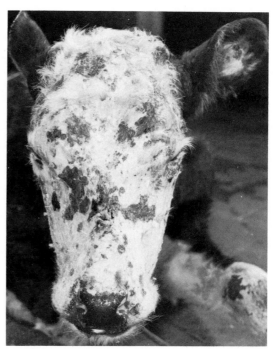

FIGURE 4–7. Bovine erythropoietic porphyria. Photodermatitis limited to the white areas of the head.

is thought to be hemolytic.[208, 211, 358] The severity of the anemia is directly correlated with erythrocyte uroporphyrin I levels. Studies have demonstrated a decreased erythrocyte lifespan, abnormal erythrocyte reduced glutathione stability and a ferrokinetic pattern compatible with intravenous hemolysis.[208–212] A maturation defect in the metarubricyte has been demonstrated in vitro, and the maturation half-time of the reticulocyte is considerably delayed (50 hours) compared with that in normal cattle (3 to 10 hours).[376] These findings suggest that high porphyrin levels adversely affect heme synthesis. This biochemical alteration is thought to be expressed as a maturation defect that results in the altered cells being more susceptible to intravascular or extravascular hemolysis.

Photodermatitis is the outstanding clinical sign. Excessive quantities of porphyrins accumulate in the skin and blood and lead to cutaneous photosensitization. Acute erythema and edema are produced in porphyric skin with UV-A (primary absorption band of the porphyrins is about 400 nm). Changes are most severe in exposed, unpigmented, hairless skin. Erythema, edema, oozing, vesicles, necrosis, ulceration, crusts, pruritus, and pain are present.

Diagnosis is based on history, physical ex-

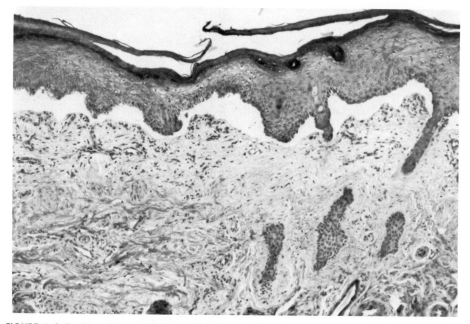

FIGURE 4–8. *Bovine erythropoietic porphyria. Subepidermal vesicular dermatitis with festooning.*

amination, Wood's light examination of teeth and urine, skin biopsy, and levels of porphyrins in urine and blood.[35, 358] Affected teeth and urine fluoresce a bright orange or red under the Wood's light. Skin biopsy reveals subepidermal vesicular dermatitis, festooning, and a homogeneous thickening of superficial dermal blood vessel walls, associated with the deposition of a hyalin-like material (Figs. 4–8 and 4–9). Inflammation is minimal to absent, unless ulceration is present. The hyalin-like material is PAS-positive. Spectrophotometric analysis of urine and blood reveals elevated levels of uroporphyrin I and coproporphyrin I.* The urine of cattle with bovine erythropoietic porphyria may contain 500 to 1000 μg/dl

*References 31, 35, 61, 118, 166, 358, 407

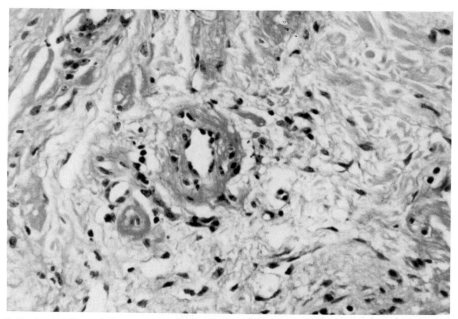

FIGURE 4–9. *Bovine erythropoietic porphyria. Deposition of PAS-positive material in and around wall of dermal blood vessel.*

uroporphyrin I and 300 to 1500 µg/dl copro-porphyrin I. Urine from normal cattle contains 1 to 2 µg/dl coproporphyrin I and no significant quantities of uroporphyrin I.

Therapy is ineffective. Affected animals and carriers should be removed from the breeding program. Heterozygous (carrier) cattle are clinically normal and can be detected only by progeny study and testing.

PHOTOSENSITIZATION OF UNKNOWN MECHANISM

There are instances of apparent photosensitization in large animals in which the pathologic mechanism is not known.* In some instances, various lush pastures have been incriminated. The photosensitization occurring in all large animals associated with ingestion of clover, alfalfa, lucerne, vetch, and oats (Trifolium spp., Vicia spp., and Avena spp.) has, in various instances, been thought to be primary, and in others hepatogenous† Photodermatitis has been seen in association with *Dermatophilus congolensis* infections of light-skinned areas of horses (see Chapter 6, discussion on dermatophilosis). The condition disappears when the dermatophilosis is cured. Photodermatitis has also been recognized in association with some cases of metritis in mares.[323]

Mycotoxicoses

The importance of fungi as poisonous agents has been appreciated for many years, but it is only recently that the scope and magnitude of the losses that they cause have become apparent. Although molds can grow on almost any organic matter, those species capable of elaborating toxic substances (mycotoxins) and consequently of producing intoxication (mycotoxicosis) are mostly pathogens and decomposers of plants. Molds grow on stored feeds and standing plants.

Mycotoxicoses with cutaneous effects are discussed later from a dermatologic standpoint. For detailed information on other clinical and pathologic aspects of these disorders, the reader is referred to several excellent textbooks.[35, 70, 421]

Ergotism

Ergotism, a mycotoxicosis caused by alkaloids produced by *Claviceps purpurea*, is characterized by dry gangrene and sloughing of distal extremities.

CAUSE AND PATHOGENESIS

Ergotism is caused by a series of active alkaloids (ergotamine, ergotoxine, ergonovine, ergocryptine, ergocornine, and so forth) contained in grains infected with the fungus *Claviceps purpurea*.[46, 49, 70, 311, 312] Ergot is the common name given to the sclerotium formed by *C. purpurea*. The sclerotium is the fungal mass that replaces the seed or kernel of the infected plant. *C. purpurea* infects over 200 grasses and cultivated cereals, especially wheat, barley, rye, and oats. Infection develops abundantly during wet seasons. The fungal alkaloids cause persistent spasm of arterioles, resulting in congestion proximal to the spasm and ischemia distal to the spasm. The vasospasm is exaggerated by cold.

CLINICAL FEATURES

Ergotism has been reported from many parts of the world.* Morbidity and mortality are usually low, and there are no apparent age, breed, or sex predilections. Clinical signs may occur as soon as seven days after exposure to contaminated food. Typically, lameness of the hind limbs is noted first, followed by fever, weight loss, poor appetite, and decreased milk production. Affected feet show swelling at the coronary band, which progresses to the fetlocks and may reach the metatarsi. The feet become necrotic, cold, and insensitive, and a distinct line separates viable from dead tissue (usually just above the coronary band) (Fig. 4–10). The front feet, ears, tail (Fig. 4–11), and teats may be similarly affected and, in severe cases, may slough.

DIAGNOSIS

The differential diagnosis includes frostbite, fescue toxicosis, traumatic or chemical gangrene, and septicemia. The definitive diagnosis is based on history, physical examination, and feed analysis.[35, 46, 49, 70, 240] The purple to black

---

*References 6, 28, 32, 35, 70, 95, 194, 229, 245, 283, 284
†References 35, 52, 53, 66, 70, 95, 138, 140, 213, 229, 283, 284

---

*References 35, 80, 95, 98, 149, 173, 200, 229, 240, 255, 281, 283, 297, 311, 312, 333, 420

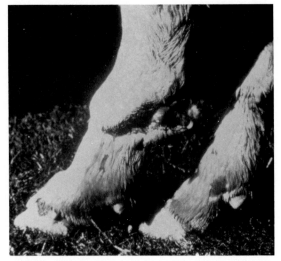

FIGURE 4–10. Ergotism in a cow. Well-demarcated necrosis and sloughing distal to fetlock. (Courtesy J. M. Kingsbury.)

ergot sclerotia can be visualized in unmilled grain. Any diet containing over 0.24 percent ergot sclerotia is potentially dangerous. Skin biopsy reveals degeneration and necrosis of vascular endothelium, thrombosis, and necrosis of surrounding tissues.[311, 312]

CLINICAL MANAGEMENT

The source of ergot must be identified and eliminated. Unless exposure continues, recovery or salvage of affected animals is usually possible. Symptomatic treatment may include hot packs and gentle cleansing to increase circulation, and antibiotics. Close grazing or cutting of pastures to prevent seed heads is recommended.

Fescue Toxicosis

Fescue toxicosis, a mycotoxicosis of cattle caused by the ingestion of tall fescue infected with *Acremonium coenophialum*, is characterized by gangrene and sloughing of extremities.

CAUSE AND PATHOGENESIS

Tall fescue (*Festuca aruninacea*) is a widely used grass in many parts of the world.* Although the pathologic mechanism is not clear, it may involve toxin(s) (ergovaline, ergosine, ergonine) produced by the fungus *Acremonium coenophialum* (*Epichloë typhina, Balansia epichloë*), resulting in vasospasm and ischemia similar to that seen with ergotism.† The condition is exaggerated by cold and is, thus, often precipitated by the onset of cold weather. Fall regrowth and the yearly accumulation of fescue are important in the toxicosis.

CLINICAL FEATURES

Fescue toxicosis may occur one week to six months after cattle are exposed.[133, 240, 418] A single animal, or most of a herd, may be affected, with a usual incidence of about 10 percent. There are no apparent age, breed, or sex predilections. Clinical signs include lameness in the rear legs, arched back, diarrhea, poor appetite, and emaciation. Cutaneous changes begin as erythema and swelling at the coronary bands and progress through swelling, necrosis, and possible sloughing of the limbs distal to the fetlocks. Affected feet are cold and insensitive. Occasionally, the front feet, ears, tail, and teats may be similarly affected.

DIAGNOSIS

The differential diagnosis includes ergotism, frostbite, traumatic or chemical gangrene, and

---

*References 70, 83, 132, 133, 145, 174a, 236a, 244a, 337, 368, 418, 421, 422
†References 15, 35, 132, 174a, 188, 193, 206, 244a, 418, 422

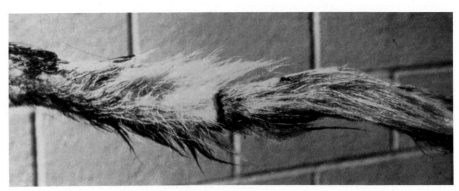

FIGURE 4–11. Ergotism in a cow. Well-demarcated necrosis and sloughing of distal tail. (Courtesy J. M. Kingsbury.)

septicemia. The definitive diagnosis is based on history and physical examination. Skin biopsy reveals degeneration and thickening of blood vessel walls, narrowing and thrombosis of vascular lumina, and necrosis of surrounding tissues.[418]

CLINICAL MANAGEMENT

Exposure to fescue must be eliminated. Symptomatic therapy may include hot packs, gentle cleansing, and antibiotics. In experimental grazing trials conducted over a period of years,[133, 244a] the following observations were made: (1) cattle receiving 2.2 to 4.4 kg ground shelled corn/head/day show milder symptoms of fescue toxicosis (high-energy feeds have a protective effect), (2) pastures of mixtures of fescue and legumes seem to cause less trouble than do pure stands, (3) rotational grazing using fescue and another grass is helpful, and (4) removal of all vegetables once a year by pasturing, cutting and baling, or clipping appears helpful. The oral administration of thiabendazole (5 gm/45 kg) before exposure to fescue and repeated every seven days was reported to be an effective preventive,[15, 35] as was 0.7 gm/45 kg/day orally.[42a]

Stachybotryotoxicosis

Stachybotryotoxicosis, a mycotoxicosis caused by toxins produced by *Stachybotrys* spp. fungi, is characterized by ulceronecrotic lesions of the mucous membranes and skin, bone marrow suppression, and hemorrhage.

CAUSE AND PATHOGENESIS

Stachybotrys spp. fungi (*S. atra, S. alternans*) grow on hay and straw and produce toxins referred to as macrocyclic tricothecenes (*Stachybotrys* toxin).* These toxins cause bone marrow suppression, resulting in profound neutropenia and thrombocytopenia as well as ulceronecrotic lesions of the skin and mucous membranes.

CLINICAL FEATURES

Stachybotryotoxicosis has been reported in horses, cattle, sheep, and swine.[35, 57, 70, 364, 381, 421] Cutaneous lesions consist of focal areas of necrosis and ulceration, especially of mucocutaneous areas. Petechiae and ulceronecrotic

---

*References 35, 57, 70, 106, 228, 364, 421

lesions are also present on visible mucous membranes. Affected animals develop hemorrhagic diathesis, hemorrhagic enteritis, septicemia, and then die.

DIAGNOSIS

Diagnosis is based on history and physical examination.

CLINICAL MANAGEMENT

Further ingestion of toxin must be prevented. Effective treatment has not been reported.

Pithomycotoxicosis

Pithomycotoxicosis (facial eczema) is a mycotoxicosis of sheep and cattle caused by the toxin sporidesmin produced by the fungus *Pithomyces chartarum*. The toxin produces hepatobiliary disease, resulting in hepatogenous photosensitization. See section on hepatogenous photosensitization for details.

Miscellaneous Mycotoxicoses

Ingestion of lupins (lupinosis) contaminated with *Phomopsis leptostromiformis* is a cause of hepatogenous photosensitization in cattle, sheep, and swine (see section on hepatogenous photosensitization).[35, 70, 421] Moldy corn disease in cattle is associated with the ingestion of T-2 toxin from *Fusarium tricinctum* and other *Fusarium* spp. (see section on hepatogenous photosensitization).[35, 70, 421] Aflatoxicosis associated with *Aspergillus flavus* is a cause of hepatogenous photosensitization in cattle and swine (see section on hepatogenous photosensitization).[35, 70, 421]

Ingestion of the mushroom *Amanita verna* is reported to cause painful defecation and matting of feces around the tail base and perineum in cattle.[35, 70, 421] Skin in the affected areas shows vesicles, papules, and necrotic foci, apparently as a result of an irritating substance(s) in the feces.

Miscellaneous Plant Toxicoses

Leucaenosis

Leucaenosis, a toxicosis resulting from the ingestion of plants and trees (jumby tree, koa haole) of the *Leucaena* genus, is characterized by alopecia in horses, cattle, sheep, and swine.* Leucaenosis has been reported from Australia, New Zealand, New Guinea, the West Indies, and Hawaii. Plants of the *Leucaena* genus (*Leucaena leucocephala* and *L. glauca*) contain the toxic amino acid mimosine, which is a potent depilatory agent.

Leucaenosis is characterized by a gradual loss of the long hairs of the mane, tail, and fetlock regions. Severely poisoned animals may shed hair and wool symmetrically and profoundly within 7 to 14 days of exposure. Hoof dystrophies and laminitis may be seen.

The differential diagnosis includes selenosis, mercurialism, arsenic toxicosis, and malnutrition. Further ingestion of *Leucaena* spp. must be prevented. The addition of 1 percent ferrous sulfate to feed is reported to reduce the severity of the toxicosis.[35, 323, 394]

Hairy Vetch Toxicosis

Hairy vetch (*Vicia villosa*) may cause toxicosis when ingested by cattle[70, 213, 216, 240, 315] and possibly horses.[7] The toxin and pathologic mechanism are not known. Toxicosis often develops two to three weeks after exposure and is most common in cattle over three years of age. Morbidity is 6 to 8 percent, and mortality may be as high as 50 percent.

Early clinical signs include cutaneous papules and plaques that ooze a yellowish puslike material, which becomes encrusted. Lesions begin on the udder, tailhead, and neck and spread to the face, trunk, and limbs. Pruritus is often marked and associated with considerable alopecia. Other clinical signs include conjunctivitis, anorexia, pyrexia, diarrhea, and weight loss.

Diagnosis is based on history, physical examination, and biopsy. Skin biopsy reveals a superficial and deep perivascular to diffuse dermatitis containing histiocytes, lymphocytes, plasma cells, multinucleated histiocytic giant cells, and eosinophils. No effective treatment has been reported. Further ingestion of hairy vetch should be prevented.

Sorghum Toxicosis

Plants from the genus *Sorghum* (Johnson, milo, and Sudan grass) produce cystitis and urinary incontinence, which results in urine scalding (primary irritant contact dermatitis) in the perineal region.[35, 226, 254, 394] The toxin is believed to be dhurrin, a cyanogenic glycoside.

It has been hypothesized that exposure to sublethal doses of hydrocyanic acid produces axonal degeneration and demyelination.[1]

ZOOTOXICOSES

Zootoxicosis is a disease caused by the bite or sting of a venomous animal.[122] Many species of snakes, arachnids, and insects have venomous bites or stings. Most lack sufficient potency to cause more than transient discomfort to large animals. Generally, the incidence of toxicity is very low in large animals, although in certain geographic areas the density of venomous snakes may result in considerable loss.

Venoms are complex organic substances composed of a wide variety of substances, including enzymes, peptides, polypeptides, amines, and glycosides. Venoms may act locally, causing tissue necrosis, vascular thrombosis, and hemorrhage, or may be transported to other sites in the body, causing hemolysis and neurotoxicity. Venoms are also allergenic, making previously sensitized animals susceptible to anaphylactic shock.

Snake Bite

In the United States, the most important venomous snake with regard to large animals is the rattlesnake.[122] There are probably thousands of large animals bitten by this snake in the United States every year.* Mortality is estimated to range between 10 and 30 percent.[300] Most bites occur during spring and summer.

Snake bites occur most commonly on the nose, head, neck, and legs. Bites around the face are potentially serious because of rapid swelling and respiratory embarrassment. The exact site of envenomation is rarely visible. Shortly after the bite, pronounced swelling obliterates the fang marks. Edema and erythema may progress to necrosis and slough. The affected area is usually painful.

Diagnosis is based on history and physical examination. Snake bites are treated according to symptoms. Animals should be kept quiet and at rest. Immediate cool hydrotherapy minimizes edema. Once the swelling has formed, warm hydrotherapy may stimulate circulation and removal of tissue fluids. Antihistamines

---

*References 35, 201, 278, 323, 343, 361, 382, 394

*References 35, 58, 69, 70, 77, 88, 237, 241, 257, 300, 302a, 321

are contraindicated. Glucocorticoids may be beneficial in reducing inflammation and pain. Broad-spectrum antibiotics are indicated, as is tetanus prophylaxis.

Specific antivenin administration is rarely warranted, except for very valuable animals or young animals, and is most useful when administered early (within two hours of the bite). If necrosis and sloughing occur, surgical débridement and routine wound care are indicated.

Hyalomma Toxicosis

Hyalomma toxicosis is a tick-borne disease of cattle and, occasionally, sheep, goats, and swine.[68, 290–293] The disease is seen in Africa and is caused by an unidentified toxin carried by certain strains of the tick *Hyalomma transiens*. The incidence of the disease is highest during warmer months. Although all ages may be affected, *Hyalomma* toxicosis is most common in cattle younger than one year of age. There are no apparent breed or sex predilections.

The popular names for *Hyalomma* toxicosis—sweating sickness, sweetsiekte, wet calf disease, la dyhydrose tropicale, schwitzkrankheit—arose from the most noticeable symptom of the disease, which was incorrectly interpreted as profuse perspiration. The disease may be peracute, acute, subacute, or mild. The incubation period varies from 4 to 11 days, and the course of the disease is usually 4 to 20 days, with a mortality of 30 to 100 percent.

Hyalomma toxicosis is characterized by a sudden onset of pyrexia (40.6 to 42.2°C), depression, hyperemia of visible mucous membranes and skin (if nonpigmented), hypersalivation, lacrimation, and nasal discharge. A moist dermatitis, appearing 48 to 72 hours later, may be confined to the ears, face, neck, axilla, flank, or groin but often is generalized. The skin is erythematous, edematous, oozing, and foul-smelling. The hair coat becomes matted and is easily epilated. When tufts of hair are epilated, the epidermis is also removed, leaving a raw surface. The skin is painful, and myiasis is a common complication. Cattle with nonpigmented hooves show distinct erythema of the coronets. In animals that do not die, the skin becomes dry, scaly, thickened, and alopecic. Recovery takes place over a period of about eight weeks.

There is no specific treatment for *Hyalomma* toxicosis. Therapy is symptomatic and supportive. Recovered animals appear to have a durable immunity.

TOXIC SYNDROMES OF UNKNOWN ETIOLOGY

Dermatitis, Pyrexia, and Hemorrhage in Dairy Cows

This syndrome has been reported in dairy cattle in the United Kingdom and the Netherlands.* Its cause is unclear and may be multifactorial. In the Netherlands, all outbreaks were associated with the feeding of pelleted concentrates containing diureidoisobutane (DUIB) at a concentration of 3 percent dry matter.[40] Affected herds developed clinical signs about two months after the concentrates were added, and no more outbreaks were seen when the concentrates were eliminated. The syndrome was reproduced in normal cattle by feeding them the concentrates. However, in the United Kingdom, outbreaks were not associated with DUIB, and a causative factor was not identified.[393]

Clinically, morbidity has varied from 10 to 90 percent, and mortality up to 25 percent.[40, 393] Initially, affected cows develop a pruritic papulocrustous dermatitis on the head, neck, back, udder, and tailhead and pyrexia (40 to 41°C). Rubbing, kicking, and licking produce excoriations and alopecia, which usually subside after a few days to several weeks. The pyrexia persists, and cows look dull and gradually lose weight. Appetite is variable. Some cows hemorrhage from the nostrils and anus.

Hemograms often reveal leukopenia early, and leukocytosis later,[392, 393] and an occasional slight anemia. Platelet counts and coagulation studies have been normal. Cultures for microorganisms, viral serology, and toxicologic studies have been unrewarding. Skin biopsy reveals superficial and deep perivascular dermatitis, with eosinophils and mononuclears.[40] Necropsy examination reveals widespread hemorrhages and mild vasculitis.[40, 393]

Therapy—including antibiotics, antihistamines, and glucocorticoids—has been of no benefit.

Dermatoses Associated with Certain Foodstuffs

A number of dermatoses that have been described in large animals in association with

---

*References 40, 97, 178, 247, 270, 392, 393, 400

the ingestion of certain foodstuffs have pathologic mechanisms that are not known.[43, 198, 199, 227] Cattle, horses, and swine that were fed potato distillery wastes developed a vesicular dermatitis on the legs, pyrexia, anorexia, lacrimation, and lameness.[35, 70, 225, 227] Horses fed corn or glucose cake developed a papulovesicular dermatitis on the distal limbs.[43, 227] Cattle and sheep fed malt or palm oil cake developed a papulovesicular dermatitis on the legs and ventrum.[227] Calves fed rice bran developed a papulovesicular dermatitis on the legs, eyelids, and feet,[227] and cattle fed sesame meal or rice flour developed a pruritic scaling and crusting eruption over the rump and neck.[184, 227] Swine fed fish meal developed a generalized papulovesicular dermatitis.

In all these poorly understood dermatoses, the affected animals recovered within two to four weeks after the offending dietary substances were eliminated.

REFERENCES

1. Adams, L. G., et al.: Cystitis and ataxia associated with sorghum ingestion by horses. JAVMA 155:518, 1969.
2. Ahmed, O. M. M., and Adams, S. E. I.: The toxicity of *Capparis tomentosa* in goats. J. Comp. Pathol. 90:187, 1980.
3. Allen, J. G., and Seawright, A. A.: The effect of prior treatment with phenobarbitone, dicophane (DDT) and β-diethylaminoethyl phenylpropyl acetate (SKF525A) on experimental intoxication of sheep with the plant *Myoporum deserti* Cunn. Res. Vet. Sci. 15:167, 1973.
4. Allen, J. G., et al.: The toxicity of *Myoporum tetrandrum* (boobialla) and myoporaceous furanoid essential oils for ruminants. Aust. Vet. J. 54:287, 1978.
5. Amoroso, E. C. R., et al.: Congenital porphyria in bovines: First living cases in Britain. Nature 180:230, 1957.
6. Amstutz, H. E.: *Bovine Medicine and Surgery II*. Santa Barbara American Veterinary Publications, Inc., 1980.
7. Anderson, C. A., and Divers, T. J.: Systemic granulomatous inflammation in a horse grazing hairy vetch. JAVMA 183:569, 1983.
8. Anderson, P., and Petaja, E.: Profound eosinophilic dermatitis in swine caused by sodium chloride. Nord. Vet. Med. 20:706, 1968.
9. Anganshakom, S., et al.: Aflatoxicosis in horses. J. Am. Vet. Med. Assoc. 197:274, 1981.
10. Araya, O. S., and Ford, E. J. H.: An investigation of the type of photosensitization caused by the ingestion of St. John's wort (*Hypericum perforatum*) by calves. J. Comp. Pathol. 91:135, 1981.
11. Argenbright, L. W., et al.: Quantitation of phototoxic hyperemia and permeability to protein. I. Inhibition by histamine (H_1 and H_2) and serotonin receptor antagonists in pig skin. Exp. Mol. Pathol. 32:154, 1980.
12. Anonymous: Leptospiral photosensitivity in calves. Surveillance 1974 4:10, 1974.
13. Anonymous: Nagaio (*Myoporum laetum*) poisoning in cattle. Surveillance 1975 3:20, 1975.
14. Anonymous: Photosensitization in calves associated with *Leptospira ballum*. Surveillance 1976 5:12, 1976.
15. Bacon, C. W., et al.: *Epichloe typhina* from toxic tall fescue grasses. Appl. Environ. Microbiol. 34:576, 1977.
16. Bagley, C. V., et al.: Photosensitization associated with exposure of cattle to moldy straw. JAVMA 183:802, 1983.
17. Bagley, C. V., and Shupe, J. L.: Sporidesmins facial eczema and pithomycotoxicosis. *In*: Howard, J. L. (ed.): *Current Veterinary Therapy. Food Animal Practice II*. Philadelphia, W. B. Saunders Co., 1980, p. 375.
18. Bailey, E. M.: Principal poisonous plants in the Southwestern United States. *In*: Howard, J. L. (ed.): *Current Veterinary Therapy. Food Animal Practice II*. Philadelphia, W. B. Saunders Co., 1986, p. 412.
19. Bakhita, A., and Adams, S. E. I.: Effects of *Acanthospermum hispidum* on goats. J. Comp. Pathol. 88:533, 1978.
20. Bath, G. F., et al.: Geeldikkop: Preservation of toxic material. J. S. Afr. Vet. Med. Assoc. 49:23, 1978.
21. Beasley, V. R.: Trichothecenes. *In*: Howard, J. L. (ed.): *Current Veterinary Therapy. Food Animal Practice II*. Philadelphia, W. B. Saunders Co., 1986, p. 372.
22. Beaton, D., et al.: An outbreak of ulcerative dermatitis in pigs. Vet. Rec. 94:611, 1974.
23. Bell, W. B.: The production of hyperkeratosis by the administration of a lubricant. Va. J. Sci. 3:71, 1952.
24. Bell, W. B.: One cause of bovine hyperkeratosis located. North Am. Vet. 33:546, 1952.
25. Bell, W. B.: The production of hyperkeratosis (X disease) by a single administration of chlorinated naphthalenes. JAVMA 124:289, 1954.
26. Bell, W. B.: Further studies of the production of bovine hyperkeratosis by the administration of a lubricant. Va. J. Sci. 3:169, 1952.
27. Bell, W. B.: The relative toxicity of the chlorinated naphthalenes in experimentally produced bovine hyperkeratosis (X-disease). Vet. Med. 48:135, 1953.
28. Berry, J. M., and Merriam, J.: Phototoxic dermatitis in a horse. Vet. Med. Small Anim. Clin. 65:251, 1970.
29. Betty, R. C., and Tikojus, V. M.: Hypericin and a non-fluorescent photosensitivity pigment from St. John's wort (*Hypericum perforatum*). Aust. J. Exp. Biol. Med. Sci. 21:175, 1943.
30. Binns, W., and James, L. F.: *Cymopterus watsonii*: A photosensitizing plant for sheep. Vet. Med. Small Anim. Clin. 59:4, 1964.
31. Black, L.: Congenital porphyria. *In*: Howard, J. L. (ed.): *Current Veterinary Therapy. Food Animal Practice*. Philadelphia, W. B. Saunders Co., 1981, p. 1124.
32. Black, L.: Photosensitization. *In*: Howard, J. L. (ed.): *Current Veterinary Therapy. Food Animal Practice*. Philadelphia, W. B. Saunders Co., 1981, p. 1125.
33. Black, L.: Gangrene. *In*: Howard, J. L. (ed.): *Current Veterinary Therapy. Food Animal Practice*. Philadelphia, W. B. Saunders Co., 1981, p. 1128.
34. Blamire, R. V., et al.: A review of some animal diseases encountered at meat inspection 1960–1968. Vet. Rec. 87:234, 1970.
35. Blood, D. C., et al.: *Veterinary Medicine VI*. London, Baillière Tindall, 1983.
36. Bourne, R. F.: Bovine hyperkeratosis (X-disease). North Am. Vet. 33:609, 1952.
37. Bourne, R. F.: Photosensitization. North Am. Vet. 34:173, 1953.
38. Boyd, C. L.: A report on XX-disease (hyperkeratosis) in Texas. JAVMA 113:463, 1948.
38a. Bracken, F. K., et al.: A condition akin to immersion foot. Vet. Med. 81:562, 1986.
39. Brenner, D. A., and Bloomer, J. R.: Comparison of human and bovine protoporphyria. Yale J. Biol. Med. 52:449, 1979.
40. Breukink, H. J., et al.: Pyrexia with dermatitis in dairy cows. Vet. Rec. 103:221, 1978.
41. Brown, J. M. M., et al.: Advances in "geeldikkop" (*Tribulosis ovis*) research. J. S. Afr. Vet. Med. Assoc. 31:179, 1960.
42. Brown, J. M. M.: Biochemical studies on geeldikkop and enzootic icterus. Onderstepoort J. Vet. Res. 35:319, 1968.
42a. Brown, J. R., et al.: The effect of various levels of continuous TBZ feeding on feedlot performance of beef calves and yearling steers previously grazing *Acremonium coenophialum*–infected tall fescue. Agri-Pract. 7:33, 1986.

43. Brownlee, A. J.: Allergy in the domestic animal. J. Comp. Pathol. Ther. 53:55, 1940.

44. Buck, W. B.: Hazardous arsenical residues associated with the use of a lawn crabgrass control preparation. Vet. Toxicol. 15:25, 1973.

45. Buck, W. B.: Copper-Molybdenum. In: Howard, J. L. (ed.): Current Veterinary Therapy. Food Animal Practice II. Philadelphia, W. B. Saunders Co., 1986, p. 437.

46. Buck, W. B., et al.: Clinical and Diagnostic Veterinary Toxicology II. 2nd ed. Dubuque, IA, Kendall/Hunt, 1976.

47. Buck, W. B.: Iodine. In: Howard, J. L. (ed.): Current Veterinary Therapy. Food Animal Practice II. Philadelphia, W. B. Saunders Co., 1986, p. 357.

48. Burdin, M. L., and Plowright, W.: Investigations into delayed toxicity due to dimidium bromide. III. Some experimental observations in ruminants. J. Comp. Pathol. 62:178, 1952.

49. Burfening, P. J.: Ergotism. JAVMA 163:1288, 1973.

50. Burell, D. M., et al.: Experimental production of dermatitis in sheep with Pseudomonas aeruginosa. Aust. Vet. J. 59:140, 1982.

51. Burell, D. M., et al.: The role of Pseudomonas aeruginosa in the pathogenesis of fleece rot and the effect of immunization. Aust. Vet. J. 58:34, 1982.

52. Cameron, R. D. A.: Skin diseases of the pig. Sydney, Proc. Univ. Post-Grad. Comm. Vet. Sci. 56:445, 1981.

53. Cameron, R. D. A.: Skin Diseases of the Pig. Sydney, Univ. Sydney Post-Graduate Foundation in Veterinary Science. Vet. Rev. No. 23, 1984.

54. Campbell, A. G.: Facial eczema. 4. Prevention of facial eczema in grazing stock. N.Z. J. Agric. 119:28, 1969.

55. Caple, I. W., et al.: Use of sulphobromophthalein liver function tests in cows with facial eczema. Aust. Vet. J. 52:192, 1976.

56. Carlton, W. W., and Krogh, P.: Sporidesmins and facial eczema. In: Howard, J. L. (ed.): Current Veterinary Therapy. Food Animal Practice. Philadelphia, W. B. Saunders Co., 1981, p. 414.

57. Carlton, W. W., and Krogh, P.: Stachybotryotoxicosis. In: Howard, J. L. (ed.): Current Veterinary Therapy. Food Animal Practice II. Philadelphia, W. B. Saunders Co., 1986, p. 379.

58. Casarett, L. J., and Doull, J.: Toxicology. New York, Macmillan Publishing Co., 1975.

59. Case, A. A., and Coffmann, J. R.: Waste oil: Toxic for horses. Vet. Clin. North Am. 3:273, 1973.

60. Case, A. A.: Principal plant problems in the Midwestern and Eastern United States. In: Howard, J. L. (ed.): Current Veterinary Therapy. Food Animal Practice II. Philadelphia, W. B. Saunders Co., 1986, p. 420.

61. Chu, T. C., and Chu, E. J. H.: Porphyrins from congenitally porphyric (pink tooth) cattle. Biochem. J. 83:318, 1962.

62. Clare, N. T.: Photosensitivity diseases in New Zealand. III. The photosensitizing agent in facial eczema. N.Z. J. Sci. Technol. 25A:202, 1944.

63. Clare, N. T.: Photosensitivity diseases in New Zealand. IV. The photosensitizing agent in Southdown photosensitivity. N.Z. J. Sci. Technol. 27A:23, 1945.

64. Clare, N. T.: A photosensitizing keratitis in young cattle following the use of phenothiazine as an anthelmintic. II. The metabolism of phenothiazine in ruminants. Aust. Vet. J. 23:340, 1947.

65. Clare, N. T., et al.: A photosensitizing keratitis in young cattle following the use of phenothiazine as an anthelmintic. III. Identification of the photosensitizing agent. Aust. Vet. J. 23:344, 1947.

66. Clare, N. T.: Photosensitization in animals. Adv. Vet. Sci. 2:182, 1955.

67. Clare, N. T.: Facial eczema. 1. The how and why of the disease. N.Z. J. Agric. 119:17, 1969.

68. Clark, R.: Observations on sweating sickness in Northern Zululand. J. S. Afr. Vet. Med. Assoc. 4:10, 1933.

69. Clarke, E. G. C., and Clarke, M. L.: Snakes and snakebite. Vet. Annu. 10:27, 1969.

70. Clarke, M, L., et al.: Veterinary Toxicology II. London, Baillière Tindall, 1981.

71. Coetzer, J. A. W., et al.: Photosensitivity in South Africa. V. A comparative study of the pathology of the ovine hepatogenous photosensitivity diseases, facial eczema and geeldikkop. Onderstepoort J. Vet. Res. 50:59, 1983.

72. Coignoue, F. L., et al.: Pathology of an ulcerative dermatitis in Belgian Landrace sows. Vet. Pathol. 22:306, 1985.

73. Copenhaver, J. S., and Bell, W. B.: The production of bovine hyperkeratosis (X-disease) with an experimentally made pellet feed. Vet. Med. 49:96, 1954.

74. Copland, R. S., and Pattie, W. A.: Fleece humidity as an indicator of susceptibility to bodystrike in Merino sheep. Aust. Vet. J. 58:38, 1982.

75. Cornelius, C. E., et al.: Hepatic pigmentation with photosensitivity. A syndrome in Corriedale sheep resembling Dubin-Johnson syndrome in man. JAVMA 146:709, 1965.

76. Cornelius, C. E., and Gronwall, R. R.: Congenital photosensitivity and hyperbilirubinemia in Southdown sheep in the United States. Am. J. Vet. Res. 29:291, 1968.

77. Crimmins, M. L.: Facts about Texas snakes and their poisons. JAVMA 71:704, 1927.

78. Crinion, R. A., and O'Connor, J. P.: Selenium intoxication in horses. Irish Vet. J. 32:81, 1978.

79. Cunningham, I. J., et al.: Photosensitivity diseases in New Zealand. I. Facial eczema: Its clinical, pathological and biochemical characterization. N.Z. J. Sci. Technol. 24:185, 1942.

80. Cunningham, I. J., et al.: The symptoms of ergot poisoning in sheep. N.Z. J. Sci. Technol. 26A:121, 1944.

81. Cunningham, I. J., and Hopkirk, C. S. M.: Experimental poisoning of sheep by ngaio (Myoporum laetum). N.Z. J. Sci. Technol. 26A:333, 1945.

82. Cunningham, I. J.: Photosensitivity diseases in New Zealand. V. Photosensitization by St. John's wort (Hypericum perforatum). N.Z. J. Sci. Technol. 29:207, 1947.

83. Cunningham, I. J.: A note on the cause of tall fescue lameness in cattle. Aust. Vet. J. 25:25, 1949.

84. Dickie, C. W., and Berryman, J. R.: Polioencephalomalacia and photosensitization associated with Kochia scoparia consumption in range cattle. JAVMA 175:463, 1979.

85. Dickie, C. W., and James, L. F.: Kochia scoparia poisoning in cattle. JAVMA 183:765, 1983.

86. Menna, M. E., and Bailey, J. R.: Pithomyces chartarum spore counts in pasture. N.Z. J. Agric. Res. 16:343, 1973.

87. Dishington, I. W.: A lveldsykens etiologi belyst ved BSP-test. Nord. Vet. Med. 28:547, 1976.

88. Ditmars, R. L.: Snake bites among domestic animals. JAVMA 94:383, 1939.

89. Dodd, D. C., and Hall, R. A.: The experimental production of hyperkeratosis in young calves by the use of a pentachlorinated naphthalene compound. N.Z. Vet. J. 1:104, 1953.

90. Dodd, D. L., and Brackenridge, D. T.: Leptospira icterohaemorrhagiae AB infection in calves. N.Z. Vet. J. 8:71, 1960.

91. Dodd, S.: Trefoil dermatitis or the sensitization of unpigmented skin to the sun's rays by the ingestion of trefoil. J. Comp. Pathol. Ther. 29:47, 1916.

92. Dollahite, J. W., et al.: Photosensitization in lambs grazing kleingrass. JAVMA 171:1264, 1977.

93. Dollahite, J. W., et al.: Photosensitization in cattle and sheep caused by feeding Ammi majus (Greater Ammi; Bishop's-weed). Am. J. Vet. Res. 39:193, 1978.

94. Done, J., et al.: The experimental intoxication of sheep with sporidesmin, a metabolic product of Pithomyces chartarum. II. Changes in some serum constituents after oral administration of sporidesmin. Res. Vet. Sci. 3:161, 1962.

95. Dunne, H. W., and Leman, A. D.: Diseases in Swine IV. Ames, Iowa State University Press, 1975.

96. Durst, H. I., et al.: Effects of PBBs on cattle. I. Clinical evaluations and clinical chemistry. Environ. Health Perspect. 23:83, 1978.

97. Dyson, D. A., and Reed, J. B. H.: Haemorrhagic syndrome of cattle of suspected mycotoxic origin. Vet. Rec. 100:400, 1977.

98. Edwards, C. M.: Ergot poisoning in young cattle. Vet. Rec. 65:158, 1953.

99. Edwards, J. R., et al.: A facial eczema outbreak in sheep. Aust. Vet. J. 57:392, 1981.

100. Edwards, J. R., et al.: An abattoir survey of the prevalence of facial eczema in sheep in Western Australia. Aust. Vet. J. 60:157, 1983.

101. Edwards, W. C., and Manin, T.: Malicious mutilation of a horse with sulfuric acid. Vet. Med. Small Anim. Clin. 77:90, 1982.

102. Edwards, W. C., and Niles, G. A.: Dermatitis induced by diesel fuel on dairy cows. Vet. Med. Small Anim. Clin. 76:873, 1981.

103. Ellis, D. J., et al.: Congenital porphyria (pink tooth) in Michigan. Mich. State Univ. Vet. 18:89, 1958.

104. Egyed, M. N., et al.: Photosensitization in dairy cattle associated with ingestion of *Ammi majus*. Refuah Vet. 31:128, 1974.

105. Eilat, A., et al.: A field outbreak of photosensitization caused by ingestion of *Ammi majus*. Refuah Vet. 31:83, 1974.

106. Eppley, R. M., and Bailey, W. J.: 12,13-Epoxy-delta 9-trichothecenes as the probable mycotoxins responsible for stachybotryotoxicosis. Science 181:758, 1973.

107. Fadok, V. A., and Wild, S.: Suspected cutaneous iodism in a horse. JAVMA 183:1104, 1983.

108. Fair, A. E., et al.: Poisoning of cattle by ganskweek (*Lasiospermum bipinnatum* (thunb.) Druce). J. S. Afr. Vet. Med. Assoc. 41:231, 1970.

109. Faulkner, L. C., et al.: Scrotal frostbite in bulls. JAVMA 151:602, 1967.

110. Fincher, M. G., and Fuller, H. K.: Photosensitization–trifoliosis–light sensitization. Cornell Vet. 32:95, 1942.

111. Fitzgerald, W. J.: Selenium toxicosis. Equine Pract. 1:6, 1979.

112. Fitzpatrick, T. B., et al.: *Dermatology in General Medicine II*. New York, McGraw-Hill Book Co., 1979.

113. Ford, E. J. H.: A preliminary investigation of photosensitization in Scottish sheep. J. Comp. Pathol. 74:37, 1964.

114. Ford, E. J. H.: Hepatogenous light sensitization in animals. *In*: Rook, A. J., and Walton, G. S.: *Comparative Physiology and Pathology of the Skin*. Oxford, Blackwell Scientific Publications, 1965, p. 351.

115. Fourie, P. J. J.: The occurrence of congenital porphyrinuria (pink tooth) in cattle in South Africa (Swaziland). Onderstepoort J. Vet. Sci. Anim. Indust. 7:535, 1936.

116. Fourie, P. J. J., and Rimington, C.: A further case of congenital porphyrinuria in a living grade Friesland cow in South Africa (Cedara case). Onderstepoort J. Vet. Sci. Anim. Indust. 10:431, 1938.

117. Fourie, P. J. J., and Rimington, C.: Living animal cases of congenital porphyrinuria. Nature 140:68, 1937.

118. Fourie, P. J. J., and Roets, G. C. S.: Quantitative studies upon porphyrin excretion in bovine congenital porphyrinuria (pink tooth). Onderstepoort J. Vet. Sci. Anim. Indust. 13:369, 1939.

119. Fourie, P. J. J.: Bovine congenital porphyrinuria (pink tooth) inherited as a recessive character. Onderstepoort J. Vet. Sci. Anim. Indust. 13:383, 1939.

120. Fourie, P. J. J.: Genetics in the diagnosis of bovine congenital porphyrinuria. Onderstepoort J. Vet. Sci. Anim. Indust. 18:305, 1943.

121. Fourie, P. J. J.: Does bovine congenital porphyria (pink tooth) produce clinical disturbances in an animal which is protected against the sun? Onderstepoort J. Vet. Sci. Anim. Indust. 26:231, 1953.

122. Fowler, M. E.: Zootoxins. *In*: Howard, J. L. (ed.): *Current Veterinary Therapy. Food Animal Practice II*. Philadelphia, W. B. Saunders Co., 1986, p. 483.

123. Fowler, M. E.: Hepatotoxic plants. *In*: Howard, J. L. (ed.): *Current Veterinary Therapy, Food Animal Practice II*. Philadelphia, W. B. Saunders Co., 1986, p. 399.

124. Fowler, M. E.: Clinical manifestations of primary hepatic insufficiency in the horse. JAVMA 147:55, 1965.

125. Fraser, I. E. B.: Observations on the microclimate of the fleece. Aust. J. Agric. Res. 8:281, 1957.

126. Frohner, E.: Case of mercurial poisoning in the horse. Vet. J. 14:448, 1907.

126a. Fubini, S. L.: Burns. *In*: Robinson, N. E. (ed.): *Current Therapy in Equine Medicine II*. Philadelphia, W. B. Saunders Co., 1986, p. 639.

127. Furr, A., and Buck, W. B.: Arsenic. *In*: Howard, J. L. (ed.): *Current Veterinary Therapy. Food Animal Practice II*. Philadelphia, W. B. Saunders Co., 1986, p. 435.

128. Gabbedy, B. J.: Toxicity in sheep associated with the prophylactic use of selenium. Aust. Vet. J. 46:223, 1970.

129. Galitzer, S. J., and Oehme, F. W.: Photosensitization: A literature review. Vet. Sci. Comm. 2:217, 1978.

130. Galitzer, S. J., and Oehme, F. W.: *Kochia scoparia* (L.) schrad toxicity in cattle: A literature review. Vet. Hum. Toxicol. 20:421, 1978.

131. Gardner, A. W., and Hall-Patch, P. K.: Molybdenosis in cattle grazing downwind from an oil refinery unit. Vet. Rec. 82:86, 1968.

132. Garner, G. B., et al.: "Fescue foot" induction from experimental pastures. J. Anim. Sci. 35:228, 1972.

133. Garner, G. B., and Cornell, C. N.: Fescue foot. *In*: Howard, J. L. (ed.): *Current Veterinary Therapy. Food Animal Practice*. Philadelphia, W. B. Saunders Co., 1981, p. 1108.

134. Geiser, D. R., and Walker, R. D.: Management of large animal thermal injuries. Compend. Cont. Ed. 7:S69, 1985.

135. Gibbons, W. J.: X-disease of cattle. Auburn Vet. 5:63, 1949.

136. Gibbons, W. J.: Photosensitization in cattle. Auburn Vet. 9:177, 1953.

137. Gibbons, W. J.: Forage poisoning. Mod. Vet. Pract. 40:43, 1959.

138. Gibbons, W. J.: Green oats intoxication and icterogenic photosensitization in cattle. Vet. Med. 53:297, 1958.

139. Glastonbury, J. R. W., et al.: A syndrome of hepatogenous photosensitization, resembling geeldikkop, in sheep grazing *Tribulus terrestris*. Aust. Vet. J. 61:314, 1984.

140. Glenn, B. L., et al.: A hepatogenous photosensitization disease of cattle: I. Experimental production and clinical aspects of the disease. Pathol. Vet. 1:469, 1964.

141. Glenn, M. W., et al.: Sodium selenate toxicosis: The effects of extended oral administration of sodium selenate on mortality, clinical signs, fertility, and early embryonic development in sheep. Am. J. Vet. Res. 25:1479, 1964.

142. Glenn, M. W., et al.: Sodium selenate toxicosis: Pathology and pathogenesis of sodium selenate toxicosis in sheep. Am. J. Vet. Res. 25:1486, 1964.

143. Gmelin, W.: Das Ekzem des Jungrindes und seine wirtschaftliche Bedeutung. Zeitschr. Hyg. Infektionskrank. 31:314, 1927.

144. Gminder, A.: Die BekampFung der Aufzuchtkrankheiten in Wurttemberg. Dtsch. Tierarztl. Wochenschr. 37:674, 1929.

145. Goodman, A. A.: Fescue foot in cattle in Colorado. JAVMA 121:289, 1952.

146. Goodrich, B. S., and Lipson, M.: Ester splitting of wool wax in fleece-rot and mycotic dermatitis. Aust. Vet. J. 54:43, 1978.

147. Gopinath, C., and Ford, E. J. H.: The effect of *Lantana camara* on the liver of sheep. J. Pathol. 99:75, 1969.

148. Gregory, R. P., et al.: Experimental production of bovine hyperkeratosis with a feed concentrate exposed to vapors of a highly chlorinated naphthalene. JAVMA 125:244, 1954.

149. Guilhan, J.: Ergotism in domestic animals. Rev. Pathol. Gen. Comp. 55:1467, 1955.

150. Gutwein, M. L.: Ear necrosis in swine. Mod. Vet. Pract. 64:143, 1983.

151. Hall, C. A., et al.: Patterns of wool moisture in Merino sheep and its association with blowfly strike. Res. Vet. Sci. 29:181, 1980.

152. Hall, C. A., et al.: The effect of a drying agent (B26) on wool moisture and blowfly strike. Res. Vet. Sci. 29:186, 1980.

153. Hallgren, W., et al.: Molybdenforgiftning ("Molybdenos") hos notkreatur i Sverige. Nord. Vet. Med. 6:469, 1954.

154. Hancock, J.: Congenital photosensitivity in Southdown sheep. A new sub-lethal factor in sheep. N.Z. J. Sci. Technol. 32A:16, 1950.

155. Hansel, W., et al.: The effects of two causative agents of experimental hyperkeratosis in vitamin A metabolism. Cornell Vet. 41:367, 1951.

156. Hansel, W., et al.: The isolation and identification of the causative agent of bovine hyperkeratosis (X-disease) from a processed wheat concentrate. Cornell Vet. 45:94, 1955.

157. Hansel, W., et al.: Bovine hyperkeratosis. Studies on a German wood preservative. Cornell Vet. 43:311, 1953.

158. Hansel, W., and McEntee, K.: Bovine hyperkeratosis (X-disease)—a review. J. Dairy Sci. 38:875, 1955.

159. Hare, T., et al.: First impressions of the beta haemolytic streptococcus infection of swine. Vet. Rec. 54:267, 1942.

160. Harrach, B., et al.: Macrocyclic thichothecenes toxins produced by a strain of *Stachybotrys atra* from Hungary. Appl. Environ. Microbiol. 41:1428, 1981.

161. Harvey, F. F.: Mercurialism in cattle. Vet. Rec. 12:328, 1932.

162. Hatch, R. C., et al.: Use of thiols and thiosulfate for treatment of experimentally induced acute arsenic toxicosis in cattle. Am. J. Vet. Res. 39:1411, 1978.

163. Haughey, K. G., and Cooper, B. S.: An outbreak of bovine hyperkeratosis in New Zealand. N.Z. Vet. J. 1:99, 1953.

164. Hay, J. B., and Mills, S. C.: Chemical changes in the wool wax of adult Merino sheep during prolonged wetting and prior to development of fleece-rot. Aust. J. Agric. Res. 33:335, 1982.

165. Hay, J. B., et al.: The effect of exposure to rainfall on white blood cell counts in sheep. Aust. Vet. J. 59:60, 1982.

166. Haydon, M.: Inherited congenital porphyria in calves. Can. Vet. J. 16:118, 1975.

167. Hayman, R. H.: Studies in fleece-rot of sheep. Aust. J. Agric. Res. 4:430, 1953.

168. Hayman, R. H.: Studies in fleece-rot of sheep. Aust. J. Agric. Res. 6:466, 1955.

169. Heard, T. W., and Jollans, J. L.: Continued observations on a closed hysterectomy-founded pig herd. Vet. Rec. 86:418, 1970.

170. Herigstad, R. R., et al.: Chronic methyl mercury poisoning in calves. JAVMA 160:173, 1972.

171. Herrmann, H. J., and Prietz, G.: Zur karzinomatosen Entdifferenzierung der Dermatitis solaris chronica des Rindes. Monat. Vet. Med. 21:826, 1966.

172. Herrmann, H. J.: Zum histochemischen und farberischen Verhatten des Koriums bei der solar dermatitis des Rindes. Pathol. Vet. 5:297, 1968.

173. Hibbs, C. M., and Wolf, N.: Ergot toxicosis in young goats. Mod. Vet. Pract. 63:126, 1982.

174. Hillman, D.: Chronic iodide toxicity in dairy cattle. Metabolic and leukocytic changes. Calif. Vet. 33:33, 1979.

174a. Hinton, D. M., et al.: The distribution and ultrastructure of the endophyte of toxic tall fescue. Can. J. Bot. 63:36, 1985.

175. Hoekstra, W. G., et al.: Production of hyperkeratosis in calves with a topically applied oil-based insecticide carrier. Am. J. Vet. Res. 15:47, 1954.

176. Hoekstra, W. G., et al.: A study on the relationship of vitamin A to the development of hyperkeratosis–X-disease in calves. J. Dairy Sci. 36:601, 1953.

177. Hoekstra, W. G., et al.: A study on the relationship of vitamin A to the development of hyperkeratosis–X-disease. Am. J. Vet. Res. 15:47, 1954.

178. Holden, A. R.: Two outbreaks of pyrexia with dermatitis in dairy cows. Vet. Rec. 106:413, 1980.

179. Hopes, R.: Skin diseases in horses. Vet. Dermatol. News. 2:4, 1976.

180. Hore, D. E.: Facial eczema. Aust. Vet. J. 36:172, 1960.

181. Horsley, C. M.: Investigation into the action of St. John's wort. J. Pharmacol. Exp. Ther. 50:310, 1934.

182. Hultine, J. D., et al.: Selenium toxicosis in the horse. Equine Pract. 1:57, 1979.

183. Hungerford, T. G.: *Diseases of Livestock VII.* Sydney, Angust Robertson, 1970.

184. Hupka, E.: Ubergehcurfte exanthematische Hauterlerankungen nach Verfutterung von Reismehl bei Kuhen. Dtsch. Tierarztl. Wochenschr. 37:183, 1929.

185. Hutchins, D. R.: Skin diseases of cattle and horses in New South Wales. N.Z. Vet. J. 8:85, 1960.

186. Ihrke, P. J.: Contact dermatitis. *In*: Robinson, N. E.: *Current Therapy in Equine Medicine.* Philadelphia, W. B. Saunders Co., 1983, p. 547.

187. Jackson, T. F., and Halbert, F. L.: A toxic syndrome associated with the feeding of polybrominated biphenyl–contaminated protein concentrate to dairy cattle. JAVMA 165:437, 1974.

188. Jacobson, D. R., et al.: Nature of fescue toxicity and progress toward identification of the toxic entity. J. Dairy Sci. 46:416, 1963.

189. James, L. F., et al.: Syndromes of *Austragalus* sp. poisoning in livestock. JAVMA 178:146, 1981.

190. James, L. F., and Shupe, J. L.: Selenium accumulators. *In*: Howard, J. L. (ed.): *Current Veterinary Therapy. Food Animal Practice II.* Philadelphia, W. B. Saunders Co., 1986, p. 394.

191. James, L. F., et al.: Principal poisonous plants in the Western United States. *In*: Howard, J. L. (ed.): *Current Veterinary Therapy. Food Animal Practice II.* Philadelphia, W. B. Saunders Co., 1986, p. 416.

192. James, P. J., and Warren, G. H.: Effect of disruption of the sebaceous layer of the sheep's skin on the incidence of fleece-rot. Aust. Vet. J. 55:335, 1979.

193. Jensen, R., et al.: Fescue lameness in cattle. I. Experimental production of the disease. Am. J. Vet. Res. 17:196, 1956.

194. Jensen, R.: *Diseases of Sheep.* Philadelphia, Lea & Febiger, 1974.

195. Jericho, K. W. F., and Church, T. L.: Cannibalism in pigs. Can. Vet. J. 13:156, 1972.

196. Johnson, A. E.: Predisposing influence of range plants on *Tetradymia*-related photosensitization in sheep. Am. J. Vet. Res. 35:1583, 1974.

197. Johnson, A. E.: Tolerance of cattle to tansy ragwort (*Senecio jacobaea*). Am. J. Vet. Res. 39:1542, 1978.

198. Johnson, A. E.: Dermatotoxic plants. *In*: Howard, J. L. (ed.): *Current Veterinary Therapy. Food Animal Practice.* Philadelphia, W. B. Saunders Co., 1981, p. 452.

199. Johnson, A. E.: Dermatotoxic plants. *In*: Howard, J. L. (ed.): *Current Veterinary Therapy. Food Animal Practice II.* Philadelphia, W. B. Saunders Co., 1986, p. 406.

200. Jones, E. B.: Ergot poisoning in young cattle. Vet. Rec. 65:158, 1953.

201. Jones, R. J., et al.: Toxicity of *Leucaena leucocephala.* Aust. Vet. J. 54:387, 1978.

202. Jorgensen, S. K., and With, T. K.: Congenital porphyria in swine and cattle in Denmark. Nature 176:156, 1955.

203. Jorgensen, S. K.: Studies on congenital porphyria in cattle in Denmark. I. Distribution of the condition and its mode of inheritance. Br. Vet. J. 117:1, 1961.

204. Jorgensen, S. K.: Studies on congenital porphyria in cattle in Denmark. II. Clinical features, morbid anatomy and chemical pathology. Br. Vet. J. 117:61, 1961.

205. Jorgensen, S. K., and With, T. K.: Congenital porphyria in animals other than man. *In*: Rook, A. J., and Walton, G. S.: *Comparative Physiology and Pathology of the Skin.* Oxford, Blackwell Scientific Publications, 1965, p. 317.

206. Julian, W. E., et al.: Feed intake in Hereford calves infused intraperitoneally with toxic fescue extract. J. Dairy Sci. 57:1385, 1974.

207. Jungherr, E. L.: Lechuguilla fever of sheep and goats; a form of swell head in West Texas. Cornell Vet. 21:227, 1931.

208. Kaneko, J. J.: Erythrokinetics and iron metabolism in bovine porphyria erythropoietica. Ann. N.Y. Acad. Sci. 104:689, 1963.

209. Kaneko, J. J., and Mattheeuws, D. R. G.: Iron metabolism in normal and porphyric calves. Am. J. Vet. Res. 27:923, 1966.

210. Kaneko, J. J., and Mills, R.: Erythrocyte enzymes, ions, fragility, and glutathione stability in bovine porphyria erythropoietica and its carrier state. Fed. Proc. 28:453, 1969.

211. Kaneko, J. J., and Mills, R.: Erythrocyte enzyme activity, ion concentrations, osmotic fragility, and glutathione stability in bovine erythropoietic porphyria and its carrier state. Am. J. Vet. Res. 30:1805, 1969.

212. Kaneko, J. J., and Mills, R.: Hematological and blood chemical observations in neonatal normal and porphyric caries in early life. Cornell Vet. 60:52, 1970.

213. Keeler, R. F., et al.: *Effects of Poisonous Plants on Livestock.* New York, Academic Press, 1978.

214. Kellerman, T. S., et al.: Photosensitivity in South Africa. I. A comparative study of *Asaemia axillaris* (Thunb.) Harv. Ex Jackson and *Lasiospermum bipinnatum* (Thunb.) Drace poisoning in sheep. Onderstepoort J. Vet. Res. 40:115, 1973.

215. Kellerman, T. S., et al.: Photosensitivity in South Africa. II.

The experimental production of the ovine hepatogenous photosensitivity disease geeldikkop (*Tribulosis ovis*) by the simultaneous ingestion of *Tribulus terrestris* plants and cultures of *Pithomyces chartanum* containing the mycotoxin sporidesmin. Onderstepoort J. Vet. Res. 47:231, 1980.

216. Kerr, L. A., and Edwards, W. C.: Hairy vetch poisoning of cattle. Vet. Med. Small Anim. Clin. 77:257, 1982.

217. Kidder, R. W., et al.: Photosensitization in cattle grazing common frosted Bermuda grass. Univ. Florida Agric. Exp. Stat. Bull. 630, Feb. 1961.

218. Kingsbury, J. M.: *Poisonous Plants of the United States and Canada.* Englewood Cliffs, NJ, Prentice-Hall, Inc., 1964.

219. Kirker-Head, C. A., and Mullowney, P. C.: Nonparasitic skin diseases of sheep. *In*: Howard, J. L. (ed.): *Current Veterinary Therapy. Food Animal Practice II.* Philadelphia, W. B. Saunders Co., 1986, p. 939.

220. Klussendorf, R. C.: Photosensitization. North Am. Vet. 35:665, 1954.

221. Knocke, K. W.: Hyperkeratose in einem Rinderbestand 13 Jahre nach Anwendungeins Holzschutzmittels. Dtsch. Tierarztl. Wochenschr. 68:701, 1961.

222. Knott, S. G., and McCray, C. W. R.: Two naturally occurring outbreaks of selenosis in Queensland. Aust. Vet. J. 35:161, 1959.

223. Kohler, D.: Zur Hyperkeratose bei Haustieren, eine Folge der Anwendung von Holzschutzmittein. Arch. Exper. Vet. 8:163, 1954.

224. Kohler, H.: Pathologisch-anatomische Befunde beider experimentellen Hyperkeratose der Haustiere. Dtsch. Tierarztl. Wochenschr. 60:316, 1953.

225. Konig, H.: Untersuchungen uber Salaninwirkung bei Rind und Schaf in Zusammenhung mit Korteffelkrant-Futterung. Schweiz. Arch. Tierheilkd. 95:97, 1953.

226. Kownacki, A. A., and Tobin, T.: Plant toxicities. *In*: Robinson, N. E.: *Current Therapy in Equine Medicine.* Philadelphia, W. B. Saunders Co., 1983, p. 595.

227. Kral, F., and Schwartzman, R. M.: *Veterinary and Comparative Dermatology.* Philadelphia, J. B. Lippincott Co., 1964.

228. LeBars, J.: La stachybotryotoxicose: Une mycotoxicose fatale due a *Stachybotrys atra* Corda. Revue. Rev. Med. Vet. 128:51, 1977.

229. Leman, A. D., et al.: *Diseases of Swine V.* Ames, Iowa State University Press, 1981.

230. Lever, W. F., and Schaumburg-Lever, G.: *Histopathology of the Skin VI.* Philadelphia, J. B. Lippincott Co., 1983.

231. Levin, E. Y.: Uroporphyrinogen III cosynthetase in bovine erythropoietic porphyria. Science 161:907, 1968.

232. Link, R. P.: Bovine hyperkeratosis. JAVMA 123:427, 1953.

233. Link, R. P., and Reber, E. F.: Observations on bovine hyperkeratosis. North Am. Vet. 35:274, 1954.

234. Lipson, M.: The significance of certain fleece properties in susceptibility of sheep to fleece-rot. Wool Technol. Sheep Breed. 26:27, 1978.

235. Lipson, M.: A technique for determining fleece wettability. Wool Technol. Sheep Breed. 24:10, 1976.

236. Lofstedt, J.: Dermatologic diseases of sheep. Vet. Clin. North Am. Large Anim. Pract. 5:427, 1983.

236a. Lyons, P. C., et al.: Occurrence of peptide and clavine ergot alkaloids in tall fescue grass. Science 232:487, 1986.

237. MacNamme, J. K.: Physiological, pathological and toxicological effects of snake bites on domesticated animals. Vet. Med. 31:376, 1936.

238. Madden, D. E., et al.: The occurrence of congenital porphyria in Holstein-Friesian cattle. J. Hered. 49:125, 1958.

239. Maddox, E. T., et al.: Ampicillin treatment of three cases of streptococcal auricular dermatosis in swine. Vet. Med. Small Anim. Clin. 68:1018, 1973.

240. Manning, T. D.: Noninfectious skin diseases of cattle. Vet. Clin. North Am. Large Anim. Pract. 6:175, 1984.

241. Mansmann, R. A., et al.: *Equine Medicine & Surgery III.* Santa Barbara, CA, American Veterinary Publications, Inc., 1983.

242. Markel, M. D. et al.: Acute renal failure associated with application of a mercuric blister in a horse. JAVMA 185:91, 1984.

243. Marsh, C. D., and Clauson, A. B.: Toxic effect of St. John's wort (*Hypericum perforatum*) on cattle and sheep. Tech. Bull. 202, U.S. Dept. Agric., Washington, DC, 1930.

244. Marsh, C. L., et al.: Observations on collagen, vitamin A, and ascorbic acid in bovine hyperkeratosis. Am. J. Vet. Res. 17:410, 1956.

244a. Martin, T., and Edwards, W. C.: Protecting grazing livestock from tall fescue toxicity. Vet. Med. 81:1162, 1986.

245. Martin, W. B.: *Diseases of Sheep.* Oxford, Blackwell Scientific Publications, 1983.

246. Mathews, F. P.: Lechuguilla (*Agave lechuguilla*) poisoning in sheep and goats. Texas Agric. Exp. Stat. Bull. 554, 1940.

247. Matthews, J. G., and Shreave, B. J.: Pyrexia/pruritus/haemorrhagic syndrome in dairy cows. Vet. Rec. 103:408, 1978.

248. McCann, P. J.: Ngaio poisoning of cattle. N.Z. J. Agric. 72:139, 1946.

249. McCormick, A. E.: Photosensitization in a yearling steer. Mod. Vet. Pract. 63:561, 1982.

250. McEntee, K., et al.: The production of hyperkeratosis (X-disease) by feeding fractions of a processed concentrate. Cornell Vet. 41:237, 1941.

251. McFarlane, D., et al.: Photosensitivity diseases in New Zealand. XIV. The pathogenesis of facial eczema. N.Z. J. Agric. Res. 3:194, 1959.

252. McGavin, M. D., et al.: Lesions in Southdown sheep with hereditary hyperbilirubinemia. Vet. Pathol. 9:142, 1972.

253. McGuirk, B., et al.: Breeding for resistance to fleece-rot and body strike—the Trangie programme. Wool Technol. Sheep Breed. 26:17, 1978.

254. McKenzie, R. A., and McMicking, L. I.: Ataxia and urinary incontinence in cattle grazing sorghum. Aust. Vet. J. 53:496, 1977.

255. McKeon, F. W., and Egan, D. A.: Lameness in cattle fed ergotized silage. Irish Vet. J. 25:67, 1971.

256. McMullan, W. C.: The skin. *In*: Mansmann, R. A., et al.: *Equine Medicine & Surgery III.* Santa Barbara, CA, American Veterinary Publications, Inc., 1982, p. 791.

257. McNellis, R.: Rattlesnake bite. JAVMA 114:145, 1949.

258. McParland, P. J., et al.: Deaths in cattle following ingestion of lead arsenate. Vet. Rec. 89:450, 1971.

259. Merritt, G. C., and Watts, J. E.: An *in vitro* technique for studying fleece-rot and fly strike in sheep. Aust. Vet. J. 54:513, 1978.

260. Merritt, G. C., and Watts, J. E.: The changes in protein concentration and bacteria of fleece and skin during the development of fleece-rot and body strike in sheep. Aust. Vet. J. 54:517, 1978.

261. Miniats, O. P., et al.: Experimental polychlorinated biphenyl toxicosis in germ free pigs. Can. J. Comp. Med. 42:192, 1978.

262. Mitchell, K. J., et al.: Factors influencing growth of *Pithomyces chartarum* in pasture. N.Z. J. Agric. Res. 14:566, 1961.

263. Mochizuki, K.: A collective outbreak of auricular dermatitis on a hog farm. J. Jpn. Vet. Med. Assoc. 36:135, 1983.

264. Mohammed, F. H. A., et al.: Hepatogenous photosensitization in horses due to *Aphis craccivora* on lucerne. Bull. Anim. Health Prod. Afr. 25:184, 1977.

265. Mangkoewidjojo, S., et al.: Pathologic features of iodide toxicosis in calves. Am. J. Vet. Res. 41:1057, 1980.

266. Monlux, A. W., et al.: Bovine hepatogenous photosensitization associated with the feeding of alfalfa hay. JAVMA 142:989, 1963.

267. Monlux, W. S., and Peckham, J. C.: Common lesions in baby pigs. Iowa State Vet. 23:137, 1961.

268. Moorehead, P. D., et al.: Effects of PBBs on cattle. II. Gross pathology and histopathology. Environ. Health Perspect. 23:111, 1978.

269. Moorehead, P. D., et al.: Pathology of experimentally induced polybrominated biphenyl toxicosis in pregnant heifers. JAVMA 170:307, 1977.

270. Morris, J., and McInnes, I. J.: Pyrexia with dermatitis in dairy cows. Vet. Rec. 102:368, 1978.

271. Morris, P.: Sporotrichosis. *In*: Robinson, N. E.: *Current Therapy in Equine Medicine.* Philadelphia, W. B. Saunders Co., 1983, p. 555.

272. Mortimer, P. H.: Intoxication of sheep with sporidesmin. Histology and histochemistry of orally dosed sheep. Res. Vet. Sci. 4:166, 1963.
273. Mortimer, P. H., and Standridge, T. A.: Excretion of sporidesmin given to sheep by mouth. J. Comp. Pathol. 78:505, 1968.
274. Mortimer, P. H.: Facial eczema. 2. Its effects within the animal. N.Z. J. Agric. 119:22, 1969.
275. Mortimer, P. H.: The experimental intoxication of sheep with sporidesmin. III. Some changes in cellular components and coagulation properties of the blood, in serum proteins and in liver function. Res. Vet. Sci. 3:269, 1962.
276. Mortimer, P. H.: The experimental intoxication of sheep with sporidesmin. I. Clinical observations and findings at post-mortem exams. Res. Vet. Sci. 3:147, 1962.
277. Muchiri, D. J., et al.: Photosensitization of sheep on kleingrass pasture. JAVMA 177:353, 1980.
278. Mullenax, C. H.: A dietary cause of hair loss in Bahamian livestock. JAVMA 131:302, 1957.
279. Mullowney, P. C., and Fadok, V. A.: Dermatologic diseases of horses. Part III. Fungal skin diseases. Compend. Cont. Ed. 6:S324, 1984.
280. Mullowney, P. C., and Baldwin, E. W.: Skin diseases of goats. Vet. Clin. North Am. Large Anim. Pract. 6:143, 1984.
281. Mullowney, P. C., and Hall, R. F.: Skin diseases of swine. Vet. Clin. North Am. Large Anim. Pract. 6:107, 1984.
282. Mullowney, P. C.: Skin diseases of sheep. Vet. Clin. North Am. Large Anim. Pract. 6:131, 1984.
283. Mullowney, P. C.: Dermatologic diseases of cattle. Part III. Environmental, congenital, neoplastic, and allergic diseases. Compend. Cont. Ed. 4:S138, 1982.
284. Mullowney, P. C.: Dermatologic diseases of horses. Part IV. Environmental, congenital, and neoplastic diseases. Compend. Cont. Ed. 7:S22, 1985.
285. Mullowney, P. C.: The pathophysiology of dermatologic diseases of food-producing animals. In: Howard, J. L. (ed.): Current Veterinary Therapy. Food Animal Practice II. Philadelphia, W. B. Saunders Co., 1986, p. 906.
286. Mullowney, P. C., and Hall, R. F.: Nonparasitic skin diseases of swine. In: Howard, J. L. (ed.): Current Veterinary Therapy. Food Animal Practice II. Philadelphia, W. B. Saunders Co., 1986, p. 946.
287. Muth, O. H., and Binns, W.: Selenium toxicity in domestic animals. Ann. N.Y. Acad. Sci. 111:583, 1964.
288. McClymont, G. L.: Possibility of photosensitization due to ingestion of aphids. Aust. Vet. J. 31:112, 1955.
289. Nay, T., and Watts, J. E.: Observation on the wool follicle abnormalities in Merino sheep exposed to prolonged wetting conducive to the development of fleece-rot. Aust. J. Agric. Res. 28:1095, 1977.
290. Neitz, W. O.: Hyalomma transiens Schulze: A vector of sweating sickness. J. S. Afr. Vet. Med. Assoc. 25:19, 1954.
291. Neitz, W. O.: Sweating sickness: A tick-borne disease transmissible to several members of the order of Artiodactyla. Bull. Epizoot. Dis. Afr. 3:125, 1955.
292. Neitz, W. O.: Studies on the aetiology of sweating sickness. Onderstepoort J. Vet. Res. 27:197, 1956.
293. Neitz, W. O.: Sweating sickness: The present state of our knowledge. Onderstepoort J. Vet. Res. 28:3, 1959.
294. Nestel, B. L.: Bovine congenital porphyria (pink tooth), with a note on 5 cases in Jamaica. Cornell Vet. 48:430, 1958.
295. Newsom, I. W.: Photosensitization in sheep. North Am. Vet. 33:38, 1952.
296. Norral, J.: Abscesses in pigs. Vet. Rec. 78:708, 1966.
297. Nyack, B., et al.: Suspected ergotism in a calf. Mod. Vet. Pract. 62:623, 1981.
298. Oehme, F. W.: Toxicoses commonly observed in horses. In: Robinson, N. E.: Current Therapy in Equine Medicine. Philadelphia, W. B. Saunders Co., 1983, p. 573.
299. Oehme, F. W.: General principles in treatment of poisoning. In: Robinson, N. E.: Current Therapy in Equine Medicine. Philadelphia, W. B. Saunders Co., 1983, p. 577.
300. Oehme, F. W.: Snake bite. In: Robinson, N. E.: Current Therapy in Equine Medicine. Philadelphia, W. B. Saunders Co., 1983, p. 587.
301. Oehme, F. W.: Phenothiazine. In: Robinson, N. E.: Current

302. Oehme, F. W.: Selenium. In: Robinson, N. E.: Current Therapy in Equine Medicine. Philadelphia, W. B. Saunders Co., 1983, p. 593.
302a. Oehme, F. W.: Snake bite. In: Robinson, N. E. (ed.): Current Therapy in Equine Medicine II. Philadelphia, W. B. Saunders Co., 1986, p. 663.
302b. Oehme, F. W.: Arsenic. In: Robinson, N. E. (ed.): Current Therapy in Equine Medicine II. Philadelphia, W. B. Saunders Co., 1986, p. 668.
302c. Oehme, F. W.: Selenium. In: Robinson, N. E. (ed.): Current Therapy in Equine Medicine II. Philadelphia, W. B. Saunders Co., 1986, p. 670.
303. Oertli, E. H., et al.: Phototoxic effects of Thamnosma texana (Dutchman's breeches) in sheep. Am. J. Vet. Res. 44:1126, 1983.
304. Olafson, P.: Hyperkeratosis (X-disease) of cattle. Cornell Vet. 37:279, 1947.
305. Olafson, J., and McEntee, K.: The experimental production of hyperkeratosis (X-disease) by feeding a processed concentrate. Cornell Vet. 41:107, 1951.
306. Olson, C., and Cook, R. H.: Attempts to produce bovine hyperkeratosis. Am. J. Vet. Res. 12:261, 1951.
307. Olson, C.: Bovine hyperkeratosis (X-disease, highly chlorinated naphthalene poisoning) historical review. Adv. Vet. Sci. 13:101, 1969.
308. Olson, C., and Cook, R. H.: Attempts to produce bovine hyperketatosis. Am. J. Vet. Res. 12:261, 1951.
309. Olson, C., and Skidmore, L. V.: Further observations on reproductive ability after recovery from bovine hyperkeratosis. Vet. Med. 49:371, 1954.
310. Olson, C., et al.: The reproductive ability of heifers recovered from bovine hyperkeratosis. JAVMA 120:186, 1952.
311. Osweiler, G. D.: Ergot (gangrenous). In: Howard, J. L. (ed.): Current Veterinary Therapy. Food Animal Practice. Philadelphia, W. B. Saunders Co., 1981, p. 404.
312. Osweiler, G. D.: Ergot (gangrenous). In: Howard, J. L. (ed.): Current Veterinary Therapy. Food Animal Practice II. Philadelphia, W. B. Saunders Co., 1986, p. 367.
313. Osweiler, G. D., and Hook, B. S.: Mercury. In: Howard, J. L. (ed.): Current Veterinary Therapy. Food Animal Practice II. Philadelphia, W. B. Saunders Co., 1986, p. 440.
314. Pace, N., and MacKinney, G.: Hypericin, the photodynamic pigment from St. John's wort. J. Am. Chem. Soc. 63:2570, 1941.
315. Panciera, R. J., et al.: A disease of cattle grazing hairy vetch pasture. JAVMA 148:804, 1966.
316. Panciera, R. J.: Serum hepatitis in the horse. JAVMA 155:408, 1969.
317. Panel Report: Skin conditions in horses. Mod. Vet. Pract. 56:363, 1975.
318. Panel Report: Skin diseases in horses. Mod. Vet. Pract. 67:43, 1986.
319. Panel Report: Dermatologic problems in cattle. Mod. Vet. Pract. 60:172, 1979.
320. Parle, J. N.: Facial eczema. 3. Fungicides and control. N.Z. J. Agric. 119:26, 1969.
321. Parrish, H. M., and Scatterday, J. E.: A survey of poisonous snakebites among domestic animals in Florida. Vet. Med. 52:135, 1957.
322. Pascoe, L.: Measurement of fleece wettability in sheep and its relationship to susceptibility to fleece-rot and blowfly strike. Aust. J. Agric. Res. 33:141, 1982.
323. Pascoe, R. R.: Equine Dermatoses. Sydney, Univ. Sydney Post-Graduate Foundation in Veterinary Science, Vet. Rev. No. 22, 1981.
324. Pearson, E. G.: Clinical manifestation of tansy ragwort poisoning. Mod. Vet. Pract. 58:421, 1977.
325. Penny, R. H. C., et al.: Foot-rot in pigs: Observations on the clinical disease. Vet. Rec. 77:1101, 1965.
326. Penny, R. H. C., et al.: Clinical observations of necrosis of the skin of suckling piglets. Aust. Vet. J. 47:529, 1971.
327. Penny, R. H. C., and Wright, A. I.: Teat necrosis in neonatal pigs. Vet. Annu. 12:79, 1972.
328. Penny, R. H. C., et al.: Tail-biting in pigs: A possible sex incidence. Vet. Rec. 91:482, 1972.

329. Penny, R. H. C., and Mullen, P. A.: Ear biting in pigs. Vet. Annu. 16:103, 1976.

330. Penny, R. H. C., and Hill, F. W. G.: Observations of some conditions in pigs at the abattoir with particular reference to tail biting. Vet. Rec. 94:174, 1974.

331. Penny, R. H. C.: Skin necrosis in suckling piglets. Vet. Dermatol. News. 3:6, 1978.

332. Percival, J. C.: Association of *Sporidesmium bakeri* with facial eczema. N.Z. J. Agric. Res. 12:1041, 1959.

333. Pierse, J. D.: An ergot-like syndrome in young calves. Irish Vet. J. 23:67, 1969.

334. Platonow, N. S., and Geissinger, H. D.: Distribution and persistence of polychlorinated biphenyls (Aroclor 1254) in growing pigs. Vet. Rec. 93:287, 1973.

335. Plonait, H.: Grossflachige Epithelablosung bei Sauen (Kurzmittelung). Dtsch. Tierarztl. Wochenschr. 79:250, 1972.

336. Pope, A. L.: A review of recent mineral research with sheep. J. Anim. Sci. 33:1332, 1971.

337. Pulsford, M. F.: A note on lameness in cattle grazing in tall meadow fescue (*Festuca arundinacea*) in South Australia. Aust. Vet. J. 26:87, 1950.

338. Quin, J. I., and Rimington, C.: Geeldikkop. J. S. Afr. Vet. Med. Assoc. 6:16, 1935.

339. Railsback, L. T.: Porphyrinuria in a yearling Hereford. Vet. Med. 34:102, 1939.

340. Rainey, J. W.: Treatment of foul-in-the-foot and acute inflammation of the skin by a Kaolin-glycerine mixture. Aust. Vet. J. 24:164, 1948.

341. Ramsey, F. K., and Howard, J. R.: Lightning strike and electrocution. *In*: Howard, J. L. (ed.): *Current Veterinary Therapy. Food Animal Practice II.* Philadelphia, W. B. Saunders Co., 1986, p. 458.

342. Rebhun, W. C.: Chemical keratitis in a horse. Vet. Med. Small Anim. Clin. 75:1537, 1980.

343. Reis, P. J., et al.: Effects of mimosine, a potential chemical defleecing agent, in wool growth and the skin of sheep. Aust. J. Biol. Sci. 28:69, 1975.

344. Rhode, E. A., and Cornelius, C. E.: Congenital porphyria (pink tooth) in Holstein-Friesian calves in California. JAVMA 132:112, 1958.

345. Richardson, J. A., et al.: Lesions of porcine necrotic ear syndrome. Vet. Pathol. 21:152, 1984.

346. Rickard, B. F.: Facial eczema: Zinc responsiveness in dairy cattle. N.Z. Vet. J. 23:41, 1975.

347. Rimington, C., and Quin, J. I.: Photosensitization in animals. VII. Nature of sensitizing agent in geeldikkop. Onderstepoort J. Vet. Sci. Anim. Indust. 3:137, 1934.

348. Rimington, C.: Some cases of congenital porphyrinuria in cattle: Chemical studies upon the living animals and post-mortem material. Onderstepoort J. Vet. Sci. Anim. Indust. 7:567, 1936.

349. Rimington, C.: Photosensitization syndromes due to porphyrins in animals and man. J. S. Afr. Vet. Med. Assoc. 36:313, 1965.

349a. Robinson, N. E. (ed.): *Current Therapy in Equine Medicine II.* Philadelphia, W. B. Saunders Co., 1986.

350. Rottgardt, A. A.: Fotosensibilizacion. Fac. Med. Vet. Univ. Natl. La Plata Annu. 7:49, 1944.

351. Ruth, G. R., et al.: Bovine protoporphyria. Proc. Am. Assoc. Vet. Lab. Diag. 21:91, 1978.

352. Ruth, G. R., et al.: Bovine protoporphyria: The first nonhuman model for this hereditary photosensitivity disease. Science 198:199, 1977.

353. Salisbury, R. H., and Barrowman, P. R.: Fleece-rot: The epidemiology and significance of the disease in sheep. J. S. Afr. Vet. Med. Assoc. 55:147, 1984.

354. Salsbury, D. L.: Pine tar irritation in a horse. Vet. Med. Small Anim. Clin. 65:60, 1970.

355. Sassa, S., et al.: Accumulation of protoporphyrin IX from D-aminolevulinic acid in bovine skin fibroblasts with hereditary erythropoietic protoporphyria. A gene-dosage effect. J. Exp. Med. 153:1094, 1981.

356. Scarratt, W. K., et al.: Cutaneous thermal injury in a horse. Equine Pract. 6:13, 1984.

357. Schwartz, S., et al.: Hereditary bovine protoporphyria, a "total body" deficiency of ferrochelatase: Some basic dis-

tinctions from hypochromic anemias. *In*: Doss, M.: *Diagnosis and Therapy of Porphyrias and Lead Intoxication.* Berlin, Springer-Verlag, 1978, p. 262.

358. Scott, D. W., et al.: Dermatohistopathologic changes in bovine congenital porphyria. Cornell Vet. 69:145, 1979.

359. Scott, D. W., et al.: Caprine dermatology. Part II. Viral, nutritional, environmental, and congenitohereditary disorders. Compend. Cont. Ed. 6:S473, 1984.

360. Seaman, J. T.: Pyrrolizidine alkaloid poisoning of horses. Aust. Vet. J. 54:150, 1978.

361. Seawright, A. A.: *Leucaena glauca* in Queensland. Aust. Vet. J. 39:211, 1963.

362. Seawright, A. A., and Watt, D. A.: Congenital porphyria in a bovine carcase. Aust. Vet. J. 48:35, 1972.

363. Seawright, A. A., and Allen, J. G.: Pathology of the liver and kidney in lantana poisoning of cattle. Aust. Vet. J. 48:323, 1972.

364. Servante, J., et al.: Stachybotryotoxicose equine: Premiere description en France. Rev. Med. Vet. 136:687, 1985.

365. Shortridge, E. H., et al.: Acute selenium poisoning in cattle. N.Z. Vet. J. 19:47, 1971.

365a. Sigmund, H. M., et al.: Udder-thigh dermatitis of cattle: Epidemiological, clinical and bacteriological investigations. Bov. Pract. 18:18, 1983.

366. Sikes, D., et al.: The experimental production of "X-disease" (hyperkeratosis) in cattle with chlorinated naphthalenes and petroleum products. JAVMA 121:337, 1952.

367. Sikes, D., and Bridges, M. E.: Experimental production of hyperkeratosis (X-disease) of cattle with a chlorinated naphthalene. Science 116:506, 1952.

368. Simpson, B. H.: Fescue poisoning in sheep. N.Z. Vet. J. 23:182, 1975.

369. Sinclair, D. P.: Thiabendazole shows promise for facial eczema control. N.Z. J. Agric. Res. 20:23, 1967.

370. Sinclair, D. P., and Howe, M. W.: Effect of thiabendazole on *Pithomyces chartarum*. N.Z. J. Agric. Res. 21:59, 1968.

371. Smalley, E. B.: T-2 toxin. JAVMA 163:1278, 1973.

372. Smith, B. L., et al.: The protective effect of zinc sulphate in experimental sporidesmin poisoning of sheep. N.Z. Vet. J. 25:124, 1977.

373. Smith, B. L., and O'Hara, P. J.: Toxicity of zinc in ruminants in relation to facial eczema. N.Z. Vet. J. 25:310, 1977.

374. Smith, B. L., and O'Hara, P. J.: Bovine photosensitization. N.Z. Vet. J. 26:2, 1978.

375. Smith, B. L., et al.: Protective effect of zinc sulphate in a natural facial eczema outbreak in dairy cows. N.Z. Vet. J. 26:314, 1978.

376. Smith, J. E., and Kaneko, J. J.: Rate of heme and porphyrin synthesis by bovine porphyric reticulocytes *in vitro*. Am. J. Vet. Res. 27:931, 1966.

377. Smith, L. P., and Austwick, P. K. C.: Effect of weather on the quality of wool in Great Britain. Vet. Rec. 96:246, 1976.

378. Smith, M. C.: Caprine dermatologic problems: A review. JAVMA 178:724, 1981.

379. Smith, M. C.: Dermatologic diseases of goats. Vet. Clin. North Am. Large Anim. Pract. 5:449, 1983.

380. Sorensen, D. K.: Chlorinated naphthalenes. *In*: Howard, J. L. (ed.): *Current Veterinary Therapy. Food Animal Practice.* Philadelphia, W. B. Saunders Co., 1981, p. 516.

381. Stankoushev, K., et al.: Stachybotryo-toxicosis in sheep. Vet. Med. Nauki 2:11, 1965.

382. Stannard, A. A.: Some important dermatoses in the horse. Mod. Vet. Pract. 53:31, 1972.

383. Stannard, A. A.: The skin. *In*: Catcott, E. J., and Smithcors, J. F.: *Equine Medicine and Surgery II.* Santa Barbara, CA, American Veterinary Publications, Inc., 1972, p. 381.

384. Stevens, G. G.: Mercurial poisoning. Cornell Vet. 28:50, 1938.

385. Stowe, H. D.: Effects of copper pretreatment upon the toxicity of selenium in ponies. Am. J. Vet. Res. 41:1925, 1980.

386. Straw, B.: Diagnosis of skin disease in swine. Compend. Cont. Ed. 7:S650, 1985.

387. Swales, W. E., et al.: Photosensitization produced in pigs by phenothiazine. Can. J. Comp. Med. Vet. Sci. 6:169, 1942.

388. Synge, R. L. M., and White, E. P.: Sporidesmin: A substance from *Sporidesmium bakeri* causing lesions characteristic of facial eczema. Chem. Indust. 1:546, 1959.

389. Taber, R. A., et al.: Isolation of *Pithomyces chartarum* in Texas. Mycologia 60:727, 1968.

390. Tanwar, R. K., et al.: Subcutaneous emphysema in goats. Mod. Vet. Pract. 64:670, 1983.

391. Teske, R. H.: Polybrominated biphenyls. *In*: Howard, J. L. (ed.): *Current Veterinary Therapy. Food Animal Practice II*. Philadelphia, W. B. Saunders Co., 1986, p. 448.

392. Thomas, G. W.: Pyrexia with dermatitis in dairy cows. Vet. Rec. 102:368, 1978.

393. Thomas, G. W.: Pyrexia with dermatitis in dairy cows. In Pract. 1:16, 1979.

394. Thomsett, L. R.: Noninfectious skin diseases of horses. Vet. Clin. North Am. Large Anim. Pract. 6:59, 1984.

395. Thornton, D. J.: Ganskweek (*Lasiospermum bipinnatum*) poisoning in cattle. J. S. Afr. Vet. Assoc. 48:210, 1977.

396. Thornton, R. H., and Percival, J. C.: Hepatotoxin from *S. bakeri* capable of producing facial eczema in sheep. Nature 183:63, 1959.

397. Tonder, E. M., et al.: Geeldikkop: Experimental induction by the plant *Tribulus terrestris* (*L. zygophyllaceae*). J. S. Afr. Vet. Assoc. 43:363, 1972.

398. Tonder, E. M., et al.: Discolouration of wool: I. Green discolouration. J. S. Afr. Vet. Assoc. 47:223, 1976.

399. Towers, N. R., and Smith, B. L.: The protective effect of zinc sulphate in experimental sporidesmin intoxication of lactating dairy cows. N.Z. Vet. J. 26:199, 1978.

399a. Traub-Dargatz, J. L., et al.: Selenium toxicity in horses. Compend. Cont. Educ. 8:771, 1986.

400. Turner, S. J., et al.: Pyrexia with dermatitis in dairy cows. Vet. Rec. 102:488, 1978.

401. Verweij, J. H. D.: Molybdeenovermaat bij het rund door luchtverontreiniging. Tijdschr. Diergeneeskd. 96:1508, 1971.

402. Vestweber, J. G. E., and Al-Ani, F. K.: Udder edema: Biochemical studies in Holstein cattle. Cornell Vet. 74:366, 1984.

402a. Vestweber, J. G. E., et al.: Udder edema in cattle: Effect of furosemide, hydrochlorothiazide, acetazolamide, or 50% dextrose on venous blood pressure. Am. J. Vet. Res. 48:673, 1987.

403. Wagener, K.: Hyperkeratosis of cattle in Germany. JAVMA 119:133, 1951.

404. Wahlstrom, R. C., et al.: The effect of arsanilic acid and 3-nitro-4-hydroxyphenylarsonic acid on selenium poisoning in the pig. J. Anim. Sci. 14:105, 1955.

405. Walker, K. H., and Kirkland, P. D.: *Senecio lautus* toxicity in cattle. Aust. Vet. J. 57:1, 1981.

406. Wass, W. M., and Hoyt, H. H.: Bovine congenital porphyria: Studies on heredity. Am. J. Vet. Res. 26:654, 1965.

407. Wass, W. M., and Hoyt, H. H.: Bovine congenital porphyria: Hematologic studies including porphyrin analyses. Am. J. Vet. Res. 26:659, 1965.

408. Watson, C. J., et al.: Some studies on the comparative biology of human and bovine erythropoietic porphyria. Arch. Intern. Med. 103:436, 1959.

409. Watts, J. E., et al.: The significance of certain skin characteristics of sheep in resistance and susceptibility to fleece rot and body strike. Aust. Vet. J. 56:57, 1980.

410. Watts, J. E., and Merritt, G. C.: Leakage of plasma proteins onto the skin surface of sheep during the development of fleece-rot and body strike. Aust. Vet. J. 57:98, 1981.

411. Watts, J. E., et al.: The ovopositional response of the Australian sheep blowfly *Lucilla cuprina* to fleece rot odors. Aust. Vet. J. 57:450, 1981.

412. Watts, J. E., et al.: Observations on fibre diameter variation of sheep in relation to fleece rot and body strike susceptibility. Aust. Vet. J. 57:372, 1981.

413. Webster, H. D., et al.: A note on vitamin-A therapy of hyperkeratosis. Michigan State Univ. Vet. 12:150, 1952.

414. Weaver, A. D.: Arsenic poisoning in cattle following pasture contamination by drift of spray. Vet. Rec. 74:249, 1962.

415. Weaver, G. A., et al.: Acute and chronic toxicity of T-2 mycotoxin in swine. Vet. Rec. 103:531, 1978.

415a. White, S. D.: Photosensitivity. *In*: Robinson, N. E. (ed.): *Current Therapy in Equine Medicine II*. Philadelphia, W. B. Saunders Co., 1986, p. 632.

416. Whittem, J. H., et al.: Bovine hyperkeratosis. Aust. Vet. J. 29:240, 1953.

417. Willett, L. B., and Durst, H. I.: Effects of PBBs on cattle. IV. Distribution and clearance of components of Five Master BP-6. Environ. Health Perspect. 23:67, 1978.

418. Williams, M., et al.: Induction of fescue foot syndrome in cattle by fractionated extracts of toxic fescue hay. Am. J. Vet. Res. 36:1353, 1975.

419. Witzel, D. A., et al.: Photosensitization in sheep fed *Ammi majus* (Bishop's weed seed). Am. J. Vet. Res. 39:319, 1978.

420. Woods, A. J., et al.: An outbreak of gangrenous ergotism in cattle. Vet. Rec. 78:742, 1966.

421. Wyllie, T. D., and Morehouse, L. G.: *Mycotoxic Fungi, Mycotoxins and Mycotoxicoses II*. New York, Marcel Dekker, Inc., 1978.

422. Yates, S. G., et al.: Detection of ergopeptine alkaloids in endophyte-infected, toxic Ky-31 tall fescue by mass spectrometry. J. Agric. Food Chem. 33:719, 1985.

CHAPTER 5

VIRAL DISEASES

Cutaneous lesions may be the only feature associated with a viral infection, or they may be part of a more generalized disease.* A clinical examination of the skin often provides valuable information that assists the veterinarian in the differential diagnosis of several viral disorders.

Many of the viral diseases discussed in this chapter do not normally occur in North America. However, to omit these diseases from consideration would be unwise. The continued freedom from major viral diseases in various areas of the world is contingent, in part, on the practicing veterinarian's recognizing them when they occur and promptly informing the appropriate veterinary authorities.

When collecting samples for the diagnosis of viral disease, it must be remembered that the clinician's suspicion that the disease is caused by a virus may be incorrect. Thus, samples should be collected for alternative diagnoses. Assuming that it is a viral disease, the following should be remembered:[106, 107, 130, 201] (1) The titer of virus is usually highest at affected sites and during the early stages of the disease, (2) viruses replicate only in living cells, and their stability is adversely affected by exposure to light, desiccation, extremes of pH, and most common disinfectants, (3) secondary bacterial or mycotic infection is a common sequela of viral disease; samples taken from the later stages of disease are less likely to contain virus.

To overcome the aforementioned problems, the samples should be protected by storage at 4°C in a virus transport medium. To avoid an erroneous or incomplete diagnosis, samples should be taken from different types of lesions and from more than one animal. When collecting a skin scraping or obtaining a biopsy for viral culture, the areas should be washed with water or saline, *not* with alcohol, as this inactivates most viruses. Scraping of the skin

and mucous membranes should be extended to the periphery and base of the lesion.

Electron microscopy is very useful in the rapid diagnosis of viral skin diseases,* but isolation of the causal virus in tissue culture is still the most widely used and most sensitive technique.

An in-depth discussion of all the viral diseases—especially their extracutaneous clinical signs and pathology and their elaborate diagnostic and control schemata—is beyond the scope of this chapter. We will concentrate on the dermatologic aspects of the diseases. The reader is referred to other excellent texts for detailed information on the extracutaneous aspects of these diseases.†

POXVIRUS INFECTIONS

The Poxviridae are a large family of DNA viruses that share group-specific nucleoprotein antigens.[23, 201, 302] The genera include Orthopoxvirus (cowpox and vaccinia), Capripoxvirus (sheep-pox, goatpox, and bovine lumpy skin disease), Suipoxvirus (swinepox), and Parapoxvirus (pseudocowpox, bovine papular stomatitis, and contagious viral pustular dermatitis). Some poxviruses—horsepox virus, the viruses of ovine viral ulcerative dermatosis, equine viral papular dermatitis, and molluscum contagiosum—remain unclassified.

Infection is usually acquired by cutaneous or respiratory routes. Poxviruses commonly gain access to the systemic circulation via the lymphatic system, although multiplication at the site of inoculation in the skin may lead to direct entry into the blood and a primary viremia. A secondary viremia disseminates the virus back to the skin and to other target organs.

---

*References 23, 77, 129, 130, 141, 142, 172, 191, 244, 253

*References 22, 54, 68, 111, 130, 131, 263
†References 23, 77, 129, 130, 141, 142, 172, 191, 244

Poxviruses induce lesions by a variety of mechanisms. Degenerative changes in epithelium are caused by virus replication and lead to vesicular lesions typical of many poxvirus infections. Degenerative changes in the dermis or subcutis may result from ischemia secondary to vascular damage. Poxvirus infections also induce proliferative lesions via epithelial hyperplasia. The host-cell DNA synthesis is stimulated before the onset of cytoplasmic virus-related DNA replication.

Pox lesions in the skin have a typical clinical evolution, beginning as erythematous macules and becoming papular, and then vesicular. The vesicular stage is well developed in some pox infections and transient or nonexistent in others. Vesicles evolve into umbilicated pustules with a depressed center and a raised, often erythematous, border. This lesion is the so-called pock. The pustules rupture and form a crust. Healed lesions often leave a scar.

Histologically, pox lesions begin with ballooning degeneration of the stratum spinosum of the epidermis (Fig. 5–1).[302] Reticular degeneration and acantholysis result in intraepidermal microvesicles. Dermal lesions include edema and a superficial and deep perivascular dermatitis. Mononuclear cells and neutrophils are present in varying proportions. Neutrophils migrate into the epidermis and produce intraepidermal microabscesses and pustules, which may extend into the dermis. There is usually marked irregular to pseudocarcinomatous epidermal hyperplasia. Poxvirus lesions contain characteristic intracytoplasmic inclusion bodies, which are single or multiple and of varying size and duration. The more prominent eosinophilic inclusions (3 to 7 μm in diameter) are called Type A and are weakly positive by the Feulgen method. They begin as small eosinophilic intracytoplasmic inclusions (Borrel's bodies) and evolve into a single, large body (Bollinger's body). The smaller basophilic inclusions are called Type B.

Diagnosis of poxvirus infections is usually based on observation of the typical clinical appearance and may be supported by characteristic histologic lesions. Demonstration of the virus by electron microscopy will confirm a poxvirus etiology but may not differentiate between morphologically similar viruses, such as the closely related orthopoxviruses. Definitive identification of specific viruses requires the isolation of the virus and its identification by serologic and immunofluorescence techniques.

Many of the poxviruses of large animals can produce skin lesions in humans: vaccinia, cowpox, goatpox, pseudocowpox, bovine papular stomatitis, horsepox, and contagious viral pustular dermatitis.* The most commonly zoo-

---

*References 15, 23, 24, 92, 108, 159, 168, 169, 179, 253, 271

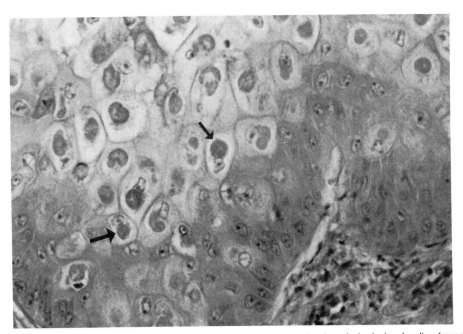

FIGURE 5–1. *Pseudocowpox. Ballooning degeneration and intracytoplasmic inclusion bodies (arrows).*

notic of these are contagious viral pustular dermatitis, pseudocowpox, and bovine papular stomatitis. In general, the clinical presentations of these diseases in humans are identical, and the presumptive diagnosis is usually made on the basis of known exposure to sheep, cattle, or goats. Because of this, it has been suggested that "farmyard pox" be used as a generic term for these human disorders, unless a more precise diagnosis is confirmed by laboratory testing.[263]

Contagious viral pustular dermatitis causes a condition in humans called ecthyma contagiosum, or "orf" (Fig. 5–2).* Humans having contact with sheep and goats (ranchers, sheep shearers, veterinarians, and veterinary students) are at risk. Transmission is by direct and indirect contact, and human-to-human transmission can occur.[290, 295] The incubation period is 4 to 14 days. Human skin lesions average 1.6 cm in diameter and usually occur singly, most commonly on a finger. However, multiple lesions or generalized eruptions can occur[3, 83, 92, 148, 263] as well as large epithelioma-like tumors, which have resulted in the finger's being amputated.[249, 263, 299] Solitary lesions may also occur on the face and legs. Regional

---

*References 16, 44, 92, 131, 133, 143, 155, 156, 164, 168, 180, 203, 204, 215, 220, 222, 227, 246, 253

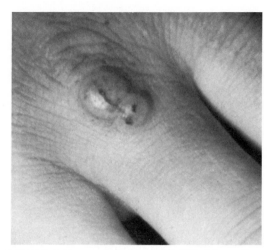

FIGURE 5–3. Human "milker's nodule." Nodule on finger after contact with a cow that had pseudocowpox.

lymphadenopathy is common, but fever, malaise, and lymphangitis are rare.

Skin lesions evolve through six stages and usually heal uneventfully in about 35 days. An elevated, erythematous papule evolves into a nodule with a red center, a white middle ring, and a red periphery. A red, weeping surface is present acutely. Later, a thin dry crust through which black dots may be seen covers the surface of the nodule. Finally, the lesion develops a papillomatous surface, a thick crust develops, and the lesion regresses. Pain and pruritus are variable.

Pseudocowpox and bovine papular stomatitis cause clinically indistinguishable syndromes in humans, called milker's nodule (Fig. 5–3).[67, 92, 96, 165, 169, 297] Humans having contact with cattle (veterinarians, veterinary students, dairy farmers, and milkers) are at risk. Transmission is by direct and indirect contact, and human-to-human transmission can occur.[270] The incubation period is 4 to 14 days. A typical human patient has a solitary, asymptomatic, or painful nodule 1 cm in diameter on the finger, hand, or forearm. Rarely, multiple lesions or lesions on other parts of the body may be seen.[92] Regional lymphadenopathy and signs of systemic illness are uncommon. The evolution and course of these lesions are identical to those previously described for contagious viral pustular dermatitis.

Vaccinia

Vaccinia is caused by an orthopoxvirus that is known to infect cattle, swine, horses, and humans.[23, 24, 77, 108, 159, 302] In cattle[24, 108, 166] and

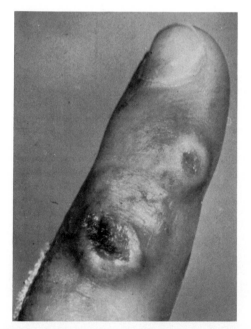

FIGURE 5–2. Human "orf." Two nodules on finger after contact with a goat that had contagious viral pustular dermatitis.

swine,[77, 172] vaccinia is clinically indistinguishable from cowpox and swinepox, respectively.

Vaccinia is caused by the virus propagated in laboratories and used for prophylactic vaccination against smallpox in humans. Infection is transmitted by contact from recently vaccinated humans to animals, whereupon it can be transmitted to other animals or susceptible humans. In view of the global eradication of smallpox, most countries of the world have now discontinued vaccination of their civilian population against the disease.

Cowpox

Cowpox, a rare disease of cattle in Europe, is caused by an orthopoxvirus.* The epidemiology of the disease is unclear. Cowpox virus is occasionally isolated from skin infections in both humans and carnivores with no history of direct contact with cattle, and it has been suggested that there exists a rodent or similar animal reservoir in which cowpox infection is probably subclinical. After the introduction of the virus into a susceptible herd of cattle, infection spreads rapidly, and within two to three weeks, the majority of the milking cattle may be affected. Transmission of the virus is probably by the teat cup of the milking machine and the milker's hands. The incubation period is about five days.

An irregular prodromal pyrexia and tenderness of the teats are followed by the typical cutaneous sequence of events leading to pocks. The classic thick, red crust, ranging in diameter from 1 to 2 cm, is said to be pathognomonic. In typical cases of cowpox, lesions are confined to the teats and udder. In severe cases, lesions may be seen on the medial thighs, perineum, vulva, scrotum of bulls, and mouth of nursing calves. In uncomplicated cases, healing takes place in about three weeks. Immunity to reinfection is said to be lifelong.

Identical clinical syndromes are produced by vaccinia and horsepox virus infections. In addition, cowpox virus may produce skin lesions in humans. Skin diseases of the bovine teat and udder are often of great economic concern and are a diagnostic challenge. The differential diagnosis of these conditions is presented in Table 5–1.

Sheep-Pox

Sheep-pox is caused by a capripoxvirus and is the most serious of the pox diseases of

TABLE 5–1. Differential Diagnosis of Bovine Teat and Udder Lesions

Viral
Vaccinia
Cowpox
Bovine lumpy skin disease
Pseudocowpox
Contagious viral pustular dermatitis
Horsepox
Bovine herpes mammillitis
Bovine pseudo–lumpy skin disease
Bovine herpes mammary pustular dermatitis
Malignant catarrhal fever
Foot-and-mouth disease
Vesicular stomatitis
Rinderpest
Blue-tongue
Papillomatosis

Bacterial
Staphylococcal impetigo
Dermatophilosis
Necrobacillosis
Atypical mycobacteriosis

Fungal
Dermatophytosis

Parasitic
Stephanofilariasis
Pelodera dermatitis
Trombiculidiasis
Chorioptic mange

Environmental
Contact dermatitis (e.g., environment, medicines)
Trauma (e.g., stepped-on teats, milking machine damage)
Thermal burns
Frostbite
Udder intertrigo
Photosensitization
Black pox
Chapping

domestic animals.* It occurs in Africa, Asia, and the Middle East, where despite attempts at vaccination, it is responsible for cycles of epidemic disease followed by periods of endemic disease with low morbidity. Sheep-pox causes severe economic losses through mortality; reduced meat, milk, and wool production; commercial inhibitions from quarantine; and the cost of disease-prevention programs. The virus is resistant to desiccation and remains viable for up to two months on wool or six months in dried crust. The incubation period is four to seven days.

There is considerable confusion and controversy surrounding the exact nosology of the sheep-pox virus.[23, 253] Sheep-pox and goatpox viruses are often considered host-specific.[23, 79,]

---

*References 23, 24, 101, 108, 128, 130, 302

*References 17, 20, 23, 130, 141, 191, 213, 214, 248, 265, 302

[81, 257, 260–262] In areas of the world where goats and sheep are herded together, however, there exist strains of virus that are *not* host-dependent.[66, 130, 260] Some investigators have suggested that, for the present, sheep-pox and goatpox be considered as caused by the same virus.[66, 130]

Sheep-pox occurs in sheep of all ages but is most severe in lambs, with morbidity reaching 75 percent and mortality reaching 80 percent. Initial clinical signs include pyrexia, depression, lacrimation, salivation, and serous nasal discharge. Skin lesions develop one to two days later, follow a typical pock evolutionary sequence, and have a predilection for the eyelids, cheeks, nostrils, ears, neck, axillae, groin, prepuce, vulva, udder, scrotum, and ventral surface of the tail. Healing takes up to six weeks. Goatpox virus infection in sheep resembles sheep-pox but is often more severe.[23]

Goatpox

Goatpox is a capripoxvirus infection of goats in Africa, Asia, parts of Europe, and the United States.* The exact nosology of the goatpox virus is controversial (see discussion on sheep-pox). Goats of all ages can be affected, but the disease is more severe in young animals. Morbidity may reach 90 percent, but mortality is usually less than 5 percent. The incubation period is 5 to 17 days.

Initial clinical signs include pyrexia, anorexia, conjunctivitis, and rhinitis. Skin lesions appear one to two days later, may or may not follow a typical pock evolutionary sequence, and have a predilection for the head, neck, ears, axillae, groin, perineum, and ventral surface of the tail. Some outbreaks are characterized by only muzzle and lip lesions, whereas others involve only the udder (Fig. 5–4), teats, scrotum, prepuce, perineum, and ventral tail. Healing usually takes place in three to four weeks. Typical poxlike lesions may develop on the hands and forearms of humans who come into contact with infected goats.[253, 271]

Bovine Lumpy Skin Disease

Lumpy skin disease *(knopvelsiekte)* is an acute to subacute infectious disease of cattle in Africa caused by a capripoxvirus (the "Neethling" poxvirus).† Although the precise

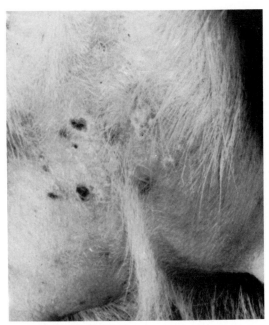

FIGURE 5–4. *Goatpox. Pocks on the udder of a goat from New York state.*

mechanism of transmission is uncertain, the theory that the disease is insect-borne is suggested by the facts that (1) the disease has the ability to traverse very long distances rapidly, (2) quarantine fails to curb the spread of the disease, (3) the disease tends to be seasonal and to coincide with the appearance of large insect populations, and (4) the virus can be isolated from *Stomoxys calcitrans*. The incubation period is about one to four weeks.

Cattle of all ages and breeds are susceptible. The initial clinical signs include pyrexia with or without lacrimation, nasal discharge, hypersalivation, and lameness. These signs are followed in about seven days by the sudden appearance of multiple papules and nodules and peripheral lymphadenopathy. The lesions, firm, well circumscribed, and flattened, are 0.5 to 5 cm in diameter and may be generalized or fairly localized. The neck, chest, back, legs, perineum, udder, and scrotum are commonly affected. Skin lesions may ulcerate. Edema of the legs and ventrum may be prominent. Although the skin lesions can persist for months to years, they usually proceed to necrosis and disappear within 4 to 12 weeks. A narrow moat forms around the lesions and separates them from normal skin. These so-called sitfasts then slough, leaving crateriform ulcers, which heal by scarring.

Morbidity varies from 5 to 90 percent, and mortality is usually low (less than 2 percent).

---

*References 11, 17, 20, 23, 79, 130, 162, 237, 240, 253, 257, 260–262, 275, 302

†References 4, 23, 41, 42, 130, 140, 170, 171, 218, 278, 294, 302

Economic losses are usually high, as a result of decreased milk production, loss of body condition, damage to hides, and abortions. Recovered cattle possess solid immunity for several months.

Diagnosis is based on history, physical examination, skin biopsy, and viral isolation. Early in the disease, skin biopsy results are characterized by vasculitis and lymphangitis with thrombosis and infarction; later fibrosing dermatitis is characteristic.[21, 34, 236, 302] Eosinophilic intracytoplasmic inclusion bodies are found in keratinocytes, macrophages, endothelial cells, pericytes, fibroblasts, and the glandular and ductal epithelial cells of apocrine sweat glands.

There is no specific treatment. Systemic antibiotics are indicated for secondary bacterial infections, and fly-strike must be prevented. Vaccination with sheep-pox virus or with modified Neethling virus is effective.

Swinepox

Swinepox occurs world wide and is endemic to areas of intensive swine production.* The

---

*References 22, 23, 49, 61, 63, 64, 77, 130, 153, 157, 172, 185, 196, 198, 219, 252, 289, 302

chief cause is a suipoxvirus; the vaccinia virus causes an identical syndrome. Swine of all ages are affected, but the disease is most common in young piglets. Neonatal piglets can be affected via transplacental infection. Morbidity may be high, but mortality is negligible. Because the disease causes very little economic loss, relatively little attention is paid to its elimination. The virus persists in dried crusts for at least one year, and once swinepox is introduced into a herd, the infection is maintained indefinitely. The hog louse *Haematopinus suis* and probably other biting insects and arthropods often act as mechanical vectors and initiators of skin trauma. The incubation period is two to six days.

Signs of systemic illness are rarely seen. Skin lesions follow the typical gross pock sequence and occur most commonly on the ventrolateral abdomen and thorax (Fig. 5–5) and the medial thighs and forelegs. Occasionally, lesions are seen on the back, sides, face (Fig. 5–6), udder, and teats. Healing usually occurs within two to four weeks. Recovery is followed by lifelong immunity. Swine that have recovered from suipoxvirus infection are still susceptible to vaccinia virus infection, and the converse is true of swine that have recovered from vaccinia infection. Suipoxvirus does *not* produce skin lesions in humans, but vaccinia virus does.

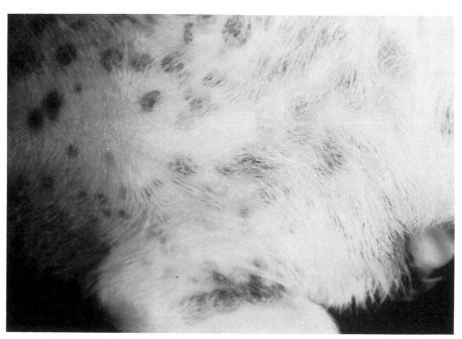

FIGURE 5–5. Swinepox. Umbilicated papules and pustules on ventral thorax.

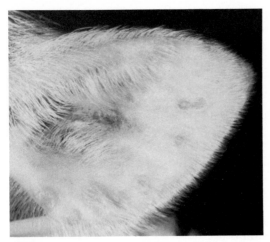

FIGURE 5–6. Swinepox. Umbilicated pustules on the pinna.

Pseudocowpox

Pseudocowpox is a common parapoxvirus infection of cattle throughout the world.* The virus appears to confer little persistent immunity, and cyclic waves of reinfection occur within a herd, frequently coinciding with muddy fall and spring months or with calving. At any time of the year, at least one or two cows within a previously affected herd will show clinical lesions of pseudocowpox, and it is probable that reinfection of the herd originates from these animals. Morbidity is about 100 percent, but usually only 5 to 10 percent of the cows are affected at any one time. Cattle of all ages are affected, and milking cows and heifers are most susceptible. In most herds, pseudocowpox appears to cause little inconvenience and is frequently overlooked. Most economic losses are associated with difficulty in milking and an increased incidence of mastitis. The incubation period is about six days.

The clinical appearance of pseudocowpox is extremely variable. There are no systemic signs of illness. Typically, the first clinical signs are focal edema, erythema, and pain of affected teats. In contrast with cowpox, bovine herpes mammillitis, and vaccinia, vesicle formation is uncommon in pseudocowpox. About 48 hours later, a small orange papule (2 to 3 mm in diameter) develops, followed by the formation of a dark-red crust (2 to 7 mm in diameter). The edges of the lesions extend peripherally, and the central crust may appear umbilicated. Peripheral extension of the lesion continues,

and the central area of the crust begins to desquamate (10 to 12 days after the onset of signs), leaving a slightly raised crust commonly called a ring or horseshoe scab (see Plate 2 *F*). This type of crust is said to be pathognomonic for pseudocowpox and can invariably be observed in an infected herd. Ulceration is rare. Healing takes place in about six weeks. Lesions occur on the teats and udder and, occasionally, the medial thighs and perineum. Parapoxvirus infection has also been reported on the scrotum of bulls.[84]

Pseudocowpox virus also causes skin lesions in humans (see discussion on poxvirus infections).

Bovine Papular Stomatitis

Bovine papular stomatitis is a cosmopolitan infectious disease of cattle caused by a parapoxvirus.* Cattle of all breeds and ages are affected, although the disease is generally more common in animals younger than one year of age. Morbidity varies from 10 to 100 percent, but mortality is rare. The incubation period is three to five days. The disease is usually of limited economic significance.

Initial lesions are erythematous macules, which evolve into papules. These papules then undergo central necrosis and become encrusted and often papillomatous. Lesions occur most commonly on the muzzle, nostrils, and lips (see Plate 3 *A*) and occasionally on the sides, abdomen, hind legs, scrotum, and prepuce. Cows nursing infected calves may develop teat lesions. Lesions may persist for weeks to months. Affected animals are otherwise healthy. Bovine papular stomatitis has also been incriminated as the cause of the so-called rat-tail syndrome in cattle.[28, 136]

Diagnosis is based on history, physical examination, skin biopsy,[117, 246] and viral isolation. Because of the mild nature of the disease, treatment is seldom required.

Bovine papular stomatitis virus also causes skin lesions (milker's nodules), especially on the fingers and hands, of humans, which are identical to those caused by the pseudocowpox and contagious viral pustular dermatitis viruses[23, 25, 45, 130, 216, 251] (see discussion on poxvirus infections).

Contagious Viral Pustular Dermatitis

Contagious viral pustular dermatitis (contagious ecthyma, contagious pustular dermatitis,

---

*References 7, 23, 48, 102, 108, 130, 132, 139, 144, 165, 205, 245, 302

*References 23, 95, 107, 115–117, 130, 146, 269

soremouth, "scabby mouth," orf) is a cosmopolitan disease of sheep and goats, and occasionally cattle, caused by a parapoxvirus.* It may cause significant economic loss through loss of condition (failure to suck or graze), mastitis, abandonment, and related deaths. Morbidity may reach 90 percent, but mortality rarely exceeds 1 percent, unless secondary infection or myiasis intervenes. The virus can overwinter in crusts and can survive in a laboratory environment at room temperature for 20 years. The disease tends to be seasonal, being most common during the lambing and kidding season and occurring within two weeks of the animal's entering a feedlot. The incubation period is 3 to 14 days.

Contagious viral pustular dermatitis is primarily a disease of lambs and kids of three to six months of age. Signs of systemic illness may include decreased feed consumption, depression, and pyrexia. Lesions usually occur on the lips, muzzle (Fig. 5–7), nostrils, and eyelids. In severe cases, they may be seen on the genitals, perineum, coronets, interdigital spaces, pasterns, fetlocks, and oral cavity. Lesions may be noted at the sites of injury, such as ear markings and tail dockings, and may also occur on the teats and udders of nursing ewes and does as well as the teats and udders of cattle. Skin lesions follow a typical pock progression but are quite proliferative. Oral mucosal lesions are raised, red or gray foci with a surrounding zone of hyperemia. Healing

usually takes place within four weeks. Recovery commonly produces a solid immunity for two to three years, but reinfection may occur within one year. However, no protective antibodies are passed in the colostrum, so that the newborn of immune dams are susceptible.

Horsepox

Horsepox is a rare benign disease of horses in Europe caused by an unclassified poxvirus.[23, 72, 80, 159, 302, 305] The horsepoxvirus is antigenically similar to the cowpoxvirus and causes lesions in cattle and humans. Three clinical expressions of the disease are described: (1) oral lesions (buccal horsepox, contagious pustular stomatitis), (2) pastern and fetlock lesions (leg horsepox, grease-heel, Jenner's horsepox), and (3) vulvar lesions (genital horsepox, coital exanthema). Cutaneous and mucosal lesions are characterized by vesicles, umbilicated pustules, and crusts. Occasional horses may have mild pyrexia, and horses with leg lesions may be lame. Most horses recover within two to four weeks. Recovery results in long-term immunity.

Ovine Viral Ulcerative Dermatosis

Viral ulcerative dermatosis (ovine venereal disease, lip and leg ulceration, infectious balanoposthitis, ulcerative vulvitis, "pizzle rot") is a cosmopolitan infectious disease of sheep caused by an unclassified poxvirus.* Transmis-

---

*References 1, 2, 6, 8, 16, 23, 27, 32, 33, 97, 113, 118, 119, 125, 130, 141, 177, 178, 181, 191, 223, 243, 253, 258, 288, 292, 296, 302

---

*References 23, 91, 93. 130, 141, 181, 191, 242, 272, 282–285, 291, 302

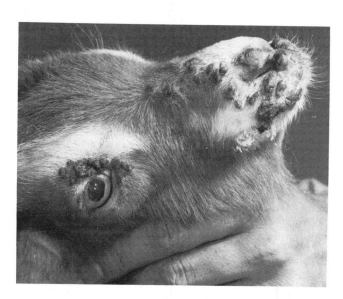

FIGURE 5–7. Contagious viral pustular dermatitis in a kid. Crusts around eye, muzzle, and lips.

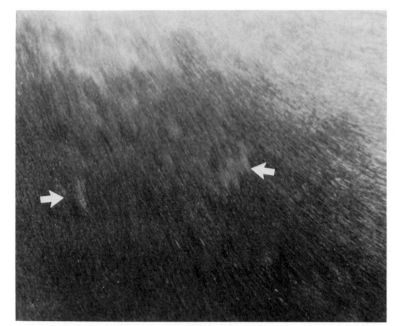

FIGURE 5–8. Equine viral papular dermatitis. Papules (arrows) on lateral thorax.

sion is by direct and indirect contact, especially during breeding, through scarified skin. The incubation period is two to seven days. Morbidity varies from 20 to 60 percent, and mortality is low if the sheep are in good health. Economic losses are usually minor. In the United States, the disease is most common in the western mountain regions.

Sheep of all ages and breeds are susceptible. The balanoposthitis-vulvitis form of the disease is most commonly seen in fall, during the breeding season. Lesions consist of granulating ulcers containing pus, adherent crusts, and edema. The lip and leg ulcer form is most commonly seen in winter. Granulating ulcers, 1 to 5 cm in diameter, containing pus and adherent crusts are present in the skin between the upper lips and nostrils, on the craniolateral aspects of the feet above the coronets, and interdigitally. Affected animals may be lame. Lesions often heal, with scarring alopecia, after a two- to six-week course.

The major differential diagnosis is contagious viral pustular dermatitis, which is characterized by proliferative lesions with thick crusts, as opposed to ulcerative lesions with thin crusts. Skin biopsy reveals an ulcerative perivascular dermatitis with ballooning degeneration and eosinophilic intracytoplasmic inclusion bodies.

Therapy is symptomatic and supportive. Infection produces a low-grade immunity, which lasts about five months. Control consists of good hygienic measures.

Equine Viral Papular Dermatitis

Viral papular dermatitis (uasin gishu disease) has been reported in horses in the United States, Australia, New Zealand, and Africa.[23, 135, 150–152, 194, 208] It is caused by an unclassified poxvirus resembling cowpox and vaccinia viruses. Horses of all ages and breeds are susceptible, and the incubation period is about seven days. Transmission presumably occurs via direct and indirect contact through scarified skin.

Clinically, viral papular dermatitis is characterized by asymptomatic papules over most of the body (Fig. 5–8), except for the head. The papules develop a crust within about seven days and then annular alopecia and scaling after about 14 days. The course of the disease varies from two to six weeks. Affected horses are otherwise healthy.

The differential diagnosis includes staphylococcal folliculitis, dermatophytosis, dermatophilosis, and demodicosis. Definitive diagnosis is based on history, physical examination, skin biopsy, and viral culture. Skin biopsy reveals hyperplastic superficial and deep perivascular dermatitis with ballooning degeneration and eosinophilic intracytoplasmic inclusion bodies.[152, 302] Mononuclear cells and plasma cells are the predominant inflammatory infiltrates.

There is no specific treatment. The disease is asymptomatic and self limiting.

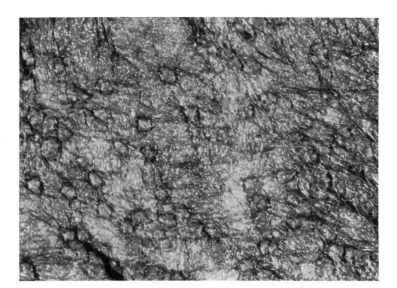

FIGURE 5–9. *Molluscum contagiosum in a horse. Multiple waxy papules in the inguinal area. (Courtesy J. A. Yager.)*

Equine Molluscum Contagiosum

Molluscum contagiosum is a mildly contagious, self-limited cutaneous infection of horses and humans caused by an unclassified poxvirus.[92, 238, 302] In horses, lesions occur on the penis, prepuce, scrotum, udder, groin, axillae, and muzzle. Initial lesions are multiple, well-circumscribed, raised, smooth, gray-white papules (Fig. 5–9), 1 to 2 mm in diameter, with a waxy surface. With time, the papules become umbilicated and develop a central pore, from which a tiny caseous plug is extruded.

Histopathologic findings in molluscum contagiosum are pathognomonic. There is well-demarcated epidermal hyperplasia and hypertrophy (Fig. 5–10). Individual keratinocytes are markedly swollen and contain large intracytoplasmic inclusions called molluscum bodies (Fig. 5–11). These occur initially as eosinophilic, floccular aggregations in the cells of the lower stratum spinosum. As the keratinocytes move toward the surface of the epidermis, these inclusions grow in size and density, compressing the cell nucleus against the cytoplasmic membrane until it is a thin crescent. Inclusions become increasingly basophilic, so

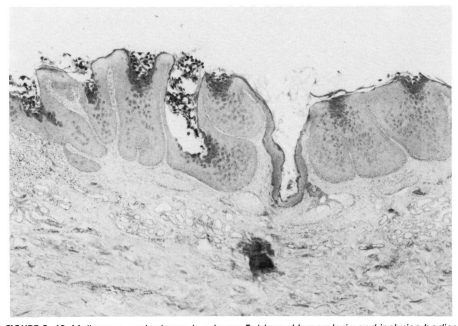

FIGURE 5–10. *Molluscum contagiosum in a horse. Epidermal hyperplasia and inclusion bodies.*

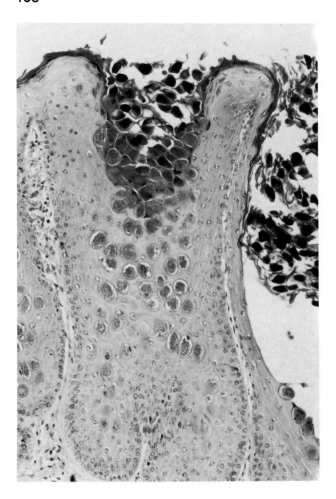

FIGURE 5–11. *Molluscum contagiosum in a horse. Intracytoplasmic inclusions ("molluscum bodies").*

that cells of the stratum corneum contain deep-purple molluscum bodies. These exfoliate through a pore that forms in the stratum corneum and enlarges into a central crater. Usually, there is no dermal reaction.

HERPESVIRUS INFECTIONS

Infectious Bovine Rhinotracheitis

Infectious bovine rhinotracheitis (infectious pustular vulvovaginitis, "rednose") is a worldwide infectious disease of cattle caused by bovine herpesvirus 1.[23, 39, 107, 130, 146] Transmission occurs by direct contact and aerosol. Cutaneous lesions include erythema, pustules, necrosis, and ulceration of the muzzle or the vulva, or both. Rarely, pustules, crusts, oozing, alopecia, and lichenification may be seen in the perineal (Fig. 5–12) and scrotal areas.

Biopsy reveals hyperplastic superficial and deep perivascular dermatitis with ballooning degeneration and epidermal necrosis.[146] Neutrophils are the predominant inflammatory cell. Cowdry's Types A and B intranuclear inclusions may be seen in epithelial cells at the periphery of lesions.

Bovine Dermatotropic Herpesviruses

A dermatotropic herpesvirus, bovine herpesvirus 2, causes two cutaneous syndromes in cattle: (1) bovine herpes mammillitis and (2) pseudo-lumpy skin disease. The factors that determine how this virus will express itself clinically in any given outbreak are unknown. In addition, bovine herpesvirus 4 has been associated with the syndrome of bovine herpes mammary pustular dermatitis.[23, 239]

Bovine Herpes Mammillitis. Bovine herpes mammillitis (bovine ulcerative mammillitis) has been reported from most parts of the world.* The exact mode of transmission is

---

*References 23, 70, 102–105, 108, 130, 173, 186–190, 234, 247, 286, 287, 293, 302

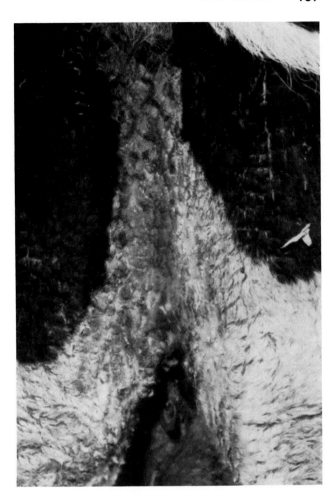

FIGURE 5–12. Infectious bovine rhinotracheitis. Crusting of the perineum and caudomedial thighs.

unclear, because (1) the disease is usually seasonal (summer and fall) and (2) exceptional efforts at hygiene and quarantine fail to curb the spread of the condition within a herd; however, it is presumed that transmission occurs via insects. It is also believed that some cattle become virus carriers and, under stress, shed infective virus. The incubation period is about three to seven days.

Bovine herpes mammillitis affects cows in milk, and heifers tend to be more severely affected than adult cows. Two epidemiologic patterns exist: (1) a disease that spreads rapidly through the majority of the herd, (2) a disease confined to newly calved heifers introduced to the herd for the first time.

Most cattle show no systemic illness. Skin lesions may be confined to one teat or involve several and may extend to the udder and perineum. Classically, the disease is sudden in onset, with swollen, tender teats. Vesicles may appear in a few hours, but in many cases, the epithelium simply sloughs and exposes an in-flamed dermis. Once the epithelium has sloughed, there is copious exudation of serum and extensive crust formation. At this stage, the painful lesions of severely affected animals cause them to refuse milking and nursing calves. The severity of the dermatitis varies from (1) lines of erythema, often in circles, which enclose dry skin or papules with occasional ulceration, to (2) annular red to blue plaques, which evolve into shallow ulcers, 0.5 to 2 cm in diameter, to (3) large areas of bluish discoloration, necrosis, slough, ulceration, and serum exudation. Rarely, suckling calves develop similar lesions on the muzzle and in the mouth.

Morbidity varies from 18 to 96 percent, but mortality is negligible. However, economic losses are severe, as a result of decreased milk production and an increased incidence of mastitis.

Diagnosis is based on history, physical examination, viral isolation, and serology.[23, 130, 302] Skin biopsy reveals hyperplastic superficial and deep perivascular dermatitis.[302] Epidermal syncytial-cell formation commences early in the stratum basale and the stratum spinosum and tends to involve the entire epidermis and the hair follicle outer root sheath. Prominent eosinophilic intranuclear inclusion bodies (Cowdry's Type A: nuclear chromatin is marginated, eosinophilic inclusions are surrounded by a clear halo) are numerous for only five days after the macroscopic lesion appears. Afterwards, the epidermis becomes necrotic and ulceration occurs.

There is no specific treatment. Routine isolation and hygienic procedures are recommended but appear to have little effect on the spread of the disease. Symptomatic treatments may include various topical agents—astringent or antiseptic soaks or emollient, antibiotic, or anesthetic creams and ointments—as indicated. Healing usually occurs within two to three weeks in mild cases but may take three months in severe cases. Recovered animals appear to have long-standing immunity, and various vaccination techniques have shown promise experimentally.[23]

Bovine Pseudo–Lumpy Skin Disease. Pseudo–lumpy skin disease has been reported in cattle throughout the world and is also caused by bovine herpesvirus 2 (the Allerton virus).* This disorder occurs in both dairy and beef cattle and is milder than true lumpy skin disease. Cutaneous lesions are similar in distribution and appearance to those of true lumpy skin disease but are located much more superficially in the skin (slightly raised plaques with a central depression and superficial necrosis). Regional lymphadenopathy and signs of systemic illness are absent. The experimental intravenous inoculation of bovine herpesvirus 2 into susceptible cattle or calves produces pyrexia, depression, peripheral lymphadenopathy, and widespread cutaneous plaques, 2 to 4 cm in diameter, with superficial epidermal necrosis.[47, 122, 173] The clinical course of pseudo–lumpy skin disease is similar to that previously described for bovine herpes mammillitis.

Diagnosis is based on history, physical examination, viral isolation, and serology. Skin biopsy reveals hydropic interface dermatitis with epidermal keratinocyte syncytial formation and eosinophilic intranuclear inclusion bodies within keratinocytes of the stratum spinosum.

Bovine Herpes Mammary Pustular Dermatitis. Bovine herpesvirus 4 has been isolated from a mammary pustular dermatitis in Holstein-Friesian cattle from the midwestern United States.[23, 127a, 239, 302] Lesions were seen only in lactating cows and were more numerous and severe in heifers. Lesions consisted of multiple vesicles and pustules, 1 to 10 mm in diameter, on the lateral and ventral aspects of the udder. The teats were not involved. In general, clinical signs were mild, and economic losses insignificant.

Biopsies revealed intraepidermal pustular dermatitis, necrotic keratinocytes, and a predominance of neutrophils. Viral isolation and serologic studies showed that the causative herpesvirus was indistinguishable from the DN599 strain of bovine herpesvirus previously isolated from cattle with respiratory tract disease.

Concern was expressed over the possible human health hazard of this bovine herpesvirus. A woman who washed udders of infected cows developed a pustule on a mildly lacerated finger. Over the next two weeks, numerous vesicles, 1 to 6 mm in diameter, occurred over the extremities and were particularly numerous on the ankles, hands, and between the toes. Unfortunately, viral isolation and serologic studies were not performed on the woman.

Bovine Malignant Catarrhal Fever

Malignant catarrhal fever (malignant head catarrh, *snotsiekte*) is a sporadic, acute, highly fatal systemic disease of cattle in most parts of the world.* The disease exists in at least two forms. The wildebeest-associated form in Africa is a result of bovine herpesvirus 3.[130, 134, 146, 232, 233] The sheep-associated form seen throughout the world is assumed to be caused by a virus, and many candidates have been isolated (syncytial virus, herpesvirus, togavirus, and enterovirus), but the precise etiology is undetermined.[57, 86, 134, 146, 149, 228] The incubation period is 18 to 73 days.

Cutaneous lesions include erythema, scaling, necrosis, and ulceration of the muzzle and face and, occasionally, the udder, teats, vulva, and scrotum (see Plate 3 *B–E*). In addition, purplish discolorations, papules, crusts, thickening, oozing, and necrosis may affect the skin in the perineal, axillary, inguinal, and back regions. Similar dermatologic lesions may occur at the coronet, horn-skin junction, and caudal pastern area and may result in sloughing of hooves or horns.

---

*References 5, 23, 62, 108, 112, 130, 173, 273, 302, 303

*References 18, 23, 65, 130, 134, 138, 146, 149, 228, 229, 256

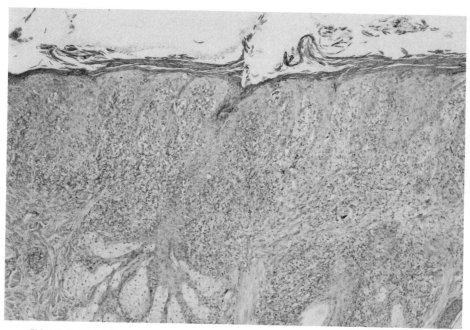

FIGURE 5–13. Malignant catarrhal fever. Hydropic and lichenoid interface dermatitis.

Skin biopsy reveals (1) hydropic and lichenoid interface dermatitis with single-cell necrosis (satellite cell necrosis) (Figs. 5–13 and 5–14) and (2) lymphohistiocytic vasculitis.[19, 146, 174–176, 256]

Equine Herpes Coital Exanthema

Equine herpes coital exanthema, a contagious venereal disease of horses in most parts of the world, is caused by equine herpesvirus 3.* In addition to transmission by coitus, transmission may also occur via insects, fomites, and inhalation. The incubation period is about seven days.

Initial lesions are papules, vesicles, and pustules, 1 to 3 mm in diameter, or larger bullae

*References 9, 23, 24a, 30, 31, 38, 58, 73, 85, 137, 161, 195, 224, 225, 264a, 274, 277

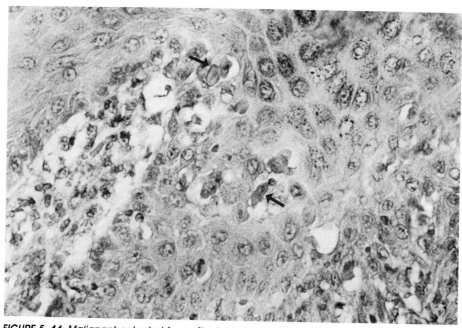

FIGURE 5–14. Malignant catarrhal fever. Single-cell necrosis of epidermal keratinocytes (arrows).

on the vulva and perineum of the mare and the penis and prepuce of the stallion. Occasionally, vesicles are found in the mouth or nostrils and on the lips. Primary lesions are usually accompanied by edema and evolve into erosions and ulcers that become encrusted. Lesions may be pruritic but are not usually painful. Macular areas of depigmentation may persist where lesions have healed. Some mares and stallions seem particularly susceptible to spontaneous or stress-related disease recurrences.

The differential diagnosis includes other genital infections, bullous pemphigoid, and horsepox. Diagnosis is based on history, physical examination, skin biopsy, and virus isolation. Biopsy reveals hyperplastic superficial and deep perivascular dermatitis with ballooning degeneration and eosinophilic intranuclear inclusion bodies (Figs. 5–15 and 15–16). The preferred treatment is abstinence from coitus for three to four weeks. Topical ointments or creams—containing emollients, antibiotics, glucocorticoids, or local anesthetics—may be used as indicated.

Pseudorabies

Pseudorabies (Aujeszky's disease, "mad itch") is an acute, rapidly fatal (24 to 72 hours) herpesvirus infection that is worldwide in distribution.* It is primarily a disease of pigs but

*References 10, 23, 77, 130, 134, 142, 149, 172, 300

occurs incidentally in most species. In ruminants and occasionally in swine, pseudorabies causes an intense, localized, unilateral pruritus with frenzied, violent licking, chewing, rubbing, and kicking at the affected area. Any part of the body may be affected, especially the head, neck, thorax, flanks, and perineum. Severe excoriations are produced, often resulting in full-thickness cutaneous defects.

The site of the itch is determined by the site of viral infection in spinal ganglia, sensory neurons of the dorsal horns, and brain stem. As neurons of the sensory ganglia degenerate, a sensation of itch is provoked in the skin innervated by these fibers.

TOGAVIRUS INFECTIONS

Equine Viral Arteritis

Equine viral arteritis is recognized in many parts of the world and is caused by a pestivirus (Togaviridae) having different strains and producing variably severe clinical signs.* Transmission occurs via coitus and inhalation. In the United States, Standardbreds are particularly affected. Clinical signs include edema of the distal limbs, scrotum, sheath, and ventrum. Histologic examination of affected tissues reveals focal or segmental fibrinoid necrosis of the media of small muscular arteries.[60, 146] A

*References 23, 53, 60, 76, 146, 193, 280

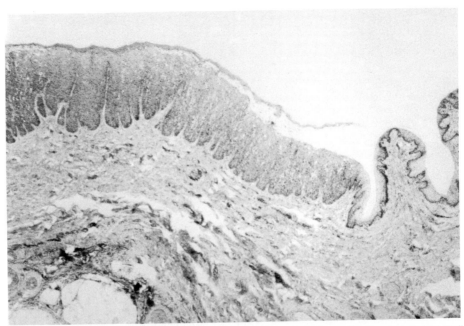

FIGURE 5–15. Equine herpes coital exanthema. Epidermal hyperplasia and ballooning degeneration.

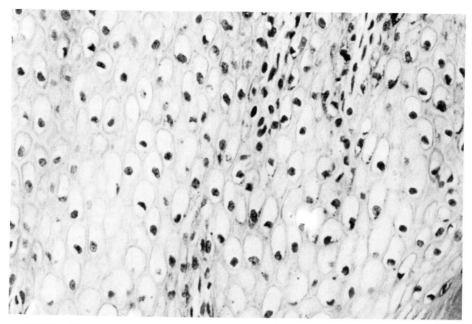

FIGURE 5–16. Equine herpes coital exanthema. Ballooning degeneration of keratinocytes.

leukocytic infiltrate is composed chiefly of lymphocytes, many of which show leukocytoclasis.

Hog Cholera

Hog cholera (swine fever, *Schweinepest, peste du porc*) is a highly infectious disease of swine caused by a pestivirus (Togaviridae).[23, 77, 130, 146] Although the disease has been eradicated in North America, the United Kingdom, and Australia, it remains a problem in South America, parts of Europe, Asia, and Africa. Transmission occurs via ingestion and inhalation.

Early cutaneous lesions consist of erythema and then purplish discoloration of the abdomen, snout, ears, and medial thighs. Areas of necrosis may develop on the pinnae, tail, and vulva. Chronically diseased swine develop a characteristic purplish blotching of the pinnae (Fig. 5–17) and generalized hypotrichosis. In utero infection of fetal swine may result in congenital alopecia.[43]

Biopsy reveals a leukocytoclastic vasculitis with edema, purpura, and thrombosis.[75, 77, 146]

Bovine Virus Diarrhea

Bovine virus diarrhea (mucosal disease) is a worldwide infectious disease of cattle caused by a pestivirus (Togaviridae).[23, 108, 130, 142, 146, 149] Transmission is by direct contact and inhala-

tion of aerosol. Cutaneous lesions begin as discrete erosions, which may coalesce and lead to necrosis of the muzzle, lips, and nostrils. Similar lesions may be present on the vulva, prepuce, coronet, and interdigital space. Occasionally, crusts, scales, and alopecia occur on the perineum, medial thighs, and neck. Infection of the bovine fetus before 150 days of gestation may result in multifocal skin necrosis or a generalized hypotrichosis that spares the head, tail, and distal limbs.[23, 46, 154]

Skin biopsy may reveal hydropic interface dermatitis with single-cell and segmental epidermal necrosis or follicular dystrophy.[46, 146, 154]

Ovine Border Disease

Border disease is a congenital infectious disease of sheep reported in most parts of the world.[23, 130, 146] The disease, caused by a pestivirus (Togaviridae), results in an abnormal fleece ("hairy shakers," "fuzzies") and frequently a darkly pigmented area of fleece on the back of the neck (see Chapter 11 for details).

PICORNAVIRUS INFECTIONS

Foot-and-Mouth Disease

Foot-and-mouth disease (aphthous fever) is a highly contagious infectious disease of cattle,

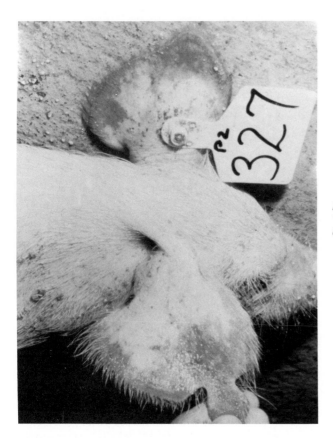

FIGURE 5-17. Hog cholera. Characteristic "blotching" of the pinnae in chronic disease. (Courtesy J. M. King.)

sheep, goats, and swine.* It is caused by an aphthovirus (Picornaviridae), which has at least seven principal antigenic types (A, O, C, SAT 1, SAT 2, SAT 3, and Asia 1), several antigenic subtypes, and variable virulence. The disease is endemic in Africa, Asia, Europe, and South America but has not been reported in the United States since 1929. Transmission occurs by contact, aerosol, and insect vectors. The incubation period is two to seven days.

Clinical signs include vesicles and bullae, which rupture to leave painful erosions in the mouth and on the muzzle, nostrils, coronet, interdigital spaces, udder, and teats. Occasionally, hooves may be sloughed. Healing is usually complete within two to three weeks, unless secondary bacterial infection intervenes. Morbidity varies from 50 to 100 percent, but mortality is usually low (less than 5 percent).

Biopsy reveals hyperplastic superficial and deep perivascular dermatitis with marked intra- and intercellular edema within the stratum spinosum.[146, 230, 304] Reticular degeneration, spongiotic microvesicles, acantholysis, and ne-

crosis of keratinocytes follow. Inflammatory cells include neutrophils, lymphocytes, and macrophages.

Vesicular Exanthema

Vesicular exanthema is an acute infectious disease of swine caused by a calicivirus (Picornaviridae).* The disease has not been reported in the United States since 1959. However, a similar if not identical virus (San Miguel Sea Lion virus), which occurs in marine fish, sea lions, and fur seals, causes a syndrome identical to vesicular exanthema when inoculated into swine.[23, 77, 146, 250, 266] Most outbreaks of vesicular exanthema were associated with feeding of raw garbage containing marine products or pork waste. The incubation period is one and one-half to three days.

Clinical signs include vesicles and painful erosions on the snout, legs, oral mucosa, coronet, interdigital spaces, and occasionally the udder and teats. Healing occurs within two weeks. Biopsy reveals hyperplastic superficial and deep perivascular dermatitis with marked

---

*References 23, 77, 78, 98, 108, 127, 130, 146, 191, 197, 199, 255, 259

*References 13, 23, 59, 77, 146, 184, 281, 298

intra- and intercellular epidermal edema.[77, 146] Reticular degeneration, spongiotic vesicles, and epidermal necrosis follow.

Swine Vesicular Disease

Swine vesicular disease is an acute infectious disease of swine in Africa, Asia, and parts of Europe caused by an enterovirus (Picornaviridae).* Transmission occurs via ingestion and direct contact. Vesicles and erosions are seen on the snout, lips, coronet, and occasionally the belly and legs.

Biopsy reveals hyperplastic superficial and deep perivascular dermatitis with marked intra- and intercellular epidermal edema.[52, 77, 146] Reticular degeneration and spongiotic vesicles are followed by epidermal necrosis. The infiltrate is mixed, containing neutrophils, eosinophils, and mononuclear cells.

MISCELLANEOUS VIRAL INFECTIONS

Vesicular Stomatitis

Vesicular stomatitis ("sore nose," "sore mouth"), an infectious disease of horses, swine, and cattle, is enzootic in North, Central, and South America.† It is caused by a vesiculovirus (Rhabdoviridae), which has two major serologic types (New Jersey and Indiana). The disease has a seasonal occurrence (summer and fall) and is believed to be transmitted by biting insects. Morbidity varies from 10 to 95 percent, but mortality is rare. The incubation period is one to three days.

Vesicles progress rapidly to painful erosions of the oral cavity, lips, muzzle, feet, and occasionally the prepuce, udder, and teats. Depigmentation may be seen in healed areas; healing usually occurs in two weeks. Rarely, hooves may be sloughed. Biopsy reveals hyperplastic superficial and deep perivascular dermatitis with marked intra- and intercellular edema of the epidermis.[50, 51, 146, 235, 241] Reticular degeneration, spongiotic microvesicles, and necrosis follow. Neutrophils are the major inflammatory cell.

Vesicular stomatitis virus can also cause disease in humans, which is characterized by influenza-like symptoms and occasional mucocutaneous vesicles and erosions.[88, 90, 123, 264]

Rinderpest

Rinderpest (cattle plague) is an acute, highly contagious systemic disease of ruminants and swine in Africa and Asia.* The causative agent is a morbillivirus (Paramyxoviridae) having many strains. Transmission occurs via direct and indirect contact and inhalation of aerosol. Cutaneous changes are characterized by erythema, papules, oozing, crusts, and alopecia over the perineum, flanks, medial thighs, neck, scrotum, udder, and teats. Occasionally, a generalized exfoliative dermatitis is seen.

Biopsy reveals hydropic interface dermatitis with single-cell necrosis and multinucleate syncytial formation within the epithelium.[146, 192]

Blue-Tongue

Blue-tongue is an insect-borne infectious disease of sheep, goats, and cattle throughout the world caused by an orbivirus (Reoviridae).† There are over 20 serotypes of the virus, and *Culicoides variipennis* is a major vector in the United States.

Sheep and goats develop erythema, edema, and occasionally ulceration of the muzzle, lips, and oral mucosa. In addition, some animals develop coronitis and lameness, with a dark-red to purple band in the skin above the coronet. Occasionally, cracking and separation of the hooves may be seen.

Cattle develop edema, dryness, cracking, and peeling of the muzzle and lips. Ulceration and crusting may be seen on the udder and teats. The neck, chest, flanks, back, and perineum may become scaly, wrinkled, alopecic, and fissured and may develop areas of moist superficial dermatitis.

Biopsy reveals a hyperplastic superficial perivascular dermatitis with ballooning degeneration and epidermal necrosis.[146, 182, 279] Superficial dermal blood vessels are dilated, engorged, often thrombosed, and surrounded by an infiltrate of neutrophils and mononuclear cells.

African Swine Fever

African swine fever is a peracute, fatal, highly contagious iridovirus infection of swine in Africa and Europe.[23, 77, 130, 146] Transmission occurs via direct and indirect contact and via

---

*References 23, 36, 40, 69, 74, 77, 130, 146, 163, 206, 217

†References 23, 37, 56, 77, 87, 89, 114, 126, 130, 147, 158, 226, 244, 276

*References 12, 14, 23, 130, 145, 146, 159, 183, 192, 200, 202, 254

†References 23, 26, 29, 55, 71, 82, 94, 130, 141, 146, 181, 191

ticks. Severely affected swine develop a red to reddish-blue to purplish discoloration of the skin of the snout, ears, belly, legs, sides, and rump. Skin biopsy reveals dilated, congested superficial dermal blood vessels with thrombi, purpura, and numerous perivascular eosinophils. Focal areas of epidermal basal cell necrosis may be seen.[77, 146]

Papillomatosis

Papillomatosis is caused by host-specific papovaviruses (see Chapter 17, discussion on papillomatosis).

Bovine Viral Leukosis

Bovine viral leukosis is caused by a retrovirus (Oncornaviridae) (see Chapter 17, discussion on lymphosarcoma).

Equine Sarcoid

Equine sarcoid may be caused by a retrovirus or bovine papovavirus 1 (see Chapter 17, discussion on equine sarcoid).

Bovine Ephemeral Fever

Bovine ephemeral fever is an insect-transmitted rhabdovirus infection of cattle in Africa, Asia, and Australia.[23, 35, 130] Clinical signs may include widespread subcutaneous emphysema and periarticular edema.

Caprine Viral Dermatitis

Caprine viral dermatitis was reported in the late 1940's in India.[120, 121] It was an acute, highly fatal disease caused by an unclassified virus. The disease could be transmitted by intravenous injection or cutaneous scarification, using blood or skin lesions from infected goats. The incubation period was seven to ten days. Cross-immunity tests with several strains of poxviruses and contagious pustular dermatitis virus revealed no immunologic relationship with the agent of caprine viral dermatitis.

Initial clinical signs included malaise and pyrexia, followed by a characteristic dermatosis. The entire cutaneous surface, including the lips, gums, and tongue, is covered with papules and nodules that become necrotic in seven to ten days and eventuate in shallow crateriform ulcers. In goats that survived, the ulcers formed crusts and healed in about three weeks. The majority of animals died within ten days.

Diagnosis was based on history, physical examination, and necropsy findings. Skin biopsy revealed a variably severe hyperplastic superficial and deep perivascular dermatitis with ballooning degeneration. Mononuclear and plasma cells were the chief inflammatory infiltrate. No inclusion bodies were seen.

Swine Parvovirus Vesicular Disease

Outbreaks of a vesicular disease were reported in swine in the midwestern United States.[160] Affected swine had vesicles and erosions on the snout and coronet and in the interdigital space and the mouth. Morbidity (13 to 100 percent) and mortality (0 to 58 percent) varied from herd to herd.

Parvovirus was isolated from the skin, serum, and many visceral organs of affected swine. In addition, parvoviral antigen was demonstrated by direct immunofluorescence testing in the outer root sheaths of hair follicles of skin adjacent to coronary band lesions. The disease was reproduced with the parvovirus in normal pigs.

Scrapie

Scrapie is a vertically and horizontally transmissible disease of sheep and goats in many parts of the world.* The disease agent is believed to be a "slow" virus, or virus-like particle (viroid). Affected animals are most commonly two to five years of age, and Suffolk sheep are commonly affected in the United States. Clinical signs include intermittent, bilaterally symmetrical pruritus, which often begins over the tailhead and progresses cranially to involve the flanks, thorax, and occasionally the head and ears. Chronic rubbing and biting lead to alopecia, excoriations, and even hematomas. Frequently, serpentine tongue movements accompany the rubbing and scratching.

Idiopathic Swine Vesicular Disease

Idiopathic swine vesicular diseases have been reported in Florida,[110] Australia,[212] and New Zealand.[221] In the Florida outbreak, affected swine had vesicles and erosions only on the feet. In Australia, affected swine had vesicles and erosions on the snout and, occasionally, the back, tail, and ears. Swine in the New Zealand outbreak had vesicles and erosions on

---

*References 23, 124, 130, 141, 146, 181, 191

the snout and feet. These three outbreaks of vesicular disease were not typical of any recognized swine vesicular disorders, and viruses were not isolated.

REFERENCES

1. Abdussalam, M.: Contagious pustular dermatitis. II. Pathological histology. J. Comp. Pathol. 67:217, 1957.
2. Abdussalam, M., and Cosslett, V. E.: Contagious pustular dermatitis virus. I. Studies on morphology. J. Comp. Pathol. 67:145, 1957.
3. Agger, W. A., and Webster, S. B.: Human orf infection complicated by erythema multiforme. Cutis 31:334, 1983.
4. Ali, B. H., and Obeid, H. M.: Investigation of the first outbreaks of lumpy skin disease in the Sudan. Br. Vet. J. 133:184, 1977.
5. Alexander, R. A., et al.: Cytopathogenic agents associated with lumpy skin disease of cattle. Bull. Epizoot. Dis. Afr. 5:489, 1957.
6. Ames, T. R., et al.: Tail lesions of contagious ecthyma associated with docking. JAVMA 184:88, 1984.
7. Asagaba, M. O.: Recognition of pseudocowpox in Nigeria. Trop. Anim. Health Prod. 14:184, 1982.
8. Aynaud, M.: La stomatite pustuleuse contagieuse des ovins (chancre du mouton). Ann. Inst. Pasteur 37:498, 1923.
9. Bagust, T. J., et al.: Studies on equine herpesvirus (3). The incidence in Queensland of three different equine herpesvirus infections. Aust. Vet. J. 48:47, 1972.
10. Baker, J. C., et al.: Pseudorabies in a goat. JAVMA 181:607, 1982.
11. Bakos, K., and Brag, S.: Studies of goat pox in Sweden. Nord. Vet. Med. 9:431, 1957.
12. Ballanini, G.: L'esantema cutaneo nella febbre catarrale maligna (FCM) del bovino. Folia Vet. Lat. 4:575, 1974.
13. Bankowski, R. A.: Vesicular exanthema. Adv. Vet. Sci. 10:23, 1965.
14. Bawa, H. S.: Rinderpest in sheep and goats in Ajmermerwara. Indian J. Vet. Sci. 10:103, 1940.
15. Baxby, D.: Is cowpox misnamed? A review of ten human cases. Br. Med. J. 1:1379, 1977.
16. Beck, C. C., and Taylor, W. B.: Orf—it's awful! Vet. Med. Small Anim. Clin. 71:1413, 1974.
17. Bennett, S. C. J., et al.: The pox disease of sheep and goats. J. Comp. Pathol. Ther. 54:131, 1944.
18. Berkman, R. N., and Barner, R. D.: Bovine malignant catarrhal fever. I. Its occurrence in Michigan. JAVMA 132:243, 1958.
19. Berkman, R. N., et al.: Bovine malignant catarrhal fever in Michigan. II. Pathology. Am. J. Vet. Res. 21:1015, 1960.
20. Bhambani, B. D., and Krishnamurty, D.: An immunodiffusion test for laboratory diagnosis of sheeppox and goat pox. J. Comp. Pathol. 73:349, 1963.
21. Bida, S. A.: Confirmation by histopathology of the probable wide spread of lumpy skin disease (LSD) in Nigeria. Bull. Anim. Health Prod. Afr. 25:317, 1977.
22. Blakemore, F., and Abdussalam, M.: Morphology of the elementary bodies and cell inclusions in swinepox. J. Comp. Pathol. Ther. 66:373, 1956.
23. Blood, D. C., et al.: *Veterinary Medicine VI.* London, Baillière-Tindall, 1983.
24. Boerner, F.: An outbreak of cow-pox, introduced by vaccination, involving a herd of cattle and a family. JAVMA 64:93, 1923.
24a. Bowen, J. M.: Venereal diseases of stallions. *In:* Robinson, N. E. (ed.): *Current Therapy in Equine Medicine II.* Philadelphia, W. B. Saunders Co., 1986, p. 567.
25. Bowman, K. F., et al.: Cutaneous form of bovine papular stomatitis in man. JAMA 246:2813, 1981.
26. Bowne, J. G., et al.: Bluetongue disease in cattle. JAVMA 153:662, 1968.
27. Broughton, I. B., and Hardy, W. T.: Contagious ecthyma (Soremouth) of sheep and goats. JAVMA 85:150, 1934.
28. Brown, L. N., et al.: "Rat-tail syndrome" of feedlot cattle

29. Browne, J. G., et al.: Bluetongue of sheep and cattle: Past, present, and future. JAVMA 151:1801, 1967.
30. Bryans, J. T., and Allen, G. P.: *In vitro* and *in vivo* studies of equine "coital exanthema." Proc. Intl. Conf. Equine Infect. Dis. 3:322, 1973.
31. Bryans, J. T.: The herpesviruses in disease of the horse. Proc. Am. Assoc. Equine Pract. 14:119, 1968.
32. Buddle, B. M., et al.: Heterogeneity of contagious ecthyma virus isolations. Am. J. Vet. Res. 45:75, 1984.
33. Buddle, B. M., et al.: Contagious ecthyma virus–vaccination failures. Am. J. Vet. Res. 45:263, 1984.
34. Burdin, M. L.: The use of histopathological examinations of skin material for the diagnosis of lumpy skin disease in Kenya. Bull. Epizoot. Dis. Afr. 7:27, 1959.
35. Burgess, G. W.: Bovine ephemeral fever: A review. Vet. Bull. 41:887, 1971.
36. Burrows, R., et al.: Swine vesicular disease. Res. Vet. Sci. 15:141, 1973.
37. Burton, A. C.: Stomatitis contagiosa in horses. Vet. J. 73:234, 1917.
38. Burki, F., et al.: Experimentelle genitale und nasale Infektion von Pferden mit dem Virus des equinen coitalen Exanthems. Zbl. Vet. Med. B21:362, 1974.
39. Bwangamoi, O., and Kaminjolo, J. S.: Isolation of IBR/IPV virus from the semen and skin lesions of bulls at Kabete, Kenya. Zbl. Vet. Med. B18:262, 1971.
40. Cameron, R. D. A.: *Skin Diseases of the Pig.* Sydney, University of Sydney Post-Graduate Foundation in Veterinary Science, Vet. Rev. 23, 1984.
41. Capstick, P. B.: Lumpy skin disease—experimental infection. Bull. Epizoot. Dis. Afr. 7:51, 1959.
42. Capstick, P. B., and Coackley, W.: Protection of cattle against lumpy skin disease. I. Trials with a vaccine against Neethling type infection. Res. Vet. Sci. 2:362, 1961.
43. Carbrey, E., et al.: Transmission of hog cholera by pregnant sows. JAVMA 149:23, 1966.
44. Carne, H. R., et al.: Infection of man by the virus of contagious pustular dermatitis in sheep. Aust. J. Sci. 9:73, 1946.
45. Carson, C. A., et al.: Bovine papular stomatitis: Experimental transmission from man. Am. J. Vet. Res. 29:1783, 1968.
46. Casaro, A. P. E., et al.: Response of the bovine fetus to bovine viral diarrhea–mucosal disease virus. Am. J. Vet. Res. 32:1543, 1971.
47. Castrucci, G., et al.: Distribution of bovid herpes 2 in calves inoculated intravenously. Am. J. Vet. Res. 39:943, 1978.
48. Cheville, N. F., and Shey, D. J.: Pseudocowpox in dairy cattle. JAVMA 150:855, 1967.
49. Cheville, N. F.: The cytopathology of swinepox in the skin of swine. Am. J. Pathol. 49:339, 1966.
50. Chow, T. L., et al.: Pathology of vesicular stomatitis in cattle. Proc. Am. Vet. Med. Assoc. 88:119, 1951.
51. Chow, T. L., and McNutt, S. H.: Pathological changes of experimental vesicular stomatitis of swine. Am. J. Vet. Res. 14:420, 1953.
52. Chu, R. M., et al.: Experimental swine vesicular disease, pathological and immunofluorescence studies. Can. J. Comp. Med. 43:29, 1979.
53. Coggins, L.: Equine viral arteritis. *In:* Robinson, N. E.: *Current Therapy in Equine Medicine.* Philadelphia, W. B. Saunders Co., 1983, p. 6.
54. Conroy, J. D., and Meyer, R. C.: Electron microscopy of swinepox virus in germ-free pigs and in cell culture. Am. J. Vet. Res. 32:2021, 1971.
55. Cornell, W. D., et al.: Bluetongue in western Kentucky cattle: A serologic survey. Vet. Med. Small Anim. Clin. 78:1257, 1983.
56. Cotton, W. E.: Vesicular stomatitis. Vet. Med. 22:169, 1927.
57. Coulter, G., and Storz, J.: Identification of a cell-associated morbillivirus from cattle affected with malignant catarrhal fever: Antigenic differentiation and cytologic characterization. Am. J. Vet. Res. 40:1671, 1979.
58. Crandell, R. A., and Davis, E. R.: Isolation of equine coital exanthema virus (equine herpesvirus 3) from the nostril of foal. JAVMA 187:503, 1985.

59. Crawford, A. B.: Experimental vesicular exanthema of swine. JAVMA 90:380, 1937.
60. Crawford, T. B., and Henson, J. B.: Viral arteritis of horses. Adv. Exp. Med. Biol. 22:175, 1972.
61. Csontos, J., and Nyiredi, S.: Untersuchungen uber die Atiologie des pockenartigen Hautausschlages der Ferkel. Dtsch. Tierarztl. Wochenschr. 41:529, 1933.
62. Dardiri, A. H., and Stone, S. S.: Serologic evidence of dermatotropic bovine herpes virus infection of cattle in the United States of America. Proc. Ann. Meet. U.S. Anim. Health Assoc. 76:156, 1972.
63. Datt, N. S.: Comparative studies of pigpox and vaccinia viruses. I. Host range pathogenicity. J. Comp. Pathol. 74:62, 1964.
64. Datt, N. S.: Comparative studies of pigpox and vaccinia viruses. II. Serological relationship. J. Comp. Pathol. 74:70, 1964.
65. Daubney, R., and Hudson, J. R.: Transmission experiments with bovine malignant catarrhal fever. J. Comp. Pathol. Ther. 49:63, 1936.
66. Davies, F. G.: Characteristics of a virus causing a pox disease in sheep and goats in Kenya, with observations on the epidemiology and control. J. Hygiene 76:163, 1976.
67. Davis, C. M., and Musil, G.: Milker's nodules: A clinical and electron microscopic report. Arch. Dermatol. 101:305, 1970.
68. Davis, C. M., et al.: Electron microscopy for the rapid diagnosis of pseudocowpox and milker's nodule. Am. J. Vet. Res. 31:1497, 1970.
69. Dawe, P. S., et al.: A preliminary investigation of the swine vesicular disease epidemic in Britain. Nature 241:540, 1973.
70. Deas, D. W., and Johnston, W. S.: An outbreak of an ulcerative skin condition of the udder and teats of dairy cattle in the east of Scotland. Vet. Rec. 78:828, 1966.
71. DeKock, G., et al.: Observations on bluetongue in cattle and sheep. Onderstepoort J. Vet. Sci. 8:129, 1937.
72. DeJong, D. A.: The relationship between contagious pustular stomatitis of the horse, equine variola (horse-pox of Jenner), and vaccinia (cow-pox of Jenner). J. Comp. Pathol. Ther. 30:242, 1917.
73. Dennis, S. M.: Perinatal foal mortality. Compend. Cont. Ed. 3:S206, 1981.
74. Dhennin, L., and Dhennin, L.: La maladie vesiculeuse du porc. Son Application en France. Bull. Acad. Vet. Fr. 46:47, 1973.
75. Dobberkau, G.: Histologische Untersuchungen de Haut bei Schweinepest. Arch. Exp. Vet. Med. 13:590, 1960.
76. Doll, E. R., et al.: Isolation of a filterable agent causing arteritis of horses and abortion of mares. Its differentiation from the equine abortion (influenza) virus. Cornell Vet. 47:3, 1957.
77. Dunne, H. D.: *Diseases of Swine IV*. Ames, Iowa State University Press, 1975.
78. Dutta, P. K., et al.: Foot-and-mouth disease in sheep and goats. Indian Vet. J. 61:267, 1984.
79. Dutta, N. K., et al.: Further studies of an outbreak of goatpox in Orissa and its diagnosis. Indian J. Anim. Health 22:121, 1983.
80. Eby, C. H.: A note on the history of horsepox. JAVMA 132:120, 1958.
81. El-Zein, A., et al.: Preparation and testing of a goat pox vaccine from a pathogenic field isolate attenuated in cell culture. Zbl. Vet. Med. B30:341, 1983.
82. Erasmus, B. J.: Bluetongue in sheep and goats. Aust. Vet. J. 51:165, 1975.
83. Erickson, G. A., et al.: Generalized contagious ecthyma in a sheep rancher: Diagnostic considerations. JAVMA 166:262, 1975.
84. Eugster, A. K., et al.: Paravaccinia infections of the scrotum of bulls. Southwest. Vet. 33:227, 1980.
85. Evermann, J. F., et al.: Equine coital exanthema virus infection. Equine Pract. 5:39, 1983.
86. Evermann, J. F.: Etiology of malignant catarrhal fever. JAVMA 178:100, 1981.
87. Federer, K. E., et al.: Vesicular stomatitis virus—the relationship between some strains of the Indiana serotype. Res. Vet. Sci. 8:103, 1967.
88. Fellows, O. N., et al.: Isolation of vesicular stomatitis virus from an infected laboratory worker. Am. J. Vet. Res. 16:623, 1955.
89. Ferris, D., et al.: Experimental transmission of vesicular stomatitis virus by Diptera. J. Infect. Dis. 96:184, 1955.
90. Fields, B. N., and Hawkins, K.: Human infection with the virus of vesicular stomatitis during an epizootic. N. Engl. J. Med. 277:989, 1967.
91. Filmer, J. F.: Ovine posthitis and balano-posthitis ("pizzle rot"): Some notes on field investigations. Aust. Vet. J. 14:47, 1938.
92. Fitzpatrick, T. B., et al.: *Dermatology in General Medicine II*. New York, McGraw-Hill Book Co., 1979.
93. Flook, W. H.: An outbreak of venereal disease among sheep (ulcerative dermatosis). J. Comp. Pathol. Ther. 16:374, 1903.
94. Foster, N. M., et al.: Transmission of attenuated and virulent bluetongue virus with *Culicoides variipennis* infected orally via sheep. Am. J. Vet. Res. 29:275, 1968.
95. Fraser, C. M., and Savan, M.: Bovine papular stomatitis—a note on its diagnosis and experimental transmission in Ontario. Can. Vet. J. 3:107, 1962.
96. Friedman-Kein, A. E., et al.: Milker's nodules: Isolation of a poxvirus from a human case. Arch. Exp. Vet. Med. 21:625, 1971.
97. Gardiner, M. R., et al.: An unusual outbreak of contagious ecthyma (scabby mouth) in sheep. Aust. Vet. J. 43:163, 1967.
98. Geering, W. A.: Foot-and-mouth disease in sheep. Aust. Vet. J. 43:485, 1967.
99. Gibbs, E. P. J., et al.: The differential diagnosis of viral skin infections of the bovine teat. Vet. Rec. 87:602, 1970.
100. Gibbs, E. P. J., et al.: Differential diagnosis of virus infection of the bovine teat skin by electron microscopy. J. Comp. Pathol. 80:455, 1970.
101. Gibbs, E. P. J., et al.: Cowpox in a dairy herd in the United Kingdom. Vet. Rec. 92:56, 1973.
102. Gibbs, E. P. J., and Osborne, A. D.: Observations on the epidemiology of pseudocowpox in South West England and South Wales. Br. Vet. J. 130:150, 1974.
103. Gibbs, E. P. J., et al.: Field observations on the epidemiology of bovine herpes mammillitis. Vet. Rec. 91:395, 1972.
104. Gibbs, E. P. J., and Collings, D. F.: Observations on bovine herpes mammillitis (BHM) virus infections of heavily pregnant heifers and young calves. Vet. Rec. 90:66, 1972.
105. Gibbs, E. P. J., et al.: Experimental studies of the epidemiology of bovine herpes mammillitis. Res. Vet. Sci. 14:139, 1973.
106. Gibbs, E. P. J.: Collecting specimens for virus disease diagnosis. In Pract. 1:21, 1979.
107. Gibbs, E. P. J.: Differential diagnosis of virus infections of the skin. *In*: Howard, J. L.: *Current Veterinary Therapy. Food Animal Practice*. Philadelphia, W. B. Saunders Co., 1981, p. 1161.
108. Gibbs, E. P. J.: Viral diseases of the skin of the bovine teat and udder. Vet. Clin. North Am. Large Anim. Pract. 6:187, 1984.
109. Gibbs, E. P. J., and Rweyemanu, M. M.: Bovine herpesvirus 2 and 3. Vet. Bull. 47:411, 1977.
110. Gibbs, E. P. J., et al.: A vesicular disease of pigs in Florida of unknown etiology. Florida Vet. J. 12:25, 1983.
111. Gibbs, E. P. J., et al.: Electron microscopy as an aid to the rapid diagnosis of virus diseases of veterinary importance. Vet. Rec. 106:451, 1980.
112. Gigstad, D. C., and Stone, S. S.: Clinical, serological, and cross-challenge response and virus isolation in cattle infected with three bovine dermatotropic herpesviruses. Am. J. Vet. Res. 38:753, 1977.
113. Glover, R. E.: Contagious pustular dermatitis of the sheep. J. Comp. Pathol. Ther. 41:318, 1928.
114. Gregg, J., et al.: Vesicular stomatitis contagiosa. Vet. Med. 12:221, 1917.
115. Griesemer, R. A., and Cole, C. R.: Bovine papular stomatitis. I. Recognition in the United States. JAVMA 137:404, 1960.
116. Griesemer, R. A., and Cole, C. R.: Bovine papular stomatitis. II. The experimentally produced disease. Am. J. Vet. Res. 22:473, 1961.

117. Griesemer, R. A., and Cole, C. A.: Bovine papular stomatitis. III. Histopathology. Am. J. Vet. Res. 22:482, 1961.
118. Guss, S. B.: Contagious ecthyma (sore-mouth, orf). Mod. Vet. Pract. 61:335, 1980.
119. Guss, S. B.: *Management and Diseases of Dairy Goats.* Scottsdale, AZ, Dairy Goat Journal Publishing Corp., 1977.
120. Haddow, J. R., and Idnani, J. A.: Goat dermatitis: A new virus disease of goats in India. Indian J. Vet. Sci. 16:181, 1946.
121. Haddow, J. R., and Idnani, J. A.: Goat dermatitis: A new virus disease of goats in India. Indian Vet. J. 24:332, 1948.
122. Haig, D. A.: Production of generalized skin lesions in calves inoculated with bovine mammillitis virus. Vet. Rec. 80:311, 1967.
123. Hanson, R. P., and Brandly, C. A.: Epizootiology of vesicular stomatitis. Am. J. Public Health 47:205, 1957.
124. Harcourt, R. A., and Anderson, M. A.: Naturally occurring scrapie in goats. Vet. Rec. 94:504, 1974.
125. Hardy, W. T., and Price, D. A.: Soremuzzle of sheep. JAVMA 120:23, 1952.
126. Heiny, F.: Vesicular stomatitis in cattle and horses in Colorado. North Am. Vet. 26:726, 1945.
127. Henderson, W. M.: Foot-and-mouth disease and related vesicular diseases. Adv. Vet. Sci. 6:19, 1960.
127a. Henry, B. E., et al.: Genetic relatedness of disease-associated field isolates of bovid herpesvirus type 4. Am. J. Vet. Res. 47:2242, 1986.
128. Hester, H. R., et al.: Studies on cowpox. I. An outbreak of natural cowpox and its relation to vaccinia. Cornell Vet. 31:360, 1941.
129. Howard, J. L.: *Current Veterinary Therapy. Food Animal Practice.* Philadelphia, W. B. Saunders Co., 1981.
130. Howard, J. L.: *Current Veterinary Therapy. Food Animal Practice II.* Philadelphia, W. B. Saunders Co., 1986.
131. Hoxtell, E., et al.: Human orf: With electron microscopic identification of the virus. Cutis 16:899, 1975.
132. Huck, R. A.: A paravaccinia virus isolated from cows' teats. Vet. Rec. 78:503, 1966.
133. Hunskaar, S.: A case of ecthyma contagiosum (human orf) treated with idoxuridine. Dermatologica 168:207, 1984.
134. Hunt, E.: Infectious skin diseases of cattle. Vet. Clin. North Am. Large Anim. Pract. 6:155, 1984.
135. Hutchins, D. R.: Skin diseases of cattle and horses in New South Wales. N.Z. Vet. J. 8:85, 1960.
136. Irwin, M. R., et al.: Association of bovine papular stomatitis with the "rat tail" syndrome of feedlot cattle. Southwest. Vet. 29:120, 1976.
137. Jacob, R. J.: Molecular pathogenesis of equine coital exanthema: Temperature-sensitive function(s) in cells infected with equine herpesviruses. Vet. Microbiol. 11:221, 1986.
138. James, M. P., et al.: An epizootic of malignant catarrhal fever. Clinical and pathological observations. N.Z. Vet. J. 23:9, 1975.
139. James, Z. H., and Povey, R. C.: Organ culture of bovine teat skin and its application to the study of herpes mammillitis and pseudocowpox infections. Res. Vet. Sci. 15:40, 1973.
140. Jansen, B. C.: Some aspects of diseases typical of ruminants in Southern Africa. Aust. Vet. J. 42:471, 1966.
141. Jensen, R., and Swift, B. L.: *Diseases of Sheep II.* Philadelphia, Lea & Febiger, 1982.
142. Jensen, R., and Mackey, D. R.: *Diseases of Feedlot Cattle III.* Philadelphia, Lea & Febiger, 1983.
143. Johannessen, J. V., et al.: Human orf. J. Cutaneous Pathol. 2:265, 1975.
144. Johnston, W. S., and Deas, D. W.: Isolation of a paravaccinia virus from bovine semen. Vet. Rec. 89:450, 1971.
145. Joshi, R. C., et al.: Occurrence of cutaneous eruptions in rinderpest outbreak among bovine. Indian Vet. J. 54:871, 1977.
146. Jubb, K. V. F., et al.: *Pathology of Domestic Animals.* New York, Academic Press, 1985.
147. Junkers, A. H.: The epizootiology of the vesicular stomatitis viruses: A reappraisal. Am. J. Epidemiol. 86:286, 1967.
148. Kahn, D., and Hutchinson, E. A.: Generalized bullous orf. Intl. J. Dermatol. 19:340, 1980.
149. Kahrs, R. F.: *Viral Diseases of Cattle.* Ames, Iowa State University Press, 1981.
150. Kaminjolo, J. S., et al.: Vaccinia-like pox virus identified in a horse with a skin disease. Zbl. Vet. Med. B21:202, 1974.
151. Kaminjolo, J. S., et al.: Isolation, cultivation and characterization of a poxvirus from some horses in Kenya. Zbl. Vet. Med. B21:592, 1974.
152. Kaminjolo, J. S., and Winquist, G.: Histopathology of skin lesions in Uasin Gishu skin disease of horses. J. Comp. Pathol. 85:391, 1975.
153. Kasza, L., and Griesemer, R. A.: Experimental swine pox. Am. J. Vet. Res. 23:443, 1962.
154. Kendrick, J. W.: Bovine viral diarrhea–mucosal disease virus. Am. J. Vet. Res. 32:533, 1971.
155. Kewish, O. K.: Sheep shearers get orf. Br. Med. J. 1:356, 1951.
156. Kim, J. C. S., and Tarrier, M.: Contagious pustular dermatitis of sheep in a veterinary student. Vet. Med. Small Anim. Clin. 72:231, 1977.
157. Kim, J. C. S., and Luong, I. C.: Ultrastructure of swine pox. Vet. Med. Small Anim. Clin. 70:1043, 1975.
158. Knight, A. P., and Messer, N. T.: Vesicular stomatitis. Compend. Cont. Ed. 5:S517, 1983.
159. Kral, F., and Schwartzman, R. M.: *Veterinary and Comparative Dermatology.* Philadelphia, J. B. Lippincott Co., 1964.
160. Kresse, J. I., et al.: Parvovirus infection in pigs with necrotic and vesicle-like lesions. Vet. Microbiol. 10:525, 1985.
161. Krogsrund, J., and Onstrad, O.: Equine coital exanthema: Isolation of a virus and transmission experiments. Acta Vet. Scand. 12:1, 1971.
162. Kuppuswamy, A. R.: Caprine variola in Province Wellesley. Indian Vet. J. 13:130, 1936.
163. Lai, S. S., et al.: Pathogenesis of swine vesicular disease in pigs. Am. J. Vet. Res. 40:463, 1979.
164. Lang, H. A.: Human orf. Br. Med. J. 2:1566, 1961.
165. Lauder, I. M., et al.: Milker's nodule virus infection and its resemblance to orf. Vet. Rec. 78:926, 1966.
166. Lauder, I. M., et al.: Experimental vaccinia infection of cattle: A comparison with other virus infections of cows' teats. Vet. Rec. 89:571, 1971.
167. Leavill, U., et al.: Ecthyma contagiosum (orf). So. Med. J. 58:239, 1965.
168. Leavill, V. W., et al.: Orf. Report of 19 human cases with clinical and pathological observations. JAMA 204:657, 1968.
169. Leavill, V. W., and Phillips, I. A.: Milker's nodules. Pathogenesis, tissue culture, electron microscopy, and calf inoculation. Arch. Dermatol. 111:1307, 1975.
170. LeFevre, P. C.: La maladie nodulaire cutanee des bovins II. Production d'un vaccin lyophilise a virus vivant. Rev. Elev. Med. Vet. Pays Trop. 32:233, 1979.
171. LeFevre, P. C., et al.: La maladie nodulaire cutana des bovins I. Situation epizotiologique actuelle en Afrique. Rev. Elev. Med. Vet. Pays Trop. 32:227, 1979.
172. Leman, A. D., et al.: *Diseases of Swine V.* Ames, Iowa State University Press, 1981.
173. Letchworth, G. J., and LaDue, R.: Bovine herpes mammillitis in two New York dairy herds. JAVMA 180:902, 1982.
174. Liggitt, H. D., et al.: Experimental transmission of malignant catarrhal fever: Gross and histopathologic changes. Am. J. Vet. Res. 39:1249, 1978.
175. Liggitt, H. D., and DeMartini, J. C.: The pathomorphology of malignant catarrhal fever. II. Multisystemic epithelial lesions. Vet. Pathol. 17:73, 1980.
176. Liggitt, H. D., and DeMartini, J. C.: The pathomorphology of malignant catarrhal fever. I. Generalized lymphoid vasculitis. Vet. Pathol. 17:58, 1980.
177. Linnabury, R. D., et al.: Contagious ecthyma (orf) in a goat herd. Vet. Med. Small Anim. Clin. 71:1261, 1976.
178. Livingston, C. W., and Hardy, W. T.: Longevity of contagious ecthyma virus. JAVMA 137:651, 1960.
179. Lloyd, G. M., et al.: Human infection with the virus of cowpox disease. Lancet 1:720, 1951.
180. Lober, C. W., et al.: Clinical and histologic features of orf. Cutis 32:142, 1983.
181. Lofstedt, J.: Dermatologic diseases of sheep. Vet. Clin. North Am. Large Anim. Pract. 5:427, 1983.

182. Luedke, A. J., et al.: Clinical and pathologic features of bluetongue in sheep. Am. J. Vet. Res. 25:963, 1964.
183. MacGregor, A. D.: A preliminary note on cutaneous rinderpest. Indian J. Vet. Sci. 14:56, 1944.
184. Madin, S. H., and Traum, J.: Experimental studies with vesicular exanthema of swine. Vet. Med. 48:395, 1953.
185. Manninger, R., et al.: Uber der Atiologie des pockenartigen Ausschlags der Ferkel. Schweiz. Arch. Tierheilkd. 75:159, 1940.
186. Martin, W. B., et al.: Ulceration of cow's teats caused by a virus. Vet. Rec. 76:15, 1964.
187. Martin, W. B., et al.: Pathogenesis of bovine mammillitis virus infection in cattle. Am. J. Vet. Res. 30:2151, 1969.
188. Martin, W. B., et al.: Bovine ulcerative mammillitis caused by a herpesvirus. Vet. Rec. 78:569, 1966.
189. Martin, W. B.: Bovine mammillitis: Epizootiologic and immunologic features. JAVMA 163:915, 1973.
190. Martin, W. B., and Scott, F. M.: Latent infection of cattle with bovine herpes virus 2. Arch. Virol. 60:51, 1979.
191. Martin, W. B.: Diseases of Sheep. Oxford, Blackwell Scientific Publications, 1983.
192. Maurer, F. D., et al.: The pathology of rinderpest. Proc. Am. Vet. Med. Assoc. 92:201, 1955.
193. McCollum, W. H., and Swerczek, T. W.: Studies of an epizootic of equine viral arteritis in racehorses. J. Equine Med. Surg. 2:293, 1978.
194. McIntyre, R. W.: Virus papular dermatitis of the horse. Am. J. Vet. Res. 10:229, 1948.
195. McMullan, W. C.: The skin. In: Mansmann, R. A., et al. (eds.): Equine Medicine & Surgery III. Santa Barbara, CA, American Veterinary Publications, 1982, p. 789.
196. McNutt, S. H., et al.: Swine pox. JAVMA 74:752, 1929.
197. McVicar, J. W.: Sheep and goats as foot-and-mouth disease carriers. JAVMA 154:40, 1969.
198. Meyer, R. C., and Conroy, J. D.: Experimental swinepox in gnotobiotic piglets. Res. Vet. Sci. 13:334, 1972.
199. Mishra, K. C., and Ghei, J. C.: A severe outbreak of foot and mouth disease of local goats of Sikkim due to "A22" virus. Indian Vet. J. 60:410, 1983.
200. Mohan, R., and Bahl, M. R.: Cutaneous eruptions of rinderpest in goats. Indian J. Vet. Sci. 23:39, 1953.
201. Mohanty, S. B., and Dutta, S. K.: Veterinary Virology. Philadelphia, Lea & Febiger, 1981.
202. Mornet, P., and Guerret, M.: Les lesions cutanees dans la peste bovine. Bull. Acad. Vet. Fr. 23:284, 1950.
203. Moore, D. M., et al.: Contagious ecthyma in lambs and laboratory personnel. Lab. Anim. Sci. 33:473, 1983.
204. Moore, R. M.: Human orf in the United States, 1972. J. Infect. Dis. 127:731, 1973.
205. Moscovici, C., et al.: Isolation of a viral agent from pseudocowpox disease. Science 141:915, 1963.
206. Mowat, G. N., et al.: Differentiation of a vesicular disease of pigs in Hong Kong from foot-and-mouth disease. Vet. Rec. 90:618, 1972.
207. Mullowney, P. C.: Dermatologic diseases of cattle, part II. Infectious diseases. Compend. Cont. Ed. 4:S3, 1982.
208. Mullowney, P. C., and Fadok, V. A.: Dermatologic diseases of horses, part II. Bacterial and viral skin diseases. Compend. Cont. Ed. 6:S16, 1984.
209. Mullowney, P. C.: Skin diseases of sheep. Vet. Clin. North Am. Large Anim. Pract. 6:131, 1984.
210. Mullowney, P. C., and Baldwin, E. W.: Skin diseases of goats. Vet. Clin. North Am. Large Anim. Pract. 6:143, 1984.
211. Mullowney, P. C., and Hall, R. F.: Skin diseases of swine. Vet. Clin. North Am. Large Anim. Pract. 6:107, 1984.
212. Munday, B. L., and Ryan, F. B.: Vesicular lesions in swine—possible association with the feeding of marine products. Aust. Vet. J. 59:193, 1982.
213. Murray, M., et al.: Experimental sheep pox. A histological and ultrastructural study. Res. Vet. Sci. 15:201, 1973.
214. Muzichin, S. I., et al.: A study of sheep pox in the Sudan. Bull, Anim. Health Prod. Afr. 27:105, 1979.
215. Nagington, J., et al.: Milker's nodule virus infections in Dorset and their similarity to orf. Nature 208:505, 1965.
216. Nagington, J., et al.: Bovine papular stomatitis, pseudocowpox and milker's nodules. Vet. Rec. 81:306, 1967.
217. Nardelli, L., et al.: A foot-and-mouth disease syndrome in pigs caused by an enterovirus. Nature 219:1275, 1968.
218. Nawathe, D. R., and Osagke, M. O.: Lumpy skin disease—experimental infection. Bull. Anim. Health Prod. Afr. 25:313, 1977.
219. Neufeld, J. L.: Spontaneous pustular dermatitis in a newborn piglet associated with a poxvirus. Can. Vet. J. 22:156, 1981.
220. Newsom, I. E., and Cross, F.: Soremouth transmitted to man. JAVMA 84:790, 1934.
221. New Zealand Veterinary Association and General News: The Temuka incident. N.Z. Vet. J. 29:55, 1981.
222. Nomland, R.: Human infection with ecthyma contagiosum, a virus disorder of sheep. Arch. Dermatol. Syphilol. 42:878, 1940.
223. Ott, R. S., and Nelson, D. R.: Contagious ecthyma in goats. JAVMA 173:81, 1978.
224. Pascoe, R. R., et al.: An equine genital infection resembling coital exanthema associated with a virus. Aust. Vet. J. 45:166, 1969.
225. Pascoe, R. R.: Equine Dermatoses. Sydney, University of Sydney Post-Graduate Foundation in Veterinary Science, Vet. Rev. 22, 1984.
226. Patterson, W. C., et al.: Experimental infections with vesicular stomatitis in swine. I. Transmission by direct contact and feeding infected meat scraps. Proc. U.S. Livestock Sanit. Assoc. 59:368, 1955.
227. Phillips, R. M.: Contagious ecthyma in a pregnant veterinary student. Vet. Med. Small Anim. Clin. 78:236, 1983.
228. Pierson, R. E., et al.: Experimental transmission of malignant catarrhal fever. Am. J. Vet. Res. 35:523, 1974.
229. Pierson, R. E., et al.: An epizootic of malignant catarrhal fever in feedlot cattle. JAVMA 163:349, 1973.
230. Platt, H.: The localization of lesions in experimental foot-and-mouth disease. Br. J. Exp. Pathol. 41:150, 1960.
231. Plowright, W., et al.: The pathogenesis of sheeppox in the skin of sheep. J. Comp. Pathol. 69:400, 1959.
232. Plowright, W.: Malignant catarrhal fever. JAVMA 152:795, 1968.
233. Plowright, W., et al.: Growth and characteristics of the virus of bovine malignant catarrhal fever in East Africa. J. Gen. Microbiol. 39:253, 1964.
234. Povey, R. C., and James, Z. H.: Bovine herpes mammillitis virus and vulvo-vaginitis. Vet. Rec. 92:231, 1973.
235. Proctor, S. J., and Sherman, K. C.: Ultrastructural changes in bovine lingual epithelium with vesicular stomatitis virus. Vet. Pathol. 12:362, 1975.
236. Prozesky, L., and Barnard, B. J. H.: A study of the pathology of lumpy skin disease. Onderstepoort J. Vet. Res. 49:167, 1982.
237. Rafyi, A., and Ramyar, H.: Goat pox in Iran. Serial passage in goats and the developing egg, and relationship with sheep pox. J. Comp. Pathol. 69:141, 1959.
238. Rahley, R. S., and Mueller, R. E.: Molluscum contagiosum in a horse. Vet. Pathol. 20:247, 1983.
239. Reed, D. E., et al.: Characterization of herpesviruses isolated from lactating dairy cows with mammary pustular dermatitis. Am. J. Vet. Res. 38:1631, 1977.
240. Renshaw, H. W., and Dodd, A. G.: Serologic and cross-immunity studies with contagious ecthyma and goat pox virus isolates from the western United States. Arch. Virol. 56:201, 1978.
241. Ribelin, W.: The cytopathogenesis of vesicular stomatitis virus infection in cattle. Am. J. Vet. Res. 19:66, 1958.
242. Roberts, R. S., and Bolton, J. F.: A venereal disease of sheep. Vet. Rec. 57:686, 1945.
243. Robinson, A. J., and Balassu, T. C.: Contagious pustular dermatitis (orf). Vet. Bull. 51:771, 1981.
244. Robinson, N. E.: Current Therapy in Equine Medicine. Philadelphia, W. B. Saunders Co., 1983.
245. Rossi, C. R., et al.: A paravaccinia virus isolated from cattle. Cornell Vet. 67:72, 1977.
246. Rucker, R. C.: Clinical picture of orf in Northern California. Cutis 20:109, 1977.
247. Rweyemamu, M. M., et al.: Bovine herpes mammillitis virus. III. Observations on experimental infection. Br. Vet. J. 124:317, 1968.

248. Sarkar, P., et al.: Application of fluorescent antibody test in the diagnosis of sheep-pox, and study of sheep-pox virus multiplication in cell-culture. Indian J. Anim. Sci. 50:428, 1980.

249. Savage, J., and Black, M. M.: "Giant" orf of finger in a patient with a lymphoma. Proc. R. Soc. Med. 65:766, 1972.

250. Sawyer, J. C.: Vesicular exanthema of swine and San Miguel sea lion virus. JAVMA 169:707, 1976.

251. Schnurrenberger, P. R., et al.: Bovine papular stomatitis incidence in veterinary students. Can. J. Comp. Med. 44:239, 1980.

252. Schwarte, L. H., and Biester, H. E.: Pox in swine. Am. J. Vet. Res. 2:136, 1941.

253. Scott, D. W., et al.: Caprine dermatology. Part II. Viral, nutritional, environmental, and congenitohereditary disorders. Compend. Cont. Ed. 6:S473, 1984.

254. Scott, G. R.: Rinderpest. Adv. Vet. Sci. 9:113, 1964.

255. Sehgal, C. L.: Studies on foot-and-mouth disease. II. Experiments on host pathogenicity of foot-and-mouth disease virus. Indian J. Anim. Sci. 39:437, 1969.

256. Selman, I. E., et al.: A clinico-pathological study of bovine malignant catarrhal fever in Great Britain. Vet. Rec. 94:483, 1974.

257. Sen, K. C., and Datt, N. S.: Studies on goat-pox virus. I. Host range pathogenicity. Indian J. Vet. Sci. 38:388, 1968.

258. Sharma, R. M., and Bhata, H. M.: Contagious pustular dermatitis in goats. Indian J. Vet. Sci. 28:205, 1959.

259. Sharma, S. K., et al.: Foot and mouth disease in sheep and goats: An iceberg infection. Indian Vet. J. 58:925, 1981.

260. Sharma, S. N., and Dhanda, M. R.: Studies on the interrelationship between sheep- and goat-pox viruses. Indian J. Anim. Sci. 41:267, 1971.

261. Sharma, S. N., and Dhanda, M. R.: Studies on sheep and goat pox viruses. Indian J. Anim. Health 11:39, 1972.

262. Sharma, S. N., et al.: A preliminary note on pathogenicity and antigenicity of sheep and goat pox viruses. Indian Vet. J. 43:673, 1966.

263. Shelley, W. B., and Shelley, E. D.: Farmyard pox: Parapoxvirus infection in man. Br. J. Dermatol. 108:725, 1983.

264. Shelokov, A. I., et al.: Prevalence of human infection with vesicular stomatitis virus. J. Clin. Invest. 40:1081, 1961.

264a. Simpson, D. J.: Venereal diseases of mares. In: Robinson, N. E.: Current Therapy in Equine Medicine II. Philadelphia, W. B. Saunders Co., 1986, p. 513.

265. Singh, I. P., and Srivastava, R. N.: Sheeppox. A review. Vet. Bull. 49:145, 1979.

266. Smith, A. W., et al.: San Miguel sea lion virus isolation, preliminary characterization and relationship to vesicular exanthema of swine virus. Nature 244:108, 1973.

267. Smith, M. C.: Caprine dermatologic problems.: A review. JAVMA 178:724, 1981.

268. Smith, M. C.: Dermatologic diseases of goats. Vet. Clin. North Am. Large Anim. Pract. 5:449, 1983.

269. Snowdon, W. A., and French, E. L.: A papular stomatitis of virus origin in Australian cattle. Aust. Vet. J. 37:115, 1961.

270. Sonck, C. E., and Penttineu, K.: Milker's nodules. Transmission from man to man. Acta Derm. Venereol. (Stockh) 34:420, 1954.

271. Sowhney, A. N., et al.: Goat-pox: An anthropozoonosis. Indian J. Med. Res. 60:683, 1973.

272. Stephenson, W. H.: Ulcerative vulvitis in ewe. Aust. Vet. J. 26:64, 1950.

273. St. George, T. D., et al.: A generalised infection of cattle with bovine herpesvirus 2. Aust. Vet. J. 56:42, 1980.

274. Studdert, M. J.: Comparative aspects of equine herpesviruses. Cornell Vet. 64:94, 1974.

275. Tantawi, H. H., et al.: Isolation and identification of the Sersenle strain of goat pox virus in Iraq. Trop. Anim. Health Prod. 11:208, 1979.

276. Theiler, S.: Eine contagiose Stomatitis des Pferdes in Sued-Afrika. Dtsch. Tierarztl. Wochenschr. 9:131, 1901.

277. Thein, P.: The association of EHV-2 with keratitis and research on the occurrence of equine coital exanthema (EHV-3) of horses in Germany. Proc. Intl. Conf. Equine Infect. Dis. 4:33, 1978.

278. Thomas, A. D., and Mare, C. V. E.: Knopvelsiekte. J. So. Afr. Vet. Med. Assoc. 16:36, 1945.

279. Thomas, A. D., and Neitz, W. O.: Further observations on the pathology of bluetongue in sheep. Onderstepoort. J. Vet. Sci. Anim. Ind. 22:27, 1947.

280. Timoney, P. J.: Equine viral arteritis. A disease of emerging significance? Equine Vet. J. 18:166, 1986.

281. Traum, J.: Vesicular exanthema of swine. JAVMA 88:316, 1936.

282. Trueblood, M. S.: Relationship of ovine contagious ecthyma and ulcerative dermatosis. Cornell Vet. 56:521, 1966.

283. Trueblood, M. S., et al.: An immunologic study of ulcerative dermatosis and contagious ecthyma. Am. J. Vet. Res. 24:42, 1963.

284. Trueblood, M. S., and Chow, T. L.: Characterization of the agents of ulcerative dermatosis and contagious ecthyma. Am. J. Vet. Res. 24:47, 1963.

285. Tunnicliffe, E. A.: Ulcerative dermatosis of sheep. Am. J. Vet. Res. 10:240, 1949.

286. Turner, A. J., et al.: Bovine herpes mammillitis of dairy cattle in Victoria. Aust. Vet. J. 52:170, 1976.

287. Turner, A. J., et al.: Isolation and characterization of bovine herpes mammillitis virus and its pathogenicity for cattle. Aust. Vet. J. 52:166, 1976.

288. Valder, W. A., et al.: Ecthyma contagiosum des Schafes-Wandel des Klinischen Bildes. Tierarztl. Umschau 34:828, 1979.

289. Velu, H.: Contribution a l'etude de l'etologie de la variole des porcelets. Rec. Med. Vet. 92:24, 1916.

290. Verdes, N., et al.: Natural transmission of contagious pustular dermatitis from sheep and goats to man and a case of person to person transmission. Rev. Pathol. Comp. Med. Exp. 70:71, 1970.

291. Vestweber, J. G., and Milleret, R. J.: Ulcerative dermatosis in sheep (a case report). Vet. Med. Small Anim. Clin. 67:672, 1972.

292. Walley, T.: Contagious dermatitis; "orf" in sheep. J. Comp. Pathol. Ther. 3:357, 1908.

293. Weaver, L. D., et al.: Bovine herpes mammillitis in New York. JAVMA 160:1643, 1972.

294. Weiss, K. E.: Lumpy skin disease virus. Virol. Monog. 3. New York, Springer Verlag, 1968.

295. Westphal, H. O.: Human to human transmission of orf. Cutis 11:202, 1973.

296. Wheeler, C. E., and Cawley, E. P.: The microscopic appearance of ecthyma contagiosum (orf) in sheep, rabbits, and man. Am. J. Pathol. 33:535, 1955.

297. Wheeler, C. E., and Cauley, E. P.: The etiology of milker's nodules. Arch. Dermatol. 75:249, 1957.

298. White, B. B.: Vesicular exanthema of swine. JAVMA 97:230, 1940.

299. Wilkinson, J. D.: Orf: A family with unusual complications. Br. J. Dermatol. 97:447, 1977.

300. Wittman, G., and Hall, S. A.: Aujeszky's Disease. Boston, Martinus Nijhoff, 1982.

301. Woods, J. A.: A skin condition of cattle. Vet. Rec. 95:326, 1974.

302. Yager, J. A., and Scott, D. W.: The skin and appendages. In: Judd, K. V.: Pathology of Domestic Animals. Vol. 1. New York, Academic Press, 1985, p. 407.

303. Yedloutschnig, R. J., et al.: Bovine herpes mammillitis–like disease diagnosed in the United States. Proc. U.S. Anim. Health Assoc. 74:208, 1970.

304. Yilma, T.: Morphogenesis of vesiculation in foot and mouth disease. Am. J. Vet. Res. 41:1537, 1980.

305. Zwick, W.: Ueber die Beziehungen der Stomatitis Pustulosa Contagiosa des Pferdes zu den Pocken der Haustiere und des Menschen. Berl. Tierarztl. Wochenschr. 40:757, 1924.

CHAPTER 6

BACTERIAL DISEASES

CUTANEOUS BACTERIOLOGY

The normal skin of healthy individuals is highly resistant to invasion by the wide variety of bacteria to which it is constantly exposed (see Chapter 1, discussion on cutaneous ecology).[114, 272] Pathogenic organisms such as co-agulase-positive staphylococci may produce characteristic lesions of impetigo, folliculitis, furunculosis, and cellulitis in the absence of any obvious impairment of host defenses. However, localized disruption of normal host defenses as produced by maceration (water, friction from skin folds, and topical treatments), physical trauma (abrasions, cuts, punctures, biting insects and arthropods, scratching, and rubbing), or the introduction of a foreign body (plant awns) may facilitate development of overt infection. Treatment with immunosuppressive agents and immunosuppressive diseases can predispose patients to infections. In cattle, neutrophil function has been reported to be suppressed by glucocorticoids,[344] progesterone,[345] and bovine virus diarrhea infection.[343] Bovine lymphocyte function is suppressed by glucocorticoids.[63, 346] Bovine immune responses are also suppressed by zinc deficiency and stress.[63]

The host-bacteria relationship in infections of the skin involves three major elements: (1) the pathogenic properties of the organism (particularly the invasive potential and the toxigenic properties), (2) the portal of entry, and (3) the host defense and inflammatory responses to bacterial invasion. Increased susceptibility to bacterial infections has been reported in cattle with suppressed neutrophil function.[139, 327] Bacterial infection involving the skin may manifest itself in either of two major forms: (1) as a primary cutaneous process or (2) as a secondary manifestation of infection elsewhere in the body. The cutaneous changes associated with systemic infection are not necessarily suppurative but may represent those of vasculitis or a hypersensitivity response.

Diagnostic Bacteriology

Identification of bacteria from skin lesions may provide important information as to the cause of cutaneous infections, whether primary or secondary to systemic processes. The presence of normal skin flora may confuse interpretation of these studies. All too often, the finding on culture of a potential pathogen, such as a coagulase-positive *Staphylococcus* species, is equated with the presence of infection. It is essential to remember that damaged skin provides a medium for proliferation of many bacteria. Only by correlating the clinical appearance of the lesion with the bacteriologic data can one reach the proper decision concerning the presence of a bacterial disease.

DIRECT SMEAR

Samples of pus or exudate from intact pustules, nodules, draining tracts, or ulcers can be smeared on glass slides, air-dried, and stained with new methylene blue, Gram's stain, or Diff-Quik for light microscopic examination. Important observations to be made include: (1) type(s) of bacteria present (cocci versus rods; gram-positive or gram-negative) and (2) the associated inflammatory response. Skin contaminants are usually recognized by being extracellular and being often clumped in microcolonies. Pathogenic bacteria are found intracellularly within neutrophils and macrophages. Thus, direct smears often provide the first clue to the specific cause of the infection and also serve as a guide in selecting appropriate culture media and antibiotic therapy.

BACTERIAL CULTURE

Because the skin of large animals is a veritable cesspool of bacteria, cultures must be carefully taken and interpreted (see Chapter 1, discussion on cutaneous ecology). Intact pustules, nodules, and abscesses are preferred lesions for culture and may be aspirated with a needle and syringe or punctured and swabbed with a culturette, after the overlying epithelium has been gently swabbed with alcohol and allowed to air-dry. Cultures of open sores (erosions, ulcers, and sinuses) and exudative surfaces often generate confusing, if not misleading, bacteriologic data.

When intact, pus-containing lesions are not available for sampling, the culturing of surgical biopsy specimens is preferred. Papules, plaques, nodules, and areas of diffuse swelling may be surgically prepared (e.g., povidone-iodine or chlorhexidine scrub) and punch or excision biopsies taken with aseptic techniques. These biopsy specimens can then be delivered to the laboratory in various transport media for culture and antibiotic sensitivity testing.

In general, samples for bacterial culture are routinely planted on blood agar and inoculated into a tube of thioglycolate broth (anaerobic). Additional media should be used as indicated by clinical findings and evaluation of direct smears.

Antibiotic Therapy

The selection of the appropriate antibiotic should be made on the basis of the appearance of the skin lesions, the characteristics of any systemic illness, direct smears or culture results, and sensitivity testing of the isolated pathogen(s). Clearly, economic and production factors are also important considerations.

STAPHYLOCOCCAL INFECTIONS

Staphylococcus species are versatile pathogens of animals and humans.* The organisms are gram-positive cocci, have a worldwide distribution, are prevalent in nature, and may gain entry to the animal host through any natural orifice and contaminated wounds. Coagulase-positive staphylococci are common large animal pathogens and produce a number of toxins, including hemotoxin, leukocidin, and dermonecrotoxin.

Until recently, all coagulase-positive staphylococci, with the possible exception of *Staphylococcus hyicus*, were identified as *Staphylococcus aureus*. However, the taxonomic unheaval to which the genus has been subjected in the last decade has resulted in the

establishment of three species: *S. aureus, S. intermedius*, and *S. hyicus*.*

Studies have been conducted on the coagulase-positive staphylococci isolated from horses, goats, sheep, and cattle.† In horses, 36 percent of the isolates were *S. intermedius*, and 64 percent were *S. aureus*. In goats, the percentages were 67 and 33, respectively. In sheep and cattle, only *S. aureus* was isolated. Differences in the antimicrobial susceptibility patterns between *S. aureus* and *S. intermedius* isolates were not significant.[52] Over 60 percent of all isolates were resistant to penicillin. Most isolates were sensitive in vitro to erythromycin, chloramphenicol, oxacillin, cephalexin, trimethoprim-sulfamethoxazole, and aminoglycosides.

Previous studies on the antimicrobial susceptibility patterns of coagulase-positive staphylococci differed from those of Biberstein and colleagues.[52] Most coagulase-positive staphylococci isolated from goats and cattle were reported to be sensitive to penicillin, ampicillin, erythromycin, methicillin, cloxacillin, cephaloridine, and kanamycin.[10, 268, 404] Most coagulase-positive staphylococci isolated from horses were found to be sensitive to penicillin, ampicillin, lincomycin, tetracycline, chloramphenicol, and sulfonamides.[358] These differences in reported antimicrobial susceptibilities may indicate regional differences.

Impetigo

Impetigo, a superficial pustular dermatitis that does not involve hair follicles, occurs commonly in goats, sheep, and cattle.‡ Predisposing factors include the stress of parturition, moist and filthy environments, and trauma. No age or breed predilections are apparent, but females appear to be predisposed.

Lesions occur most commonly on the udder (Fig. 6–1), with the base of the teats and the intramammary sulcus most often affected. Occasionally, lesions may spread to the teats, ventral abdomen, medial thighs, perineum, and ventral surface of the tail. Superficial vesicles rapidly become pustular, rupture, and leave erosions and yellow-brown crusts. Pruritus and pain are rare, and affected animals usually suffer no systemic disturbance unless staphylococcal mastitis ensues.

---

*References 60, 75, 166, 169, 208, 246, 248

*References 52, 91–93, 95, 140–142, 203, 352
†References 9, 10, 52, 97, 140–142, 195, 203, 211, 296, 303, 352, 365
‡References 60, 135, 159, 248, 283, 360, 375, 404

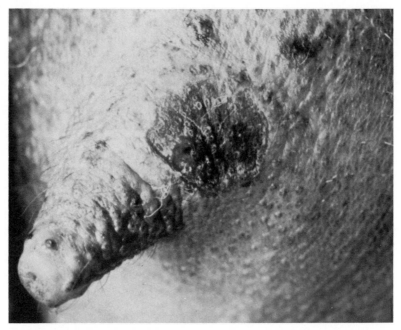

FIGURE 6–1. Ovine impetigo. Pustules and annular erosions on udder.

The differential diagnosis includes other bacterial infections, dermatophilosis, dermatophytosis, stephanofilariasis, and viral infections. The definitive diagnosis is based on history, physical examination, direct smears, skin biopsy, and culture. Skin biopsy reveals subcorneal pustular dermatitis, with cocci often visible within the pustules (Fig. 6–2).

Therapy with daily topical medicaments (chlorhexidine, iodophors) usually results in rapid healing within a few days. Systemic antibiotics are rarely needed, but penicillin and ampicillin have been effective. In recurrent, chronic, or epizootic situations, autogenous bacterins may be helpful.[59, 159, 360, 375]

Impetigo may be spread by the milker to

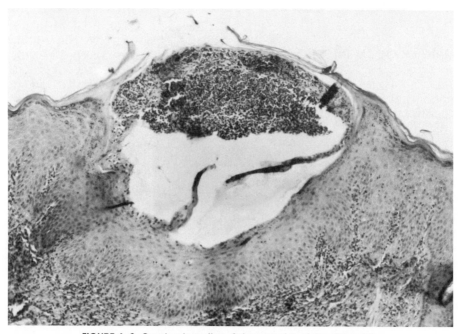

FIGURE 6–2. Caprine impetigo. Subcorneal pustular dermatitis.

other cattle and goats.[59, 159, 360, 375] Thus, affected animals should be milked last, single-service paper towels should be used, and the hands of the milker should be washed after contact with infected animals. Additionally, infection may be transmitted to the exposed skin of humans.[59, 117, 360, 375]

Exudative Epidermitis

Exudative epidermitis is an acute, generalized, exudative, vesicopustular disease of suckling pigs caused by *Staphylococcus hyicus*.* Synonyms for this disorder in the older veterinary literature include impetigo contagiosa, contagious pyoderma, seborrhea oleosa, greasy pig disease, dermatitis crustosa, marmite disease, and watery eczema.†

Exudative epidermitis is caused by *S. hyicus* subspecies *hyicus*.‡ This organism was formerly named *S. hyos*, *Micrococcus hyicus*, and *M. epidermitis*. The disease has been reproduced in conventional and gnotobiotic pigs by administering the bacteria orally, intranasally, intravenously, intramuscularly, and intracutaneously by skin scarification and by direct contact.§ Amtsberg[23] found that the route of infection determined the disease syndrome produced in specific pathogen-free pigs: (1) infection by skin scarification produced the typical cutaneous syndrome, (2) intramuscular injection produced septicemia, polyarthritis, and generalized skin disease with necrosis of ears and tail and abscesses, and (3) intravenous administration resulted in polyarthritis. It has been reported that biotin-deficient pigs infected with *S. hyicus* healed much more slowly than did normal pigs.[383]

S. hyicus was administered intracutaneously to rabbits and a calf, resulting in an exfoliative exudative dermatosis similar to porcine exudative epidermitis.[24, 26] Considering the experimental and clinical data and the associated dermatohistopathologic findings,[353] Amtsberg speculated that porcine exudative epidermitis might be analogous to the staphylococcal scalded skin syndrome in humans.[24, 114] A bacteria-free, concentrated culture supernatant from five different *S. hyicus* strains was injected subcutaneously into pigs, resulting in the production of typical exudative epidermitis.[24] Thus, it would appear that porcine exudative epidermitis may be caused not by *S. hyicus* infection per se but by some toxin(s) elaborated by the microorganism. This is quite similar to the staphylococcal scalded skin syndrome in humans, in which certain strains of staphylococci elaborate exfoliative toxins (exfoliatins) that produce a widespread subcorneal cleavage within the stratified squamous epithelium of skin and oral mucosa.[114]

Because *S. hyicus* can be isolated from the skin, ears, and nostrils of most normal pigs,[22, 92, 93, 144, 174] most authors believe that clinical disease requires some combination of the bacteria and predisposed piglets (skin trauma, inadequate nutrition, other diseases, or stress).[60, 72, 103, 217, 398]

Exudative epidermitis has a worldwide distribution.* The incidence is not high, but the disease can be a severe problem on individual farms. It is most commonly seen in suckling pigs of one to seven weeks of age, with no breed or sex predilections. Morbidity varies from 10 to 90 percent, and mortality from 5 to 90 (average 20) percent. The disease is nonseasonal, and hygiene and management are often good in affected herds. The incubation period is three to four days.

Clinically, exudative epidermitis has been divided into peracute, acute, and subacute forms.† In the peracute form, a dark-brown greasy exudate appears periocularly (Fig. 6–3), followed by a vesicopustular eruption on the nose, lips, tongue, gums, and coronets. Red-brown macules then appear behind the ears and on the ventral abdomen and medial thighs. The entire body is then covered by erythema, a moist, greasy exudate, and thick brown crusts. The feet are frequently affected with erosions of the coronary band and heel. Conjunctivitis is common, and excessive exudation may result in the adherence of eyelids and blindness. The piglets show progressive depression, anorexia, and polydipsia and usually die within three to five days. Pruritus, pain, and fever are usually absent.

The acute form follows the general pattern of the peracute form. The skin becomes thicker and wrinkled. The total body exudate

*References 59, 60, 72, 73, 103, 174, 186, 187, 213, 217, 277

†References 60, 103, 161, 198, 199, 232, 331, 332, 353, 376, 386

‡References 22, 23, 92, 93, 143, 194, 316

§References 21–23, 62, 143, 187, 213–216, 254, 355, 356, 383, 384, 396, 398

*References 21, 47, 59, 60, 62, 72, 103, 147, 154, 161, 163, 174, 195, 213, 217, 312, 348

†References 28, 60, 72, 73, 103, 217, 398

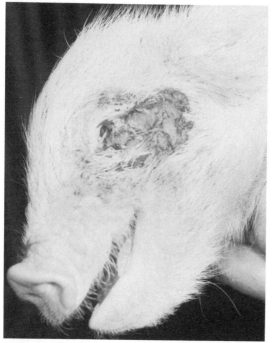

FIGURE 6–3. Exudative epidermitis. Periocular waxy crusts.

then becomes hardened and cracked, resulting in a furrowed appearance (Figs. 6–4 and 6–5). Death often occurs within four to eight days. In the subacute form, skin lesions are often confined to the head and ears and are less exudative. The piglets are usually healthy otherwise and recover spontaneously. Additional disorders described in porcine exudative epidermitis include subcutaneous abscesses,

necrosis of the ears and tail, and polyarthritis.[22, 23, 217, 316]

Because of the losses attributable to death, weight loss, stunting, and medical bills, exudative epidermitis can be a significant economic problem.[60, 217, 312]

The differential diagnosis of exudative epidermitis includes swine parakeratosis, streptococcal pyoderma, biotin deficiency, and viral infections. The definitive diagnosis is based on history, physical examination, skin biopsy, and culture. Skin biopsy reveals subcorneal vesicular-to-pustular dermatitis (Fig. 6–6).[62, 254, 291, 292, 353] A mild to moderate degree of acantholysis may be seen. With special stains, gram-positive cocci may be seen within the vesicles and pustules. *S. hyicus* may be cultured from vesicopustules and, consistently, from the conjunctiva.[195, 254, 396–398] *S. hyicus* is usually white in colony color, nonhemolytic, and coagulase variable.[92, 93, 163, 384]

Moderate neutrophilia has been found in pigs with exudative epidermitis.[254] No significant differences in serum protein fractions between affected and normal pigs were detected by cellulose acetate electrophoresis.[405] Necropsy findings in pigs with exudative epidermitis include (1) dilatation of ureters and renal pelvices as a result of ureteral obstruction caused by edema, cellular infiltration, and hyperplasia and mucoid degeneration of ureteral epithelium, (2) serous lymphadenitis, and (3) mild catarrhal gastroenteritis.*

---

*References 186–188, 214, 254, 353, 396–398

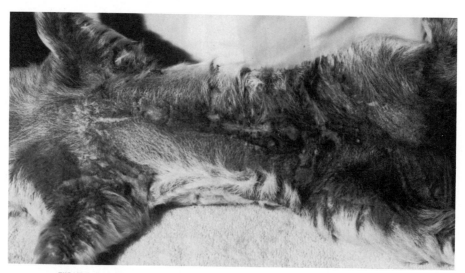

FIGURE 6–4. Exudative epidermitis. Total body dermatitis and waxy crusts.

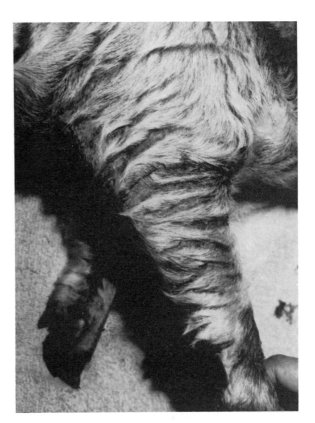

FIGURE 6–5. Exudative epidermitis. Furrowed appearance of leg.

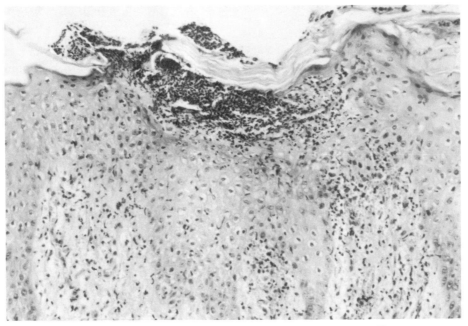

FIGURE 6–6. Exudative epidermitis. Subcorneal pustular dermatitis.

The efficacy of any treatment for exudative epidermitis is inversely proportional to the duration and severity of the infection.[60, 72, 103, 217, 398] Hence, the literature is replete with great cures and conflicting claims. Medicaments such as vitamin A, zinc, fatty acids, and a plethora of topical agents have been praised but ultimately shown to be of little or no value.* However, clinical and experimental evidence suggests that vitamin B (especially biotin) supplementation is helpful in therapy and prevention.[72, 126, 217, 232, 317, 383] This may reflect a prior nutritional deficiency in affected pigs rather than a therapeutic effect of vitamin B.

Antimicrobial susceptibility tests on numerous *S. hyicus* isolates indicate that most are sensitive to oxacillin, methicillin, neomycin, and novobiocin and are resistant to lincomycin, erythromycin, and streptomycin.[96, 163, 312] Susceptibility to penicillin, ampicillin, and tylosin has been variable, with most Belgian isolates being resistant[96] and most British and New Zealand isolates being sensitive.[163, 312] This discrepancy may represent true regional differences in antibiotic resistance.

Clinically, early treatment with penicillin (5000 IU/kg twice daily) given intramuscularly for three to five days is effective.† In addition, tylosin (8 mg/kg) given intramuscularly for two to three days has been reported to be beneficial.[60, 103, 217, 402] One author reported good success with a single injection of oxytetracycline (11 to 18 mg/kg) followed by oxytetracycline in the feed (300 gm/T).[73] Topical treatment with cleansing, degreasing, and antimicrobial agents is also helpful, when feasible. If conjunctivitis is severe, an antibiotic eye ointment is helpful. It is recommended that affected piglets be isolated from the rest and that exposed piglets be treated as well, when feasible.[216, 398] Other supportive measures include improving hygiene, nutrition, and other management practices, when indicated.

Amtsberg[25] reported that immunization was effective in the prevention of experimentally induced exudative epidermitis. Inoculation with a formalinized vaccine or with the exfoliative toxin protected pigs and their suckling piglets against later intraocular challenge with live *S. hyicus*. These immunization procedures did *not* prevent the development of polyarthritis after intravenous administration of live *S. hyicus*, however.

Folliculitis and Furunculosis

Staphylococcal folliculitis and furunculosis are common in horses, goats, and sheep and uncommon in cattle and swine.* These infections are usually believed to be secondary to cutaneous trauma and various physiologic stresses.

Folliculitis is an inflammation of hair follicles. When the inflammatory process breaks through the hair follicles and extends into the surrounding dermis and subcutis, the process is called furunculosis. When multiple areas of furunculosis coalesce, the resultant focal area of induration and fistulous tracts is called a carbuncle (boil).

The primary skin lesion of folliculitis is a follicular papule. Pustules may arise from these papules. Frequently one first notices erect hairs over a 2- to 3-mm papule that is more easily felt than seen. These lesions can regress spontaneously but often progressively enlarge. Some lesions enlarge to 6 to 10 mm in diameter, develop a central ulcer that discharges a purulent or serosanguineous material, and then become encrusted. The chronic or healing phase is characterized by progressive flattening of the lesion and a static or gradually expanding circular area of alopecia and scaling. Hairs at the periphery of these lesions are often easily epilated. It is extremely important to remember that in the chronic or healing stage, all folliculitides, regardless of cause, are often characterized by circular areas of alopecia and scaling (so-called classic ringworm lesion).

Some lesions progress to furunculosis. This stage is distinguished by varying combinations of nodules, draining tracts, ulcers, and crusts. Large lesions are often associated with severe inflammatory edema and may assume an edematous plaque or urticarial appearance. Scarring, leukoderma, and leukotrichia may follow.

In the horse, staphylococcal folliculitis and furunculosis (acne, heat rash, summer rash, summer scab, sweating eczema of the saddle region, saddle scab, saddle boils) are common.† No age, breed, or sex predilections are evident. About 90 percent of the cases begin in spring and early summer. This period coincides with shedding, heavy riding and work schedules, higher environmental temperature

---

*References 47, 62, 103, 147, 216, 348, 382, 396, 398
†References 60, 72, 103, 147, 216, 217, 396, 398

*References 208, 217, 229, 248, 309, 359, 360
†References 164, 176, 208, 253, 273, 304, 307, 309, 358, 359, 389

and humidity, and increased insect population densities. Poorly groomed horses may be at risk.

Skin lesions initially affect the saddle and tack areas in about 90 percent of cases (Fig. 6–7). The lesions are painful in up to 70 percent of cases, rendering the horse unfit for riding or work, but are rarely pruritic. Whether or not immunity develops is unclear, but cases of chronically recurrent lesions are well known.

Less frequent manifestations of equine staphylococcal folliculitis and furunculosis are the so-called pastern folliculitis and tail pyoderma. Pastern folliculitis affects the caudal aspect of the pastern and fetlock regions, with involvement of one or more limbs.[253, 273, 359] This disorder must be considered in the differential diagnosis of "grease heel" (see Chapter 15, discussion on equine pastern dermatitis). Recently, *S. hyicus* was isolated from horses with pastern folliculitis.[98] Experimentally, the *S. hyicus* isolate caused dermatitis in normal horses. Tail pyoderma may follow the cutaneous trauma produced by tail rubbing provoked by insect bites, mange, pinworms, lice, food allergy, and vice.[253, 273] The dorsal surface of the tail is particularly affected. Occasionally, coagulase-positive staphylococci are associated with a severe cellulitis of one or more legs in thoroughbred racehorses.[246a]

In goats, staphylococcal folliculitis and furunculosis (acne) are also common.[44, 117, 135, 159, 360, 375] No age, breed, or sex predilections are evident. Predisposing factors include stress of parturition, moist and filthy environments, and trauma.

Skin lesions are most commonly seen on the udder, ventral abdomen, medial thighs, perineum, face, pinnae, and distal limbs (Fig. 6–8). Deeper lesions are often warm and painful. Severe infections, especially with secondary mastitis, may produce pyrexia, anorexia, depression, and septicemia.

Staphylococcal folliculitis and furunculosis are also common in sheep.* They may occur as benign pustular dermatitis (plooks) in otherwise healthy three- to four-week-old lambs, especially on the lips and perineum, which spontaneously regresses within three weeks. The condition also occurs as a severe facial dermatitis (facial or periorbital eczema, eye scab) in sheep of all ages (Fig. 6–9) but especially in adult ewes just prior to lambing. Pustules, nodules, ulcers, and black scabs develop on the face, pinnae, and horn base. This facial form appears to be contagious, and spread through a flock has been attributed to infection of head abrasions while animals are feeding at troughs or fighting. Staphylococcal dermatitis has also been reported on the legs of sheep pastured in a field containing thistles.[385]

---

*References 42, 120, 149, 229, 248, 303, 350, 361

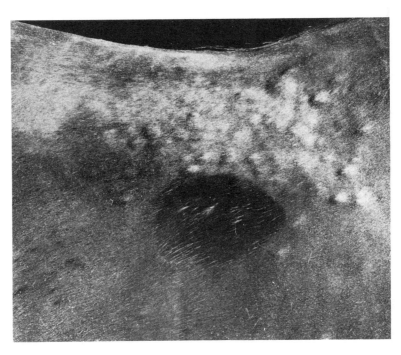

FIGURE 6–7. Equine staphylococcal folliculitis. Multiple papules in saddle area.

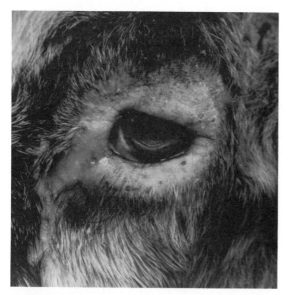

FIGURE 6–8. Caprine staphylococcal folliculitis. Periocular alopecia and crusts.

Staphylococcal folliculitis and furunculosis (acne, tail worm, perianal furunculosis) are uncommon in cattle.[112, 208, 221, 326, 364] Although cattle of any age, breed, or sex may be affected, the condition is particularly common in young bulls; 10 to 27 percent of artificial insemination center animals may be affected.[221, 326, 364] Trauma and poor hygiene are believed to be initiating factors. Lesions are most commonly found on the tail and perineum (Fig. 6–10) and less commonly on the scrotum and face. Pruritus and pain are variable. Recently, diffuse gangrene of the hind limbs associated with *S. aureus* infection was reported in a calf.[250]

In swine, staphylococcal folliculitis and furunculosis are uncommon.[124, 208, 217] No breed or sex predilections are apparent. The condition is most frequently seen in pigs less than eight weeks of age. An asymptomatic, erythematous pustular dermatitis covers much of the body, especially the hindquarters, abdomen, and chest (Fig. 6–11). The dermatosis usually regresses spontaneously within three weeks. Less commonly, a facial dermatitis is seen in young growing pigs, secondary to cutaneous trauma from needle-sharp canine teeth.

The differential diagnosis of staphylococcal folliculitis and furunculosis on the general body surface includes other bacterial infections (especially *C. pseudotuberculosis* in horses, dermatophilosis, dermatophytosis, demodicosis, and Pelodera dermatitis. For equine pastern folliculitis and tail pyoderma, the differentials must also include the grease heel complex (see Chapter 15, discussion on equine pastern dermatitis) and the various causes of tail rubbing and dermatitis (see Chapter 3, discussion on regional diagnoses). Definitive diagnosis is based on history, physical examination, direct smears, skin biopsy, and culture. Skin biopsy reveals varying degrees of perifolliculitis, folliculitis (Figs. 6–12, 6–13), and furunculosis (Fig. 6–14), with extensive tissue eosinophilia

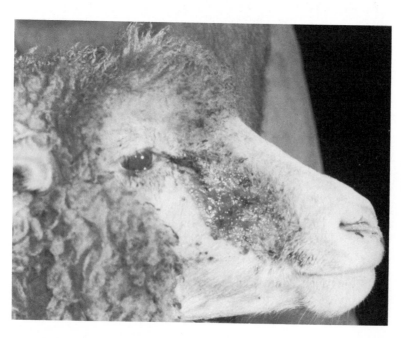

FIGURE 6–9. Ovine staphylococcal furunculosis. Facial ulceration and crusting.

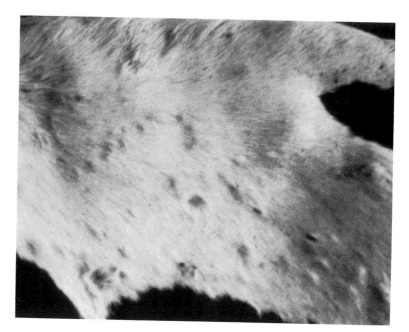

FIGURE 6–10. Bovine staphylococcal folliculitis. Papules and crusts over rump.

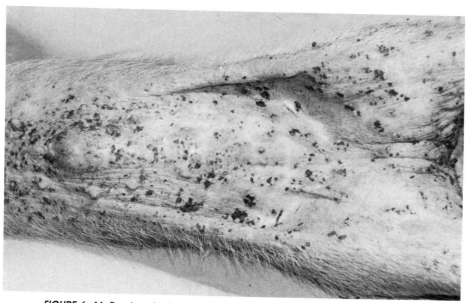

FIGURE 6–11. Porcine staphylococcal folliculitis. Pustules and crusts on ventrum.

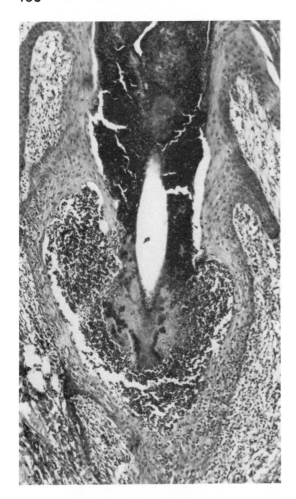

FIGURE 6–12. Porcine staphylococcal folliculitis. Suppurative folliculitis.

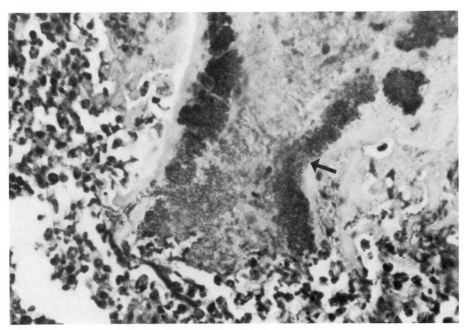

FIGURE 6–13. Porcine staphylococcal folliculitis. Numerous cocci within follicular pus (arrow).

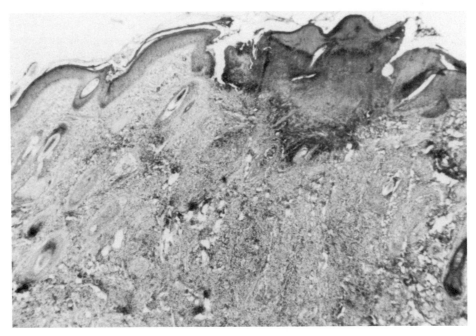

FIGURE 6-14. *Equine staphylococcal furunculosis. Nodular area of pyogranulomatous dermatitis associated with ruptured hair follicles.*

often accompanying furunculosis. Bacteria may be visible with tissue Gram's stain or with Brown and Brenn's stain.

Therapy for staphylococcal folliculitis and furunculosis varies with the severity and stage of the disease, the natural course of the infection, and economic factors. Mild cases in all species may resolve spontaneously.[208, 217, 248, 359] More severe cases may require topical cleansing, drying, and antibacterial therapy.* Daily applications of aqueous iodophors and chlorhexidine are usually performed for five to seven days, then twice weekly until the infection is resolved. Severe or progressive cases require systemic antibiotics in addition to topical therapy. The choice of systemic antibiotics is best made on the basis of culture and sensitivity testing. In horses, goats, and cattle, procaine penicillin (22,000 IU/kg twice daily) given intramuscularly for seven to ten days has been reported to be effective in many cases.† Healing is usually complete within four weeks. However, in severe chronic cases of tail pyoderma in horses and cattle, all forms of treatment may fail.[253, 273, 326] Staphylococcal dermatitis on the legs of sheep was successfully treated with parenteral injections of long-acting oxytetracycline (10 to 20 mg/kg).[385]

Control measures include proper hygiene and management. Cutting or removing the canine teeth of piglets at birth may be helpful. In horses with recurrent infections, antimicrobial shampoos before and after work have been reported to be an effective preventive measure.[307, 359] In recurrent or epizootic situations, autogenous bacterins have been reported to be helpful in goats and horses.[44, 159, 233, 307, 360, 375]

It must be remembered that staphylococci are also common human pathogens.[169] The prevalence and epidemiologic significance of cross-infections are poorly defined. However, certain strains have been reported to be transmitted from infected cattle and goats to humans[59, 169, 360, 364] who come into contact with these animals.

STREPTOCOCCAL INFECTIONS

Streptococcus species are numerous and associated with variable clinical manifestations[60, 75, 103, 165, 217, 246] The organisms are gram-positive cocci, worldwide in distribution, and prevalent in nature and may gain entry to the animal host through any natural orifice and contaminated wounds.

In horses, streptococci have been isolated from individuals with ulcerative lymphangitis,[60, 80, 208, 301, 409] folliculitis and furunculosis,[208,

---

*References 112, 124, 248, 304, 307, 358–360
†References 253, 304, 307, 309, 358–360, 364, 407

[389] and abscesses in foals.[39] *Streptococcus equi* is the cause of equine strangles, an acute contagious upper respiratory disease characterized by pyrexia, mucopurulent nasorrhea, and abscess formation in mandibular or retropharyngeal lymph nodes.[40, 59, 75, 246] Streptococcal hypersensitivity associated with *S. equi* infection has been the alleged pathologic mechanism of urticaria, dermatitis, and purpura hemorrhagica (see Chapter 10, discussion on Vasculitis) seen in conjunction with equine strangles.

In swine, β-hemolytic streptococci, especially *S. zooepidemicus* and *S. equisimilis*, have been isolated from *subcutaneous abscesses*[103, 185, 209, 217, 258, 259] and porcine ear necrosis.[240] Beta-hemolytic streptococci (principally Lancefield Group C) have also been reported to cause so-called contagious pustular dermatitis in suckling pigs.[60, 72, 73, 150, 208] Piglets have premonitory signs of fever, anorexia, and depression, which are followed by erythema with or without petechiation over the ventrum and periocular area. Pustules then develop, especially on the groin, medial thighs, periocular and dorsal lumbosacral areas, lips, pinnae, and tail. Circular crusts are the healing phase of the disease and are often associated with pruritus. Similar lesions may be seen on the udder and teats of sows. In some cases, abscesses and ulcers occur, especially on the snout, cheeks, tail, legs, and feet. Treatment with penicillin (11,000 IU/kg) or tetracyclines (20 mg/kg) is effective. Suggestive control measures including minimizing cutaneous injuries (clipping of needle teeth, and so on) and improved hygiene. Autogenous bacterins were reported to be helpful in problem herds.[161] In general, streptococcal cross-infections in animals and humans have been poorly studied. At present, the major concerns are *S. pyogenes* and *S. equisimilis* infections, which may produce sore throats or scarlet fever in humans.[169]

CORYNEBACTERIAL INFECTIONS

Corynebacterium species are gram-positive, pleomorphic short rods. In general, (1) these bacteria require various predisposing factors to become established as an infection, (2) manipulation of the immune response by natural or artificial methods is not adequate for producing resistance to these bacteria, and (3) good management practices may be the most important means of controlling infections with these bacteria.[35, 60, 75] *Corynebacterium pseudotuberculosis* (*C. ovis*, Preisz-Nocard bacillus) causes caseous lymphadenitis in sheep and goats; deep-seated subcutaneous abscesses in horses, cattle, sheep, and goats; folliculitis and furunculosis in horses; and ulcerative lymphangitis in horses and cattle.* *C. pyogenes* causes abscesses and wound infections in all large animal species.[35, 60, 73, 277] *Rhodococcus equi* causes ulcerative lymphangitis and subcutaneous abscesses in horses.† *C. pseudotuberculosis*, *C. pyogenes*, and *R. equi* are all capable of producing infections in humans.[169]

Corynebacterium pseudotuberculosis Abscesses in the Horse

C. pseudotuberculosis is a cause of deep subcutaneous abscesses ("Wyoming strangles," false strangles, bastard strangles, "pigeon breast") in horses‡ and, rarely, cattle, sheep, and goats.[145, 146, 360] Most of the reports of this disorder have come from the western United States, especially California, although the condition has also been recognized in Brazil.[83] Two biotypes of the organism have been described: isolates from sheep and goats (nitrate-negative biotype) and isolates from horses and cattle (nitrate-positive biotype).[51, 64]

C. pseudotuberculosis is believed to be spread by biting flies, especially horn flies, and inoculated through fly bites during the summer time. Subsequent lymphatic spread and abscess formation occur. Fly bites seem uniquely susceptible, as *C. pseudotuberculosis* rarely contaminates lacerations, wire cuts, abrasions, and so forth. Although *C. pseudotuberculosis* is capable of living in soil and fomites for long periods of time (up to 55 days),[30] it has usually not been isolated from the soil on premises where infected horses are kept. However, ticks can harbor the organism, and dipterids have been experimentally contaminated and were mechanical vectors for three days. In addition, the seasonal patterns of ventral midline dermatitis (see Chapter 9, discussion on equine ventral midline dermatitis) and *C. pseudotuberculosis* abscesses are similar.

There are no apparent age, breed, or sex predilections, although infection is rare in

---

*References 35, 48, 60, 75, 145, 358, 360
†References 38, 80, 99, 106a, 110, 342, 370, 372
‡References 69, 75, 146, 170, 204, 241, 249, 257, 273, 325, 412

horses younger than one year of age. Neither do husbandry practices appear to be important. The condition has a seasonal occurrence, with peak incidences in late summer, fall, and early winter. The highest incidence of disease is seen following winters of above average rainfall, which result in optimal breeding conditions for insects in the following summer and fall.

Clinically, the condition is characterized by single or multiple slowly or rapidly developing deep subcutaneous abscesses. About 50 percent of these abscesses occur in the pectoral and ventral abdominal areas. Additionally, abscesses can occur on the thorax, shoulder, neck, and head. The purulent discharge is usually creamy to caseous and whitish to greenish. These abscesses are often associated with pitting edema, ventral midline dermatitis, depression, fever, and lameness. Untoward sequelae, consisting of prolonged or chronic suppurative discharge, multiple abscesses, internal abscesses, and abortion, were not uncommon in cases of marked or prolonged fever and in cases of cutaneous abscesses in areas other than the typical pectoral or ventral abdominal regions.[75, 171, 257, 273, 347] Purpura hemorrhagica may be a sequela in some long-standing refractory cases.[273]

The differential diagnosis includes other bacterial, fungal, and foreign body abscesses. Definitive diagnosis is based on history, physical examination, direct smears, and culture. In smears, C. pseudotuberculosis appears as small gram-positive rods with a typical "Chinese-letter" configuration. However, the organisms are often present in too small a number to be detected in smears. Serologic techniques have value as epidemiologic tools, but titers are not accurate for detecting active clinical disease.[204, 205]

Treatment is best accomplished by allowing the subcutaneous abscesses to come to a head and then surgically incising and draining them. Healing is usually complete within two to three months. Warm soaks may help bring slowly developing abscesses to a head. Using systemic antibiotics before the abscesses have come to a head is usually ineffective and is commonly followed by exacerbations when the drugs are stopped.[75, 257, 273] When drainage is not feasible, high doses of procaine penicillin (20,000 to 50,000 IU/kg/day) for prolonged periods (up to six months) may be effective.[75, 255, 273, 347]

Attempts to use bacterins and toxoids for prevention have not been successful.[75, 204] Any

immunity produced by natural or artificial means is very transitory. Good sanitation and fly control should help to decrease the incidence of disease.

C. pseudotuberculosis is also capable of producing infections in humans.[169] The sudden onset of a mildly painful regional lymphadenopathy that proceeds to rupture and drain a greenish, creamy, odorless pus is the typical clinical picture. Thus, caution should be exercised when handling infected materials.

Ulcerative Lymphangitis

Ulcerative lymphangitis is a bacterial infection of the cutaneous lymphatics in horses and cattle and, rarely, sheep and goats.* The condition is most commonly associated with poor hygiene and management and insect transmission and is infrequently seen today.

The most commonly isolated organism from all species is C. pseudotuberculosis, with staphylococci, streptococci, C. pyogenes, C. equi, Pasteurella haemolytica, Pseudomonas aeruginosa, Fusobacterium necrophorum (Fusiformis necrophorus), and Actinobacillus equuli being less frequently found.† Mixed infections as well as negative cultures have been described. These infections are thought to arise from wound contamination.

In horses, cases of ulcerative lymphangitis are sporadic, with no apparent age, breed, or sex predilections.‡ Lesions are most commonly found on a hind limb, especially the fetlock, and rarely above the hock (Fig. 6–15). Lesions consist of hard to fluctuant nodules, which abscess, ulcerate, and develop draining tracts (Fig. 6–16). Individual ulcers tend to heal within one to two weeks, but new lesions continue to develop. The regional lymphatics are often corded. In C. pseudotuberculosis infections, edema and fibrosis are usually striking. Lameness and debilitation may be seen. Rarely, lymph node involvement or systemic spread may occur.

In cattle, ulcerative lymphangitis is very uncommon and has no apparent age, breed, or sex predilections.[37, 60, 118, 176, 208, 322] Lesions are the same as those previously described for horses and may be found on the fetlock, feet, neck, shoulders, forelegs, and flanks. Heat,

---

*References 11, 37, 60, 80, 208, 253, 273, 307, 309
†References 37, 38, 60, 75, 80, 99, 110, 208, 253, 260, 273, 301, 307, 322, 342
‡References 1, 60, 75, 80, 253, 262, 273, 301, 307, 368

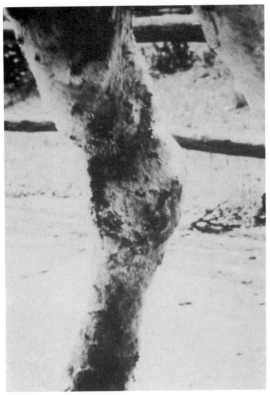

FIGURE 6–15. Ulcerative lymphangitis in a horse. Marked swelling of hind leg, with multiple ulcers and draining tracts.

pain, and lameness are variable, but regional lymphadenopathy and marked edema are very common.

The differential diagnosis includes glanders, sporotrichosis, equine histoplasmosis, and my-cobacterial infections. Definitive diagnosis is based on history, physical examination, direct smears, and culture. Skin biopsy reveals superficial and deep perivascular dermatitis to diffuse dermatitis (Fig. 6–17). The dermatitis may be suppurative or pyogranulomatous. Edema and fibrosis are often marked. It may be possible to see the organism with tissue Gram's stain or Brown and Brenn's stain.

Although ulcerative lymphangitis is rarely fatal, debilitation and disfigurement can occur. In early equine cases, hydrotherapy, exercise, surgical drainage, and high doses of procaine penicillin (20,000 to 80,000 IU/kg twice daily) for prolonged periods (over 30 days) may be effective.[75, 80, 273, 309] However, once significant fibrosis occurs, there is virtually no chance for cure. Therapeutic recommendations for cattle include hydrotherapy, exercise, surgical drainage, and a 20 percent solution of NaI given intravenously (16.5 ml/50 kg) once in conjunction with procaine penicillin (44,000 IU/kg once daily) and streptomycin (11 mg/kg twice daily) given subcutaneously for ten days.[37]

Although early workers[206, 208] claimed success with bacterins in the treatment of *C. pseudotuberculosis* ulcerative lymphangitis, recent investigators have not had good results.[75, 80, 204] Good hygiene and management practices as well as early wound treatment and fly control should be helpful control measures.

Equine Folliculitis and Furunculosis

Bacterial folliculitis and furunculosis is a common equine dermatosis. *C. pseudotuber-*

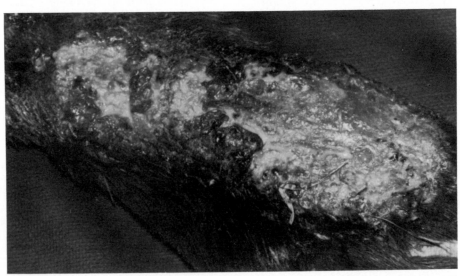

FIGURE 6–16. Ulcerative lymphangitis in a horse. Linear area of ulceration and draining tracts on medial aspects of hock.

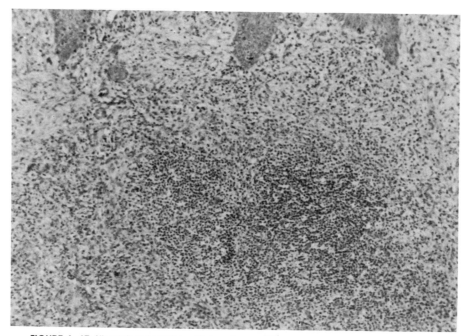

FIGURE 6–17. Ulcerative lymphangitis in a horse. Diffuse pyogranulomatous dermatitis.

culosis (Canadian horsepox, contagious acne, contagious pustular dermatitis) is a rare cause of this condition.* There are no apparent age, breed, or sex predilections.

C. pseudotuberculosis folliculitis and furunculosis is most commonly seen in spring and summer and may be precipitated by various forms of cutaneous trauma (riding, work, heat, moisture). Lesions consist of follicular papules and nodules, which are often painful and occur most commonly over the saddle and tack areas. These lesions tend to ulcerate and drain a creamy, greenish-white pus.

Diagnosis and treatment of equine folliculitis and furunculosis are discussed in the section on staphylococcal infections.

Caseous Lymphadenitis

Caseous lymphadenitis, a common disease of sheep and goats caused by *C. pseudotuberculosis*, is the most frequent cause of abscesses in these animals. As a general rule, any abscess associated with a lymph node of a sheep or goat should be assumed to be due to *C. pseudotuberculosis* until proved otherwise.

Lesions of caseous lymphadenitis are characterized by abscesses of lymph nodes and nodules and draining tracts in the skin (Fig. 6–18).[208, 275, 276, 360] The purulent discharge is

usually thick, creamy or cheesy, and yellowish, greenish, or tan.

Diagnosis is based on history, physical examination, direct smears, and culture. Skin biopsy reveals nodular to diffuse dermatitis associated with tuberculoid granulomatous inflammation (Fig. 6–19). There is typically a

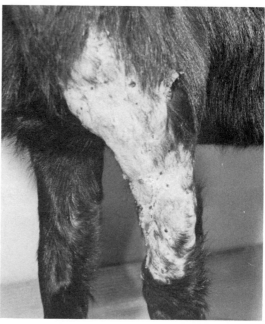

FIGURE 6–18. Caseous lymphadenitis in a goat. Abscess formation and draining tracts on the leg.

*References 75, 176, 208, 253, 307, 309, 358, 359

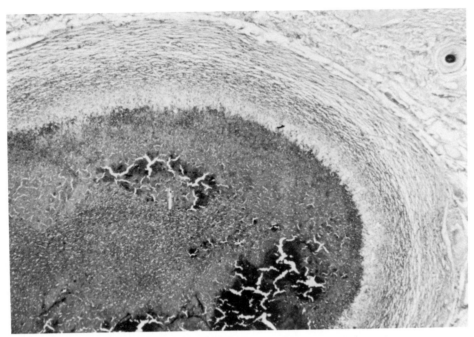

FIGURE 6-19. Caseous lymphadenitis in a goat. Tuberculoid granuloma.

central area of neutrophilic infiltration and caseous necrosis that is surrounded by a layer of macrophages, which is in turn surrounded by a layer of lymphocytes and plasma cells. An outer fibrovascular capsule is usually present. It may be possible to identify the organism with tissue Gram's or Brown and Brenn's stain.

Details of diagnosis, treatment, and control are discussed in other texts and articles.[36, 60, 135, 275, 360]

ACTINOMYCETIC INFECTIONS

Large animals are susceptible to infection with a number of actinomycetes (filamentous or fungus-like bacteria). Examples of such infections include dermatophilosis, actinomycosis, actinobacillosis, and nocardiosis.

With many of these infections, except dermatophilosis, the resultant lesions are often called mycetomas (fungal tumors).[77, 114, 272, 360] Clinically, the triad of tumefaction, draining tracts, and "grains" always suggests mycetoma. The grains, or granules, are pinpoint in size and variable in color and represent microorganisms coated with host immunoglobulin and fibrin.

Naturally occurring mycetomas were reported in three goats.[133] Two goats had a mycetoma on the hind leg, and one had a mycetoma on the scapula. The discharges from these lesions were gray and watery and contained red, orange, or purple grains. All three goats were emaciated, and one died. Cultures were performed on two of the goats, and *Actinomadura madurae* was isolated. In the other goat, only a histopathologic examination was performed, and an organism consistent with *Actinomadura pelletierii* was seen. Skin biopsies from all three goats revealed nodular to diffuse dermatitis resulting from pyogranulomatous inflammation. Basophilic tissue grains and branching hyphae were readily demonstrated.

Experimentally, normal goats were inoculated subcutaneously with *A. madurae*, *A. pelletierii*, and *Nocardia brasiliensis*.[134] Only those goats inoculated with *A. pelletierii* developed draining tracts.

In humans and small animals, the therapy of mycetoma varies with the causative organism and can include surgical excision or amputation, sulfonamides, penicillin, inorganic iodides, amphotericin B, 5-fluorocytosine, and ketoconazole.[114, 272] Successful therapy of caprine mycetoma has not been reported.

Dermatophilosis

Dermatophilosis is a common infectious, superficial, pustular, and crusting dermatitis of horses, cattle, sheep, and goats caused by *Dermatophilus congolensis.*

Cause and Pathogenesis

Dermatophilus congolensis is a gram-positive, facultative anaerobic actinomycete.[60, 77, 189, 225, 351] Prior incorrect synonyms for the organism include *Actinomyces dermatonomus, Nocardia dermatonomus, Dermatophilus dermatonomus, D. pedis, Polysepta pedis,* and *Rhizopus.* The disease itself has also been branded with numerous names, some reflecting obsolete conceptions of the etiologic agent, others being descriptive of the clinical appearance: streptothricosis, mycotic dermatitis, cutaneous actinomycosis, aphis, Senkobo skin disease, lumpy wool, rain scald, rain rot, and strawberry foot-rot.

The natural habitat of *D. congolensis* is unknown.[2, 189, 192, 196, 351, 381] Attempts to isolate it from soil have been unsuccessful.* *D. congolensis* has been isolated only from the integument and crusts of various animals and is thought to exist in quiescent form in clinically inevident but chronically infected carrier animals until climatic conditions are favorable for its infectivity.†

There is probably a multiplicity of factors in operation for the initiation, development, and propagation of dermatophilosis, and to consider one factor in isolation is probably unrealistic.‡ Research workers have failed to reproduce the disease as it is seen in nature, and field work in different parts of the world aimed at elucidating the reasons for the pronounced seasonal variations in occurrence and for the disease's various manifestations has led to apparently conflicting results.

The two most important factors in the initiation and development of dermatophilosis are skin damage and moisture.§ It is virtually impossible to establish infection and lesions on intact, undamaged skin, even with very heavy, pure cultures of *D. congolensis.* Moisture causes the release of the infective, motile, flagellated zoospore form of the organism. These zoospores are attracted to low concentrations of carbon dioxide but repelled by high concentrations.[337–340, 351] The high concentrations of carbon dioxide produced in wet crusts by dense populations of zoospores accelerate their escape to the skin surface, whereas the respiratory efflux of low concentrations of carbon dioxide from the skin attracts zoospores to susceptible areas on the skin surface.

Important sources of skin damage include biting flies and arthropods, prickly vegetation, and maceration.* The distribution of clinical lesions often mirrors these environmental insults. *D. congolensis* can survive on the mouthparts of ticks for many months and can be transmitted by biting and nonbiting flies for up to 24 hours after they have fed on donor lesions.† The importance of moisture is evidenced by the markedly increased incidence of disease during periods of heavy rainfall.‡

Other, more controversial proposed predisposing factors in the pathogenesis of dermatophilosis include high ambient temperature, high relative humidity, poor nutrition, poor hygiene, and various debilitating or stressful conditions.§ In mice with experimentally induced dermatophilosis, concurrent administration of glucocorticoids increased the severity of the lesions.[5] Chronic dermatophilosis has been associated with a wide range of circumstances that all produce a reduction of the host's immune responses, such as poor nutrition, heavy intestinal parasite burden, bovine trypanosomiasis and rinderpest, and localized reductions in immunity in the area of an arthropod bite.[85, 381] The thickness of the skin and stratum corneum were not found to be important predisposing factors.[16, 183, 362] In any particular herd or group of animals, all the animals are presumably exposed, yet often only a few become infected. Additionally, of those that do become clinically affected, some have a very mild disease, whereas others are severely diseased. This has caused investigators to postulate an intrinsic factor(s) that favors or hinders the development of dermatophilosis.[20, 153, 225, 248, 295, 351] By the same token, apparent breed differences in susceptibility to disease have raised the question of genetic factors in resistance.‖

---

*References 189, 192, 196, 225, 334, 351, 358, 381
†References 2, 225, 229, 248, 273, 274, 295, 351, 358, 378, 381
‡References 2, 6, 60, 123, 189, 225, 273, 274, 295, 351a, 381
§References 2, 31, 60, 189, 219, 225, 229, 248, 255, 273, 295, 297, 358, 378, 381

*References 2, 225, 229, 235–237, 239, 248, 255, 273, 295, 297, 307, 308, 328, 378, 381
†References 2, 60, 225, 234, 235–237, 297, 328, 381
‡References 2, 31, 60, 122, 219, 225, 229, 255, 273, 297, 358, 360, 381
§References 2, 6, 59, 115, 225, 228, 255, 273, 295, 351, 381
‖References 17, 31, 102, 153, 225, 248, 351

It has been hypothesized that *D. congolensis* can be eliminated from normal skin, but if the processes involved in elimination are inhibited, the lesion produced by the bacterium becomes chronic.[84, 85] Guinea pigs were sensitized to dinitrochlorobenzene and infected with *D. congolensis* at the site of a subsequent application of this chemical.[85] The bacterium was recovered from the skin over a longer period of time in sensitized individuals than in non-sensitized control subjects. However, the lesions produced at the site of infection did not become chronic.

Studies have shown that zoospores can remain viable within crusts, at a temperature of 28 to 31°C, for up to 42 months.[225, 297, 358, 360] In addition, zoospores within crusts can resist drying and can withstand heating at 100°C when dried.[225, 297, 358, 360] Therefore, crusts on animals and in the environment are important potential sources of infection and reinfection.[225, 273, 297, 358, 360] Dermatophilosis is a contagious disease. The incubation period averages about two weeks but may be as short as 24 hours or as long as 34 days.*

Clinical Features

The cutaneous syndromes attributable to dermatophilosis are truly protean. It is best to consider any crusting dermatosis to be dermatophilosis until proved otherwise. In general, there are no age, breed, or sex predilections. Infections in any one group of animals may involve a single individual or up to 80 percent of the herd.

The primary lesions in dermatophilosis are follicular and nonfollicular papules and pustules. These lesions rapidly coalesce and become exudative, which results in large ovoid groups of hairs becoming matted together (paintbrush effect). Close examination shows the proximal portions of these hairs to be embedded in dried exudate. When these paintbrushes are plucked off, ovoid areas of eroded to ulcerated, often bleeding and pustular skin are revealed (see Plate 3F). Active lesions contain a thick, creamy, whitish, yellowish, or greenish pus, which adheres to the skin surface and to the undersurface of the crusts. The undersurface of the crusts is usually concave, with the roots of the hairs protruding. Acute, active lesions of dermatophilosis are often painful, but the disease is rarely pruritic. The

healing or chronic stage of the disease is characterized by dry crusts, scaling, and alopecia (ringworm-like lesions).

In horses, these exudative, crusted lesions are commonly found over the (1) rump and topline (rain scald) (Figs. 6–20 and 6–21), (2) saddle area, (3) face and neck (Fig. 6–22), and (4) pasterns, coronets, and heels (grease heel, scratches, mud fever) (Fig. 6–23).* Lesions of the distal limbs may be associated with edema, pain, and lameness.[231, 253, 273, 304–308, 381] Infections on white-skinned and haired areas, especially the muzzle and distal limbs, are often associated with severe erythema (dew poisoning) and may represent a type of photodermatitis caused by *D. congolensis*.[115, 273, 307, 308] In other horses, the infection may be isolated to the cranial aspect of the hind cannon bones (resembling cannon keratosis)[306, 307] or may become generalized.[115, 307, 308, 358, 381] Severely affected animals may show depression, lethargy, poor appetite, weight loss, fever, and lymphadenopathy.

In goats, the lesions of dermatophilosis are commonly seen on the pinnae and tail of kids and the muzzle, dorsal midline (Fig. 6–24), and scrotum of adults.† Lesions may be limited to the distal limbs, resembling the strawberry foot-rot form of dermatophilosis seen in sheep.[360] Occasionally, cutaneous horns of 1 mm in diameter by 12 mm in length are seen on the scrotum, ventral abdomen, or medial thighs.[279] Chronic lymphadenitis has been reported.[371] Double infections with dermatophilosis and contagious ecthyma have been reported.[280]

In sheep, the most common clinical forms of dermatophilosis are (1) crusts on the ears, nose, and face of lambs, (2) pyramidal crusts over the topline and flanks (lumpy wool), and (3) crusts from coronets to tarsi and carpi, with underlying bleeding, fleshy masses of tissue (strawberry foot-rot).‡ Fine-wooled breeds, such as Suffolk and Romney, are most susceptible. Dermatophilosis also produces various abnormalities that detract from the value of sheep wool and hide, including (1) hide thickening (coarse grain), (2) unevenness of hide (spread cockle), (3) permanent enlargement of wool follicles (pinhole), and (4) secretory staining of wool (yellow wool).[31, 45, 87–89, 153, 225]

---

*References 60, 111, 189, 219, 225, 248, 255, 273, 274

*References 69, 115, 189, 192, 196, 231, 238, 251, 253, 273, 304–309, 358, 379, 381
†References 70, 200, 256, 279, 300, 360, 375
‡References 60, 104, 225, 229, 248, 255, 275, 300, 351

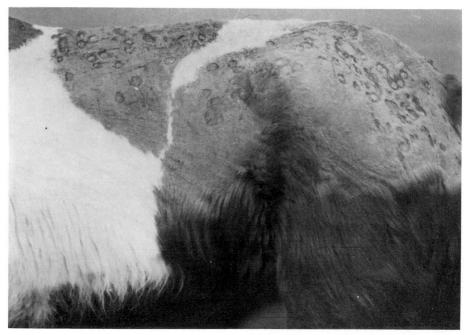

FIGURE 6–20. Equine dermatophilosis. Multiple crusts over top line (area has been clipped).

FIGURE 6–21. Equine dermatophilosis. Multiple crusts over rump (area has been clipped).

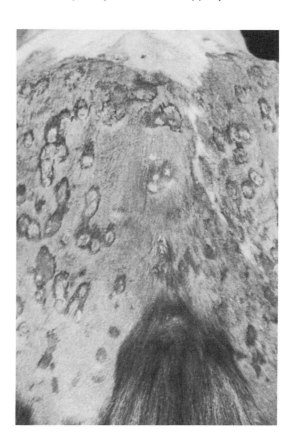

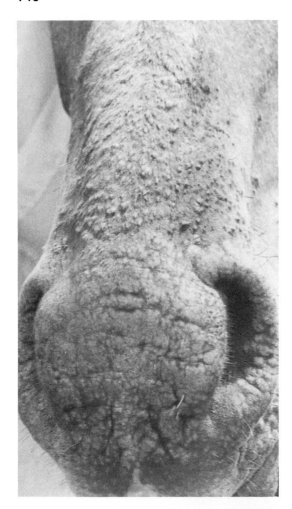

FIGURE 6–22. Equine dermatophilosis. Crusts on muzzle.

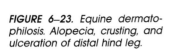

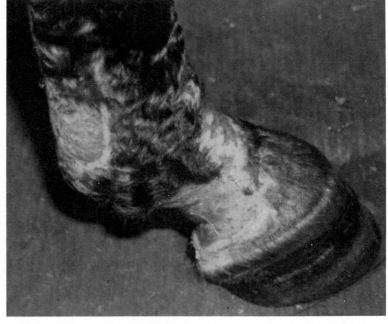

FIGURE 6–23. Equine dermatophilosis. Alopecia, crusting, and ulceration of distal hind leg.

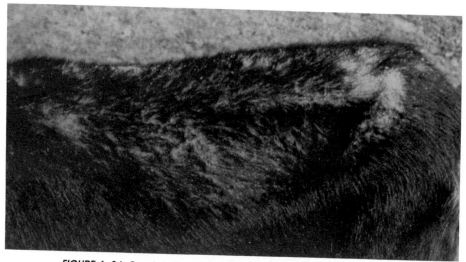

FIGURE 6–24. Caprine dermatophilosis. Alopecia and crusts over back.

Dual infections with dermatophilosis and contagious ecthyma have been reported.[82, 248, 280] In addition, subcutaneous abscesses and nodules, and lymphangitis and lymphadenitis, have rarely been reported in ovine dermatophilosis.[264, 264a, 395]

In cattle, common clinical forms of dermatophilosis include (1) face and ears (especially calves [milk scald] and bulls), (2) rump and topline (Fig. 6–25), (3) brisket, axillae, and groin, (4) udder and teats, or scrotum and prepuce (Fig. 6–26), (5) distal limbs (Fig. 6–27), and (6) perineum and tail (leproid form).* Focal lesions may be seen on the pinnae, and cutaneous horns may arise from skin lesions at any site.[225, 231, 351] Subcutaneous and lymph node granulomas have been reported.[125] Animals with over 50 percent of their body affected often show rapid weight loss and dehydration and die.[60, 274, 295]

Dermatophilosis is very rare in swine.[230, 377, 381] Affected pigs have a generalized exudative, crusting dermatitis. Dual infections with *D. congolensis* and *Staphylococcus hyicus* have been reported.[230]

Dermatophilosis can be an economically devastating disease, leading to (1) loss of production of hides, wool, meat, and milk, (2) losses resulting from culling or death in severe infections (with or without secondary infection or myiasis), and (3) losses because of veterinary expenses.†

In addition, dermatophilosis is a zoonosis. Human infections are characterized by pitted keratolysis or an erythematous, pruritic or painful, pustular dermatitis in contact areas that lasts two weeks to two months without treatment.* An unusual case of granulomatous dermatophilosis was reported in an immunodeficient child.[14]

Diagnosis

The differential diagnosis is extensive, including dermatophytosis, staphylococcal folliculitis and furunculosis, viral infections, zinc-responsive dermatoses, and pemphigus foliaceus. Definitive diagnosis is based on history, physical examination, direct smears, skin biopsy, and culture. Direct smears of pus or saline-soaked and minced crusts may be stained with new methylene blue, Diff-Quik, or Gram's stains. *D. congolensis* appears as fine-branching and multiseptate hyphae, which divide transversely and longitudinally to form cuboidal packets of coccoid cells arranged in two to eight parallel rows within branching filaments (railroad track appearance) (Fig. 6–28). In the healing or dry chronic stages of the disease, direct smears are rarely positive.

Skin biopsy usually reveals varying degrees of folliculitis, intraepidermal pustular dermatitis, and superficial perivascular dermatitis.† Intracellular edema (vacuolar alteration) of keratinocytes is often striking (Fig. 6–29). Sur-

---

*References 2, 19, 60, 173, 210, 225, 231, 255, 274, 295, 297, 319, 351, 381, 416
†References 60, 71, 122, 224, 225, 248, 274, 286, 290, 351, 381

*References 55, 115, 177, 190, 191, 248, 273, 274
†References 16, 18, 54, 70, 188, 225, 255, 256, 295, 297, 336, 358, 378

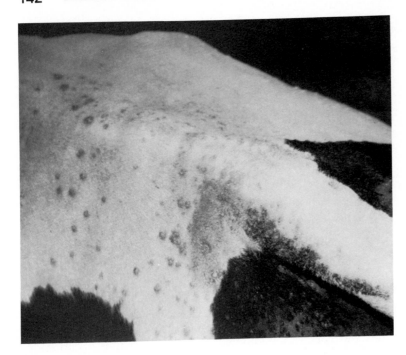

FIGURE 6–25. Bovine dermatophilosis. Multiple crusts over
rump.

FIGURE 6–26. Bovine dermatophilosis. Multiple crusts on
perineum, scrotum, and caudomedial thighs. (Courtesy
J. Edwards.)

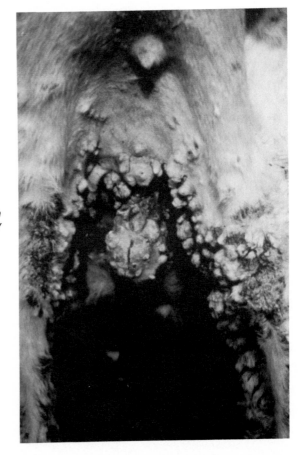

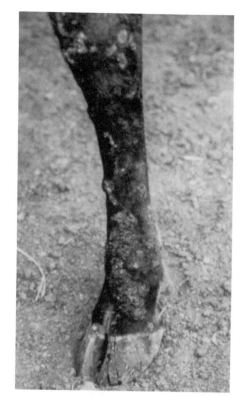

FIGURE 6–27. Bovine dermatophilosis. Crusts on leg. (Courtesy J. Edwards.)

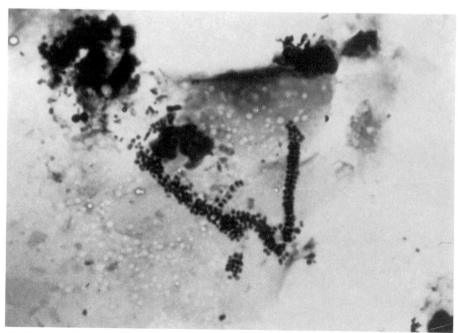

FIGURE 6–28. Dermatophilosis. Typical "railroad tracks" appearance of Dermatophilus congolensis in a direct smear.

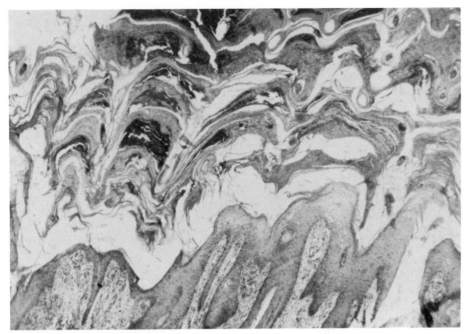

FIGURE 6–29. Dermatophilosis. Typical "palisading" crust.

face crust is characterized by alternating layers of keratin (ortho- or parakeratotic) and leukocytic debris (palisading crust) (Fig. 6–30). *D. congolensis* is usually seen in the keratinous debris on the surface of the skin and within hair follicles (see Plate 4 *A*). The organism can be seen in sections stained with H & E but is better visualized with Giemsa's, Brown and Brenn's, or acid orcein–Giemsa (AOG) stains. *D. congolensis* has also been occasionally seen in sebaceous glands and the superficial dermis.[16, 225] A nodular to diffuse dermatitis resulting from granulomatous inflammation may be seen occasionally.[4, 7, 125, 264, 294, 295] Tissue granules containing *D. congolensis* and covered with Splendore-Hoeppli material are rare.[125]

D. congolensis grows well on blood agar when incubated in a microaerophilic atmosphere with increased carbon dioxide.[127, 189, 225, 295, 351] However, the culture can be unsatisfactory as a result of rapid overgrowth of secondary invaders and contaminating saprophytes and in the chronic nonexudative stage.* In such instances, special, often complicated isolation techniques may be helpful.[3, 4, 351, 351a] On blood agar, *D. congolensis* is dry, filamentous, whitish, and hemolytic in a microaerophilic atmosphere at 37°C and is moist, coccoid,

nonhemolytic, and generally bright orange at 22°C.

Serologically, there are no cross-reactions between *D. congolensis* and *Actinomyces* or *Nocardia* species,[127] and agar gel precipitin and passive hemagglutination tests were found to be inaccurate for the diagnosis of active disease.[244, 329] A specific fluorescent antibody technique was reported to be rapid and specific for the diagnosis of dermatophilosis.[329]

Clinical Management

Differences in management practices, climate, and economic considerations make a standard therapeutic protocol unrealistic and make "doing the best we can under the circumstances" mandatory. For example, treatment regimens recommended for temperate areas of the world are often unsuccessful in subtropical and tropical regions.[60, 136, 153, 179, 225, 248] General therapeutic guidelines are as follows: (1) most cases spontaneously regress within four weeks if the animals can be kept dry,* (2) keeping the animals dry is very important,† (3) crust removal and disposal and topical treatments

---

*References 2–4, 192, 225, 273, 308, 329, 351, 363

*References 20, 115, 189, 225, 229, 231, 248, 273, 274, 295, 297, 307, 308, 351, 358, 360, 378, 379, 381
†References 115, 189, 225, 229, 295, 297, 307, 308, 351, 358, 360, 378, 379, 381

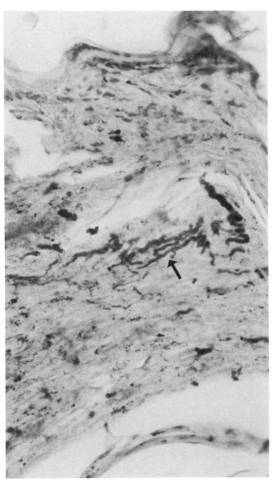

FIGURE 6–30. Dermatophilosis. D. congolensis branching "railroad tracks" (arrow) in surface keratin.

are also very important,* and (4) systemic therapy is often needed for severe, generalized, or chronic infections.†

In horses, goats, sheep, and cattle in temperate regions of the world, commonly used topical solutions include iodophors, 2 to 5 percent lime sulfur, 0.5 percent zinc sulfate, 0.2 percent copper sulfate, and 1 percent potassium aluminum sulfate (alum).‡ In general, the topical solutions are applied as total body washes, sprays, or dips for three to five consecutive days, then weekly until healing has occurred. It must be remembered that iodo-

phors, lime sulfur, and copper sulfate stain hair and wool. For severely crusted and cracked focal lesions in horses, the daily topical application of 0.25 to 0.5 percent chloramphenicol in cod liver oil for five to seven days is reported to be very effective.[253, 304–308] In problem flocks of sheep when elimination of dermatophilosis is impractical, routine summer and fall protective dips with 0.5 percent zinc sulfate or 1 percent potassium aluminum sulfate are reported to be effective.[229, 248] However, another investigator reported that the routine dipping of weaner sheep from flocks in which the disease was known to occur was undesirable, as it resulted in more lesions and less wool.[410] This same author recommended powders (which are more laborious and are less practical to use).

In vitro, *D. congolensis* is sensitive to many drugs.[4, 57, 225, 289, 400] In temperate regions of the world, the most commonly used systemic antibiotics are penicillin and streptomycin.* Frequently used regimens are as follows: (1) for horses, 22,000 IU/kg procaine penicillin G and 11 mg/kg streptomycin twice daily for seven days, (2) for cattle, sheep, and goats, 5000 IU/kg procaine penicillin G and 5 mg/kg streptomycin daily for four days, and (3) for sheep, a single injection of 70,000 IU/kg procaine penicillin and 70 mg/kg streptomycin. For cattle, anecdotal reports have suggested that inorganic iodides may be effective in severe cases.[20, 105, 175]

In Africa, where standard therapeutic protocols are often unsuccessful, encouraging results were reported in cattle and sheep with oxytetracycline.[136, 179] A single intramuscular injection of long-acting oxytetracycline (20 mg/kg) was reported to be curative in over 90 percent of the animals treated. However, another study indicated that results obtained with intramuscular penicillin (70,000 IU/kg) and streptomycin (70 mg/kg) daily for three treatments were superior to those obtained with long-acting oxytetracycline.[122]

Other recommendations for therapy and control of dermatophilosis include improved hygiene, nutrition, and management practices; biting insect and arthropod control measures; isolation or culling of affected animals; avoidance of mechanical trauma to skin.†

*References 189, 225, 229, 248, 253, 273, 274, 308, 358, 360, 381
†References 56, 57, 69, 136, 179, 225, 248, 253, 273, 274, 307–309, 351, 358, 360, 381
‡References 57, 60, 151, 152, 225, 229, 248, 273, 274, 307, 308, 351, 351a, 358, 360, 381

*References 19, 20, 57, 58, 60, 69, 220, 229, 248, 253, 265, 273, 274, 307, 333, 351, 351a, 358
†References 60, 225, 229, 234, 248, 273, 274, 381

Previously infected animals do not develop a significant immunity to reinfection.* Attempts to immunize animals with several *D. congolensis* antigens were unsuccessful.[197] However, intradermal vaccination of cattle in Africa with a nonlyophilized *D. congolensis* preparation was reported to be quite effective.[320] Intradermal vaccination was reported to induce increased serum IgG levels and increased levels of IgG, IgA, and IgM in skin surface washings.[227]

Actinomycosis

Actinomycosis is an infectious, suppurative to granulomatous disease of cattle, sheep, swine, horses, and goats caused by *Actinomyces* species.

Cause and Pathogenesis

Actinomycosis is worldwide in distribution and, in the United States, is seen most commonly in the west and midwest. *Actinomyces* species are normal inhabitants of the oral cavity, upper respiratory tract, and digestive tract of domestic animals and humans.† Although the exact pathogenesis of actinomycosis is not clear, these gram-positive, filamentous anaerobes are probably opportunistic invaders of damaged oral mucosa and skin. Predilection factors include mucosal damage done by dietary roughage (thorns, awns), exposure of dental alveoli when deciduous teeth are shed, and penetrating wounds of the skin.

In cattle, the causative organism is *A. bovis*. In swine, based on biochemical reactions and an agar gel precipitin test, the name *A. suis* has been proposed for this apparently swine-specific strain of *Actinomyces*.[119]

Clinical Features

Actinomycosis is most commonly seen in cattle, with the basic lesion being a rarefying osteomyelitis.[12, 19, 60, 168, 175] The mandible and maxilla are commonly affected (lumpy jaw), especially at the level of the third or fourth molar. The disease is most commonly seen in two- to five-year-old cattle (shedding of deciduous teeth), with no apparent breed or sex predilections. Firm, variably painful, immovable bony swellings extend to the overlying skin, resulting in nodules, abscesses, and fistulae. The exudate is honey-like and contains hard yellowish-white granules (sulfur granules) that are the size and consistency of sand. The course may be rapid or progress slowly over a period of years, eventuating in anorexia and progressive emaciation. The infection may occasionally involve the palatine and turbinate bones, esophageal groove, reticulum, udder, and testicles.

In swine, actinomycosis is characterized by a suppurative, granulomatous, fibrous enlargement of the udder.* Fistulae drain a yellowish pus containing the characteristic sulfur granules. Mechanical trauma and tooth wounds from suckling piglets are thought to be important predisposing factors. The disease may occasionally involve the spleen, liver, kidney, and lung.

Actinomycosis is apparently rare in horses, sheep, and goats and mimics the bovine disease.[60, 65, 132, 168, 175, 208]

Diagnosis

The differential diagnosis includes other bacterial and fungal granulomatous diseases, especially botryomycosis, actinobacillosis, mycetoma, and coccidioidomycosis. Definitive diagnosis is made by direct smears, biopsy, and culture. The sulfur granules may be squashed on a glass slide and shown to consist of gram-positive filamentous organisms. Skin biopsy reveals a nodular to diffuse suppurative or pyogranulomatous dermatitis, in which the organisms may be seen individually or in granules (grains) (Fig. 6–31). These granules contain masses of the organism, usually surrounded by an eosinophilic covering of material that has a radiating or clublike appearance (Splendore-Hoeppli phenomenon). The organisms are best visualized in sections stained with Gram's or Grocott's methenamine silver stain.

The sulfur granules may also be collected, rinsed with sterile saline, and used for culture (anaerobic). The simple swabbing of a fistula often results in other organisms being cultured as well, especially *Corynebacterium pyogenes* and coagulase-positive staphylococci.

---

*References 2, 196, 197, 225, 248, 255, 256, 334, 351, 387
†References 19, 60, 77, 114, 168, 188, 272

---

*References 50, 60, 103, 119, 130, 217, 242, 277, 403

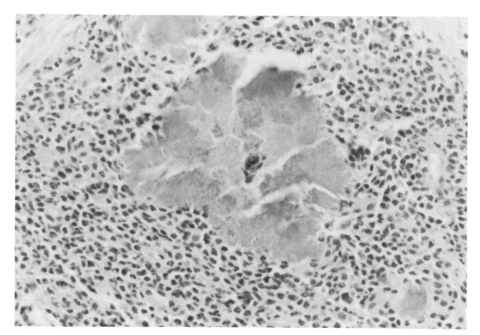

FIGURE 6–31. Bovine actinomycosis. Granulomatous dermatitis surrounding a tissue grain.

Clinical Management

The literature on the therapy of bovine actinomycosis is confusing and contradictory. Some authors report good success with parenteral or intralesional penicillin, with or without streptomycin and proteolytic enzymes,[202, 222, 357] but others have reported this to be ineffective.[19, 168, 175] Some authors have reported good success with parenteral inorganic iodides,[113, 288] while still others have found this to be ineffective.[19, 168, 175] Isoniazid given at 6 to 10 mg/kg orally s.i.d. for two to three weeks was reported to be beneficial.[60, 168, 406] One report suggested giving the isoniazid in conjunction with inorganic iodides.[168] Radiation therapy was reported to be of little permanent benefit.[168]

It would appear that there is no easy, inexpensive, commonly effective therapy for bovine actinomycosis. When bony lesions are severe, the most that can be expected from any treatment is to arrest further growth. This is probably best accomplished with surgical excision or drainage and parenteral inorganic iodides.

In swine and horses, reports of therapy for actinomycosis are few and difficult to evaluate. One report indicated that, in swine, surgical excision was 100 percent curative and penicillin (1 million IU) and streptomycin (1 gm/50 kg) were 95 percent curative when one half was given intramuscularly and one half was given intratumorally, and this was repeated in six to seven days.[50] Another report indicated that, in two horses, surgical drainage and parenteral therapy with penicillin and streptomycin were curative.[175]

Nocardiosis

Nocardiosis is an infectious disease of horses and cattle caused by actinomycetes of the genus *Nocardia*.[60, 77] These organisms are environmental saprophytes, which gain entry to the host via wound contamination. The organisms are gram-positive, partially acid-fast, filamentous bacteria. Rarely, *Nocardia asteroides* has been reported to cause dermatitis in the horse.[27, 53, 299]

Bovine farcy was originally thought to be caused only by *N. farcinica*.[32–34, 60, 226, 269, 270] However, an identical syndrome in Africa has been reported to be caused by *Mycobacterium farcinogenes*.[76, 107] Bovine farcy is geographically restricted to Africa, Asia, and South America. *N. farcinica* is a soil saprophyte and can be harbored by ticks for several months. Skin lesions are characterized by firm, painless, slow-growing subcutaneous nodules, which can occur anywhere on the body, especially the head, neck, shoulder, and limbs. The lesions may ulcerate and discharge a thick, odorless, grayish-white or yellowish material. Corded lymphatics (lymphangitis and regional lymphadenopathy) are usually present. Bovine farcy may have a prolonged course with no general health effects or may become generalized (to the lungs, liver, kidneys, or peritoneum) and result in emaciation and death. The differential diagnosis includes ulcerative lymphangitis and atypical mycobacteriosis (skin tuberculosis). Dermatohistopathologic findings include nodular to diffuse suppurative pyogranulomatous or granulomatous dermatitis, in which the gram-positive and partially (beaded) acid-fast organisms may be seen singly or within granules (rosettes). *N. farcinica* grows aerobically at 37°C on blood agar or Löwenstein-Jensen medium. Although therapy is not usually attempted, the parenteral administration of inorganic iodides has been recommended. In dogs, cats, and humans, sulfonamides are often effective for the treatment of nocardial infections.[114, 272]

ACTINOBACILLOSIS

Actinobacillosis is an infectious, suppurative to granulomatous disease of cattle, sheep, and rarely swine and horses caused by *Actinobacillus lignieresii*.

Cause and Pathogenesis

Actinobacillosis is worldwide in distribution, and, in the United States, is seen most commonly in the west and southwest. *A. lignieresii* may be isolated from the saliva and alimentary tract of healthy cattle and sheep and from manure and soil.*

Although the exact pathogenesis of actinobacillosis is not clear, these gram-negative, aerobic coccobacilli apparently cannot invade healthy tissues and require antecedent trauma (sharp awns, stickers, or oral and cutaneous wounds).

Clinical Features

Actinobacillosis is most commonly seen in cattle, in whom the disease is characterized by thick-walled abscesses of the soft tissues of the head (big head).[19, 60, 74, 167] Ninety percent of the animals have involvement of cervical lymph nodes, and 10 percent have tongue involvement (wooden tongue). Affected lymph

nodes enlarge and abscess but are not hot and painful. The nodes eventually rupture to discharge a viscid, odorless, white to slightly green pus that contains brown-white grains (sulfur granules). Multiple mobile head and neck abscesses and fistulae may be present. Primary cutaneous involvement is apparently rare (Fig. 6–32).[157, 302] The soft tissues of the pharynx and larynx may be involved (dysphagia, dyspnea), and occasional hematogenous spread can result in lesions in the liver, lungs, gastrointestinal tract, and peritoneum (usually fatal). Animals with tongue involvement show progressive drooling and inability to properly prehend and masticate feed. Eventually, the tongue becomes enlarged, firm, immobile, and protruding.

In sheep, actinobacillosis is rare and is characterized by soft tissue abscesses of the head and neck (Fig. 6–33).[60, 121, 156, 167, 229, 247] The tongue is not affected.

In swine, actinobacillosis is also rare and is distinguished by udder abscesses in sows (*A. lignieresii*)[167] and multiple cutaneous hemorrhages (especially of the ears and belly) with or without necrosis of the tail and the skin over the joints (*A. equuli, A. suis*).[243, 411]

In horses, actinobacillosis (*A. equuli*) is usually a highly fatal septicemic disease in newborn foals (shigellosis).[60, 90] The author has recognized two cases of botryomycosis in adult horses, in which *A. equuli* was isolated in pure culture (see the section on botryomycosis). Recently, *A. lignieresii* was isolated from the enlarged tongue of a horse.[43]

Diagnosis

The differential diagnosis includes other bacterial and fungal granulomatous diseases. Definitive diagnosis is made by direct smears, biopsy, and culture. The sulfur granules may be squashed on a glass slide and shown to consist of gram-negative coccobacilli. Skin biopsy reveals a nodular to diffuse suppurative or pyogranulomatous dermatitis, in which the organisms may be seen individually or in granules. These granules contain masses of the organism, usually surrounded by an eosinophilic covering of material that has a radiating or clublike appearance (Splendore-Hoeppli phenomenon). The organisms are best visualized in sections stained with Gram's stain or Grocott's methenamine silver stain.

The sulfur granules may also be collected, rinsed with sterile saline, and used for culture (aerobic). The simple swabbing of a fistula

---

*References 19, 60, 74, 121, 167, 188, 223, 229, 313–315

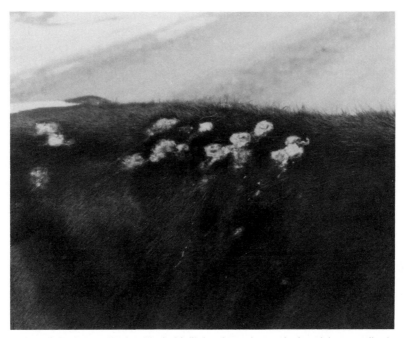

FIGURE 6–32. Bovine actinobacillosis. Multiple alopecic, crusted nodules over the back.

often results in other organisms being cultured as well, especially *Corynebacterium pyogenes* and coagulase-positive staphylococci.

Tube agglutination tests were reported to be ineffective in the diagnosis of bovine actinobacillosis.[74, 315]

Clinical Management

Bovine actinobacillosis usually responds well to surgical excision or drainage and parenteral inorganic or organic iodides.[19, 60, 74, 167, 302] Sodium iodide is administered as a 10 to 20 percent aqueous solution intravenously at a dosage of 1 gm/15 kg. Two or three injections are given at 10- to 14-day intervals. Potassium iodide may be given as an oral drench at a dosage of 6 to 10 gm/head/day for seven to ten days. Ethylenediamine dihydroiodide (EDDI) may be used in the feed at a dosage of 15 to 30 gm/head/day for two to three weeks. Treat-

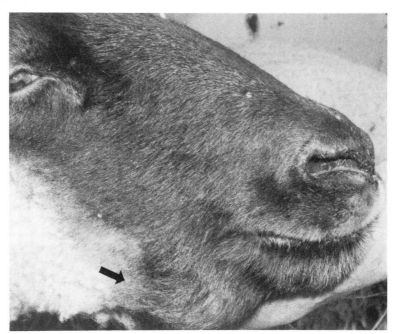

FIGURE 6–33. Ovine actinobacillosis. Abscess on mandible (arrow).

ment should be discontinued if signs of iodism (anorexia, lacrimation, nasorrhea, or dry or scaly skin and coat) appear. Although warnings against the use of these compounds in pregnant cows (abortions, premature births) and breeding bulls (temporary sterility) have been issued,[19, 60, 113, 167] these side effects are apparently rare.

Isolates of *A. lignieresii* from cattle have shown in vitro susceptibility to penicillin, streptomycin, tetracycline, chloramphenicol, and ampicillin.[74] Clinically, bovine actinobacillosis has been reported to respond favorably to triple sulfa (sulfanilamide, sulfapyridine, sulfathiazole) given intravenously at a dosage of 1 gm/7 kg for five to six days and to streptomycin.[19, 60, 74, 167]

In sheep, actinobacillosis is usually treated with surgical drainage and 80 mg/kg or 20 to 25 ml/kg of a 10 percent aqueous solution of sodium iodide given intravenously or subcutaneously and repeated weekly for four to five weeks.[60, 121, 167, 229] It has been reported that EDDI given in the feed at a dosage of 7.5 to 15 gm/head/day for two to three weeks is also beneficial.[167, 229] Streptomycin given intramuscularly at a dosage of 20 mg/kg/day for five to seven days has also been reported to be effective[229] but works best when combined with systemic iodide therapy.

In swine, actinobacillosis (*A. equuli*) has been reported to respond favorably to tetracycline.[411]

Important control measures in the management of actinobacillosis include the isolation or destruction of affected animals, the isolation of animals being treated, and appropriate sanitation.[167]

ABSCESSES

Abscesses, circumscribed subcutaneous accumulations of pus, are seen fairly commonly in large animals.* They usually follow bacterial contamination of skin wounds (from accidents, fighting, surgery, infections, foreign bodies, or ectoparasites).

In swine, abscesses are most commonly caused by *Corynebacterium pyogenes* and β-hemolytic streptococci, and then *Fusobacterium* (*Sphaerophorus*) *necrophorum* and *Bac-*

teroides and *Clostridium* species.* They occur most commonly on the shoulders, neck, ears, flank, tail, and feet (Fig. 6–34). An epizootic of subcutaneous streptococcal abscesses reported in weaned feeder pigs resulted in 30 percent mortality.[258, 259] The pigs were infested with lice, and the abscesses followed the development of swinepox lesions by two to three weeks. *Staphylococcus hyicus* subspecies *hyicus* has also been reported to cause subcutaneous abscesses in swine (see the section on exudative epidermitis).[22, 23]

In horses, subcutaneous abscesses are usually caused by *Corynebacterium pseudotuberculosis*, *Clostridium* species, and β-hemolytic streptococci.† In cattle, subcutaneous abscesses are usually caused by *Corynebacterium pyogenes*,[35, 60, 188] whereas in sheep and goats, they are caused by *C. pseudotuberculosis* and *C. pyogenes*.[35, 60, 188, 248, 275, 360] Sporadic abscesses in sheep and goats can be initiated by anything that traumatizes the skin, such as shearing, clipping, vaccination, ear tagging, rough hay racks or milking stanchions, overcrowding, fighting, and foreign bodies (notably plant awns and thorns).[121, 178] These various forms of trauma are then contaminated by resident skin bacteria, soil and fecal bacteria, or by oral bacteria from licking the wound.

The therapy for subcutaneous abscesses in all animals includes surgical drainage and débridement, flushing or packing with topical antimicrobials, and, occasionally, appropriate systemic antibiotics.

PORCINE SPIROCHETOSIS

Spirochetosis is an ulcerative or granulomatous dermatosis of swine caused by the interplay of *Borrelia suilla*, poor hygiene, and cutaneous wounds.

Cause and Pathogenesis

The cause and pathogenesis of porcine spirochetosis (ulcerative granuloma of swine) are poorly understood.[13, 58, 60, 72, 148, 298] The spirochete, *B. suilla*, is believed to be a secondary invader often associated with poor hygiene and skin trauma (abrasions, lacerations, fight wounds, surgical sites). Bilateral ulcerative spirochetosis of the ears is often associated with

---

*References 19, 35, 60, 72, 75, 103, 121, 217, 246, 248, 282a, 322a, 360

*References 49, 60, 73, 103, 185, 209, 217, 287, 394
†References 38, 39, 60, 75, 246, 273, 309

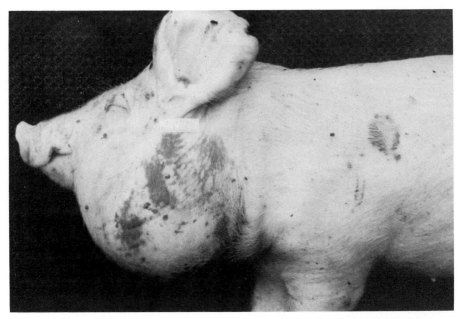

FIGURE 6–34. *Corynebacterial abscess on the neck of a pig. (Courtesy J. M. King.)*

the trauma of sarcoptic mange or the vice of ear biting.[73]

Clinical Features

Young pigs (especially two to three weeks post weaning) are most commonly affected.[13, 58, 72, 73, 148, 277] Although any region of the body may be involved, lesions are most frequently seen on the head (Fig. 6–35), ears, gums, shoulders, side of the body, and scrotum (after castration). The lesions are characterized by initial erythema and edema, which are followed by necrosis and ulceration or tumefaction and fistulae. A grayish-brown, glutinous pustular discharge is typical. The central area of large tumors often sloughs out. Ear lesions frequently begin bilaterally at the base of the pinnae, extend distally, and slough off, leaving a ragged bleeding margin (Fig. 6–36).

Diagnosis

The differential diagnosis includes other infectious granulomas, foreign body granuloma, neoplasia, and various forms of necrosis (pressure, septicemia).[46, 60, 72, 217] Definitive diagnosis is based on direct smears, biopsy, and culture. Direct smears or darkfield illumination of wet preparations from lesions reveals spirochetes. Skin biopsy reveals variable degrees of necrosis, ulceration, granulation tissue, granulomatous inflammation, and vasculitis.[58, 148, 178] Me-

dial fibroplasia, thrombosis, and recanalization of affected vessels have been described. Spirochetes may be visualized with silver stains.

Clinical Management

Porcine spirochetosis has been reported to respond to (1) several days of injectable peni-

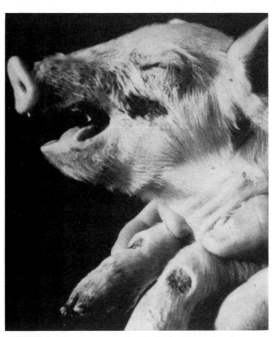

FIGURE 6–35. *Porcine spirochetosis. Necrotic ulcers on cheek and carpi. (Courtesy R. D. Cameron.)*

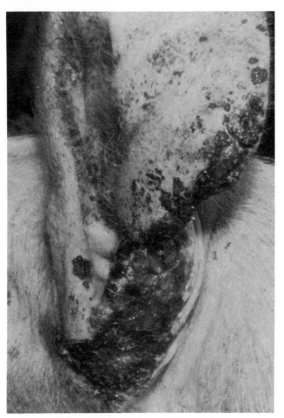

FIGURE 6–36. *Porcine spirochetosis. Necrosis and ulceration of pinna. (Courtesy R. D. Cameron.)*

cillin,[72, 73] (2) three to five days of oral or injectable sulfonamides,[72, 73, 172] or (3) several days of potassium iodide given orally at a dosage of 1 gm/35 kg, up to 3 gm total dose.[72, 73, 172] Ulcerative lesions on the pinnae are reported to respond rapidly to topical tetracycline.[72, 73] Control measures should include improved sanitation and management.

NECROBACILLOSIS

Necrobacillosis, an uncommon necrotizing and ulcerative dermatosis of cattle and swine, is associated with wound contamination by *Fusiformis necrophorus.*

Cause and Pathogenesis

Fusiformis (Sphaerophorus) necrophorus is a common inhabitant of soil and manure.[19, 60, 217, 369] This anaerobic, filamentous, gram-negative rod is assumed to cause disease by wound contamination. Although necrobacillosis is often associated with poor hygiene and man-

agement, it can occur even when husbandry methods are excellent.

Clinical Features

In cattle, necrobacillosis is reported to complicate all kinds of wounds: postsurgical, traumatic, toxic, and infectious.[19, 60] Thus, the disease may complicate cutaneous damage caused by viral infections, ectoparasitism, ergotism, fescue poisoning, photodermatitis, and intertrigo (skin folds between udder forequarters or between the udder and hind limbs). Wherever they occur, the skin lesions are characterized by a diffuse, moist, necrotizing, and ulcerative dermatitis that has a fetid odor. Infection can spread to joints and tendons, resulting in significant economic losses because of lameness, weight loss, decreased milk production, and reduced fertility in bulls.

In swine, necrobacillosis is also reported to complicate all kinds of wounds, especially those induced by the sharp canine teeth of suckling piglets.[73, 103, 129, 172, 217, 277] Morbidity is usually low. The disorder is most commonly seen in large litters, especially in the weaker piglets and when milk let-down is slow.[73] Lesions frequently occur bilaterally on the cheeks (facial pyemia) (Fig. 6–34) and, if severe, may make it difficult for the piglet to open its mouth, resulting in starvation. Less commonly, similar lesions may occur on the lips, gums, tongue, legs, and body of suckling piglets. They may also occur on the teats of sows and on the feet of swine of any age. The lesions are characterized by necrosis, ulceration, thick, adherent brown or black crusts, and a fetid odor. Severely affected pigs may become toxemic, febrile, and listless, may be reluctant to move, and may lose weight.

Diagnosis

The differential diagnosis includes infectious dermatoses, especially exudative epidermitis and porcine spirochetosis. Definitive diagnosis is based on history, physical examination, direct smears, and culture (anaerobic).

Clinical Management

The general principles of therapy include drainage and débridement, local wound care, and systemic medicaments. In cattle, sulfonamides, tetracyclines, and penicillin-streptomycin have been reported to be effective.[19, 60] In severe chronic situations, ethylene diamine-dihydroiodide (EDDI) at 200 to 400 mg/head/day and chlortetracycline at 75 mg/head/day have been reported to be effective as feed additives in reducing the incidence of bovine necrobacillosis.[19, 60]

In swine, localized cases of necrobacillosis usually respond to débridement and topical medicaments. If severe or systemic, injectable sulfonamides or penicillin-streptomycin for three to four days is reported to be effective.[172, 217]

Control measures include improved hygiene and management. Cutting or removing the canine (milk) teeth of piglets at birth is reported to be effective in reducing the incidence of porcine necrobacillosis.[73, 172, 217]

BOTRYOMYCOSIS

Botryomycosis is a bacterial granulomatous disorder of the skin and, rarely, viscera.

Cause and Pathogenesis

The term botryomycosis is technically erroneous.[77, 137] It comes from the Greek word botrys, which means a bunch of grapes, and the original misinterpretation that the disease was caused by a fungus (mycosis). The pathogenesis of botryomycosis (bacterial pseudomycosis) is unclear.[100, 137, 272, 273] Most cases are initiated by local trauma, with or without an associated foreign body. The granulomatous reaction presumably develops because a delicate balance exists between the virulence of the organism and the response of the host. The host is able to isolate and contain the infection but is unable to eradicate it.

Clinical Features

Botryomycosis has been reported in horses[61, 208, 253, 273] and cattle.[100] In horses, botryomycosis has most frequently followed wound contamination on the limbs and scrotum. The lesions are characterized by poorly circumscribed firm, nonpruritic nodular to tumorous growths (Fig. 6–37). Draining tracts and ulcerations are usually present. Small whitish to yellowish granules (grains) may be visible in the purulent discharge. In cattle, botryomycosis has occurred as crusted nodules and ulcers on the udders of 17 of 60 Holstein-Friesians.[100]

Diagnosis

The differential diagnosis includes other bacterial and fungal granulomas, habronemiasis (horse), granulation tissue, and neoplasia. Definitive diagnosis is based on history, physical examination, skin biopsy, and culture. Coagulase-positive staphylococci are most com-

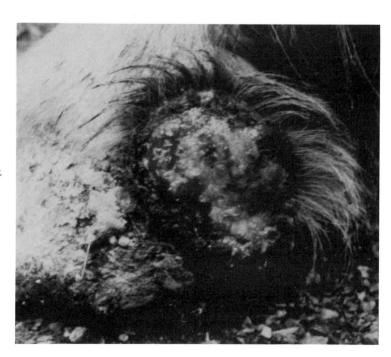

FIGURE 6–37. Equine botryomycosis. Ulcerated tumor above coronet.

monly isolated; however, other bacterial and mixed infections can occur.[77, 137, 208, 253, 272, 273] In Holstein-Friesian cattle,[100] *Pseudomonas aeruginosa* was isolated in pure culture. In two cases of equine botryomycosis studied by the author, *Actinobacillus equuli* was isolated in pure culture.

Histopathologically, there is a nodular to diffuse dermatitis or panniculitis, or both, with tissue granules surrounded by a granulomatous to pyogranulomatous cellular infiltrate (Fig. 6–38). The edges of the granules (masses of bacteria) may show clubbing and may be eosinophilic with H & E stain (Splendore-Hoeppli phenomenon). Bacteria within the tissue granules are best demonstrated with tissue Gram's or Brown and Brenn's stain (Fig. 6–39).

Clinical Management

Simple surgical drainage or systemic antibiotic therapy, or both, are usually ineffective. The matrix that covers the tissue granules and the surrounding granulomatous tissue reaction appear to impede antibiotic penetration of the lesions. The best therapeutic results are obtained with complete surgical excision, or radical surgical debulking followed by prolonged systemic antibiotic therapy based on in vitro antibiotic sensitivity testing.[208, 253, 272, 273]

Treatment of the Holstein-Friesians with *P.*

aeruginosa botryomycosis involved individual washing and drying of infected udders and removal of prickly pigweed from the pasture to reduce mechanical abrasions.[100] The lesions regressed over a four-month period.

CLOSTRIDIAL INFECTIONS

Clostridium species are ubiquitous, anaerobic, spore-forming, gram-positive rods.[60, 75, 273, 374] They produce a wide variety of toxins (hemolytic, necrotizing, and lethal) and diseases.

Malignant edema (gas gangrene) is an acute wound infection (from trauma, injections, or surgery) of cattle, sheep, horses, and swine caused by *Clostridium* species, including *C. septicum*, *C. sordellii*, and *C. perfringens* (*welchii*).* Clinical signs appear within 12 to 48 hours of infection. There is always a local lesion at the site of infection consisting of a soft, doughy swelling (pitting edema) with marked local erythema. Later, the swelling becomes tense and, occasionally, hot and painful, and the skin becomes dark and taut and sloughs (Fig. 6–40). Emphysema (crepitus) may or may not be present. Lesions may occur

---

*References 19, 60, 72, 73, 79, 103, 108, 109, 181, 184, 188, 201, 217, 229, 248, 252, 267, 273, 323, 324, 373, 399, 408, 415

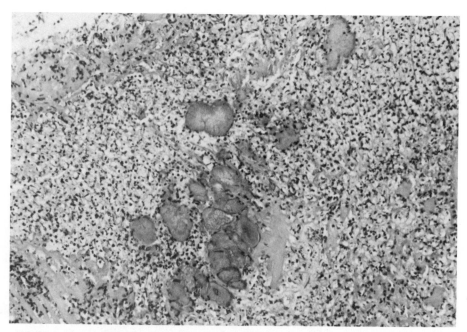

FIGURE 6–38. Equine botryomycosis. Pyogranulomatous dermatitis surrounding tissue grains.

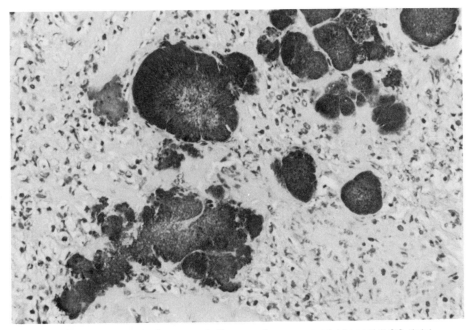

FIGURE 6–39. Equine botryomycosis. Tissue grains composed of cocci (AOG stain).

anywhere, especially in the inguinal, abdominal, cervical, shoulder, and head areas. A high fever is usually present. Affected animals are weak and depressed, may show muscle tremors and lameness, and usually die within 24 to 48 hours.

Blackleg is an acute infectious disease of cattle, sheep, horses, and swine caused by *C. chauvoei* (*feseri*).* Clinical signs appear within 12 to 48 hours of infection. The early lesion is a hot, painful swelling, which progresses to a cold, painless, edematous and emphysematous swelling. The skin is discolored and becomes dry and cracked. Lesions occur most commonly on an upper limb, the rump, and the neck. Affected animals have a high fever, are depressed and anorectic, and often die within 48 hours.

Clostridial swelled head (big head) is an acute wound infection of sheep and goats caused by *C. novyi*.† It is usually seen in rams and bucks of one to two years of age, especially in the summer and early fall when fighting is common. The disease has a rather restricted geographic distribution—Australia, South Africa, and parts of the western United States.

Lesions begin around the eyes and head, may spread to the neck, and consist of subcutaneous edema and fluid exudation. Emphysema is rarely seen. Affected animals are pyrexic and toxemic and usually die within 48 to 72 hours.

Dermatohistopathologic findings in these clostridial infections include diffuse subcuta-

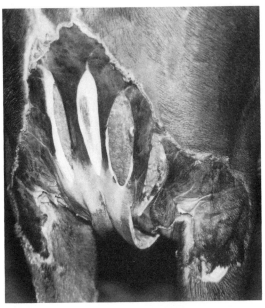

FIGURE 6–40. Equine clostridial infection. Extensive necrosis and sloughing over chest. (Courtesy W. C. Rebhun.)

*References 19, 60, 106, 131, 184, 188, 217, 246, 267, 281, 380

†References 60, 67, 86, 121, 184, 188, 201, 229, 248, 276

neous and dermal edema and cellulitis with large numbers of degenerate neutrophils and bacteria (Gram's stain). Septic thrombi may be seen in subcutaneous blood vessels.

Early surgical drainage and débridement and administration of high levels of penicillin (50,000 IU/kg) or tetracycline (10 to 20 mg/kg) can be attempted but are often futile. In endemic areas, it is recommended that cattle and sheep be vaccinated and that they be excluded from pastures known to be heavily contaminated.

MYCOBACTERIAL INFECTIONS

Tuberculosis, caused by *Mycobacterium bovis*, *M. avium*, and *M. tuberculosis*, has been reported in all domestic animals and humans.* Skin involvement, rare in domestic animals, is characterized by nodules and ulcers, which often involve the ventral thorax and abdomen, medial thighs, and perineal regions.† Dermatohistopathologic findings include tuberculoid granulomas with or without caseation and mineralization. The organisms are often small in number and difficult or impossible to find. Details of diagnosis and control may be found elsewhere.‡

Atypical mycobacteriosis is a worldwide cause of skin disease (skin tuberculosis) in cattle.§ The frequent occurrence of lesions on the lower limbs suggests cutaneous wounds as the probable portal of entry for the atypical mycobacteria, which are ubiquitous environmental saprophytes. Although gram-positive, acid-fast organisms can often be found in smears and biopsy specimens from these lesions, the precise species involved is not clear in most cases. *M. kansasii* has been isolated from the lesions of some cattle with atypical mycobacteriosis.[182, 245, 414] Skin lesions begin as papules and nodules on the distal limbs (Fig. 6–41) and often spread to the thighs, shoulders, and even the abdomen. The lesions may be single or multiple and are often in chains connected by corded lymphatics. The lesions may rupture and discharge a thick, cream to yellow to grayish pus. Regional lymph nodes

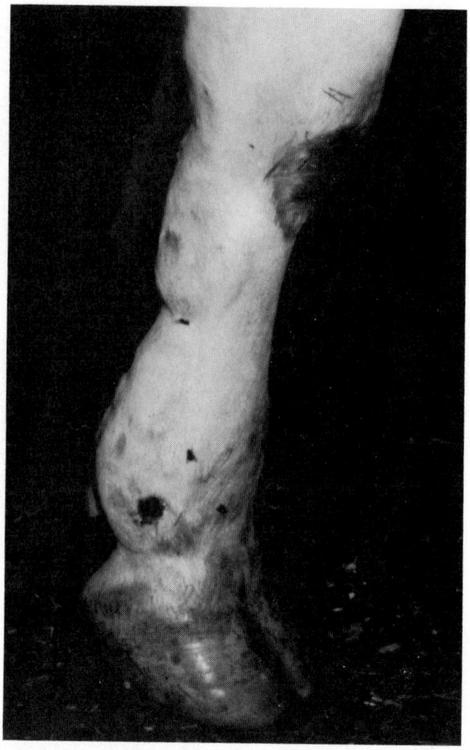

FIGURE 6–41. Atypical mycobacteriosis in a cow. Nodules on the leg. (Courtesy W. C. Rebhun.)

are usually not involved. The differential diagnosis includes ulcerative lymphangitis and bovine farcy. The lesions of atypical mycobacteriosis cause little inconvenience, but they are unsightly, and affected cattle may give a suspicious or positive reaction to the tuberculin test. Dermatohistopathologic findings are as previously described for tuberculosis, but the organisms are usually easy to find (Fig. 6–42). Treatment or control measures are usually not instituted, although surgical removal may be undertaken for cosmetic reasons.

Although the atypical mycobacterioses are not thought to be contagious, humans are susceptible to many of the known organisms (including *M. kansasii*).[114, 169] Cutaneolymphatic and even pulmonary infections can occur as a result of wound contamination.

Another atypical mycobacterium, *M. farcinogenes*, has been reported to cause the syndrome referred to as bovine farcy in Africa (see the section on nocardiosis).[76, 107]

ERYSIPELAS

Erysipelas is an infectious disease of swine caused by *Erysipelothrix insidiosa* (*rhusiopa-*

---

*References 19, 60, 75, 103, 169, 188, 207, 208, 217, 246, 248, 311, 360
†References 29, 41, 66, 101, 176, 208, 212, 285, 318, 367, 388
‡References 19, 60, 207, 217, 246, 248, 311, 360
§References 19, 60, 138, 155, 158, 188, 261, 321. 391–393

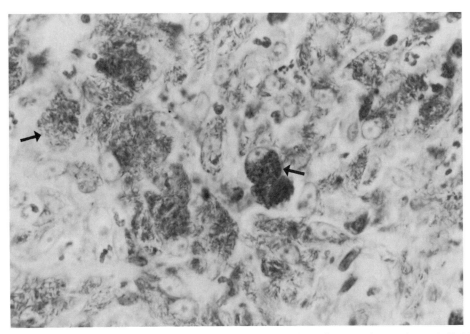

FIGURE 6–42. Atypical mycobacteriosis in a cow. Acid-fast bacilli in dermal macrophages (arrows) (Ziehl-Neelsen stain).

thiae). * The organism is a gram-positive, pleomorphic facultative anaerobe. Erysipelas is worldwide in distribution and of serious economic importance in swine operations.

Erysipelas occurs in acute, subacute, and chronic clinical forms. In the acute form, fever, depression, anorexia, and lameness are accompanied by bluish to purplish discoloration of the skin, especially the abdomen, ears, and extremities. Pinkish to red macules and papules may also be seen. In the subacute phase, erythematous papules (see Plate 4 *B*) and wheals (urticaria) enlarge and assume square, rectangular, or rhomboidal shapes (so-called diamond-skin disease; see Plate 4 *C*). These lesions often develop a purplish center and either regress spontaneously or progress to the chronic phase. The chronic phase is characterized by necrosis and sloughing, resulting in dark, dry, firm areas of skin, which peel away. Occasionally, the ears, tail, and feet may slough as well. Dermatohistopathologic findings include marked dermal vascular dilatation and engorgement in the acute phase and a neutrophilic vasculitis (arteritis) and suppurative hidradenitis in the subacute and chronic phases.[81, 128, 188, 349, 354] The organisms may occasionally be visualized in sections stained with Gram's stain. Penicillin (11,000 IU/kg/day) is the antibiotic of choice for treatment.

_____
*References 60, 73, 103, 162, 188, 217, 218, 277

Humans are susceptible to infections with *E. insidiosa*.[114, 169] The disorder is an occupational disease in people who come into contact with animals, such as veterinarians and workers in fisheries and rendering plants. Wound contamination results in a dermatologic disorder referred to as erysipeloid. Lesions are most commonly seen on the hands and fingers and consist of a slowly progressive, discrete, violaceous to erythematous cellulitis. Erysipeloid is usually painful, but pruritus is variable.

ANTHRAX

Anthrax is an acute infectious disease characterized by septicemia, sudden death, and the exudation of tarry blood from body orifices.[60, 193, 199] The specific cause is *Bacillus anthracis*, a gram-positive spore-forming bacillus. In cattle and sheep, massive edematous swellings may be seen in the neck, brisket, flanks, abdomen, and perineum.[19, 60, 208, 263] Necrosis and sloughing may occur in some areas in more subacute cases. In swine, facial and cervical edema and cutaneous hyperemia and formation of petechiae are seen.[60, 73, 103, 208, 217, 284] In horses, hot, painful, rapidly developing inflammatory edema is seen on the neck, sternum, abdomen, prepuce, and udder.[60, 75, 78, 193, 208, 246] Dermatohistopathologic findings include diffuse subcutaneous and dermal edema with numerous extravasated erythrocytes but few inflammatory cells. Bacteria can usually be identified with Gram's stains, and blood vessel walls may show degenerative changes.

In humans, anthrax is considered an occupational disease, being more commonly recognized in people handling animal products and having close contact with infected animals (e.g., veterinarians, farmers, and butchers).[114, 169] Humans develop cutaneous, respiratory, and intestinal forms of anthrax. The cutaneous lesions occur in exposed skin (wound contamination) and are characterized by variably pruritic, erythematous macules and papules, which become edematous and vesicular and develop central necrosis and a characteristic black eschar.

GLANDERS

Glanders (farcy) is a contagious disease of horses caused by the gram-negative, facultative anaerobic rod, *Pseudomonas* (*Actinobacillus*, *Malleomyces*) *mallei*.[60, 75, 188, 208, 246] The disease is highly fatal and of major importance in any affected horse population. It is restricted geographically to Eastern Europe, Asia, and North Africa.

Glanders occurs in acute and chronic forms and is characterized by nodules or ulcers, or both, in the respiratory tract and the skin. The skin lesions may occur anywhere on the body, but especially on the medial aspect of the hocks. They begin as subcutaneous nodules, which rapidly ulcerate and discharge a honeylike exudate. Corded lymphatics (lymphangitis) and regional lymphadenopathy are frequently seen. Dermatohistopathologic findings include nodular to diffuse suppurative or pyogranulomatous dermatitis. The causative bacterium may be seen with Gram's stains. Details on diagnosis and control may be found in other texts.[60, 75]

Humans are susceptible to glanders, and the infection is usually fatal.[114, 169] Humans are infected via inhalation, ingestion, and wound contamination and develop acute respiratory disease, septicemia, and multiple cutaneous eruptions.

SALMONELLOSIS

Salmonella species are ubiquitous gram-negative rods that cause enteric and septicemic diseases in many species.* In swine, septicemic salmonellosis, usually associated with *S. choleraesuis*, may result in a bluish to purplish discoloration of the skin, especially of the ears, ventral abdomen, snout, and tail.† This is due

---

*References 19, 60, 75, 103, 160, 184, 188, 217, 246
†References 60, 72, 73, 103, 188, 217, 310

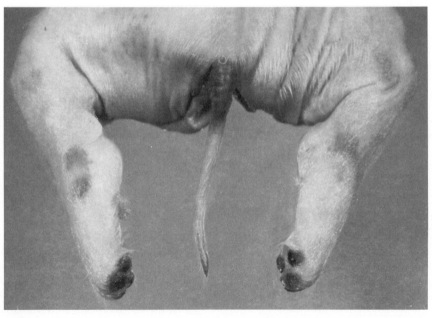

FIGURE 6–43. Sloughing of feet and multiple ecchymoses in a piglet with salmonellosis.

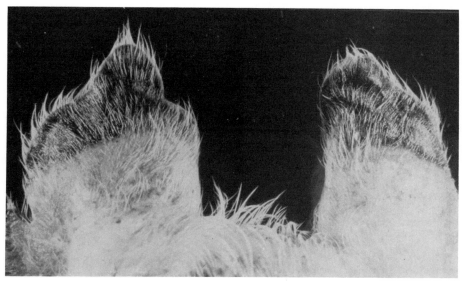

FIGURE 6–44. Necrosis of the pinnae of a piglet with salmonellosis.

to intense dermal capillary dilatation and engorgement. Some animals develop thrombosis, which may lead to necrosis and sloughing either in patches of the skin mentioned previously or of the feet, tail, and ear margins (Figs. 6–43 and 6–44).

In cattle, *S. dublin* infections have been associated with gangrene of the distal extremities, tail, and pinnae (Fig. 6–45).[271, 293, 330, 341] Histopathologic studies of some calves[341] have revealed intimal thickening, thrombosis of arteries and veins, and perivascular inflammation.

In humans, infection with a number of *Salmonella* species may produce a variety of responses, from asymptomatic carriage to enteric disease or septicemia.[169]

PASTEURELLOSIS

Pasteurella species are ubiquitous gram-negative rods, which gain entry to the animal host

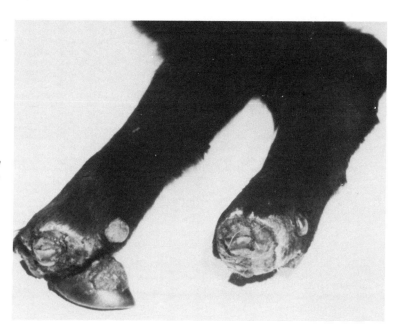

FIGURE 6–45. Sloughing of feet in a calf with Salmonella *septicemia.*

by aerosol and wound contamination.[60, 169] In swine, *Pasteurella multocida* has been reported to cause an acute, diffuse swelling of the cervical and pharyngeal areas, with diffuse bluishred discoloration of the skin, especially on the neck, snout, ears, flanks, and abdomen.[103, 282] In horses, *P. haemolytica* has been reported to cause ulcerative lymphangitis.[260]

In humans, *P. multocida* has produced wound abscesses and infections of the respiratory and urinary tracts.[114, 169] *P. haemolytica* has been very rarely associated with wound abscesses.[169]

EDEMA DISEASE

Edema disease occurs in weaner and grower pigs and is believed to be an enterotoxemia associated with hemolytic *E. coli*.[60, 73, 103, 188, 217] In addition to progressive ataxia and paralysis, affected pigs have subcutaneous edema of the eyelids, face, ears, and neck. Dermatohistopathologic findings include diffuse subcutaneous and dermal edema, occasionally mural edema, hyalin degeneration, fibrinoid necrosis, and inflammation of arterioles and arteries.

REFERENCES

1. Abu-Samra, M. T., et al.: Ulcerative lymphangitis in a horse. Equine Vet. J. 12:149, 1980.
2. Abu-Samra, M. T.: *Dermatophilus* infection: The clinical disease and diagnosis. Zbl. Vet. Med. B 25:641, 1978.
3. Abu-Samra, M. T., and Walton, G. S.: Modified techniques for the isolation of *Dermatophilus* spp. from infected material. Sabouraudia 15:23, 1977.
4. Abu-Samra, M. T., et al.: *Dermatophilus congolensis*. A bacteriological, *in vitro* antibiotic sensitivity and histopathological study of natural infection in Sudanese cattle. Br. Vet. J. 132:627, 1976.
5. Abu-Samra, M. T.: The effect of prednisolone trimethylacetate in the pathogenicity of *Dermatophilus congolensis* to white mice. Mycopathologia 66:1, 1978.
6. Abu-Samra, M. T.: The epizootiology of *Dermatophilus congolensis* infection (a discussion article). Rev. Elev. Med. Vet. Pays Trop. 33:23, 1980.
7. Abu-Samra, M. T., and Imbabi, S. E.: Experimental infection of domesticated animals and fowl with *Dermatophilus congolensis*. J. Comp. Pathol. 86:157, 1976.
8. Abu-Samra, M. T., and Walton, G. S.: The inoculation of rabbits with *Dermatophilus congolensis* and the simultaneous infection of sheep with *D. congolensis* and orf virus. J. Comp. Pathol. 91:324, 1981.
9. Adamson, P. J., et al.: Susceptibility of equine bacterial isolates to antimicrobial agents. Am. J. Vet. Res. 46:447, 1985.
10. Adegoke, G. O., and Ojo, M. O.: Biochemical characterization of staphylococci isolated from goats. Vet. Microbiol. 7:463, 1982.
11. Addo, P. B.: Role of the common housefly (*Musca domestica*) in the spread of ulcerative lymphangitis. Vet. Rec. 113:496, 1983.
12. Albiston, H. E., and Pullar, E. M.: A short note on actinomycotic granulomata. Aust. Vet. J. 10:146, 1934.
13. Albiston, H. E.: Spirochetal granuloma of swine. *In:* Hungerford, T. G.: *Diseases of Domestic Animals in Australia II*. Canberra, Commonweath Bureau of Health, 1965, p. 5.
14. Albrecht, R., et al.: *Dermatophilus congolensis* chronic nodular disease in man. Pediatrics 53:902, 1974.
15. Amakiri, S. F.: Alkaline phosphatase activity in normal and *Dermatophilus congolensis* infected bovine skin. Nigerian Vet. J. 1:46, 1972.
16. Amakiri, S. F.: Anatomical location of *Dermatophilus congolensis* in bovine cutaneous streptothricosis. *In:* Lloyd, D. H., and Sellers, K. C.: *Dermatophilus Infection in Animals and Man*. New York, Academic Press, 1976, p. 163.
17. Amakiri, S. F.: Electrophoretic studies of serum proteins in healthy and streptothricosis-infected cattle. Br. Vet. J. 133:106, 1977.
18. Amakiri, S. F., and Nwufoh, K. J.: Changes in cutaneous blood vessels in bovine dermatophilosis. J. Comp. Pathol. 91:439, 1981.
19. Amstutz, H. E.: *Bovine Medicine and Surgery II*. Santa Barbara, CA, American Veterinary Publications, Inc., 1980.
20. Amstutz, H. E.: Bovine skin conditions: A brief review. Mod. Vet. Pract. 60:821, 1979.
21. Amtsberg, G., et al.: Bakteriologische, serologische und tierexperimentelle Untersuchungen zur Atiologischen Bedeutung von *Staphylococcus hyicus* beim Nassendem Ekzemdes Schweines. Dtsch. Tierarztl. Wochenschr. 80:493, 1973.
22. Amtsberg, G.: Untersuchungen zum Vorkommen von *Staphylococcus hyicus* beim Schwein bzw von *Staphylococcus epidermidis* Biotyp 2 bei anderen Tierarten. Dtsch. Tierarztl. Wochenschr. 85:385, 1978.
23. Amtsberg, G.: Tierexperimentelle Untersuchungen zur Pathogenese des lokalen und generalisierten Nassenden Ekzems sowie der durch *Staphylococcus hyicus* verursachten Polyarthritis der Schweine. Dtsch. Tierarztl. Wochenschr. 85:433, 1978.
24. Amtsberg, G.: Nachweis von Exfoliation auslosenden substanzen in Kulturen von *Staphylococcus hyicus* des Schweines und *Staphylococcus epidermidis* Biotyp 2 des Rindes. Zbl. Vet. Med. B 26:257, 1979.
25. Amtsberg, G.: Infections versuche mit *Staphylococcus hyicus* an aktiv und passiv immunisierten Schweinen. Berl. Munch. Tierarztl. Wochenschr. 91:201, 1978.
26. Amtsberg, G.: Vergleichende experimentelle Untersuchungen zum Nachweis der Pathogenitat von *Staphylococcus hyicus* des Schweines bzw. *Staphylococcus* epidermidis Biotyp 2 des Rindes an gnotobiotischen Ferkeln und Kaninchen. Berl. Munch. Tierarztl. Wochenschr. 91:299, 1978.
27. Andreatta, J. N., and Fernandez, E. J.: Equine dermatitis due to *Nocardia* sp. Rev. Agron. Vet. Argent. 2:16, 1975.
28. Andrews, J. J.: Ulcerative glossitis and stomatitis associated with exudative epidermitis in suckling pigs. Vet. Pathol. 16:432, 1979.
29. Antepioglu, H.: Skin tuberculosis in a horse. Fak. Vet. Derg. 10:399, 1963.
30. Augustine, J. L., and Renshaw, H. W.: Survival of *Corynebacterium pseudotuberculosis* in axenic purulent exudate on common barnyard fomites. Am. J. Vet. Res. 47:713, 1986.
31. Austwick, P. K. C.: The probable relationship of rainfall to *Dermatophilus congolensis* infection in sheep. *In:* Lloyd, D. H., and Sellers, K. C.: *Dermatophilus Infection in Animals and Man*. New York, Academic Press, 1976, p. 87.
32. Awad, F. I., and Karib, A. A.: Studies on bovine farcy (nocardiosis) among cattle in the Sudan. Zbl. Vet. Med. 5:265, 1958.
33. Awad, F. I.: The interrelationship between tuberculosis and bovine farcy. J. Comp. Pathol. 68:324, 1960.
34. Awad, F. I.: Nocardiosis of the bovine udder and testis. Vet. Rec. 72:341, 1960.
35. Ayers, J. L.: Corynebacterial infections. *In*: Howard, J. L. (ed.): *Current Veterinary Therapy. Food Animal Practice*. Philadelphia, W. B. Saunders Co., 1981, p. 658.

36. Ayers, J. L.: Caseous lymphadenitis. *In*: Howard, J. L. (ed.): *Current Veterinary Therapy. Food Animal Practice*. Philadelphia, W. B. Saunders Co., 1981, p. 660.

37. Ayers, J. L., and McClure, A.: Ulcerative lymphangitis of cattle. *In*: Howard, J. L. (ed.): *Current Veterinary Therapy. Food Animal Practice*. Philadelphia, W. B. Saunders Co., 1981, p. 662.

38. Bain, A. M.: *Corynebacterium equi* infections. Aust. Vet. J. 39:116, 1963.

39. Bain, A. M.: Common bacterial infections of foetuses and foals and association of the infection with the dam. Aust. Vet. J. 39:413, 1963.

40. Baker, G. J.: Strangles. *In*: Robinson, N. E.: *Current Therapy in Equine Medicine*. Philadelphia, W. B. Saunders Co., 1983, p. 24.

41. Baker, J. R.: A case of generalized avian tuberculosis in a horse. Vet. Rec. 93:105, 1973.

42. Barakat, A. A., et al.: Field observations on recurrent skin lesions in sheep caused by *Staphylococcus aureus*. Assiut Vet. Med. J. 2:203, 1975.

43. Baum, K. H., et al.: Isolation of *Actinobacillus lignieresii* from enlarged tongue of a horse. JAVMA 185:792, 1984.

44. Baxendell, S. A.: Caprine udder conditions. Univ. Sydney Post-Grad. Comm. Vet. Sci. Proc. 52:241, 1980.

45. Baxter, M., et al.: Investigations into "cockle," a skin disease of sheep. IV. Mycological aspects. N.Z. J. Agric. Res. 23:403, 1980.

46. Beaton, D., et al.: An outbreak of ulcerative dermatitis in pigs. Vet. Rec. 94:611, 1974.

47. Behrens, H.: Vitamin-A-Bestimmungen bei Ferkelen mit seborrhoischem Ekzem. Dtsch. Tierarztl. Wochenschr. 72:386, 1965.

48. Benham, C. L., et al.: *Corynebacterium pseudotuberculosis* and its role in disease of animals. Vet. Bull. 32:645, 1962.

49. Benno, Y., and Mitsuoka, T.: Susceptibility of *Bacteroides* from swine abscesses to 13 antibiotics. Am. J. Vet. Res. 45:2631, 1984.

50. Bethke, M.: Mammary actinomycosis of the sow: Comparison of treatment with antibiotics plus enzymes, penicillin plus streptomycin, and surgical treatment. Vet. Bull. 43:497, 1971.

51. Biberstein, E. L., et al.: Two biotypes of *Corynebacterium pseudotuberculosis*. Vet. Rec. 89:691, 1971.

52. Biberstein, E. L., et al.: Species distribution of coagulase-positive staphylococci in animals. J. Clin. Microbiol. 19:610, 1984.

53. Biberstein, E. L., et al.: *Nocardia asteroides* infection in horses: A review. JAVMA 186:273, 1985.

54. Bida, S. A., and Dennis, S. M.: Sequential pathological changes in natural and experimental dermatophilosis in Bunaji cattle. Res. Vet. Sci. 22:18, 1977.

55. Binford, C. H., et al.: *Pathology of Tropical and Extraordinary Diseases*. Washington, D. C., Armed Forces Institute of Pathology, 1978.

56. Blancou, J. M.: Traitement de la Streptothricose bovine par une injection unique d'antibiotiques a haute dose. Rev. Elev. Med. Vet. Pays Trop. 22:35, 1969.

57. Blancou, J. M.: The treatment of infection by *Dermatophilus congolensis* with particular reference to the disease in cattle. *In*: Lloyd, D. H., and Sellers, K. C.: *Dermatophilus Infection in Animals and Man*. New York, Academic Press, 1976, p. 246.

58. Blandford, T., et al.: Suspected porcine ulcerative spirochaetosis in England. Vet. Rec. 90:15, 1972.

59. Blood, D. C., and Jubb, K. V.: Exudative epidermitis of pigs. Aust. Vet. J. 33:126, 1957.

60. Blood, D. C., et al.: *Veterinary Medicine VI*. Philadelphia, Lea & Febiger, 1983.

61. Bollinger, O.: Mycosis der lunge beim pferde. Virchows Arch. Pathol. Anat. 49:583, 1870.

62. Bollwahn, W., et al.: Experimentelle untersuchungen sur Atiologie des nassenden Eksems des Schweine. Dtsch. Tierarztl. Wochenschr. 77:601, 1970.

63. Brown, J. R.: Immonosuppression in the bovine species. Agri-Pract. 6:7, 1985.

64. Brown, C. C., et al.: Serologic response and lesions in goats experimentally infected with *Corynebacterium pseudotuberculosis* of caprine and equine origins. Am. J. Vet. Res. 46:2322, 1985.

65. Burns, R. H. G., and Simmons, G. C.: A case of actinomycotic infection in a horse. Aust. Vet. J. 28:34, 1952.

66. Buss, W.: Hauttubaerkulose des Pferdes als Ursache menschlicher Hauttuberkulose. Tierarztl. Umschau 9:164, 1954.

67. Bull, L. B.: "Swell head" or "big head" in rams due to localized infection by *Clostridium oedematiens*. J. Comp. Pathol. Ther. 48:21, 1935.

68. Butler, W. J.: Chest abscess disease. Rep. Montana Livestock Sanit. Board, Helena, 1939, p. 194.

69. Bussieras, J., et al.: La dermatophilose equine en Normandie. Rec. Med. Vet. 157:415, 1981.

70. Bwangamoi, O.: *Dermatophilus* infection in cattle, goats, and sheep in East Africa. *In*: Lloyd, D. H., and Sellers, K. C.: *Dermatophilus Infection in Animals and Man*. New York, Academic Press, 1976, p. 49.

71. Bwangamoi, O.: Economic aspects of streptothricosis in livestock in East Africa. *In*: Lloyd, D. H., and Sellers, K. C.: *Dermatophilus Infection in Animals and Man*. New York, Academic Press, 1976, p. 292.

72. Cameron, R. D. A.: Skin diseases of the pig. Univ. Sydney Post-Grad. Comm. Vet. Sci. Proc. 56:445, 1981.

73. Cameron, R. D. A.: *Skin Diseases of the Pig*. Sydney, University of Sydney Post-Graduate Foundation in Veterinary Science, Veterinary Review No. 23, 1984.

74. Campbell, S. G., et al.: An unusual epizootic of actinobacillosis in dairy heifers. JAVMA 166:604, 1975.

75. Catcott, E. J., and Smithcors, J. F.: *Equine Medicine and Surgery II*. Wheaton, American Veterinary Publications, 1972.

76. Chamoiseau, G.: *Mycobacterium farcinogenes*, agent causal du farcin du boeuf en Afrique. Rev. Elev. Med. Vet. Pays Trop. 27:61, 1974.

77. Chandler, F. W., et al.: *Color Atlas and Text of the Histopathology of Mycotic Diseases*. Chicago, Year Book Medical Publishers, Inc., 1980.

78. Cohen, M.: Anthrax. *In*: Robinson, N. E.: *Current Therapy in Equine Medicine*. Philadelphia, W. B. Saunders Co., 1983, p. 17.

79. Cohen, M.: Malignant edema. *In*: Robinson, N. E.: *Current Therapy in Equine Medicine*. Philadelphia, W. B. Saunders Co., 1983, p. 21.

80. Cohen, M.: Ulcerative lymphangitis. *In*: Robinson, N. E.: *Current Therapy in Equine Medicine*. Philadelphia, W. B. Saunders Co., 1983, p. 31.

81. Collins, D. H., and Goldie, W.: Observations on polyarthritis and an experimental *Erysipelothrix* infection of swine. J. Pathol. Bacteriol. 50:323, 1940.

82. Cooper, B. S., et al.: An outbreak of contagious pustular dermatitis associated with *Dermatophilus congolensis* infection. N.Z. Vet. J. 18:199, 1970.

83. Cury, R., and Penha, A. M.: Observacoes sobre a infeccao porbacilo de Preisz-Nocard no estado de Sao Paulo. Bol. Soc. Paul. Med. Vet. 8:43, 1948.

84. Davis, D.: An *in vivo* method of assay for *Dermatophilus congolensis*. J. Comp. Pathol. 93:115, 1983.

85. Davis, D.: Infection *Dermatophilus congolensis* at a contact hypersensitivity site and its relevance to chronic streptothricosis lesions in the cattle of West Africa. J. Comp. Pathol. 94:25, 1984.

86. DeKock, G.: Swelled head, big-head, or dikkopsiekte in rams. J. S. Afr. Vet. Med. Assoc. 1:39, 1928.

87. Dempsey, M., et al.: Investigations into "cockle," a skin disease of sheep. I. Some factors and a possible cause. N.Z. J. Agric. Res. 15:741, 1972.

88. Dempsey, M., et al.: Investigations into "cockle," a skin disease of sheep. II. A preventive treatment and its effect on weight gain. N.Z. J. Agric. Res. 17:423, 1974.

89. Dempsey, M., et al.: Investigations into "cockle," a skin disease of sheep. III. Further investigations into preventive treatment and weight gain. N.Z. J. Exp. Agric. 3:305, 1975.

90. Derksen, F. J.: Actinobacillosis. *In*: Robinson, N. E.: *Current Therapy in Equine Medicine*. Philadelphia, W. B. Saunders Co., 1983, p. 14.

91. Devriese, L. A., and Oeding, P.: Coagulase and heat-resistant nuclease producing *Staphylococcus epidermidis* strains from animals. J. Appl. Bacteriol. 39:197, 1975.

92. Devriese, L. A.: Isolation and identification of *Staphylococcus hyicus*. Am. J. Vet. Res. 38:787, 1977.

93. Devriese, L. A., et al.: *Staphylococcus hyicus* (sompolinsky 1953) comb nov and *Staphylococcus hyicus* subsp chromogenes subsp nov. Intl. J. Syst. Bacteriol. 28:482, 1978.

94. Devriese, L. A., and Derycke, J.: *Staphylococcus hyicus* in cattle. Res. Vet. Sci. 26:356, 1979.

95. Devriese, L. A., and Oeding, P.: Characteristics of *Staphylococcus aureus* strains isolated from different animal species. Res. Vet. Sci. 21:284, 1976.

96. Devriese, L. A.: Gevoeligheid tegenover antibiotica van *Staphylococcus hyicus* stammen geisoleerd uit gevallen van exudatieve epidermitis bij biggen. Vlaams Diergeneeskd. Tijdschr. 46:43, 1976.

97. Devriese, L. A., et al.: Identification and characterizing of staphylococci isolated from lesions and normal skin of horses. Vet. Microbiol. 10:269, 1985.

98. Devriese, L. A., et al.: *Staphylococcus hyicus* in skin lesions of horses. Equine Vet. J. 15:263, 1983.

99. Dewes, H. F.: *Strongyloides westeri* and *Corynebacterium equi* in foals. N.Z. Vet. J. 20:82, 1972.

100. Donovan, G. A., and Gross, T. L.: Cutaneous botryomycosis (bacterial granulomas) in dairy cows caused by *Pseudomonas aeruginosa*. JAVMA 184:197, 1984.

101. Dukie, B., and Putrik, M.: Tuberculosis of the skin of the abdomen in a horse. Acta Vet. (Belgr.) 21:135, 1971.

102. Dumas, R., et al.: Note sur la sensibilité héréditaire des bovins à la streptothricose. Rev. Elev. Med. Vet. Pays Trop. 24:349, 1971.

103. Dunne, H. W., and Leman, A. D.: *Diseases of Swine IV*. Ames, Iowa State University Press, 1975.

104. Edwards, J. R., et al.: A survey of ovine dermatophilosis in Western Australia. Aust. Vet. J. 62:361, 1985.

105. Egerton, J. R.: Mycotic dermatitis of cattle. Aust. Vet. J. 40:144, 1964.

106. Eggleston, E. L.: Blackleg in swine. Vet. Med. 45:253, 1950.

106a. Ellenberger, M. A., and Genetzky, R. M.: *Rhodococcus equi* infections: Literature review. Compend. Cont. Educ. 8:S414, 1986.

107. El Sanousi, S. M., and Salih, M. A. M.: Miliary bovine farcy experimentally induced in a Zebu calf. Vet. Pathol. 16:372, 1979.

108. Erid, C. H.: Malignant edema infection in a horse. Calif. Vet. 8:30, 1955.

109. Estola, T., and Stenberg, H.: On the occurrence of *Clostridia* in domestic animals and animal products. Nord. Vet. Med. 15:35, 1963.

110. Etherington, W. G., and Prescott, J. F.: *Corynebacterium equi* cellulitis associated with *Strongyloides* penetration in a foal. JAVMA 177:1025, 1980.

111. Ezeh, A. O., and Makinde, A. A.: Case of *Dermatophilus congolensis* infection in a two-day-old calf. Vet. Rec. 114:321, 1984.

112. Fantinati, L.: Estesa foruncolosi in bovini importati dalla Polonia. Riv. Zootec. Vet. 6:557, 1976.

113. Farquharson, J.: Intravenous use of sodium iodide in actinomycosis. JAVMA 91:551, 1937.

114. Fitzpatrick, T. B., et al.: *Dermatology in General Medicine II*. New York, McGraw-Hill Book Co., 1979.

115. Ford, R. B., et al.: Equine dermatophilosis: A two-year clinicopathologic study. Vet. Med. Small Anim. Clin. 69:1557, 1974.

116. Fontanelli, E.: Pustular dermatitis of the udder in sheep and goats associated with *Corynebacterium*. Zooprofilassi 7:261, 1952.

117. Fontanelli, E., and Caparrin, W.: Pustular dermatitis of the udder in sheep and goats in the Viterboprovince. Zooprofilassi 10:603, 1955.

118. Fouad, K., et al.: Further investigations on the so-called "oedematous-skin disease of buffaloes and cattle." Egypt. Vet. Med. Assoc. J. 33:154, 1973.

119. Franke, F.: Aetiology of actinomycosis of the mammary gland of the pig. Zbl. Bakteriol. Parasitenkd. 223:111, 1973.

120. Fraser, J., et al.: Experimental reinfection of the skin of sheep with *Staphylococcus aureus*. Vet. Rec. 111:485, 1982.

121. Fubini, S. L., and Campbell, S. G.: External lumps on sheep and goats. Vet. Clin. North Amer. Large Anim. Pract. 5:457, 1983.

122. Gbode, T. A., and Hdife, L.: Some observations on chemotherapy of bovine dermatophilosis. Br. Vet. J. 138:288, 1982.

123. Gbodi, T. A.: Serum mineral status of normal and *Dermatophilus congolensis*–infected Friesian calves. Bull. Anim. Health Prod. Afr. 28:348, 1980.

124. Gibbons, W. J.: Skin diseases. Mod. Vet. Pract. 43:76, 1962.

125. Gibson, J. A., et al.: Subcutaneous and lymph node granulomas due to *Dermatophilus congolensis* in a steer. Vet. Pathol. 20:120, 1983.

126. Gillespie, T. G.: Biotin supplementation in greasy pig disease. Mod. Vet. Pract. 63:724, 1982.

127. Gordon, M. A.: Characterization of *Dermatophilus congolensis*: Its affinities with the *Actinomycetales* and differentiation from *Geodermatophilus*. *In:* Lloyd, D. H., and Sellers, K. C.: *Dermatophilus Infection in Animals and Man*. New York, Academic Press, 1976, p. 187.

128. Godgluck, G., and Wellmann, G.: Rotlaufbakterien in der Haut und in Blut bei experimentell mit Rotlauf infizierten Schweinen. Dtsch. Tierarztl. Wochenschr. 60:537, 1953.

129. Golovin, V. I.: Outbreak of cutaneous necrobacillosis in swine. Veterinariya (Moscow) 54:56, 1977.

130. Grasser, R.: Mikroaerophile actinomyceten aus Gesaugeaktinomykosen des Schweines. Vet. Bull. 32:2971, 1962.

131. Gualandi, G. L.: L'infezione da *"Clostrium chauvoei"* nel suino. Arch. Vet. Ital. 6:57, 1955.

132. Guard, W. F.: Actinomycosis in a horse. JAVMA 93:198, 1938.

133. Guma, S. A., et al.: Mycetoma in goats. Sabouraudia 16:217, 1978.

134. Guma, S. A., and Abu-Samra, M. T.: Experimental mycetoma infection in the goat. J. Comp. Pathol. 91:341, 1981.

135. Guss, S. B.: *Management and Diseases of Dairy Goats*. Scottsdale, AZ, Dairy Goat Journal Publishing Corporation, 1977.

136. Gyang, E. O., et al.: Treatment of ovine dermatophilosis with long-acting oxytetracycline. Vet. Rec. 106:106, 1980.

137. Hacker, P.: Botryomycosis. Intl. J. Dermatol. 22:455, 1983.

138. Hagan, W. A.: Subcutaneous lesions which sometimes induce tuberculin hypersensitiveness in cattle. Cornell Vet. 19:173, 1929.

139. Hagemoser, W. A., et al.: Granulocytopathy in a Holstein heifer. JAVMA 183:1093, 1983.

140. Hajek, V., and Marsalek, E.: *Staphylokokken ausserhalb* des Krankenhauses. *Staphylococcus aureus* bei Schafen. Zbl. Bakteriol. Parasitenkd. Infektionskr. Hyg. 161B:455, 1976.

141. Hajek, V., et al.: A study of staphylococci isolated from the upper respiratory tract of different animal species. Zbl. Bakteriol. Parasitenkd. Infektionskr. Hyg. 229A:429, 1974.

142. Hajek, V.: *Staphylococcus intermedius*, a new species isolated from animals. Intl. J. Syst. Bacteriol. 26:401, 1976.

143. Hajsig, D., et al.: Eksudativni epidermitis (EE) u prasadi I. Prikaz bolesti i prvo objektivno utvrdivanje u jugoslaviji. Vet. Archiv. 48:185, 1978.

144. Hajsig, D., et al.: Exudative epidermitis in piglets. II. Distribution of *Staphylococcus hyicus subsp. hyicus* findings in healthy piglets. Vet. Archiv. 55:45, 1985.

145. Hall, I. C., and Stone, R. V.: The diphtheroid bacillus of Preisz-Nocard from equine, bovine, and ovine abscesses. J. Infect. Dis. 18:195, 1916.

146. Hall, I. C., and Fisher, C. W.: Suppurative lesions in horses and a calf of California due to the diphteroid bacillus Preisz-Nocard. JAVMA 48:18, 1915.

147. Hanson, L. J.: Studies on parakeratosis and exudative epidermitis in swine. Thesis, Univ. of Minnesota, 1962.

148. Harcourt, R. A.: Porcine ulcerative spirochaetosis. Vet. Rec. 92:647, 1973.

149. Hardy, W. T., and Price, D. A.: Staphylococcic dermatitis of sheep. JAVMA 119:445, 1951.

150. Hare, T., et al.: First impressions of the beta-haemolytic *Streptococcus* infection of swine. Vet. Rec. 54:267, 1942.

151. Hart, C. B., et al.: Mycotic dermatitis in sheep. II. *Dermatophilus congolensis* and its reaction to compounds in vitro. Vet. Rec. 81:623, 1967.

152. Hart, C. B., and Tyszkiewicz, K.: Mycotic dermatitis in sheep. III. Chemotherapy with potassium aluminum sulphate. Vet. Rec. 82:272, 1968.

153. Hart, C. B.: *Dermatophilus* infection in the United Kingdom. *In:* Lloyd, D. H., and Sellers, K. C.: *Dermatophilus Infection in Animals and Man.* New York, Academic Press, 1976, p. 72.

154. Hasitscha, R.: Ein Beitrag zur Therapie der ruffartigen Dermatose der Saugferkel. Wien. Tierarztl. Monatsschr. 50:703, 1963.

155. Hastings, E. G., et al.: No-lesion and skin-lesion tuberculin-reacting cattle. JAVMA 66:36, 1924.

156. Hayston, J. T.: Actinobacillosis in sheep. Aust. Vet. J. 24:64, 1948.

157. Hebeler, H. F., et al.: Atypical actinobacillosis in a dairy herd. Vet. Rec. 73:517, 1961.

158. Hestrom, H.: Studies on so-called skin tuberculosis in cattle, concerning its prevalence in Sweden, its diagnosis, etiology, and allergy to tuberculin. Nord. Vet. Med. 2:83, 1950.

159. Heindrick, H. J., and Renk, W.: *Diseases of the Mammary Glands of Domestic Animals.* Philadelphia, W. B. Saunders Co., 1967.

160. Hibbs, C. M., and Kennedy, G. A.: Salmonellosis. *In:* Howard, J. L. (ed.): *Current Veterinary Therapy. Food Animal Practice.* Philadelphia, W. B. Saunders Co., 1981, p. 703.

161. Hjarre, A.: Kontagios pyodermi hos svin (impetigo contagiosa). Skand. Vet. Tidskr. 38:662, 1948.

162. Hogg, A.: Swine erysipelas. *In:* Howard, J. L. (ed.): *Current Veterinary Therapy. Food Animal Practice.* Philadelphia, W. B. Saunders Co., 1981, p. 670.

163. Holland, J. T. S., and Hodges, R. T.: Bacteriological observations on exudative epidermitis of pigs in New Zealand. N.Z. Vet. J. 29:57, 1981.

164. Hopes, R.: Skin diseases in horses. Vet. Dermatol. News. 1:4, 1976.

165. Howard, J. L.: Streptococcal diseases. *In:* Howard, J. L. (ed.): *Current Veterinary Therapy. Food Animal Practice.* Philadelphia, W. B. Saunders Co., 1981, p. 663.

166. Howard, J. L.: Staphylococcal diseases. *In:* Howard, J. L. (ed.): *Current Veterinary Therapy. Food Animal Practice.* Philadelphia, W. B. Saunders Co., 1981, p. 666.

167. Howard, J. L.: Actinobacillosis. *In:* Howard, J. L. (ed.): *Current Veterinary Therapy. Food Animal Practice.* Philadelphia, W. B. Saunders Co., 1981, p. 667.

168. Howard, J. L.: Actinomycosis. *In:* Howard, J. L. (ed.): *Current Veterinary Therapy. Food Animal Practice.* Philadelphia, W. B. Saunders Co., 1981, p. 668.

169. Hubbert, W. T., et al.: *Diseases Transmitted From Animals to Man VI.* Springfield, IL, Charles C. Thomas Publishers, 1975.

170. Hughes, J. P., and Biberstein, E. L.: Chronic equine abscesses associated with *Corynebacterium pseudotuberculosis.* JAVMA 135:559, 1959.

171. Hughes, J. P., et al.: Two cases of generalized *Corynebacterium pseudotuberculosis* infections in mares. Cornell Vet. 52:51, 1962.

172. Hungerford, T. G.: *Diseases of Livestock VII.* Sydney, Angus and Robertson, 1970.

173. Hunt, E.: Infectious skin diseases of cattle. Vet. Clin. North Am. Large Anim. Pract. 6:155, 1984.

174. Hunter, D., et al.: Exudative epidermitis of pigs. Br. Vet. J. 126:225, 1970.

175. Hutchins, D. R.: Skin diseases of cattle and horses in New South Wales. N.Z. Vet. J. 8:85, 1960.

176. Hutyra, F., et al.: *Special Pathology and Therapeutics of the Diseases of Domestic Animals V.* Chicago, Alexander Eger, 1946.

177. Hyslop, N. G.: Dermatophilosis (streptothricosis) in animals and man. Comp. Immunol. Micribiol. Infect. Dis. 2:389, 1980.

178. Ilchmann, G., et al.: Gehauftes Auftreten multipler Unterhautabszesse in einem Mastlammerbestand infolge perkutanen Eindringens von Gerstengrannen. Mh. Vet. Med. 35:252, 1980.

179. Ilemobade, A. A., et al.: Cure of *Dermatophilus congolensis* infection in cattle by long-acting oxytetracycline. Res. Vet. Sci. 27:302, 1979.

180. Istvan, S., et al.: Pikkelyezo-porkos borelvaltozas es orrhurut (stachybotryotoxicosis) sertesallomanyokban. I. Klinikai megfigyelesek es oktani vizsgalatok. Magy. Allatorv. Lapja 25:21, 1970.

181. Jaartsveld, F. H. J., et al.: *Clostridium* infectie bij biggen. Tijdschr. Diergeneeskd. 87:768, 1962.

182. Jarnagin, J. L., et al.: Isolation of *Mycobacterium kansasii* from lymph nodes of cattle in the United States. Am. J. Vet. Res. 44:1853, 1983.

183. Jenkinson, D. M.: The skin surface: An environment of *Dermatophilus congolensis.* *In:* Lloyd, D. H., and Sellers, K. C.: *Dermatophilis Infection in Animals and Man.* New York, Academic Press, 1976, p. 146.

184. Jensen, R.: *Diseases of Sheep.* Philadelphia, Lea & Febiger, 1974, p. 285.

185. Jones, J. E. T.: Observations on the bacterial flora of abscesses in pigs. Br. Vet. J. 146:343, 1980.

186. Jones, L. D.: Exudative epidermitis of pigs. Am. J. Vet. Res. 17:19, 1956.

187. Jones, L. D.: Observations on exudative epidermitis. Vet. Med. 56:95, 1961.

188. Jubb, K. V., and Kennedy, P. C.: *Pathology of Domestic Animals.* New York, Academic Press, 1970.

189. Jungerman, P. F., and Schwartzman, R. M.: *Veterinary Medical Mycology.* Philadelphia, Lea & Febiger, 1972.

190. Kaminski, G. W., and Suter, I. I.: Human infection with *Dermatophilus congolensis.* Med. J. Aust. 1:443, 1976.

191. Kaplan, W.: Dermatophilosis in primates. *In:* Lloyd, D. H., and Sellers, K. C.: *Dermatophilus Infection in Animals and Man.* New York, Academic Press, 1976, p. 128.

192. Kaplan, W., and Johnston, W. J.: Equine dermatophilosis (cutaneous streptothricosis) in Georgia. JAVMA 149:1162, 1966.

193. Kaufmann, A. F.: Anthrax. *In:* Howard, J. L. (ed.): *Current Veterinary Therapy. Food Animal Practice.* Philadelphia, W. B. Saunders Co., 1981, p. 677.

194. Kawano, J., et al.: Isolation of phages for typing of *Staphylococcus intermedius* isolated from horses. Jpn. J. Vet. Sci. 43:933, 1981.

195. Kawano, J., et al.: Bacteriophage typing of *Staphylococcus hyicus* subspecies *hyicus* isolates from pigs. Am. J. Vet. Res. 44:1476, 1983.

196. Kelly, D. C.: *Dermatophilus* infections in the United States. *In:* Lloyd, D. H., and Sellers, K. C.: *Dermatophilus Infection in Animals and Man.* New York, Academic Press, 1976, p. 116.

197. Kelly, D. C.: Immunological studies of antigenic components of *Dermatophilus congolensis.* *In:* Lloyd, D. H., and Sellers, K. C.: *Dermatophilus Infection in Animals and Man.* New York, Academic Press, 1976, p. 229.

198. Kernkamp, H. C.: Seborrhea oleosa in pigs. North Am. Vet. 29:438, 1948.

199. Kernkamp, H. C.: Weeping skin disease of baby pigs—seborrhea oleosa. North Am. Vet. 33:116, 1952.

200. King, N. B.: Diseases of goats. Univ. Sydney Post-Grad. Comm. Vet. Sci. Proc. 39:53, 1978.

201. King, N. B.: Clostridial diseases. Univ. Sydney Post-Grad. Comm. Vet. Sci. Proc. 52:217, 1980.

202. Kingman, H. E., and Palen, J. S.: Streptomycin in the treatment of actinomycosis. JAVMA 118:28, 1951.

203. Kloos, W. E.: Natural populations of the genus *Staphylococcus.* Annu. Rev. Microbiol. 34:559, 1980.

204. Knight, H. D.: Corynebacterial infections in the horse: Problems of prevention. JAVMA 155:446, 1969.

205. Knight, H. D.: A serologic method for the detection of *Corynebacterium pseudotuberculosis* infection in horses. Cornell Vet. 68:220, 1978.

206. Knowles, R. H.: Treatment of ulcerative lymphangitis by vaccines made from the Preisz-Nocard bacillus prepared with ethylchloride. J. Comp. Pathol. Ther. 31:262, 1918.

207. Konyha, L. D.: Tuberculosis. *In:* Howard, J. L. (ed.): *Current Veterinary Therapy. Food Animal Practice.* Philadelphia, W. B. Saunders Co., 181, p. 742.

208. Kral, F., and Schwartzman, R. M.: *In:* Kral, F., and Schwartzman, R. M.: *Veterinary and Comparative Dermatology.* Philadelphia, J. B. Lippincott Co., 1964.

209. Krantz, G. E., and Dunne, H. W.: An attempt to classify

streptococci isolated from domestic animals. Am. J. Vet. Res. 26:951, 1965.

210. Kumi-Diaka, J., et al.: Effect of scrotal streptothricosis on spermatogenesis in the bull. Vet. Rec. 107:525, 1980.

211. Langlois, B. E., et al.: Identification of *Staphylococcus* species of bovine origin with the API Staph-Ident System. J. Clin. Microbiol. 18:1212, 1983.

212. Laszlo, F.: Beitrag zur Hauttuberkulose. Dtsch. Tierarztl. Wochenschr. 43:196, 1935.

213. L'Ecuyer, C.: Exudative epidermitis in pigs. Clinical studies and preliminary transmission trials. Can. J. Comp. Med. 30:9, 1966.

214. L'Ecuyer, C., and Jericho, K.: Exudative epidermitis in pigs. Etiological studies and pathology. Can. J. Comp. Med. 30:94, 1966.

215. L'Ecuyer, C.: Exudative epidermitis of pigs. Bacteriological studies on the causative agent, *Staphylococcus hyicus*. Can. J. Comp. Med. 31:243, 1967.

216. L'Ecuyer, C., and Alexander, D. C.: Exudative epidermitis in pigs. Treatment trials. Can. Vet. J. 10:227, 1969.

217. Leman, A. D., et al.: *Diseases of Swine V*. Ames, Iowa State University Press, 1981.

218. Lenz, W.: Seltenes Zusammentreffen von Hautnekrose und spetikamischer Endocarditis valvularis beim Schwein. Wien. Tierarztl. Monatsschr. 61:343, 1974.

219. Le Riche, D. D.: The transmission of dermatophilosis in sheep. Aust. Vet. J. 44:64, 1968.

220. Le Roux, D. J.: The treatment of "lumpy wool," *Dermatophilus congolensis* infection in Merino sheep, with streptomycin and penicillin. J. So. Afr. Vet. Med. Assoc. 39:87, 1968.

221. Lewandowski, M., and Karpinski, J.: Epidemiological factors in the dissemination of purulent infections at cattle breeding centers. Med. Weter. 34:490, 1978.

222. Lewis, E. F.: Penicillin therapy in actinomycosis in cattle. Vet. Rec. 59:435, 1947.

223. Lignieresi, J., and Spitz, G.: L'actinobacillose. Rec. Vet. Med. 79:487, 1902.

224. Lloyd, D. H.: The economic effects of bovine streptothricosis. *In:* Lloyd, D. H., and Sellers, K. C.: *Dermatophilus Infection in Animals and Man*. New York, Academic Press, 1976, p. 274.

225. Lloyd, D. H., and Sellers, K. C.: *Dermatophilus Infection in Animals and Man*. New York, Academic Press, 1976.

226. Lloyd, D. H.: Bovine farcy. *In:* Howard, J. L. (ed.): *Current Veterinary Therapy. Food Animal Practice*. Philadelphia, W. B. Saunders Co., 1981, p. 1136.

227. Lloyd, D. H., Jenkinson, D. M.: Serum and skin surface antibody response to intradermal vaccination of cattle with *Dermatophilus congolensis*. Br. Vet. J. 137:601, 1981.

228. Lloyd, D. H., and Jenkinson, D. M.: The effect of climate on experimental infection of bovine skin with *Dermatophilus congolensis*. Br. Vet. J. 136:122, 1980.

229. Lofstedt, J.: Dermatologic diseases of sheep. Vet. Clin. North Am. Large Anim. Pract. 5:427, 1983.

230. Lomax, L. G., and Cole, J. R.: Porcine epidermitis and dermatitis associated with *Staphylococcus hyicus* and *Dermatophilus congolensis* infections. JAVMA 183:1091, 1983.

231. Londero, A. T.: *Dermatophilus* infection in the subtropical zone of South America. *In:* Lloyd, D. H., and Sellers, K. C.: *Dermatophilus Infection in Animals and Man*. New York, Academic Press, 1976, p. 110.

232. Luke, D., and Gordon, W. A. M.: Observations on some pig diseases. Vet. Rec. 62:179, 1950.

233. Lynch, J. A.: Successful bacterin therapy in a case of chronic equine staphylococcal infection. Can. Vet. J. 24:224, 1983.

234. Macadam, I.: Some observations on *Dermatophilus* infection in the Gambia with particular reference to the disease in sheep. *In:* Lloyd, D. H., and Sellers, K. C.: *Dermatophilus Infection in Animals and Man*. New York, Academic Press, 1976, p. 33.

235. Macadam, I.: Observations on the effects of flies and humidity on the natural lesions of streptothricosis. Vet. Rec. 76:194, 1964.

236. Macadam, I.: Bovine streptothricosis: Production of lesions by the bites of the tick *Amblyomma variegatum*. Vet. Rec. 74:643, 1962.

237. Macadam, I.: The effects of ectoparasites and humidity on natural lesions of streptothricosis. Vet. Rec. 76:354, 1964.

238. Macadam, I.: Streptothricosis in Nigerian horses. Vet. Rec. 76:420, 1964.

239. Macadam, I.: Some observations on bovine cutaneous streptothricosis in Northern Nigeria. Trop. Anim. Health Prod. 2:131, 1970.

240. Maddox, E. T., et al.: Ampicillin treatment of three cases of streptococcal auricular dermatitis in swine. Vet. Med. Small Anim. Clin. 68:1018, 1973.

241. Maddy, K. T.: *Corynebacterium pseudotuberculosis* infection in a horse. JAVMA 122:367, 1953.

242. Magnussen, H.: The commonest forms of actinomycosis in domestic animals and their etiology. Acta Pathol. Microbiol. Scand. 5:170, 1928.

243. Mair, N. S.: *Actinobacillus suis* infection in pigs: A report of four outbreaks and two sporadic cases. J. Comp. Pathol. 84:113, 1974.

244. Makinde, A. A.: The reverse single radial immunodiffusion technique for detecting antibodies to *Dermatophilus congolensis*. Vet. Rec. 106:383, 1980.

245. Mallman, W. L., et al.: A study of pathogenicity of Runyon group III organisms isolated from bovine and porcine sources. Am. Rev. Respir. Dis. 92:82, 1965.

246. Mansmann, R. A., et al.: *Equine Medicine and Surgery III*. Santa Barbara, CA, American Veterinary Publications, Inc., 1982.

246a. Markel, M. D., et al.: Cellulitis associated with coagulase-positive staphylococci in racehorses: Nine cases (1975–1984). JAVMA 189:1600, 1986.

247. Marsh, H., and Wilkins, H. W.: Actinobacillosis in sheep. JAVMA 94:363, 1939.

248. Martin, W. B.: *Diseases of Sheep*. Oxford, Blackwell Scientific Publications, Inc., 1983.

249. Mayfield, M. A., and Martin, M. T.: *Corynebacterium pseudotuberculosis* in Texas horses. Southwest. Vet. 32:133, 1979.

250. Mbassa, G.: Diffuse gangrene of the hind limb associated with umbilicus infection in a calf. Vet. Rec. 116:662, 1985.

251. McCaig, J.: "Mud fever" in horses. Vet. Rec. 81:173, 1967.

252. McKay, R. J., et al.: *Clostridium perfringens* associated with a focal abscess in a horse. JAVMA 175:71, 1979.

253. McMullan, W. C.: The skin. *In:* Mansmann, R. A., et al. (eds.): *Equine Medicine and Surgery III*. Santa Barbara, CA, American Veterinary Publications, Inc., 1982, p. 789.

254. Mebus, C. A., et al.: Exudative epidermitis: Pathogenesis and pathology. Pathol. Vet. 5:146, 1968.

255. Memery, G., and Thiery, G.: La streptothricose cutanée. I. Etude de la maladie naturelle et experimentale des bovins. Rev. Elev. Med. Vet. Pays Trop. 13:123, 1960.

256. Memery, G.: La streptothricose cutanee. II. Sur quelques cas spontanes chez des caprins dans la region de Dakar. Rev. Elev. Med. Vet. Pays Trop. 13:143, 1960.

257. Miers, K. C., and Ley, W. B.: *Corynebacterium pseudotuberculosis* infection in the horse: Study of 117 clinical cases and consideration of etiopathogenesis. JAVMA 117:250, 1980.

258. Miller, R. B., and Olson, L. D.: Epizootic of concurrent cutaneous streptococcal abscesses and swinepox in a herd of swine. JAVMA 172:676, 1978.

259. Miller, R. B., and Olson, L. D.: Experimental induction of cutaneous streptococcal abscesses in swine as a sequela to swinepox. Am. J. Vet. Res. 41:341, 1980.

260. Miller, R. M., and Dresher, L. K.: Equine ulcerative lymphangitis caused by *Pasteurella haemolytica* (2 case reports). Vet. Med. Small Anim. Clin. 76:1335, 1981.

261. Mitchell, C. A.: Bovine subcutaneous tuberculosis. JAVMA 73:493, 1928.

262. Mitchell, C. A., and Walker, R. V. L.: Preisz-Nocard disease. Study of a small outbreak occurring among horses. Can. J. Comp. Med. Vet. Sci. 8:3, 1944.

263. Mohiyuddeen, S., and Rao, N. S. K.: An epidemic of cutaneous anthrax among bovines in North Kanara District. Indian Vet. J. 35:55, 1958.

264. Momotani, E., et al.: Granulomatous subdermal lesions in sheep inoculated with *Dermatophilus congolensis*. J. Comp. Pathol. 94:33, 1984.

264a. Momotani, E., et al.: Experimental subcutaneous granulomas in sheep with *Dermatophilus*-like microorganisms from porcine tonsil. Mycopathologia 91:143, 1985.

265. Moreira, E. C., and Barbosa, M.: Dermatophilosis in tropical South America. *In:* Lloyd, D. H., and Sellers, K. C.: *Dermatophilus Infection in Animals and Man.* New York, Academic Press, 1976, p. 102.

266. Morgan, C. O.: Blackleg. *In:* Howard, J. L. (ed.): *Current Veterinary Therapy. Food Animal Practice.* Philadelphia, W. B. Saunders Co., 1981, p. 684.

267. Morgan, C. O.: Malignant edema and braxy. *In:* Howard, J. L. (ed.): *Current Veterinary Therapy. Food Animal Practice.* Philadelphia, W. B. Saunders Co., 1981, p. 688.

268. Morrison, S. M., et al.: *Staphylococcus aureus* in domestic animals. Publ. Health Rep. 76:673, 1961.

269. Mostafa, I. E.: Studies of bovine farcy in the Sudan. I. Pathology of the disease. J. Comp. Pathol. 77:223, 1967.

270. Mostafa, I. E.: Studies of bovine farcy in the Sudan. II. Mycology of the disease. J. Comp. Pathol. 77:231, 1967.

271. Mouwen, J. M. V. M., et al.: Perifere weefselnecrose bij het kalf. Tijdschr. Diergeneeskd. 92:1282, 1967.

272. Muller, G. H., et al.: *Small Animal Dermatology III.* Philadelphia, W. B. Saunders Co., 1983.

273. Mullowney, P. C., and Fadok, V. W.: Dermatologic diseases of horses. Part II. Bacterial and viral skin diseases. Comp. Cont. Ed. 6:S16, 1984.

274. Mullowney, P. C.: Dermatologic diseases of cattle. Part III. Infectious diseases. Comp. Cont. Ed. 4:S3, 1982.

275. Mullowney, P. C., and Baldwin, E. W.: Skin diseases of goats. Vet. Clin. North Am. Large Anim. Pract. 6:143, 1984.

276. Mullowney, P. C.: Skin diseases of sheep. Vet. Clin. North Am. Large Anim. Pract. 6:131, 1984.

277. Mullowney, P. C., and Hall, R. F.: Skin diseases of swine. Vet. Clin. North Am. Large Anim. Pract. 6:107, 1984.

278. Munce, T. W.: Swine erysipelas. North Am. Vet. 23:161, 1942.

279. Munro, R.: Caprine dermatophilosis in Fiji. Trop. Anim. Health Prod. 10:221, 1978.

280. Munz, E.: Double infection of sheep and goats in Kenya with orf virus and dermatophilosis. *In:* Lloyd, D. H., and Sellers, K. C.: *Dermatophilus Infection in Animals and Man.* New York, Academic Press, 1976, p. 57.

281. Murphy, D. B.: *Clostridium chauvoei* as the cause of malignant edema in a horse. Vet. Med. Small Anim. Clin. 75:1152, 1980.

282. Murty, D. K., and Kaushik, P. K.: Studies on an outbreak of acute swine pasteurellosis due to *Pasteurella multocida* type B (Carter 1955). Vet. Rec. 77:411, 1965.

282a. Nguhiu-Mwangi, J. A., and Gitao, C. G.: Acute cellulitis as a complication of footrot in cattle. Mod. Vet. Pract. 68:110, 1987.

283. Nicholls, T. J., and Rubira, R. J.: Staphylococcal dermatitis and mastitis. Aust. Vet. J. 57:54, 1981.

284. Nieberle, K., and Stolpe, B.: Zur Kenntnis des metastatischen Hautmilzbrandes beim Schwein. Dtsch. Tierarztl. Wochenschr. 35:281, 1927.

285. Nieland, H.: Haut und Nasenscheidewand-tuberkulose beim Pferd. Dtsch. Tierarztl. Wochenschr. 46:98, 1938.

286. Nobel, T. A., et al.: Cutaneous streptothricosis (dermatophilosis) of cattle in Israel. *In:* Lloyd, D. H., and Sellers, K. C.: *Dermatophilus Infection in Animals and Man.* New York, Academic Press, 1976, p. 70.

287. Norval, J.: Abscesses in pigs. Vet. Rec. 78:708, 1966.

288. Nusbaum, S. R.: A practitioner's experience with intravenous sodium iodide–mercuric nitrate therapy in *Actinomyces bovis* infection. Vet. Med. 60:888, 1965.

289. Nwufoh, K. J., et al.: The pattern of sensitivity of a *Dermatophilus congolensis (D. congolensis)* strain to various antibiotics *in vitro* in Nigeria. Rev. Elev. Med. Vet. Pays Trop. 34:19, 1982.

290. Obeid, H. M. A.: Cutaneous streptothricosis in Sudanese cattle. *In:* Lloyd, D. H., and Sellers, K. C.: *Dermatophilus Infection in Animals and Man.* New York, Academic Press, 1976, p. 44.

291. Obel, A. L.: Epithelial changes in porcine exudative epidermitis. The light microscopical picture. Pathol. Vet. 5:253, 1968.

292. Obel, A. L., and Nicander, L.: Epithelial changes in porcine exudative epidermitis. An ultrastructural study. Pathol. Vet. 7:328, 1970.

293. O'Connor, P. J., et al.: On the association between salmonellosis and the occurrence of osteomyelitis and terminal dry gangrene in calves. Vet. Rec. 90:459, 1972.

294. Oduye, O. O.: Histopathological changes in natural and experimental *Dermatophilus congolensis* infection of the bovine skin. *In:* Lloyd, D. H., and Sellers, K. C.: *Dermatophilus Infection in Animals and Man.* New York, Academic Press, 1976, p. 172.

295. Oduye, O. O.: Bovine streptothricosis in Nigeria. *In:* Lloyd, D. H., and Sellers, K. C.: *Dermatophilus Infection in Animals and Man.* New York, Academic Press, 1976, p. 2.

296. Oeding, P., et al.: A comparison of antigenic structure and phage pattern with biochemical properties of *Staphylococcus aureus* strains isolated from horses. Acta Pathol. Microbiol. Scand. B 82:899, 1974.

297. Oppong, E. N. W.: Epizootiology of *Dermatophilus* infection in cattle in the Accra plains of Ghana. *In:* Lloyd, D. H., and Sellers, K. C.: *Dermatophilus Infection in Animals and Man.* New York, Academic Press, 1976, p. 17.

298. Osborne, H. G., and Ensor, C. R.: Some aspects of the pathology, aetiology, and therapeutics of foot-rot in pigs. N.Z. Vet. J. 3:191, 1955.

299. Otcenasek, M., et al.: *Nocardia asteroides* vyvolaratelem superficialni dermatozy kone. Veterinarstvi 25:29, 1975.

300. Oyejide, A., et al.: Prevalence of antibodies to *Dermatophilus congolensis* in sheep and goats in Nigeria. Vet. Quart. 6:44, 1984.

301. Page, E. H.: Common skin diseases of the horse. Proc. Am. Assoc. Equine Pract. 18:385, 1972.

302. Parihar, N. S., et al.: Cutaneous actinobacillosis in a bull. Indian Vet. J. 54:431, 1977.

303. Parker, B. N. J., et al.: Staphylococcal dermatitis in unweaned lambs. Vet. Rec. 113:570, 1983.

304. Pascoe, R. R.: The nature and treatment of skin conditions observed in horses in Queensland. Aust. Vet. J. 49:35, 1973.

305. Pascoe, R. R.: An outbreak of mycotic dermatitis in horses in South-Eastern Queensland. Aust. Vet. J. 47:112, 1971.

306. Pascoe, R. R.: Further observations on *Dermatophilus* infections in horses. Aust. Vet. J. 48:32, 1972.

307. Pascoe, R. R.: *Equine Dermatoses.* Sydney, University of Sydney Post-Graduate Foundation in Veterinary Science, Veterinary Review No. 22, 1981.

308. Pascoe, R. R.: Dermatophilosis. *In:* Robinson, N. E.: *Current Therapy in Equine Medicine.* Philadelphia, W. B. Saunders Co., 1983, p. 553.

309. Pascoe, R. R.: Infectious skin diseases of horses. Vet. Clin. North Am. Large Anim. Pract. 6:27, 1984.

310. Pay, M. G.: The effect of disease on a large pig-fattening enterprise. Vet. Rec. 87:648, 1970.

311. Peel, J. E.: Tuberculosis. *In:* Robinson, N. E.: *Current Therapy in Equine Medicine.* Philadelphia, W. B. Saunders Co., 1983, p. 29.

312. Pepper, T. A., and Taylor, D. J.: The effect of exudative epidermitis on weaner production in a small pig herd. Vet. Rec. 101:204, 1977.

313. Phillips, J. E.: The commensal role of *Actinobacillus lignieresii*. J. Pathol. Bacteriol. 82:205, 1964.

314. Phillips, J. E.: Commensal actinobacilli from the bovine tongue. J. Pathol. Bacteriol. 87:442, 1964.

315. Phillips, J. E.: Antigenic structure and serological typing of *Actinobacillus lignieresii*. J. Pathol. 93:463, 1967.

316. Phillips, W. E., et al.: Isolation of *Staphylococcus hyicus* subspecies *hyicus* from a pig with septic polyarthritis. Am. J. Vet. Res. 41:274, 1980.

317. Piercy, D. W.: Greasy pig disease. Vet. Rec. 78:477, 1966.

318. Pinkiewicz, A., et al.: Skin tuberculosis in a horse. Med. Weter. 19:692, 1963.

319. Plowright, W.: Cutaneous streptothricosis of cattle. Vet. Rec. 68:350, 1956.

320. Provost, A., et al.: Vaccination trials against bovine dermatophilosis in Southern Chad. *In:* Lloyd, D. H., and Sellers, K. C.: *Dermatophilus Infection in Animals and Man.* New York, Academic Press, 1976, p. 260.

321. Puhringer, H.: Tuberkulose der Uterhaut beim Rinde. Wien. Tierarztl. Monatsschr. 17:778, 1930.

322. Purchase, H. S.: An outbreak of ulcerative lymphangitis in cattle caused by *Corynebacterium ovis*. J. Comp. Pathol. Ther. 54:238, 1944.

322a. Rakestraw, J., and Edwards, A. J.: The effect of swim vat dipping on the incidence of ear implant abscesses in yearling feedlot steers. Agri-Pract. 8:22, 1987.

323. Rebhun, W. C., et al.: Malignant edema in horses. JAVMA 187:732, 1985.

324. Reef, V. B.: *Clostridium perfringens* cellulitis and immune-mediated hemolytic anemia in a horse. JAVMA 182:251, 1983.

325. Reid, C. H.: Habronemiasis and *Corynebacterium* "chest" abscess in California horses. Vet. Med. Small Anim. Clin. 60:233, 1965.

326. Remes, E., and Koiranen, L.: Stafylokokkien aiheuttama furukuloosi ks-sonneilla. Suomen Elain. 80:8, 1974.

327. Renshaw, H. W., et al.: Leukocyte dysfunction in the bovine homologue of the Chédiak-Higashi syndrome of humans. Infect. Immun. 10:928, 1974.

328. Richard, J. L., and Pier, A. C.: Transmission of *Dermatophilus congolensis* by *Stomoxys calcitrans* and *Musca domestica*. Am. J. Vet. Res. 27:419, 1966.

329. Richard, J. L., et al.: Comparison of antigens of *Dermatophilus congolensis* isolates and their use in serological tests in experimental and natural infections. *In:* Lloyd, D. H., and Sellers, K. C.: *Dermatophilus Infection in Animals and Man.* New York, Academic Press, 1976, p. 216.

330. Richardson, A.: Osteomyelitis in calves caused by *Salmonella dublin*. Vet. Rec. 90:410, 1972.

331. Rieder, L.: Das polybakterielle Pemphigoid der Ferkel. Tierarztl. Umschau 20:180, 1965.

332. Ristic, M., et al.: Seborrhea oleosa in pigs. Vet. Med. 51:421, 1956.

333. Roberts, D. W.: Chemotherapy of epidermal infection with *Dermatophilus congolensis*. J. Comp. Pathol. Ther. 77:129, 1967.

334. Roberts, D. S.: *Dermatophilus* infection. Vet. Bull 37:513, 1967.

335. Roberts, D. S.: Barriers to *Dermatophilus dermatonomus* infection on the skin of sheep. Aust. J. Agric. Res. 14:492, 1963.

336. Roberts, D. S.: The histopathology of epidermal infections with the actinomycete *Dermatophilus congolensis*. J. Pathol. Bacteriol. 90:213, 1965.

337. Roberts, D. S.: The influence of carbon dioxide on the growth and sporulation of *Dermatophilus dermatonomus*. Aust. J. Agric. Res. 14:412, 1963.

338. Roberts, D. S.: Synergistic effects of salts and carbon dioxide on *Dermatophilus dermatonomus*. J. Gen. Microbiol. 37:403, 1964.

339. Roberts, D. S.: The release and survival of *Dermatophilus dermatonomus* zoospores. Aust. J. Agric. Res. 14:386, 1963.

340. Roberts, D. S.: Chemotactic behavior of the infective zoospores of *Dermatophilus dermatonomus*. Aust. J. Agric. Res. 14:400, 1963.

341. Rogers, P. A. M.: Terminal dry gangrene in young calves. Irish Vet. J. 23:126, 1969.

342. Rooney, J. R.: Corynebacterial infections in foals. Mod. Vet. Pract. 47:43, 1966.

343. Roth, J. A., et al.: Effects of bovine viral diarrhea virus infection on bovine polymorphonuclear leukocyte function. Am. J. Vet. Res. 42:244, 1981.

344. Roth, J. A., and Kaeberle, M. L.: Effects of *in vivo* dexamethasone administration on *in vitro* bovine polymorphonuclear leukocyte infection. Infect. Immun. 33:434, 1981.

345. Roth, J. A., et al.: Effect of estradiol and progesterone on lymphocyte and neutrophil function in steers. Infect. Immun. 35:997, 1982.

346. Roth, J. A., and Kaeberle, M. L.: Effect of levamisole on lymphocyte blastogenesis and neutrophil function in dexamethasone-treated cattle. Am. J. Vet. Res. 45:1781, 1984.

347. Rumbaugh, G. E.: Internal abdominal abscesses in the horse: A study of 25 cases. JAVMA 172:304, 1978.

348. Sandbu, E. H.: Impetigo contagiosa. En del undersokelser over sjukdommens-araksforhold. Nord. Veterinarmotet. 8:85, 1959.

349. Satoh, H., et al.: Histopathological investigations on acute swine erysipelas. Jpn. J. Vet. Res. 1:111, 1953.

350. Savey, M., et al.: Identification de la dermatite staphylococcique du mouton. Rec. Med. Vet. 159:701, 1983.

351. Scanlan, C. M., et al.: *Dermatophilus congolensis* infections of cattle and sheep. Comp. Cont. Ed. 6:S4, 1984.

351a. Scheidt, V. J., and Lloyd, D. H.: Dermatophilosis. *In:* Robinson, N. E. (ed.): *Current Therapy in Equine Medicine II.* Philadelphia, W. B. Saunders Co., 1986, p. 630.

352. Schleifer, K.H., et al.: Chemical and biochemical studies for the differentiation of coagulase-positive staphylococci. Arch. Microbiol. 110:263, 1976.

353. Schmidt, U., et al.: Das nassende Ekzem des Schweines. Pathologisch-anatomische Befunde. Berl. Munch. Tierarztl. Wochenschr. 85:181, 1972.

354. Schulz, L., et al.: Durch Blutgerinnnungsstorungen gekennzeichnete Mikroangiopathien beim septikamischen Rotlauf. Dtsch. Tierarztl. Wochenschr. 78:563, 1971.

355. Schultz, W.: Untersuchungen zur Aetiologie der exudativen Epidermitis der Ferkel unter besonderer Berucksichtigung des *Staphylococcus hyicus*. Arch. Exp. Veterinaermed. 23:415, 1969.

356. Schultz, W.: Die Exsudative Epidermitis der Ferkel-Untersuchungen zur Atiologie und Pathogenese unter besonderer berucksichtigung des *Staphylococcus hyicus*. Monat. Vet. Med. 25:428, 1970.

357. Schwobel, W. P.: Enzyme-antibiotic treatment for bovine actinomycosis. Mod. Vet. Pract. 44:64, 1963.

358. Scott, D. W., and Manning, T. O.: Equine folliculitis and furunculosis. Equine Pract. 2:11, 1980.

359. Scott, D. W.: Folliculitis and furunculosis. *In:* Robinson, N. E.: *Current Therapy in Equine Medicine.* Philadelphia, W. B. Saunders Co., 1983, p. 542.

360. Scott, D. W., et al.: Caprine dermatology. I. Normal skin and bacterial and fungal disorders. Comp. Cont. Ed. 6:S190, 1984.

361. Scott, F. M. M., et al.: Staphylococcal dermatitis of sheep. Vet. Rec. 107:572, 1980.

362. Searcy, G. P., and Hulland, T. J.: *Dermatophilus* dermatitis (streptothricosis) in Ontario. I. Clinical observations. Can. Vet. J. 9:7, 1968.

363. Searcy, G. P., and Hulland, T. J.: *Dermatophilus* dermatitis (streptothricosis) in Ontario. II. Laboratory findings. Can. Vet. J. 9:16, 1968.

364. Sertic, V.: O pojavi i znacenju duboke stafilodermije repa u bikova. Vet. Archiv. 42:265, 1972.

365. Shimizu, A., and Kato, E.: Bacteriophage typing of *Staphylococcus aureus* isolated from horses in Japan. Jpn. J. Vet. Sci. 41:409, 1979.

366. Shores, S. A.: Dermatitis in a colt. Southwest. Vet. 18:68, 1964.

367. Sickmuller, E.: Hauttuberkulose des Rindes. Dtsch. Tierarztl. Wochenschr. 37:330, 1929.

368. Simmons, J.: A case of ulcerative lymphangitis. Southwest. Vet. 18:235, 1965.

369. Simon, P. C., and Stovell, P. L.: Diseases of animals associated with *Sphaerophorus necrophorus*: Characteristics of the organism. Vet. Bull. 39:311, 1969.

370. Simpson, R.: *Corynebacterium equi* in adult horses in Kenya. Bull. Epizoot. Dis. Afr. 12:303, 1964.

371. Singh, V. P., and Murty, D. K.: An outbreak of *Dermatophilus congolensis* infection in goats. Indian Vet. J. 55:674, 1978.

372. Smith, B. P., and Jang, S.: Isolation of *Corynebacterium equi* from a foal with an ulcerated leg wound and a pectoral abscess. JAVMA 177:623, 1980.

373. Smith, L. D. S., et al.: *Clostridium sordelli* infection in sheep. Cornell Vet. 52:62, 1962.

374. Smith, L. D. S.: *The Pathogenic Anaerobic Bacteria II.* Springfield, IL, Charles C. Thomas Publisher, 1975.

375. Smith, M. C.: Caprine dermatologic problems: A review. JAVMA 178:724, 1981.

376. Sompolinsky, D.: De l'impetigo contagiosa suis et du *Micrococcus hyicus*. Schweiz. Arch. Tierheilkd. 95:302, 1953.

377. Stankusheve, K., et al.: Mycotic dermatitis in pigs. Veterinarna Sbirka 65:3, 1968.
378. Stannard, A. A., and Jang, S. S.: Dermatophilosis in a lamb. JAVMA 163:1161, 1973.
379. Stannard, A. A.: Equine dermatology. Proc. Am. Assoc. Equine Pract. 22:273, 1976.
380. Sterne, M., and Edwards, J. B.: Blackleg in pigs caused by *Clostridium chauvoei*. Vet. Rec. 67:314, 1955.
381. Stewart, G. H.: Dermatophilosis: A skin disease of animals and man. Parts I and II. Vet. Rec. 91:537, 555, 1972.
382. Stubenrauch, L.: Zur Behandlung der ruffartigen Dermatose derm Saugferkel mit Glukokortikoiden. Wien. Tierarztl. Monatsschr. 48:277, 1961.
383. Stuker, G., and Glattli, H. R.: Besteht ein zusammenhang zwischen der Biotinversorgung der Ferkel und dem Auftreten von Epidermitis exsudativa? Schweiz. Arch. Tierheilkd. 118:305, 1976.
384. Stuker, G., and Bertschinger, H. U.: *Staphylococcus hyicus*: Kulturell-biochemische Charakterisierung, serologische Typisierung und Pathogenitatsnachweis im Tierversuch. Zbl. Vet. Med. B 23:733, 1976.
385. Synge, B. A., et al.: Dermatitis of the legs of sheep associated with *Staphylococcus aureus*. Vet. Rec. 116:459, 1985.
386. Terpstra, J. I., and Akkermans, J. P. W. M.: De dermatitis crustosa van het Varken. Tijdschr. Diergeneeskd. 81:755, 1956.
387. Thiery, G., and Memery, G.: La streptothricose cutanée. IV. Etiologie, traitement, prophylaxie. Rev. Elev. Med. Vet. Pays Trop. 14:413, 1961.
388. Thomann, H.: Untersuchungen uber das Vorkommen der "skin-lesion" beim schweizerischen Braunvieh. Schweiz. Arch. Tierheilkd. 91:237, 1949.
389. Thomsett, L. R.: Skin diseases of the horse. In Pract. 1:15, 1979.
390. Traum, J.: Case reports of lymphangitis in cattle caused by an acid-alcoholic fast organism. JAVMA 49:254, 1916.
391. Traum, J.: Further report on lymphangitis in cattle caused by acid-alcohol fast organism. JAVMA 55:639, 1919.
392. Traum, J.: Lymphangitis in cattle, caused by acid-fast organism. Cornell Vet. 13:240, 1923.
393. Traum, J.: The relation of acid-fast skin infections of cattle to bovine tuberculosis and other acid-fast infections. JAVMA 74:553, 1929.
394. Udea, S., et al.: An outbreak of suppurative disease caused by *Corynebacterium pyogenes* on a pig farm. J. Jpn. Vet. Med. Assoc. 25:125, 1972.
395. Ulvund, M. J.: Dermatophilose hos sau. En oversikt med beskrivelse av to atypiske kasus. Norsk. Vet. Tidsshrift. 87:537, 1975.
396. Underdahl, N. R., et al.: Experimental transmission of exudative epidermitis of pigs. JAVMA 142:754, 1963.
397. Underdahl, N. R., et al.: Porcine exudative epidermitis: Characteristics of bacterial agent. Am. J. Vet. Res. 26:617, 1965.
398. Underdahl, N. R.: Exudative epidermitis (XE) of pigs. *In*: Howard, J. L. (ed.): *Current Veterinary Therapy. Food Animal Practice*. Philadelphia, W. B. Saunders Co., 1981, p. 1159.
399. Valberg, S. J., and McKinnar, A. O.: Clostridial cellulitis in the horse: A report of five cases. Can. Vet. J. 25:67, 1984.
400. Vanbreuseghem, R., et al.: Some experimental research on *Dermatophilus congolensis*. *In*: Lloyd, D. H., and Sellers, K. C.: *Dermatophilus Infection in Animals and Man*. New York, Academic Press, 1976, p. 202.
401. Van Meurs, G. K.: De diagnostiek van smeer pokken. Tijdschr. Diergeneeskd. 94:1683, 1969.
402. Van Os, J. L.: Een nieuwe therapie voor dermatitis crustosa van biggen. Tijdschr. Diergeneeskd. 92:662, 1967.
403. Vawter, L. R.: Pulmonary actinomycosis in swine. JAVMA 109:198, 1946.
404. Verma, B. B., et al.: A note on impetigo in goats. Indian Vet. J. 61:895, 1984.
405. Watanabe, T., et al.: An outbreak of exudative dermatitis in swine. J. Jpn. Vet. Med. Assoc. 29:217, 1976.
406. Watts, T. C., et al.: Treatment of bovine actinomycosis with isoniazid. Can. Vet. J. 14:23, 1973.
407. West, J. E., et al.: Postparturient pectoral abscess in a mare. Mod. Vet. Pract. 67:531, 1986.
408. Westman, C. W., et al.: Clostridial infection in a horse. JAVMA 174:725, 1979.
409. Wegmann, E.: Lymphangitis from *Streptococcus pyogenes* infection in a foal. Mod. Vet. Pract. 67:735, 1986.
410. Wilkinson, F. C.: Dermatophilosis of sheep association with dipping and effects on production. Aust. Vet. J. 55:74, 1979.
411. Windsor, R. S.: *Actinobacillus equuli* infection in a litter of pigs and a review of previous reports on similar infections. Vet. Rec. 92:178, 1973.
412. Wisecup, W. G., et al.: *Corynebacterium pseudotuberculosis* associated with rapidly occurring equine abscesses. JAVMA 144:152, 1964.
413. Woolcock, J. B., et al.: Selective medium for *Corynebacterium equi*. J. Clin. Microbiol. 9:640, 1979.
414. Worthington, R. W., et al.: Isolation of *Mycobacterium kansasii* from bovines. J. S. Afr. Med. Assoc. 35:29, 1964.
415. Zeller, M.: Enzootischer Pararuschbrand in einer Schweinemastanstalt. Tierarztl. Umschau 11:406, 1956.
416. Zlotnik, I.: Cutaneous streptothricosis in cattle. Vet. Rec. 67:613, 1955.

CHAPTER 7

FUNGAL DISEASES

CUTANEOUS MYCOLOGY

Fungi are omnipresent in the environment. Of the thousands of different fungal species, only a few have the ability to cause disease in animals. The great majority of fungi are either soil organisms or plant pathogens. However, more than 300 species of fungi have been reported to be animal pathogens.[64, 106, 175, 224, 333] A mycosis is a disease caused by a fungus. A dermatophytosis is an infection of the keratinized tissues, nail, hair, and stratum corneum that is caused by a species of *Microsporum, Trichophyton,* or *Epidermophyton.* A dermatomycosis is a fungal infection of hair, nail, or skin that is caused by a nondermatophyte. Fungi, however, are not nearly as common a cause of skin disease as is generally supposed, and many nonspecific, pruritic or nonpruritic dermatoses, especially if associated with target or ringworm-like lesions, are diagnosed as dermatomycoses on inadequate evidence. On the other hand, many true fungal infections probably are not diagnosed, because of the great variability of clinical presentations.

Dermatophytoses can be transmitted from animals to humans, from animals to animals, and from humans to animals. Zoophilic fungi prefer animals as hosts but often cause acute inflammatory reactions when they invade humans. This inflammation is unfavorable to the invading fungus, thereby limiting the progress of the infection. Zoophilic fungal infections rarely cause an acute inflammatory reaction in animals, so that the dermatophyte is able to exist in a continuing relationship with its host.

Characterization of Pathogenic Fungi

Fungi pathogenic to plants are distributed throughout all divisions of the fungi, but those pathogenic to animals are found primarily in the Fungi Imperfecti and Ascomycota groups.

The term fungus includes yeasts and molds. A yeast is a unicellular budding fungus that forms blastoconidia, whereas a mold is a filamentous fungus. Some pathogenic fungi, such as *Histoplasma capsulatum, Coccidioides immitis, Sporothrix schenckii,* and *Blastomyces dermatitidis,* are dimorphic. Dimorphic fungi are capable of existing in two different morphologic forms. For example, at 37° C in enriched media or in vivo, *B. dermatitidis* exists as a yeast, but at 25 or 30° C, it grows as a mold. *C. immitis* is unique because at 37° C or in tissue, spherules containing endospores are formed. Some fungi such as *Aspergillus* form true hyphae in tissue and are a mold at either 30 or 37° C. Another manifestation of fungal growth in tissue is the presence of granules (grains) that are organized in masses of hyphae in a crystalline or amorphous matrix. These granules, characteristic of the mycotic infection, mycetoma, are the result of interaction between the host tissue and the fungus.

Culture and Examination of Fungi

To ascertain the cause of a dermatophytosis, proper specimen selection and collection, isolation, and correct identification are necessary.

Wood's Light

One aid used to assist in specimen collection is the Wood's light, an ultraviolet light with a 253.7 nm light wave filtered through a cobalt or nickel filter.

Before being used to examine an animal, the Wood's light should be allowed to warm up for five to ten minutes. The animal should be examined in a dark room or enclosure. When exposed to the Wood's light, hairs invaded by *M. canis* and *M. equinum*[258, 302] may fluoresce yellow-green, as a result of tryptophan metabolites produced by the fungus. This metabolite is produced only by actively growing hair and cannot be elicited from an in vitro infection of hair. Fluorescence is not present in scales or crusts or in cultures of dermatophytes. Although the distinctness of *M. equinum* has long been debated,* recent studies using reference antigens, monospecific antisera, and mating experiments have demonstrated that it is a unique species.[316, 317] Other less common dermatophytes that may fluoresce include *M. distortum*, *M. audouinii*, and *T. schoenleinii*.[258, 324, 333]

Many factors influence fluorescence. Medications may destroy it. Bacteria such as *Pseudomonas aeruginosa* and *Corynebacterium minutissimum* may produce fluorescence, but of a different color. Keratin, soaps, petroleum, and other medications and debris may fluoresce and give false-positive reactions. If the short stubs of hair are producing fluorescence, the proximal end of hairs extracted from the follicles should fluoresce. These fluorescing hairs should be selected with a forceps and used for inoculating fungal media and for microscopic examination.

Unfortunately, in large animal dermatophytoses, the Wood's light examination is rarely positive.

Specimen Collection

Hair is the specimen most commonly collected for the isolation of dermatophytes. Using forceps, hairs should be selected that appear stubbled and broken, especially at the advancing periphery of an active, nonmedicated lesion. In addition, surface keratin may be gathered by forceps or skin scrapings from similar areas and inoculated onto the culture medium.

The hair and surface keratin of large animals are veritable cesspools of saprophytic fungi and bacteria (see Chapter 1, discussion on cutaneous ecology). Hence, it is essential to cleanse the skin prior to taking samples for culture. This may be done by *gently* cleasing the area to be sampled with a mild soap and water, or 70 per cent alcohol, and allowing it to air-dry.

Impression Smear

A stained smear can be made by obtaining a skin scraping, needle aspirate, or direct touch impression from suspected lesions. These slides can be stained with new methylene blue or Diff-Quik. This method is especially useful for yeasts.

Direct Microscopic Examination of Hair and Keratin

This procedure requires practice and expertise. Because most animal fungal infections are ectothrix, clearing techniques are not as necessary as in the common endothrix infections involving humans. Thus, hair and keratin from animal dermatophytoses can often be successfully examined by simply suspending the specimens in mineral oil (Fig. 7–1).

When clearing is desirable, several methods have been utilized.* Several drops of 20 per cent potassium hydroxide (KOH) may be applied to microscope slides onto which hair and keratin have been placed. A coverslip is added to the slide, and the slide is gently heated for 15 to 20 seconds (avoid boiling) or allowed to stand for 30 minutes at room temperature. Another procedure is to add one part of 1.2 percent dye solution of Permanent Black Super Quink (Parker Pen Company) or India ink to two parts of 20 percent KOH. The addition of this dye may aid in the interpretation of the KOH preparation by staining the hyphae and conidia. Another commonly used clearing solution is called chlorphenolac. This solution is made by adding 50 gm chloral hydrate to 25 ml liquid phenol and 25 ml liquid lactic acid. Slides cleared with this solution can be read almost immediately.

Artifacts such as threads, wisps of cotton, fiber glass or elastic fibers, early KOH crystal formations from overheated or dried-out slide preparations, and keratinized cell wall "skeletons" may be confused with fungal hyphae and conidia.

In ectothrix invasion of hair, arthroconidia are on the hair shaft, with hyphae penetrating and invading the hair shaft. Conidia may accumulate in masses or in a mosaic pattern on the hair. Endothrix invasion is characterized by conidia formation within the hair shaft. Endothrix invasion is rarely seen in animals.

Fungal Culture

Sabouraud's dextrose agar has been used traditionally in veterinary mycology for isola-

---

*References 62, 71, 114, 283, 302, 306, 384

*References 106, 141, 175, 224, 258, 260, 302, 324, 333, 371, 383

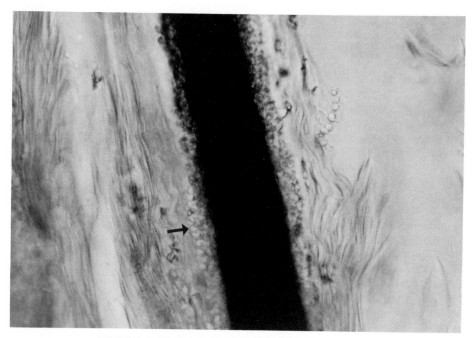

FIGURE 7–1. Arthroconidia (arrow) on a hair in mineral oil.

tion of fungi; however, other media are available with bacterial and fungal inhibitors, such as Dermatophyte Test Medium (DTM), potato dextrose agar, and rice grain medium.* Mycosel and Mycobiotic agar are formulations of Sabouraud's dextrose agar with cycloheximide and chloramphenicol added to inhibit fungal and bacterial contaminants. If a medium with cycloheximide is used, fungi sensitive to it will not be isolated. Some organisms sensitive to cycloheximide include *Cryptococcus neoformans,* many members of the Zygomycota, some *Candida* species, *Aspergillus* species, *Pseudoallescheria boydii,* and many agents of phaeohyphomycosis. DTM is essentially Sabouraud's dextrose agar containing cycloheximide, gentamicin, and chlortetracycline as antifungal and antibacterial agents and to which the pH indicator phenol red has been added. Dermatophytes utilize protein in the medium first, with alkaline metabolites turning the medium red (Fig. 7–2). Most other fungi utilize carbohydrate first, giving off acid metabolites, which do not produce a red color change. These saprophytic fungi will later use the protein in the medium, resulting in a red color change. However, this usually occurs only after a prolonged incubation (10 to 14 days or more). Consequently, DTM cultures should be

examined daily for the first ten days. Fungi such as *B. dermatitidis, S. schenckii, H. capsulatum, C. immitis, P. boydii,* some *Aspergillus* species, and others cause a red color change in DTM, so microscopic examination is essential to avoid an erroneous presumptive diagnosis.[165, 258, 341] Since DTM may depress development of conidia, mask colony pigmentation, and inhibit some pathogens, fungi recovered on DTM should be transferred to plain Sabouraud's dextrose agar for identification. It has been recommended that 1 to 2 drops of a sterile injectable B complex vitamin preparation be added to culture plates when culturing horses, as one strain of *T. equinum (T. equinum* var. *equinum)* has a unique niacin requirement.

Skin scrapings and hair should be inoculated onto Sabouraud's dextrose agar and DTM and incubated at 30° C with 30 percent humidity. A pan of water in the incubator will usually provide enough humidity. Cultures should be checked every day for growth. DTM may be incubated for 14 days, but cultures on Sabouraud's agar should be allowed 30 days to develop.

Some dermatophytes that cause disease in large animals have special nutritional or incubation requirements. Many strains of *T. verrucosum* grow best at 37° C. A common dermatophyte of horses, *T. equinum* var. *equinum,* has a special niacin requirement. If

*References 41, 106, 141, 175, 224, 258, 260, 302, 324, 333, 371, 383

such special requirements are not heeded, fungal cultures will be falsely negative.

Microscopic Examination of Fungi

Fungal structures can often be determined by a slide preparation.[106, 141, 224, 333] Hyphae and conidia from mature colonies may be teased apart and spread on a microscope slide. The slide is flooded with water containing a wetting agent such as Tween 80 or lactophenol cotton blue stain, covered with a coverslip, and examined.

An alternative method is the acetate tape method. Preparations by this method are easily made with pressure-sensitive tape from stationery stores. Number 800 clear acetate-backed tape (Minnesota Mining and Manufacturing Company) preserves the preparation longer, but other tapes are adequate for most purposes. To make the preparation, a "flag of tape" 1 cm by 1 cm is fastened to the end of a wooden applicator stick or wire needle or grasped in forceps, and the sticky surface of the flag is touched to the surface of the colony just proximal to the advancing periphery. The tape is then pressed, sticky side down, on a slide with a drop of water or lactophenol cotton blue stain and examined under the microscope.

DERMATOMYCOSES

Superficial Mycoses. These are fungal infections that involve the skin and hair. The organisms may be dermatophytes such as *Microsporum* and *Trichophyton*, which are able to use keratin. However, other fungi such as *Candida* may also produce superficial mycoses.

Subcutaneous Mycoses. These are fungal infections that have invaded the viable tissues of the skin. These infections are usually acquired by traumatic implantation of organisms that normally exist in soil or vegetation. The lesions are chronic and, in most cases, remain localized. The terminology used in reference to subcutaneous mycoses has been confusing and contradictory. The term phaeohyphomycosis includes subcutaneous and systemic diseases caused by fungi that develop in the host tissue in the form of dark-walled (dematiacious) septate mycelial elements. *Chromoblastomycosis* is characterized by sclerotic bodies (chromobodies, Medlar's bodies), which are large dark-walled cells 4 to 12 μm in diameter located in subcutaneous microabscesses. Chromomycoses are mycotic infections characterized by the presence of dematiacious fungal elements in tissue. Since this general term includes both chromoblastomycosis and phaeohyphomycosis, it is more precise to use the specific terms. In contrast with phaeohyphomycosis and chromoblastomycosis, a mycetoma is a unique fungal infection characterized by granules (grains), tumefaction, and draining tracts (sinuses). Mycetomas may be either eumycotic mycetomas or actinomycotic mycetomas. The etiologic agents of eumycotic mycetomas are fungi, whereas actinomycotic mycetomas are caused by members of the

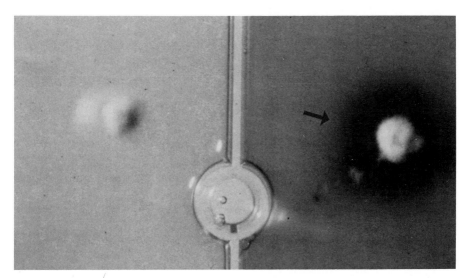

FIGURE 7–2. Early color change of dermatophyte test medium surrounding Trichophyton equinum *colony (arrow).*

Actinomycetales such as *Actinomyces, Nocardia,* and *Actinobacillus,* which are bacteria. Other terms such as *Madura* foot, maduromycosis, maduromycetoma should be discouraged.

Another term that creates confusion is phycomycosis. Zygomycosis is now the preferred name for this disease. The class Phycomycetes no longer formally exists. Some members of the class are members of the kingdom Prostista, and some are members of either the division Zygomycota or Chytridiomycota. Included in Zygomycota are the orders Mucorales and Entomophthorales. Diseases caused by members of these two orders are often called mucormycosis and entomophthoromycosis, respectively. For simplicity, the term zygomycosis is preferred.

Diseases and infective agents in this group include (1) sporotrichosis *(S. schenckii),* (2) phaeohyphomycosis *(Drechslera spicifera, D. rostrata, Peyronellaea glomerata, Phaeosclera dematioides),* (3) rhinosporidiosis *(Rhinosporidium seeberi),* (4) zygomycosis *(Basidiobolus haptosporus, Conidiobolus coronatus),* (5) eumycotic mycetoma *(Curvularia geniculata, P. boydii),* (6) prototheosis *(Prototheca wickerhamii),* and (7) pythiosis *(Pythium* spp).

Systemic Mycoses. These are fungal infections that usually involve internal organs but may involve the skin by hematogenous spread. When skin is involved, fistulas or nodules called infectious granulomas are produced. These infections are usually not contagious, since the animal inhales or contacts conidia from a specific ecologic niche. The systemic mycoses will be discussed only briefly here, and the reader is referred to texts on mycology and infectious diseases for additional information. Fungi that cause systemic mycoses are divided into primary and secondary pathogens.

Primary pathogens are organisms that are able to invade a normal healthy host. Clinical syndromes ranging from asymptomatic to severe infection may result from inhalation of conidia.

Primary Pathogen	Usual Habitat
B. dermatitidis	Unknown
C. immitis	Soil of semiarid areas
H. capsulatum	Soil contaminated by feces of birds, bats, and poultry
H. farciminosum	Unknown

Secondary pathogens may be found in animals or the environment but usually initiate infection only when the host's resistance is compromised.

Secondary Pathogen	Usual Habitat
Aspergillus spp.	Vegetation and soil
Candida spp.	Gastrointestinal and reproductive tracts
C. neoformans	Soil and pigeon droppings

Superficial Mycoses

Dermatophytosis

The dermatophytes that most frequently infect animals are *Microsporum* and *Trichophyton.* These genera can be divided into three groups on the basis of their natural habitat: geophilic, zoophilic, and anthropophilic. Geophilic dermatophytes, such as *M. gypseum, M. nanum,* and *T. (Keratinomyces) ajelloi,* normally inhabit the soil. Zoophilic dermatophytes, such as *M. canis* and *T. equinum,* have become adapted to animals and are only rarely isolated from soil. Anthropophilic dermatophytes, such as *M. audouinii,* have become adapted to humans and will not survive in the soil.

Although a large number of fungi have been reported to cause dermatophytosis in large animals (Table 7–1), the most commonly isolated are *T. equinum, T. mentagrophytes,* and *M. gypseum* (horse); *T. verrucosum* (cow, goat, and sheep); and *M. nanum* (pig).

The incidence of dermatophytosis and the fungi most commonly isolated vary with the climate and natural reservoirs. A higher incidence of dermatophytosis is observed in a hot, humid climate than in a cold, dry climate.

This text will discuss the five major dermatophytes of large animals. For identification of other fungi, the reader is referred to mycology texts in the reference list.[106, 141, 224, 324, 333]

MICROSPORUM GYPSEUM

M. gypseum infections have been reported in horses, cattle, sheep, goats, pigs, and humans.* Sporadic outbreaks appear to be due to the worldwide distribution of *M. gypseum* in soil. The organism is frequently isolated from soil and may be found as a contaminant of normal animal skin and hair. In animals, thick, well-circumscribed, tightly adherent gray to yellowish-brown crusts are typical clinical lesions.

*References 106, 175, 197, 224, 302, 324, 333, 352

TABLE 7-1. Fungi Reported to Cause Dematophytosis in Large Animals and Humans*

Fungus	Horse	Cow	Sheep	Goat	Pig	Human
Microsporum canis	+	+	+	+	+	+
M. cookei	+	+				+
M. equinum	+					+
M. gypseum	+	+	+	+	+	+
M. nanum		+			+	+
Trichophyton ajelloi	+	+	+			+
T. equinum	+	+				+
T. megnini		+				+
T. mentagrophytes	+	+	+	+	+	+
T. quinckeanum	+	+	+			+
T. rubrum	+	+	+		+	+
T. schoenleinii	+		+	+		+
T. terrestre	+	+				+
T. tonsurans	+				+	+
T. verrucosum	+	+	+	+	+	+
T. violaceum		+				+
Epidermophyton floccosum				+		+

*References:
  Horse: 13, 15, 40a, 41, 48, 53, 61, 62, 63, 74, 99, 114, 147, 159, 166, 176, 182, 206, 237, 283, 284, 290, 302, 306, 310, 331, 373, 379, 384, 385, 389, 396
  Cow: 2, 3, 10, 40a, 61, 88, 131, 132, 161, 175, 176a, 178, 202, 252, 289, 290, 325, 330, 349, 373, 381, 395a
  Sheep: 3, 40a, 61, 77, 128, 129, 175, 200, 207, 222, 336, 355, 364
  Goat: 8, 32, 43, 86, 131, 132, 175, 200, 287, 289, 293, 306, 364, 373, 380
  Pig: 21, 40a, 60, 61, 85, 89, 98, 118, 131, 175, 190, 197, 200, 211, 234, 281, 319, 338a, 373
  Human: 15, 28, 37, 38, 43, 52, 94, 104, 112, 113, 142, 169, 174, 176a, 183, 188, 209, 220–222, 256, 259, 269, 282, 290, 318, 324, 333, 338a, 339, 340, 346, 367, 378, 389, 390, 395a

Colony Morphology. On Sabouraud's dextrose agar, *M. gypseum* colonies are rapid-growing, with flat to granular texture and a buff to cinnamon-brown color. Sterile, white mycelia may develop in time. The reverse pigmentation is pale yellow to tan.

Microscopic Morphology. Echinulate, ellipsoid macroconidia contain up to six cells with relatively thin walls.

MICROSPORUM NANUM

M. nanum infections have been reported in swine, cattle, and humans. The fungus is worldwide in distribution and has been isolated from the soil.[16, 175, 224, 324, 333] Clinical lesions are usually characterized by a circular brownish appearance.

Colony Morphology. A thin-spreading colony with a more or less powdery dark-buff surface is produced. The reverse pigmentation is frequently reddish brown.

Microscopic Morphology. Characteristic rough-walled macroconidia are produced. They are egg-shaped and consist of only one to three cells. Microconidia are clavate.

TRICHOPHYTON EQUINUM

T. equinum infections have been reported in horses, cattle, and humans.* The fungus is worldwide in distribution and has been isolated from many fomites. Clinical lesions are usually characterized by a typical ringworm-like appearance or by follicular papules.

Colony Morphology. A flat colony with a white to cream-colored, powdery surface is produced. The center of the colony is frequently reddish. The reverse pigmentation is usually deep yellow. The most common American and European strains (*T. equinum* var. *equinum*) have a special nutritional requirement for niacin (nicotinic acid),[115, 175, 302, 324, 333] whereas the common Australian and New Zealand strains (*T. equinum* var. *autotrophicum*) do not.[175, 302, 324, 333, 366, 368] Because commercial fungal media such as DTM do not support the growth of *T. equinum* var. *equinum,* two drops of injectable vitamin B complex should be applied to the media.[36, 229]

Microscopic Morphology. Typically pyriform to spherical, stalked microconidia are seen along the hyphae. Less frequently, the microconidia are clustered with clavate macroconidia.

TRICHOPHYTON MENTAGROPHYTES

T. mentagrophytes infections have been reported in horses, cattle, swine, sheep, goats, and humans.† Sporadic outbreaks appear to be due to the worldwide distribution of *T. mentagrophytes* in soil. Wild animals, especially rodents, may serve as a reservoir for this fungus. It is commonly isolated from soil and may be found as a contaminant of normal animal skin and hair. Clinical lesions may be characterized by the typical ringworm-like appearance or highly inflammatory follicular papules and nodules.

Colony Morphology. The zoophilic form of *T. mentagrophytes* produces a flat colony with

---

*References 2, 72, 113, 115, 183, 282, 302, 324, 333, 366, 367, 376
†References 175, 210, 252, 302, 324, 333, 352, 354

a white to cream-colored, powdery surface. The reverse pigmentation is usually brown to tan but may be dark red.

Microscopic Morphology. The zoophilic form of *T. mentagrophytes* produces globose microconidia that may be arranged singly along the hyphae or in grapelike clusters. Macroconidia, if present, are cigar-shaped, with thin smooth walls. Some strains produce spiral hyphae, which may also be seen in other dermatophytes.

TRICHOPHYTON VERRUCOSUM

T. verrucosum infections have been reported in cattle, goats, sheep, horses, swine, and humans. The fungus is worldwide in distribution and has been isolated from soil, dung, and numerous fomites.* Clinical lesions are usually characterized by thick, well-demarcated, tightly adherent, grayish crusts.

Colony Morphology. Usually, a white, very slow-growing glabrous colony is produced that is heaped-up and button-like in appearance. Two variants also occur: a flat, yellow, glabrous colony (*T. verrucosum* var. *ochraceum*), and a flat, slightly downy gray-white colony (*T. verrucosum* var. *discoides*). All strains require thiamine, may require inositol, and many grow best at 37°C.[151, 175, 324, 333]

Microscopic Morphology. On Sabouraud's dextrose agar, tortuous hyphae with antler-like branching are seen. Tear-shaped microconidia and rat tail– or string bean–shaped macroconidia are characteristic.

CAUSE AND PATHOGENESIS

When dermatophytes contact the skin, the fungi (1) may be brushed off mechanically, (2) may not be able to establish residence because of inability to compete with normal flora, (3) may establish residence on the skin but not produce recognizable lesions (asymptomatic carrier state), or (4) may establish residence and cause disease.[175] Since dermatophytes do not invade living tissue, the only mechanism by which they may produce disease is by elaborating or excreting toxins (irritants) or allergens. These substances penetrate the living epidermis and enter the dermis, where blood vessels are capable of responding to the challenge of toxic or allergenic materials through an inflammatory reaction. Thus, dermatophytosis is often described as a type of biologic contact dermatitis.[175]

In addition to meeting the other challenges dermatophytes face to maintain their existence on the skin, their survival largely depends on *not* evoking a severe inflammatory reaction. Thus, through a long-term evolutionary process, dermatophytes have adapted to survive on the skin of a particular host and, under ideal parasitic conditions, elaborate minimal amounts of toxins or allergens. When zoophilic dermatophytes contact human skin, a violent eruption often ensues that may eliminate the fungi.

It has been shown that dermatophytes elaborate penicillin-like substances that result in the increased isolation of penicillin-resistant bacteria from affected skin.[33, 34] This could be important in the development of clinical antibiotic resistance and secondary pyodermas.

The invasion of hair by dermatophytes has been studied extensively.[158, 194, 195, 212, 311] Hair is always invaded in both ectothrix and endothrix infections. The endothrix fungi do not form masses of external conidia. Fungal elements deposited on the skin surface reach the follicle orifice in a couple of days and penetrate the hair shaft by working under the cuticle, lifting it away from the shaft, and growing downward. Fungal elements reach Adamson's fringe by the seventh to eighth day. Fungi do not penetrate the mitotic region of the hair, and when hair growth terminates, fungal growth ceases and the clinical infection resolves spontaneously. "Club," or dead telogen, hairs are resistant to infection. In humans, it has been shown that dermatophytes may be isolated in cultures from normal-looking skin up to 6 cm from the margins of the clinical lesions.[196]

Dermatophytosis is transmitted by direct and indirect contact. Contaminated objects (e.g., housing, fencing, grooming equipment, riding and working gear, and dung) are extremely important in the natural dissemination of the disease.* Fungal spores may remain viable under natural conditions for years.† The incubation period between exposure and clinical disease varies from one to six weeks.‡

---

*References 17, 65, 106, 150, 152, 211, 301, 302, 312, 352, 354

†References 17, 72, 88, 106, 152, 211, 231, 232, 301, 302, 352, 354

‡References 17, 58, 59, 88, 102, 118, 119, 150, 152, 175, 198, 199, 200, 229, 299, 302

---

*References 89, 152, 175, 302, 324, 326, 333, 354, 371

Dermatophytosis is common in cattle, horses, goats, and swine but is uncommon in sheep.* It may be seen in animals of any age but is most common in those younger than one year of age.† There are no breed or sex predilections. Although dermatophytosis is seen at all times of the year, it is especially common in fall and winter, particularly in confined animals.‡ Other authors have noticed frequent outbreaks of equine dermatophytosis during moist, warm weather, when there are large populations of stable flies and mosquitoes[298, 299, 302] and when horses are brought together for training and racing purposes.[154, 160, 302, 309, 376, 387]

The predisposing factors in dermatophytosis include age (young), immunity (prior exposure or immunosuppression), environment (contamination, crowding, high humidity, poor ventilation, or darkness), and poor condition (poor nutrition or debilitating diseases).§ Studies in cattle[292] and horses[298, 302, 344] have suggested that the increased susceptibility of the young is due not to age per se but to lack of previous exposure to the dermatophytes.

The immunology of dermatophytosis has been studied extensively in humans and laboratory rodents.[12, 171, 317] Cell-mediated immunity and the delayed-type hypersensitivity reaction appear to be the main sources of immunity to dermatophytes. Thus, individuals with reduced T-cell function, either drug- or disease-induced, are more susceptible to dermatophytosis than are normal individuals. In cattle, the ability to eliminate *T. verrucosum* infection and to resist reinfection with the same fungus correlated well with the ability to mount a gross and histologic delayed-type hypersensitivity reaction.[212, 213] Cattle that have recovered from experimental or natural *T. verrucosum* infections may be resistant to reinfection for up to one year or more after the resolution of primary lesions.‖ Horses having recovered from *T. equinum* or *M. gypseum* infections also showed enhanced resistance to reinfection.[298, 299, 302, 344]

Dermatophytosis is a self-limited disease in large animals.* The duration of clinical infection is one to four months. Reinfection is uncommon. With animals suffering from severe, chronic, or recurrent dermatophytosis, significant environmental (filth, moisture, or crowding) or immunosuppressive (underlying diseases or deficiencies) factors should be suspected.

CLINICAL FEATURES

The gross appearance of dermatophytosis (ringworm, tinea, girth itch) is quite variable. The classic ringworm-like lesion is characterized by an annular area of alopecia, stubbled hairs, and variable amounts of scaling, crusting, and dermatitis. However, this type of gross lesion is far from diagnostic and may be produced by other disorders, including staphylococcal dermatitis, dermatophilosis, demodicosis, and pemphigus foliaceus. In addition, the alopecia may be patchy, and either scaling or crusting may predominate in the absence of much alopecia. Folliculitis and furunculosis are also common manifestations of dermatophytosis. In such cases, the predominant lesions may include varying combinations of papules, nodules, ulcers, and sinuses. A kerion is a localized, severe inflammatory lesion that is nodular and boggy and oozes pus.

In cattle, *T. verrucosum* (*T. album, T. discoides, T. faviforme*) is the most common cause of dermatophytosis, with *T. mentagrophytes, T. equinum, M. gypseum, M. nanum, M. canis,* and others being less commonly isolated (Table 7–1).† Lesions are most commonly seen on the head, neck, and pelvis and vary from discrete circular areas of alopecia to severe scaling, crusting, suppuration, and ulceration (Fig. 7–3). Pruritus and pain are variable. In two large studies of trichophytosis in cattle,[270, 291] the site of lesions was found to be sex- and age-dependent. Characteristic locations of lesions were the periocular region for calves, the thorax and limbs for cows and heifers, and the dewlap and intermaxillary space for bulls. It was postulated that these site differences were basically associated with behavioral differences between the different

---

*References 17, 59, 77, 85, 106, 175, 200, 216, 222, 229, 302, 312, 352, 354

†References 9, 17, 58, 66, 85, 102, 106, 126, 152, 177, 200, 229, 289, 302, 306, 312, 356

‡References 17, 66, 77, 88, 90, 102, 106, 118, 120, 126, 133, 140, 177, 229, 231, 232, 289, 302, 306, 356, 374

§References 17, 85, 106, 126, 142, 152, 177, 200, 212, 213, 229, 289, 302, 326, 352–354

‖References 150, 186, 188, 212, 213, 356, 393

*References 9, 17, 19, 58–60, 77, 85, 88, 102, 106, 152, 175, 211, 212, 216, 222, 229, 232, 302, 352, 354, 356, 374

†References 9, 15, 17, 106, 132, 152, 161, 175, 177, 200, 275, 306, 312, 326

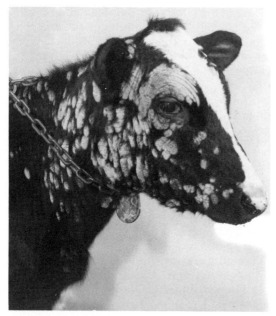

FIGURE 7–3. Bovine dermatophytosis. Multiple thick crusts associated with Trichophyton verrucosum infection.

sex and age groups. In herd outbreaks of dermatophytosis due to *T. mentagrophytes* and *T. equinum* in adult cattle, lesions consisted of generalized areas of circular alopecia with minimal scaling or crusting.[202, 252] In addition, combined infections with *T. verrucosum* and *T. mentagrophytes*,[3, 131] or *T. verrucosum* and *T. violaceum*,[131] have been recorded.

In horses, *T. equinum (T. equinum* var. *equinum* or *T. equinum* var. *autotrophicum)* is the most common cause of dermatophytosis, with *T. mentagrophytes*, *M. gypseum*, *M. canis*, *T. verrucosum*, and others being less commonly isolated.* Lesions are most commonly seen on the saddle and tack areas (thorax, head, and shoulders) and vary from discrete circular areas of alopecia to severe scaling, crusting, suppuration, and ulceration (Figs. 7–4 and 7–5; see Plate 4). The primary skin lesion is a follicular papule, and the initial clinical finding may be erect hairs over a 2 to 3 mm papule. Occasionally, an urticarial eruption will precede the more typical follicular dermatosis by 24 to 72 hours.[354, 371] Lesions may be limited to the posterior pastern region (scratches, mud fever or grease heel–like) and may wax and wane (analogous to athlete's foot in humans) with stress, local irritation, mois-

ture, and unsanitary conditions.[153, 229, 260, 302, 354, 371] Dermatophytosis may also manifest as multifocal to generalized scaling (seborrhea sicca) without significant alopecia.[354, 371] Pruritus and pain vary from severe to absent. Combined infections with *T. equinum* and *T. mentagrophytes* have been recorded.[41]

In goats, *T. verrucosum* is the most common cause of dermatophytosis, with *T. mentagrophytes*, *M. canis*, and others being less commonly isolated.* Lesions are most commonly seen on the face, pinnae, neck, and limbs and include circular to uneven to diffuse areas of alopecia, scaling, erythema, and yellowish-gray crusts (Fig. 7–6). Pruritus and pain are rare. An outbreak of presumptive tinea versicolor was reported in a herd of milking goats.[40] The lesions consisted of annular areas of hypo- or hyperpigmentation with scaling margins on the teats and udder. The causal fungus of tinea versicolor in humans (*Malassezia furfur*, or *Pityrosporum orbiculare*) could not be cultured.

In sheep, *T. verrucosum* is the most common cause of dermatophytosis, with *T. mentagro-*

---

*References 32, 68, 175, 192, 200, 293, 352, 380

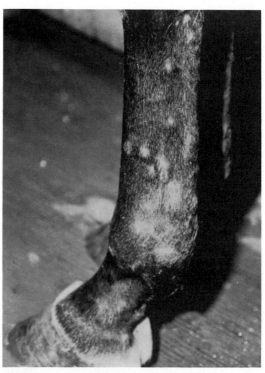

FIGURE 7–4. Crusted papules on the leg of a horse resulting from Trichophyton equinum.

---

*References 13, 14, 40, 41, 48, 61, 62, 147, 159–161, 200, 206, 229, 260, 283, 284, 302, 354, 384, 385, 396

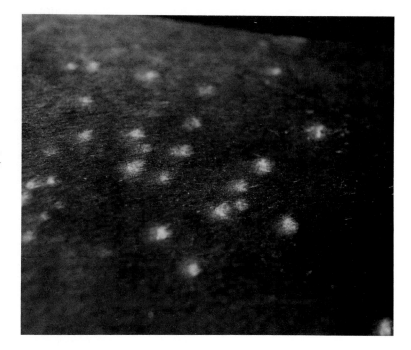

FIGURE 7–5. Annular areas of alopecia and crusting over thorax of a horse due to Trichophyton mentagrophytes.

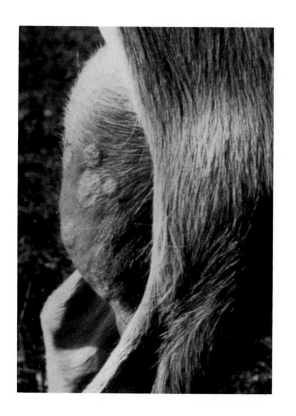

FIGURE 7–6. Caprine dermatophytosis. Multiple annular crusts on the udder, associated with Trichophyton verrucosum infection.

phytes, M. gypseum, M. canis, and others being less commonly isolated.* Lesions are most commonly seen on the face, neck, thorax, and back and are characterized by circular areas of alopecia and thick grayish crusts. Combined infections with *T. verrucosum* and *T. rubrum* have been reported.[3]

In swine, *M. nanum* is the most common cause of dermatophytosis, with *T. mentagrophytes, T. verrucosum, M. canis,* and others being less commonly isolated.† Lesions may be seen anywhere but are especially common behind the ears and on the trunk (Fig. 7–7). They are characterized by annular areas of red to brown discoloration of the skin and superficial, dry, brown to orange crusts. Alopecia and pruritus are rare. Chronic infections may be established behind the ears of adult swine.

Dermatophytosis usually has no effect on animal growth rate or other measures of productivity, unless the eyes or muzzle are severely affected, or secondary bacterial infection occurs.‡ Economic losses may arise because of hide damage or the animal's inability to work or show.

---

*References 3, 77, 90, 128, 129, 175, 185, 187, 200, 207, 216, 222, 304, 306, 336, 355
†References 21, 58–60, 61a, 73, 78, 84, 85, 106, 118, 120, 175, 190, 211, 219, 257, 281, 369
‡References 15, 17, 85, 106, 203, 211, 229, 302

Dermatophytosis in all large animal species is a significant public health hazard.* Humans may acquire infections via direct or indirect contact, and the animal dermatophytes often produce severe inflammatory reactions in human skin (Fig. 7–8). Needless to say, great care should be exercised when handling animals suspected of having dermatophytosis.

DIAGNOSIS

The major differential diagnoses include staphylococcal dermatitis, dermatophilosis, demodicosis, zinc-responsive dermatosis (ruminants), and pemphigus foliaceus (horses and goats). Definitive diagnosis is based on microscopic examination of hairs and surface debris, fungal culture, and skin biopsy.

Histopathology. The histopathologic features of dermatophytosis are as variable as the clinical lesions. There is no diagnostic histopathologic appearance characteristic of dermatophytosis. The most common histopathologic patterns observed in dermatophytosis are (1) perifolliculitis, folliculitis, and furunculosis (Fig. 7–9), (2) superficial perivascular derma-

---

*References 28, 37, 38, 52, 77, 94, 104, 112, 113, 142, 169, 174, 175, 187, 188, 209, 220, 221, 256, 261, 269, 306, 318, 324, 339, 340, 346, 352

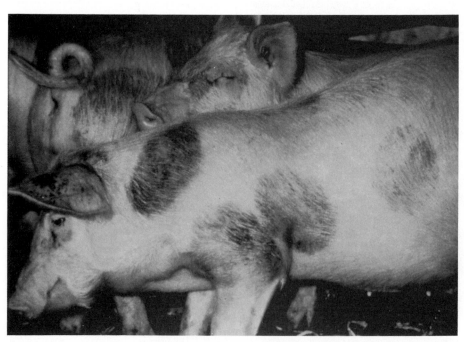

FIGURE 7–7. Porcine dermatophytosis. Large annular areas of dermatitis from Microsporum nanum. *(Courtesy R. D. Cameron.)*

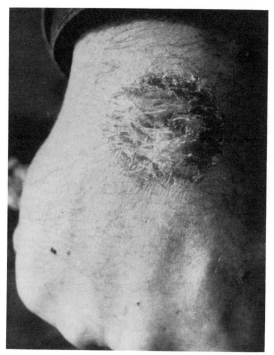

FIGURE 7–8. Dermatophytosis on the hand after contact with a calf having Tricophyton verrucosum *infection.*

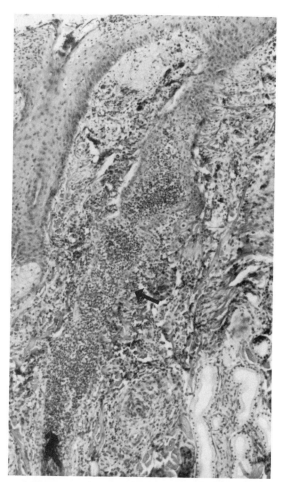

FIGURE 7–9. Equine dermatophytosis. Suppurative folliculitis (arrow).

titis (spongiotic or hyperplastic) with orthokeratotic or parakeratotic hyperkeratosis of the epidermis and hair follicles, and (3) intraepidermal vesicular (spongiotic) or pustular dermatitis. A rare histopathologic pattern is that of nodular or diffuse dermatitis (suppurative, pyogranulomatous, or granulomatous), with the fungus present as grains and hyphae within the dermis or subcutis or both. Such unusual tissue reactions to dermatophytes are often referred to as Majocchi's granuloma or pseudomycetoma.[332] Septate fungal hyphae and spherical to oval conidia may be present within surface keratin and crust, within the hair follicles, or in and around the hairs. The number of fungal elements present is usually inversely proportional to the severity of the inflammatory response. Dermatophytes are often visible in sections stained with H&E (Fig. 7–10) but are more readily detected with periodic acid–Schiff (PAS), Gomori's methenamine silver (GMS), or acid orcein–Giemsa (AOG) stains (Fig. 7–11).

CLINICAL MANAGEMENT

Dermatophytosis in all species is usually a self-limiting disease, with spontaneous remission occurring within one to four months.[*] Because of this, a veritable plethora of therapeutic agents have been espoused as ringworm cures.[†] Controlled studies documenting the efficacy of this "sea of antifungal agents" in the dermatophytoses of large animals are virtually nonexistent.

Because of the current lack of efficacious antifungal agents that are economically feasible and practical in terms of administration, the goal of therapy in dermatophytosis, in most instances, is to reduce contagion to the environment, other animals, and humans while

*References 9, 17, 40a, 48, 59, 77, 85, 88, 102, 118, 119, 138, 150, 152, 175, 177, 216, 222, 229, 231, 260, 302, 312, 354, 356, 371
†References 8, 9, 14, 15, 17, 26, 40a, 48, 59, 83, 85, 122, 130, 131, 152, 156, 161, 162, 167, 175, 184, 200, 203, 204, 204a, 211, 233, 251, 260, 264, 271, 272, 286, 295, 296, 302, 304, 374, 382, 391, 394, 396

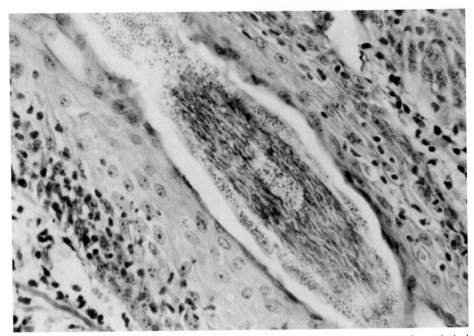

FIGURE 7–10. Equine dermatophytosis (arrow). Perifolliculitis and arthroconidia surrounding a hair shaft.

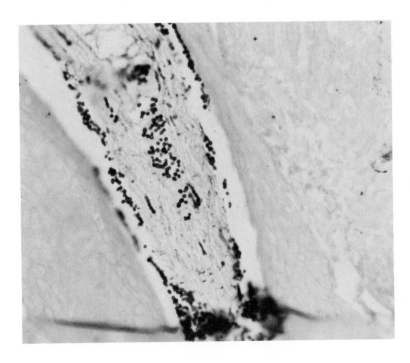

FIGURE 7–11. Equine dermatophytosis. Arthroconidia associated with a hair shaft (GMS stain).

waiting for spontaneous regression. Topical antifungal agents are the most suitable medicaments in such cases. The most commonly used topical antifungal agents are 2 to 5 percent lime sulfur (Orthorix, Lime Sulfur), 3 percent captan (Orthocide), iodophors (Weladol, Betadine), and 0.5 percent sodium hypochlorite (Clorox).* These agents should be applied as total body sprays and dips for five consecutive days and repeated once weekly thereafter until clinical cure is apparent, when feasible. For cattle, spray applications of 1.5 gallons per animal of 400 to 450 pounds pressure have been recommended.[17, 26, 152]

Captan is a heterocyclic nitrogen compound. It is fungicidal, possibly via inhibition of synthesis of certain amino compounds or inactivation of coenzyme A and other thiols.[253, 312, 351] It is *not* approved for use on food animals. In addition, it is a potent contact sensitizer in humans. Thus, care should be taken to avoid contact with the skin of humans.

Lime sulfur is a potent fungicidal agent, with pentathionic acid thought to be the active ingredient.[351] Its shortcomings include a rotten egg odor and a tendency to stain and discolor jewelry. It can be drying and irritating to the skin.

Iodophors are strong fungicidal agents, with elemental iodine being the active ingredient.[351] They tend to be more expensive than the other commonly used topical antifungal agents. In addition, iodophors are occasionally irritating to the skin of horses and goats.

Sodium hypochlorite is a potent fungicidal halogenated agent, with hypochlorous acid thought to be the active ingredient.[351] It is economical and nonirritating. Prolonged or repeated exposure may cause pitting and rusting of metals, including stainless steel.[20]

Topical solutions of 1 to 5 percent thiabendazole, a fungistatic imidazole,[39, 337, 338] were reported to be beneficial in bovine and equine trichophytoses.[110, 184, 203, 260, 267, 294] In cattle, the solutions were applied to lesions every three days, with healing occurring much faster than in untreated controls. Natamycin (pimaricin), a broad-spectrum fungicidal agent,[321] was applied topically as a 100 ppm aqueous solution by spray (about 1 L/cow) twice, at three- to four-day intervals, to hundreds of cattle with trichophytosis.[125, 276, 277, 278, 350, 370] More than 90

percent of the animals were reported to be cured within 12 weeks after the second spray application. Natamycin was also reported to be beneficial in equine dermatophytosis.[260, 279]

Whichever topical antifungal agent is used, it is important to (1) treat *all* in-contact animals (clinically affected or normal), (2) treat the environment and fomites, and (3) dispose of infectious materials (crusts, hair, bedding, and so on) when feasible.* Recommended products for treatment of the environment and fomites include 5 percent lime sulfur, 5 percent sodium hypochlorite, 5 percent formalin, 3 percent captan, and 3 percent cresol.

Systemic treatment for dermatophytosis in large animals is controversial. Again, most of the confusion and controversy surrounding the efficacy of systemic antifungal agents in large animals stems from the frequently ignored high incidence of spontaneous recovery.

Oral thiabendazole (50 to 100 mg/kg) has been used in cattle and goats with no benefit.[39, 203, 267, 314] Intravenous sodium iodide has been long touted as a beneficial medicament for severe dermatophytosis in cattle and horses.† Although this information is purely anecdotal, the author has had good results with two intravenous injections of 10 to 20 percent sodium iodide (1 gm/14 kg) at weekly intervals in severely affected calves and adult cattle. Systemic iodides may cause abortion and should not be used in pregnant animals.

The oral administration of griseofulvin has been frequently recommended for the treatment of dermatophytosis in large animals.‡ The results of such therapy have often been contradictory and anecdotal with treatment being conducted under poorly controlled circumstances. The most convincing data have been accumulated for cattle. Doses varying from 7.5 to 60 mg/kg, administered orally (by drenching, or mixed in feed or milk) for 7 to 20 days, were shown to produce marked improvement or complete healing within one to seven weeks in treated cattle; untreated controls remained infected.§ In addition, griseofulvin administered orally at 60 mg/kg/day for five weeks was reported to prevent the experimental production of *T. verrucosum* infection in calves.[210]

---

*References 17, 18, 26, 40a, 58, 59, 77, 131, 152, 175, 200, 211, 253, 260, 264, 272, 295, 296, 302, 312, 353, 354, 371

*References 17, 19, 40a, 85, 152, 211, 229, 260, 276, 301, 302, 312, 354, 371
†References 17, 18, 152, 156, 260, 286, 295, 302
‡References 17, 40a, 148, 149, 211, 222, 229, 260, 302, 312, 327
§References 19, 69, 87, 148, 189, 210, 251, 305, 388

In swine, recommended dosages for oral griseofulvin are approximately 1 gm/100 kg/day for 7 to 40 days.[40a, 58, 60, 190] In horses, recommendations for oral griseofulvin vary from 5 to 10 mg/kg/day for seven to ten days or longer[145, 149, 229, 302, 354, 384] to 6.25 to 17.5 gm/horse by tube once a week (repeated once or twice).[229, 260, 296, 354] However, the actual minimum dose of griseofulvin effective in horses is apparently not known, and many authors have found no evidence that this product is efficacious.[154, 353, 354, 371] Sheep and goats have been treated with 10 mg/kg orally.[327]

The current expense associated with the therapeutic use of griseofulvin in large animals, when considered in light of the high incidence of spontaneous recovery from dermatophytosis, makes the routine use of this drug impractical and unnecessary. Griseofulvin appears to be free of side effects in large animals, although it is a known teratogen when administered to pregnant cats and dogs.[258, 302] However, it is *not* licensed for use in food animals. At present, it appears that griseofulvin will probably be used only in valuable show stock or breeders on an individual basis.

Adjunctive therapeutic measures in the treatment of dermatophytosis include correcting predilecting or aggravating factors.* Such measures encompass assurance of good nutrition, good general health, and a clean, dry, sunny environment, when feasible. There is no indication that vitamin and mineral preparations are of any benefit in most cases.†

A modified live (apathogenic) *T. verrucosum* vaccine has been used successfully to prevent bovine trichophytosis in the Soviet Union and Scandinavia.‡ In two studies,[1, 125a] 400,000 cattle were vaccinated and evaluated. It was found that intramuscular injections of calves at one and three weeks of age conferred nearly 100 percent protection. Common side effects of vaccination were a localized noninfective lesion at the site of injection that healed in two weeks and a slight increase in rectal temperature (0.2 to 0.7°C) that occurred at three to ten days after injection and lasted one to two days. Other side effects were rare: A few calves developed transient restlessness, dyspnea, and diarrhea, and a few calves developed fatal anaphylactoid reactions after the first or second vaccination. Immunity lasted at least four to five years. However, the vaccine was not protective against other dermatophytes, as epizootics of *M. canis* and *T. equinum* occurred in vaccinated herds.[125a]

Candidiasis

Candidiasis is a rare infection of the skin with candidal yeasts.

CAUSE AND PATHOGENESIS

Candida species are yeasts characterized by the formation of blastoconidia, pseudohyphae, and, occasionally, true hyphae in culture and in tissue.[215, 313, 333] They are considered to be part of the normal microflora of the intestinal and reproductive tracts. With lowered host resistance caused by prolonged maceration, antibiotics, glucocorticoids, or immunosuppressive therapy or by inherent or disease-induced immunologic defects, serious local or systemic infections may be produced by *Candida* species.

CLINICAL FEATURES

Cutaneous infection with *Candida* species (moniliasis, thrush) is rarely diagnosed in large animals. *C. albicans* was reported as the cause of a moist, exudative dermatitis of the distal limbs, medial thighs, and abdomen in 40 percent of 450 garbage-fed feeder pigs. The constant maceration from their lying in garbage was thought to be the initiating factor.[329] The surface exudate was gray, and the underlying skin was lichenified and bluish. *C. albicans* was isolated in culture and visualized in skin biopsy specimens. Dry housing resulted in healing in a few weeks.

C. guilliermondii was reported as the cause of a generalized nodular skin disease with mastitis and pyrexia in an adult mare.[268] The cutaneous nodules were firm and tender. Skin biopsy revealed a granulomatous dermatitis containing budding yeasts. *C. guilliermondii* was isolated in pure culture. Oral candidiasis was reported in eight immunodeficient foals.[223]

A generalized exfoliative dermatitis in protein-deficient goats was associated with a yeast infection resembling candidiasis.[352] The goats had a fairly symmetric nonpruritic dermatitis characterized by alopecia, scaling, crusting, greasiness, and lichenification (Figs. 7–12 and

---

*References 17, 40a, 152, 198, 200, 201, 229, 260, 302, 352–354, 371

†References 17, 18, 260, 295, 302, 354, 371

‡References 1, 44, 101, 125a, 137, 214, 263, 307, 323, 340a, 386a, 392

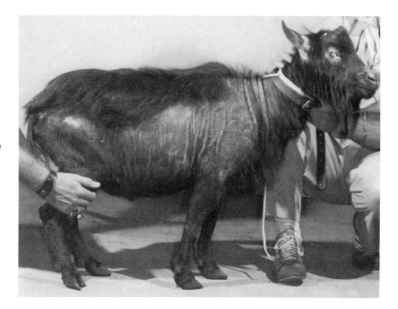

FIGURE 7–12. Yeast dermatitis in a goat. Extensive alopecia.

7–13). Numerous budding yeasts and pseudo-hyphae were seen in direct smears and skin biopsy specimens, but cultures were negative.

DIAGNOSIS

Diagnosis of candidiasis is based on direct smears, cultures, and skin biopsies. Direct smears stained with new methylene blue or Diff-Quik reveal blastoconidia (budding cells) and pseudohyphae. Skin biopsy may reveal superficial perivascular dermatitis or folliculitis, or both (Fig. 7–14). The organisms may be seen in histologic sections as blastoconidia (ovoid cells that are often budding and range from 3 to 5 μm in diameter), as pseudohyphae, and, occasionally, as hyphae. *Candida* species are easily visualized in sections stained with H

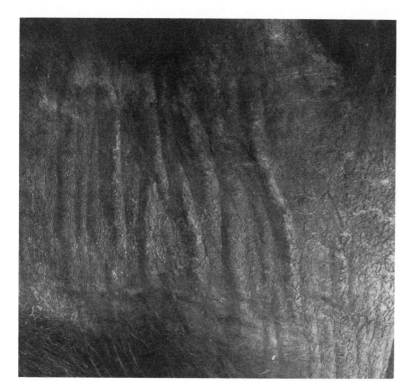

FIGURE 7–13. Yeast dermatitis in a goat. Alopecia, scaling, crusting, and lichenification.

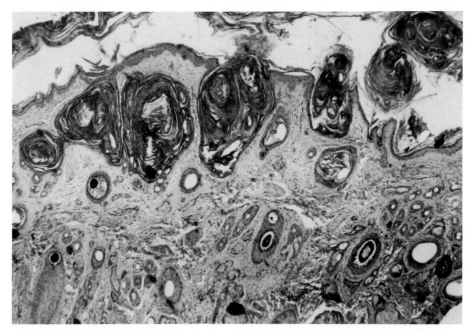

FIGURE 7–14. Yeast dermatitis in a goat. Marked hyperkeratosis of hair follicles and surface epithelium.

& E but may be highlighted with AOG, PAS, or GMS stains (Fig. 7–15). *Candida* organisms must be demonstrated invading tissue to confirm the diagnosis. Cultures should be performed in Sabouraud's dextrose agar and should be incubated in 30°C. *Candida* species appear as soft, cream-colored colonies.

CLINICAL MANAGEMENT

In the treatment of candidiasis, correction of predisposing causes is fundamental. Correction of immunodeficiency states or avoidance of immunosuppressive drugs may be most helpful. Excessive moisture must be avoided.

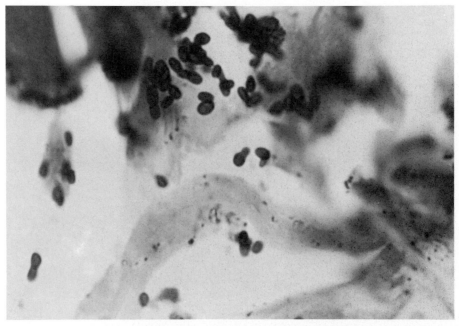

FIGURE 7–15. Yeast dermatitis in a goat. Budding yeasts and pseudohyphae formation in hair follicle (PAS stain).

In humans and small animals, topical therapy with nystatin (Mycostatin), miconazole (Conofite), clotrimazole (Lotrimin), potassium permanganate (1:3000 in water), or gentian violet (1:10,000 in 10 percent alcohol) is often effective in mild cases. Severe cases are usually managed with oral ketoconazole or intravenous amphotericin B. The benefits of such therapies in large animals are not known.

Piedra

Piedra is a rare fungal infection confined to hair shafts and resulting in the formation of nodules.

CAUSE AND PATHOGENESIS

There are two varieties of piedra, black and white, caused by *Piedraia hortae* and *Trichosporon beigelii* (*T. cutaneum*), respectively.[180, 200] The diseases tend to be most common in temperate and tropical areas of the world. The fungi have been isolated from a variety of natural substrates (e.g., soil and vegetation). These fungi invade beneath the hair cuticle, proliferate, and break out to surround the hair shaft. Nodules (black or white) are thus formed on the hair shaft; they are composed of tightly packed septate hyphae held together by a cement-like substance.

CLINICAL FEATURES

White piedra (*T. beigelii*) has been reported in horses.[96, 200, 260] Only the long hairs of the mane, tail, and forelock were affected. The hairs were characterized by the presence of whitish nodules or thickenings along the shafts. Affected hairs were often split or broken off.

DIAGNOSIS

The differential diagnosis of piedra includes trichorrhexis nodosa. Definitive diagnosis is based on microscopic examination of affected hair shafts and fungal culture. Microscopic examination reveals a mass of closely packed, branching, septate hyphae (2 to 4 μm in diameter), held together by a cement-like substance, surrounding the hair shaft. *T. beigelii* grows rapidly on Sabouraud's dextrose agar and is characterized by a creamy and wrinkled surface, which later becomes deeply furrowed and folded.

CLINICAL MANAGEMENT

Clipping the hair effects a cure. To prevent recurrence, antifungal preparations such as iodophors may be applied topically after clipping.

Subcutaneous Mycoses

Mycetoma

Mycetomas (fungal tumors) are chronic subcutaneous infections characterized by tumefaction, draining tracts (sinuses and fistulae), and tissue granules (grains).

CAUSE AND PATHOGENESIS

Actinomycotic mycetomas are caused by bacteria of the Actinomycetales (see Chapter 6, discussion on actinomycosis). Eumycotic mycetomas are caused by fungi that normally inhabit soil and vegetation and gain entrance to animal tissues by traumatic implantation.[64, 258, 333] *Curvularia geniculata* and *Pseudoallescheria boydii* have been isolated from mycetomas in the horse. *P. boydii* is the perfect stage of *Monosporium apiospermum* and is the currently accepted name for *Allescheria boydii* or *Petriellidium boydii*. Granules from *C. geniculata* mycetomas are brown to black, whereas those from *P. boydii* mycetomas are white to yellow.

CLINICAL FEATURES

Black-grain mycetomas due to *C. geniculata* have been reported in horses (Fig. 7–17).[42, 238] Two horses had ulcerated nodules localized to the external nares[238] and commissure of the lips,[238] respectively. Two others had a large subcutaneous tumor on the ventral thorax[42] and multiple black papillomatous growths over the neck, shoulders, and proximal front limbs,[42] respectively.

White-grain mycetoma due to *P. boydii* was reported on the tail of a horse.[348]

DIAGNOSIS

Diagnosis is based on history, physical examination, skin biopsy, and culture.

Skin biopsy reveals diffuse or nodular dermatitis (suppurative, pyogranulomatous, or granulomatous). Fungal elements present as a granule, or grain, within the tissues (Fig.

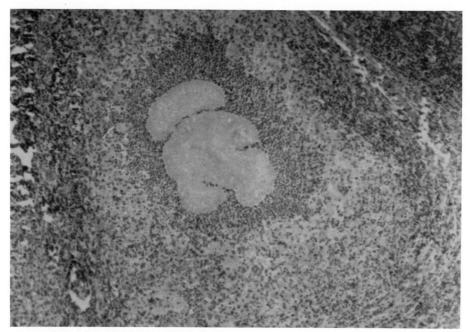

FIGURE 7–16. Equine mycetoma due to Pseudoallescheria boydii. *Tissue grain surrounded by pyogranuloma.*

7–16). These granules consist of septate branching hyphae, vesicles, and a cementing matrix and may be round, horseshoe-shaped, or scroll-like in appearance. The fungal elements may be pigmented or nonpigmented. Hyphae are often visualized in sections stained with H & E but are highlighted by AOG, PAS, GMS, and Gridley's stains.

The exudate or granules should be cultured on Sabouraud's dextrose agar without cycloheximide. *C. geniculata* grows rapidly with a colony surface changing from tannish brown to gray then to black. The reverse pigmentation is brown at first, changing to black with concentric circles. Microscopically, there are numerous tan to brown conidia, which are ellipsoid and contain three to four cross walls. *P. boydii* grows rapidly and has a colony surface changing from cottony white to smoky gray. The reverse pigmentation is colorless at first, then changes to gray. Microscopically, there are numerous light-brown, unicellular, oval to pyriform conidia.

CLINICAL MANAGEMENT

In humans and small animals, surgical excision and amputation are the only commonly successful therapeutic measures.

Phaeohyphomycosis

Phaeohyphomycosis is a chronic subcutaneous and systemic infection caused by dematiaceous (dark, pigmented) fungi. This disease differs from mycetomas in that the fungus in tissues is not organized into granules but is present as septate hyphae.

CAUSE AND PATHOGENESIS

The dematiaceous fungi are soil and vegetation inhabitants that gain access to animal tissues by traumatic implantation.[64] *D. spicifera* and *Hormodendrum* species have been isolated from phaeohyphomycosis in horses, *D. rostrata* and *Phaeosclera dematioides* in cattle, and *Peyronellaea glomerata* in goats.

CLINICAL FEATURES

D. spicifera was isolated from cutaneous lesions in a horse.[179] The lesions were scattered over the body and were characterized as black, denuded plaques studded with pustules and papules. *Hormodendrum* was isolated from multiple nodules on the ventral neck and thorax of a horse.[358] Other cases of equine phaeohyphomycosis were misdiagnosed as eumycotic (maduromycotic) mycetomas due to

Helminthosporium (Brachycladium) speciferum.[179] Two of these horses had multiple generalized cutaneous nodules,[46, 143] and three others had lesions restricted to the rump.[347] thorax,[54] and foot.[45]

D. rostrata was isolated in culture and was demonstrated histologically in tissues from a cow with multiple ulcerated, oozing nodules in the skin over the rump and thighs and in the nasal mucosa.[320] The cow was also dyspneic and cachectic. Phaeohyphomycosis probably due to *D. spicifera* (reported as *H. speciferum*) was reported in a cow with multiple cutaneous nodules on the pinnae, tail, vulva, and thighs.[303] The cow also exhibited nasal stertor and epistaxis in association with phaeohyphomycotic nodules in the nasal mucosa. *D. rostrata* and *D. dematioides* were isolated from nasal granulomas in cattle.[225, 226]

Peyronellaea glomerata was isolated from hyperkeratotic skin lesions on the pinnae of wild goats in Scotland and England.[82] Skin biopsy revealed orthokeratotic and parakeratotic hyperkeratosis, epidermal hyperplasia, intra- and intercellular epidermal edema, neutrophilic exocytosis, and congestion of dermal blood vessels and lymphatics. Brown septate hyphae were present in the surface keratin and adjacent to congested dermal vessels.

DIAGNOSIS

Diagnosis is based on history, physical examination, skin biospy, and culture.

Histologically, phaeohyphomycosis is characterized by diffuse or nodular dermatitis (suppurative, pyogranulomatous, or granulomatous). Fungal elements are present as pigmented, septate hyphae, with occasional pigmented vesicles (Fig. 7–17). The organisms are best visualized with H & E stain to determine their diagnostic dematiacious nature. The Splendore-Hoeppli phenomenon may be seen.

Exudates or tissues are cultured on Sabouraud's dextrose agar, *without* cycloheximide or antibiotics, at 30°C or room temperature. *D. spicifera* grows rapidly, and the colony surface color changes from off-white to brownish gray to blackish brown. The surface is flat and velvety, and the reverse pigmentation is black. Microscopic examination of the colony reveals dematiacious hyphae. The light to dark-brown conidiophores are solitary or grouped, flexuose, geniculate, 4 to 9 μm in width, and up to 300 μm in length. Conidia are abundant, straight and oblong, smooth-walled, constantly pseudoseptate, and 30 to 40 μm by 9 to 14 μm.

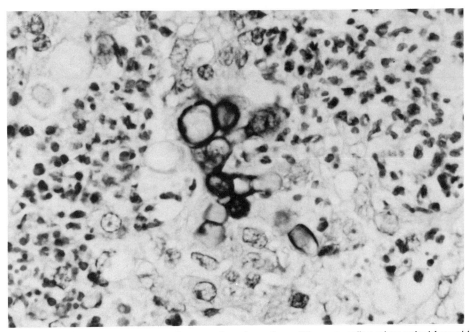

FIGURE 7–17. Equine phaeohyphomycosis. Pyogranulomatous dermatitis surrounding pigmented fungal hyphae.

CLINICAL MANAGEMENT

In humans and small animals, surgical excision, amphotericin B, 5-fluorocytosine, ketoconazole, and local hyperthermia have all had variable results in the treatment of phaeohyphomycosis.[258] No such treatments have been reported in large animals.

Sporotrichosis

Sporotrichosis is a chronic cutaneolymphatic, cutaneous, or systemic infection caused by *Sporothrix schenckii*.

CAUSE AND PATHOGENESIS

Sporothrix schenckii, a dimorphic fungus, is a soil and vegetation inhabitant.[64, 175, 255] It gains entrance to its host by wound contamination, especially in puncture wounds from thorns, wood slivers, or bites. Its geographic distribution is universal, but *S. schenckii* is most common along the coastal regions and river valleys of the southern United States or in countries with similar climates.

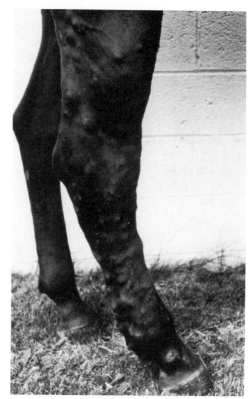

FIGURE 7–18. Equine sporotrichosis. Multiple nodules and draining tracts on hind leg.

CLINICAL FEATURES

Sporotrichosis has been most frequently reported in the horse.* In this species, the cutaneolymphatic form is the most common. After inoculation into the skin, a primary lesion occurs on an exposed part of the body, usually a limb and less commonly a part of the upper body, such as the shoulder, hip, or perineal region. Progressively, hard subcutaneous nodules develop along the lymphatics draining the region (Figs. 7–18 and 7–19). The lymphatics may become corded, and the large nodules may abscess, ulcerate, and discharge a small amount of thick, brown-red pus or serosanguineous fluid. Regional lymph nodes are usually not involved. Occasionally, the primary cutaneous form is seen with no lymphatic involvement.

Humans are also susceptible to sporotrichosis.[258, 333] Cutaneolymphatic and primary cutaneous infections are most commonly reported. Thus, caution is in order when handling infected animals and discharges.

---

*References 36, 40a, 80, 100, 116, 172, 175, 193, 200, 227, 229, 255, 286, 386

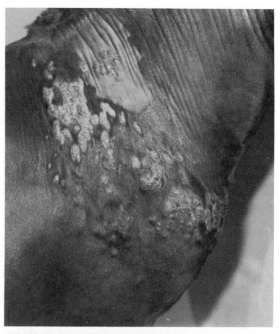

FIGURE 7–19. Equine sporotrichosis. Multiple nodules and crusted plaques over shoulder.

DIAGNOSIS

Differential diagnosis includes various bacterial and fungal granulomatous disorders. Diagnosis is based on history, physical examination, skin biopsy, and culture. Skin biopsy is characterized early by hyperplastic perivascular dermatitis and later by diffuse or nodular dermatitis (suppurative, pyogranulomatous, or granulomatous) (Fig. 7–20). Intraepidermal microabscesses and pseudocarcinomatous epidermal hyperplasia may be seen. *S. schenckii* is present as round to oval cells producing buds that range from 3 to 6 μm in diameter (Fig. 7–21). The classic "cigar bodies" (4 to 8 μm in length, 1 to 2 μm in diameter) are less commonly observed. *S. schenckii* is often impossible to find in histologic sections, even with special stains. Asteroid bodies that are the result of antigen-antibody complexes formed from the fungal cell wall may be seen. However, this host-parasite interaction is not unique to sporotrichosis.

Direct culture from exudate or tissues is reliable, and organisms grow readily on Sabouraud's dextrose agar at 30°C. *S. schenckii* is a dimorphic fungus, growing as a yeast in tissues and on medium at 37°C but as a mold on Sabouraud's dextrose agar at 25 to 30°C. The colony is white initially, changing to gray, and finally black with a white periphery.

Mouse inoculation, fluorescent antibody techniques, and indirect immunoperoxidase staining methods have also been helpful in diagnosis but require special equipment.

CLINICAL MANAGEMENT

In humans and small animals, the cutaneous and cutaneolymphatic forms of sporotrichosis respond well to oral doses of inorganic iodides,[258] In addition, local hyperthermia (e.g., hot packs) applied several times daily may be beneficial adjunctive therapy.[258] The disseminated form of sporotrichosis does not usually respond to iodide therapy, but good results have been achieved with intravenous doses of amphotericin B.

In horses, the cutaneous and cutaneolymphatic forms of sporotrichosis respond well to iodide therapy.[200, 227, 229, 255, 260, 286] The inorganic iodides, sodium or potassium iodide, or the organic iodide, ethylenediamine dihydroiodide (EDDI), can be utilized.

Sodium iodide is often used as a 20 percent solution and administered intravenously (20 gm, or 40 mg/kg) for two to five days, and then orally once daily until cured.* Potassium

---

*References 80, 100, 193, 200, 227, 229, 255, 260, 286

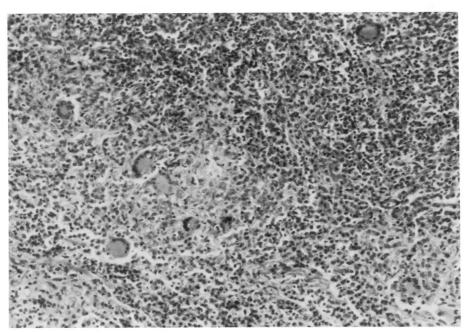

FIGURE 7–20. Equine sporotrichosis. Granulomatous dermatitis with multinucleated histiocytic giant cells.

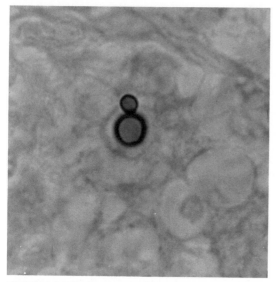

FIGURE 7–21. Equine sporotrichosis. Budding yeast (GMS stain).

iodide is administered orally at 1 to 2 mg/kg s.i.d. or b.i.d. for one week, then 0.5 to 1 mg/kg s.i.d. until cured.[255] Potassium iodate is administered orally in a fashion identical to that for potassium iodide.[255] EDDI may offer some advantages over the inorganic iodides because the iodine in EDDI may be retained in tissues longer.[255] EDDI is administered orally in a fashion identical to that for potassium iodide. The oral iodides are usually administered with sweet feed or mixed with molasses and administered by syringe. Therapy should be continued until three to four weeks after lesions disappear.

Tolerance to iodide therapy varies, and some horses may show signs of iodism, such as scaling and alopecia, depression, anorexia, fever, coughing, lacrimation, serous nasal discharge, salivation, nervousness, or cardiovascular abnormalities.[95, 255, 260] In such cases, the dosage may be reduced or therapy temporarily discontinued. Additionally, systemic iodides may cause abortion in mares[260] and should not be used during pregnancy.

Zygomycosis

Zygomycosis is a chronic fungal infection that is cutaneous, subcutaneous, systemic, or rhinocerebral.

CAUSE AND PATHOGENESIS

Zygomycosis is a polymorphic disease of multiple etiology.[64] Infections caused by the

various zygomycetes have, in the course of time, been given a wide variety of names: phycomycosis, mucormycosis, entomophthoromycosis, hyphomycosis, basidiobolomycosis, and oomycosis. The general term zygomycosis was adopted to replace the various names, since fundamental changes in the classification of fungi have been made.

Regardless of the clinical expression of zygomycosis, the unifying diagnostic hallmark of the disease is the form assumed by the etiologic agents in tissue. The invasive form is mycelial and is infrequently septate and significantly broader than any of the fungi with a filamentous tissue form (*Aspergillus* species, the agents of phaeohyphomycosis). Fungi reported to cause cutaneous zygomycosis in large animals include *Basidiobolus haptosporus* (horse), *Conidiobolus coronatus* (horse), and *Rhizopus oryzae* (pig). These fungi are environmental saprophytes and presumably cause infection via traumatic implantation.[242, 245]

CLINICAL FEATURES

Basidiobolomycosis is an ulcerative granulomatous equine skin disease caused by *B. haptosporus*.[75, 240, 241, 245, 285] There are no apparent age, breed, or sex predilections, and cases occur regularly throughout the year. Most lesions are found on the chest, trunk, head, and neck, where they are often located on the more lateral aspects of the body. Large (up to 60 cm in diameter), circular, ulcerative granulomas with a serosanguineous discharge are characteristic (see Plate 5A). Solitary lesions are the rule, and pruritus is usually noted. The leeches that characterize pythiosis are not always seen in basidiobolomycosis but, if present, are smaller and of no characteristic shape.

Conidiobolomycosis (entomophthoromycosis or rhinophycomycosis) is an ulcerative granulomatous equine skin disease caused by *C. coronatus* (*Entomophthora coronata*).* There are no apparent age, breed, or sex predilections, and cases occur regularly throughout the year. Most lesions are found on the external nares or in the nasal passage or both. Lesions may be single or multiple and unilateral or bilateral, and those of the external nares appear grossly similar to those of basidiobolomycosis. Lesions in the nasal passages are firm nodules covered by an edematous,

---

*References 47, 51, 67, 78, 92, 105, 144, 157, 236, 241, 245, 246, 262, 302, 328

focally ulcerated mucosa. Leeches are usually present but are often smaller than 0.5 mm. Horses often develop a hemorrhagic nasal discharge and dyspnea due to nasal blockage.

Zygomycosis caused by *R. oryzae* was reported in feeder pigs.[342] Affected animals had gastric and lymph node granulomas and occasional subcutaneous granulomas with draining tracts.

DIAGNOSIS

The differential diagnosis includes other fungal and bacterial granulomas, habronemiasis, exuberant granulation tissue, and various neoplasms (especially sarcoid and squamous cell carcinoma). In the United States, basidiobolomycosis and conidiobolomycosis are most commonly seen in states along the Gulf of Mexico. Diagnosis is based on biopsy and culture. Biopsy reveals granulomatous to pyogranulomatous dermatitis with large numbers of eosinophils and plasma cells. A wide cuff of eosinophilic material surrounds fungal hyphae (Splendore-Hoeppli phenomenon). The fungi are easily seen in sections stained with H & E. *B. haptosporus* hyphae are 5 to 20 μm in diameter, thin-walled, rarely branching, and commonly septate.[249] *C. coronatus* hyphae are 5 to 13 μm in diameter, thin-walled, rarely branching, and commonly septate.[249]

Both *B. haptosporus* and *C. coronatus* grow well on Sabouraud's dextrose agar incubated at 37°C. Leeches should be collected from the lesions, vigorously washed in water, and implanted into the agar. The fungi are classified by hyphal morphology and the morphology of asexual and sexual spores.[191, 323, 324]

CLINICAL MANAGEMENT

Treatment of equine basidiobolomycosis and conidiobolomycosis should be attempted as soon as possible after diagnosis, because chronic lesions have a poorer prognosis. Surgery is curative if all diseased tissue is removed.[229, 230, 245, 285, 302] Systemic antifungal therapy has variable success and has not been carefully evaluated. Sodium iodide (1 gm/15 kg intravenously twice weekly) and potassium iodide (0.5 to 1.2 gm/30 kg/day orally) have been recommended.[157, 245, 285, 296, 299, 302] The combination of surgery, systemic iodides, systemic antibiotics, and appropriate wound care may be the most successful approach.[239, 245, 302] Immunotherapy utilizing a phenolized vaccine prepared from cultures of a *Pythium* species was of no benefit in horses with basidiobolomycosis.[244]

Alternariosis

Alternaria species are common saprophytic fungi found in the environment and on the skin of animals and humans (see Chapter 1, discussion on cutaneous ecology).[258, 333] *A. tenuis* was consistently isolated from the tissues of an adult horse with asymptomatic papules and nodules scattered over the head, chest, and legs.[70] The horse was otherwise healthy. Skin biopsy revealed pyogranulomatous dermatitis with myriad branching, septate hyphae, and chlamydospores.

Systemic Mycoses

Systemic mycoses are fungal infections of internal organs that may disseminate secondarily to the skin. Rarely, primary cutaneous infections may be established by local inoculation. Fungi that cause systemic mycoses exist in soil and vegetation and are rare pathogens. In endemic regions, many animals are exposed to these fungi without developing clinical disease.

Infections with *B. dermatitidis*, *C. immitis*, *Cryptococcus neoformans*, and *H. capsulatum* have been reported in large animals.[17, 35, 40a, 47, 175, 200] However, most infections either were asymptomatic or did not involve the skin. A sternal abscess was associated with disseminated coccidioidomycosis in a horse.[76] Cutaneous granulomas of the lip were reported in a horse with cryptococcosis.[395] Multiple granulomas and abscesses were found around the perineum and udder of a mare with blastomycosis.[29]

Histologically, the systemic mycoses are initially characterized by perivascular dermatitis, which progresses to diffuse or nodular dermatitis (suppurative, pyogranulomatous, or granulomatous). Intraepidermal microabscesses and pseudocarcinomatous epidermal hyperplasia are frequent findings. The diagnostic feature is the presence of the fungi, which are usually easily found both within macrophages and giant cells and free within the dermis. *B. dermatitidis* appears as spherical to oval, thick-walled (double-contoured) cells, with broad-based budding, that range from 8 to 15 μm in diameter. *C. immitis* appears as spherical, thick-walled spherules that range from 10 to

80 μm in diameter. The spherule contains a granular cytoplasm or spherical endospores (2 to 10 μm in diameter). *C. neoformans* is present as spherical to oval cells that may be budding and range from 4 to 12 μm in diameter. *C. neoformans* blastoconidia may be surrounded by a thick, clear capsule. *H. capsulatum* is present as spherical to oval cells that range from 2 to 4 μm in diameter. All of the fungi causing systemic mycoses can be seen in sections stained with H & E but they may be highlighted with AOG, PAS, GMS, or Gridley's stains. The gelatinous capsule of *C. neoformans* contains acid polysaccharides and thus stains metachromatically purple with alcian blue, and red with mucicarmine.

Diagnosis is confirmed by culturing the fungi from exudates and tissues. In humans and small animals, the systemic mycoses have been treated with amphotericin B, ketoconazole, and 5-fluorocytosine.[258] Such treatments have not been reported in large animals.

Histoplasmosis Farciminosi

Histoplasmosis farciminosi (epizootic lymphangitis, pseudoglanders, African farcy, equine blastomycosis, equine cryptococcosis) is a chronic cutaneolymphatic infection of horses that can also involve other organs.

CAUSE AND PATHOGENESIS

Histoplasmosis farciminosi is endemic in Africa, Asia, and Eastern Europe.* It is caused by the dimorphic fungus. *H. (Cryptococcus, Zymonema, Saccharomyces) farciminosum.* Except for extremely rare reports in humans[266] and pigs,[274] infections with *H. farciminosum* appear to be limited to equines (horse, mule, donkey).[4-6] The disease may be transmitted by intracutaneous, subcutaneous, oral, or respiratory inoculation. Trauma appears to be an essential prerequisite for infection to take place. Mosquitoes and biting and nonbiting flies are able to serve as vectors for the disease. The fungus survives for eight to ten weeks in soil and water at 26°C.[7] The environmental niche of *H. farciminosum* is unknown. The average incubation period for clinal infections is 35 days, with a range of 4 to 72 days.

CLINICAL FEATURES

Infection with *H. farciminosum* has no apparent age, breed, or sex predilections.* Initial lesions consist of unilateral nodules, 15 to 25 mm in diameter, in the skin of the face, head, neck, and rarely the limbs. Initially, the nodules are firm; then they become fluctuant and eventually rupture to discharge a light-green, blood-tinged exudate. Resultant ulcers increase in size because of the formation of granulation tissue, occasionally reaching 10 cm in diameter. In some animals, nodules develop in a chain along enlarged and tortuous lymphatics, resulting in a corded or knotted appearance. After a period of 8 to 12 weeks, infection often spreads to the other side of the body, especially the medial thigh and prepuce. General health is usually unaltered.

Infections on the limbs may involve joints, resulting in purulent synovitis.[4-6] Lacrimal, conjunctival, nasal cavity, pulmonary, and other organ infections have been reported.† Spontaneous recovery sometimes occurs, and complete immunity results.[40a, 175] The impact of histoplasmosis farciminosi in endemic areas is serious.[4-6, 40] Economic losses through condemnation and slaughter of livestock are significant.

H. farciminosum infections are apparently rare in humans. An accidentally acquired infection was described in a veterinarian who contaminated an open wound with pus from an infected horse.[240] He developed painful migratory cutaneolymphatic nodules and abscesses as well as pyrexia.

DIAGNOSIS

The differential diagnosis includes other mycotic and bacterial infections, especially sporotrichosis, ulcerative lymphangitis, and glanders. Definitive diagnosis is based on direct smears, biopsy, and culture. Owing to difficulties in culturing the organisms (cultures positive in only 58 percent of the horses in one large study),[4-6] demonstration of the yeast phase in tissues by smears or biopsies is still considered the most reliable means of laboratory diagnosis.[4-6, 56, 57, 64] Direct smears stained with Giemsa or Diff-Quik reveal macrophages containing an average of four to six round, unicellular organisms, 1 to 5 μm in diameter.

---

*References 4–6, 40a, 64, 175, 360–363

*References 4, 25, 31, 40a, 164, 175, 315, 335, 360, 362
†References 30, 31, 40a, 91, 97, 103, 360–362

Skin biopsy reveals nodular to diffuse dermatitis (pyogranulomatous or granulomatous).[64, 362] *H. farciminosum* is found as a round to oval yeast, primarily within macrophages. The organism produces single, narrow-based buds. It is morphologically and tinctorially indistinguishable from *H. capsulatum.*

On Sabouraud's dextrose agar incubated at 26°C, growth of the fungus is not evident before two to three weeks.[4-6] Colonies are few in number, dry, dull gray, and 2 to 4 mm in diameter. Over the following three weeks of incubation, the colonies turn brown and develop a folded cerebriform appearance.

Encouraging preliminary investigations have suggested that tube and passive hemagglutination tests, intradermal skin testing with a histoplasmin, and a fluorescent antibody technique may be useful diagnostic tools.[5, 107, 108]

CLINICAL MANAGEMENT

Histoplasmosis farciminosi is a reportable disease and is managed by strict isolation and slaughter. An effective treatment has not been developed. The organism is sensitive to amphotericin B and nystatin in vitro.[109]

Aspergillosis

Aspergillus species, ubiquitous in soil and vegetation, are extremely rare causes of skin disease in large animals.[40a, 64, 117, 136, 258] *Aspergillus terreus* was isolated from a subcutaneous granuloma in a Holstein-Friesian cow.[79] Skin lesions characterized by multiple generalized plaques were reported in an aborted bovine fetus in association with *Aspergillus* species infection.[136] A papular dermatitis from which an *Aspergillus* species was isolated in culture was reported in swine.[375] Aspergillosis was reported in an 18-month-old Black Benga male goat.[127] The animal presented with granulomatous lesions on the scrotum and medial thighs. *A. fumigatus* was cultured from the skin lesions and produced granulomas when inoculated into the skin of the medial thighs of a normal Black Benga goat.

Histologically, aspergillosis is characterized by diffuse or nodular dermatitis (suppurative, pyogranulomatous, or granulomatous) or by necrosis with minimal inflammation. *Aspergillus* species may be present in large numbers as septate hyphae that may branch at an acute angle and show terminal bulbous dilatations. The organisms are usually visualized in sections stained with H & E but are highlighted with PAS, GMS, AOG, and Gridley's stains. Diagnosis is confirmed by isolating the organisms in culture or Sabouraud's dextrose agar from exudates or tissues.

In humans and small animals, aspergillosis has been treated with inorganic iodides, 5-fluorocytosine, thiabendazole, ketoconazole, and amphotericin B with varying results.[258] Such therapy has not been reported in large animals.

Pythiosis

Pythiosis is a chronic subcutaneous fungal infection that usually affects the legs or ventrum and rarely becomes systemic.

CAUSE AND PATHOGENESIS

Equine pythiosis (phycomycosis, hyphomycosis, bursatti, swamp cancer, Florida horse leeches, Gulf Coast fungus, oomycosis) is caused by a *Pythium* species (*Hyphomyces destruens*).[24, 64, 163, 242, 357] Members of the genus *Pythium* are properly classified in the kingdom Protista in the phylum Oomycetes. They are not members of the division Zygomycetes in the kingdom Fungi. *Pythium* is an aquatic fungus that probably relies on an aquatic plant or organic substrate for its normal life cycle. The zoospores of *Pythium* show chemotaxis toward damaged plant or animal tissues. This probably explains why most lesions are located on the legs and ventral abdomen, areas in the most frequent prolonged contact with water.

CLINICAL FEATURES

There are no apparent age, breed, or sex predilections for equine pythiosis.[123, 227, 229, 241, 245] Pythiosis has recently been reported in cattle.[250] Environmental conditions are probably the most influential factors governing the occurrence of oomycosis. *Pythium* requires warm temperatures and moisture for reproduction. Thus, most cases are seen during the summer and fall in tropical and temperate areas of the world, such as the Gulf Coast region of the United States, Australia, and South America.

Most lesions are found on the distal extremities and the ventral abdomen and chest.* Lesions are usually single and unilateral but

---

*References 24, 47, 50, 123, 146, 170, 227, 229, 230, 302

may be multiple and bilateral. Large (up to 45 cm in diameter), roughly circular, ulcerative granulomas with a serosanguineous discharge are characteristic (see Plate 5). A thick (serous, hemorrhagic, mucoid, and/or purulent) exudate fills the sinuses permeating the lesions and covers the surface. Numerous elongated, gritty, gray-white to yellowish, coral-like bodies are present in the sinus tracts (see Plate 5). These bodies are composed of fungal hyphae and reactive host tissue. Because of their gross appearance, these bodies were originally described as "kunkers," leeches, or roots.

The lesions often arise explosively at the site of a previous, apparently insignificant wound and are usually intensely pruritic. Limb edema, tendon sheath involvement, joint involvement, lameness, and regional lymphadenopathy may be seen. Internal spread is rare, with lesions of lymph nodes, trachea, lungs, and stomach being described.[75, 121, 135, 230, 245, 261]

DIAGNOSIS

The differential diagnosis includes other fungal and bacterial granulomas, habronemiasis, exuberant granulation tissue, and various neoplasms (especially sarcoid and squamous cell carcinoma). Diagnosis is based on biopsy and culture. Biopsy reveals granulomatous to pyogranulomatous dermatitis with large numbers of eosinophils (Figs. 7–22 and 7–23). Large, focal eosinophilic areas of necrotic eosinophils

and neutrophils, collagenolysis, and fungal hyphae are seen within the granulomatous inflammation. These correspond to the leeches seen grossly. Hyphae of *Pythium* are 2.6 to 6.4 μm in diameter, thick-walled, irregularly branching, occasionally septate, and easily seen in sections stained with H & E, GMS, or Gridley's stains (Fig. 7–24).[249]

Culture of the fungus is not difficult.[242, 245] Leeches should be collected from the lesion, vigorously washed in water, implanted into vegetable extract agar, and incubated at 37°C. Identification is based on hyphal morphology and asexual reproduction involving zoospores.

Hematologic studies of horses with pythiosis revealed a frequent occurrence of microcytic, hypochromic anemia with moderate leukocytosis and absolute neutrophilia and eosinophilia.[247] Immunologic studies on horses with pythiosis showed that 64 percent of clinically infected horses, 100 percent of recovered horses, and 31 percent of normal in-contact horses, respectively, had evidence of cellular immunity to *Pythium* as assessed by delayed-type hypersensitivity reactions to the intradermal injection of a *Pythium* species preparation.[243]

CLINICAL MANAGEMENT

Treatment of equine pythiosis should be instituted as soon as possible after diagnosis, because chronic lesions have a poorer prog-

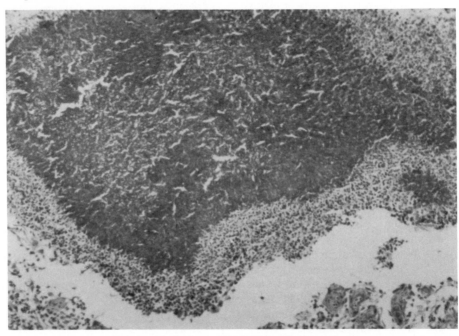

FIGURE 7–22. *Equine pythiosis. Palisading granuloma.*

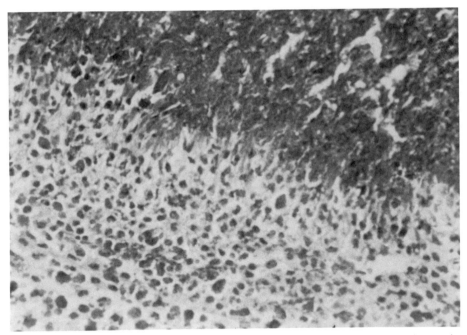

FIGURE 7–23. Equine pythiosis. Eosinophilic palisading granuloma bordering area of necrosis.

nosis.[124, 227, 229, 230, 245, 302] Surgery is curative if all diseased tissue is removed. However, even with radical surgical extirpation, recurrence is frequent. Repeat surgery is indicated as soon as new foci of infection are noted. These are first apparent as dark red to black hemorrhagic spots, 1 to 5 mm in diameter, in the new granulation bed. One major surgical procedure and two to three minor "retrims" are customary in the average case.[230]

Topical antifungal agents have been used and recommended but are of uncertain benefit.[229, 230, 245, 302] Both iodophors and amphotericin B (gauze dressing pads soaked in a solution

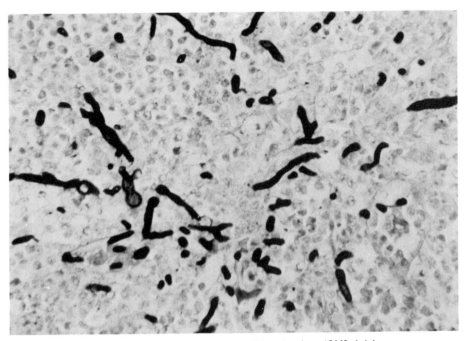

FIGURE 7–24. Equine pythiosis. Pythium hyphae (GMS stain).

of 50 mg of amphotericin B in 10 ml sterile water and 10 ml dimethyl sulfoxide [DMSO]) have been used.

Systemic treatment with amphotericin B has been reported to be useful when combined with surgical excision.[227–230, 245] The starting dose is 150 mg of amphotericin B per 450 kg added to 1 L of 5 percent dextrose given intravenously with a 16-gauge 5-cm needle to prevent perivascular injection. Every third day, the dose is increased by 50 mg until a maximum of 400 mg/day is reached, which is then continued on a daily or alternate-day schedule for a total treatment interval of 30 days. The blood urea nitrogen (BUN) and packed cell volume (PCV) should be monitored weekly. If the patient becomes severely depressed or anorectic or if the BUN exceeds 40 mg/dl, therapy should be temporarily discontinued. A major limiting factor with amphotericin B therapy is expense. Amphotericin B has been suspected of causing abortions in horses[173, 260] and was administered to six pregnant mares,[229] that had five normal foals and one stillborn foal with arthrogryposis.

Immunotherapy using a phenolized, ultrasonicated preparation from cultures of *Pythium* has been reported to be effective in the treatment of equine pythiosis.[244, 245] The vaccine was administered subcutaneously on a weekly basis for at least three weeks. Fifty-three percent of the horses were cured after vaccination, while another 33 percent showed clinical improvement. Success was greatest when lesions were less than two months' duration, particularly when vaccination was used in conjunction with unsuccessful primary surgery. Most horses tolerated the vaccination well. In all cases, there was a moderate to severe reaction at the site of subcutaneous injection that subsided within 96 hours. In approximately 30 percent of the injections, a sterile abscess formed at the site but responded promptly to treatment.

Five horses with pythiosis of the limbs were treated unsuccessfully by surgery or topical application of amphotericin B, or both.[248] Follow-up immunotherapy with the aforementioned *Pythium* vaccine resulted in only one horse's responding favorably. Three horses were cured of the fungal infection but developed osteitis or deep-seated laminitis, which necessitated their destruction. The remaining horse, which had severe anemia, died before the course of vaccination was completed.

REFERENCES

1. Aamodt, O., et al.: Vaccination of Norwegian cattle against ringworm. Zbl. Vet. Med. B 29:451, 1982.
2. Abdallah, I. S., and Abd el Hamid. Y. M.: Experimental infections of *Trichophyton equinum* in calves. Mykosen 16:61, 1973.
3. Abou-Gabal, M., et al.: Animal ringworm in upper Egypt. Sabouraudia 14:33, 1976.
4. Abou-Gabal, M., et al.: Study of equine histoplasmosis "epizootic lymphangitis." Mykosen 26:1983.
5. Abou-Gabal, M., and Kahifa, K.: Study of the immune response and serological diagnosis of equine histoplasmosis "epizootic lymphangitis." Mykosen 26:89, 1983.
6. Abou-Gabal, M., et al.: Study of equine histoplasmosis farciminosi and characterization of *Histoplasma farciminosum*. Sabouraudi 21:121, 1983.
7. Abou-Gabal, M., and Hennager, S.: Study on the survival of *Histoplasma farciminosum* in the environment. Mykosen 26:481, 1983.
8. Abu-Samra, M. T., and Hago, B. E. D.: Experimental infection of goats and guinea pigs with *Microsporum canis* and trials on treatment with Canesten cream and Neguvon solution. Mycopathologia 72:79, 1980.
9. Abu-Samra, M. T., et al.: An abnormal outbreak of ringworm among Sudanese calves. Zbl. Vet. Med B 23:171, 1976.
10. Abu-Samra, M. T., et al.: *Microsporum canis* infection in calves. Sabouraudia 13:154, 1975.
11. Abu-Samra, M. T.: Some skin diseases of domestic animals in the Sudan with special reference to cutaneous streptothricosis. M.V.Sc. Thesis, University of Khartoum, Sudan, 1975.
12. Ahmed, A. R.: Immunology of human dermatophyte infections. Arch. Dermatol. 118:521, 1982.
13. Aho, R.: Studies on fungal flora in hair from domestic and laboratory animals suspected of dermatophytosis. Acta Pathol. Microbiol. Scand. B 88:79, 1980.
14. Ainsworth, G. C., and Austwick, P. K C.: A survey of animal mycoses in Britain: General aspects. Vet. Rec. 67:88, 1955.
15. Ainsworth, G. C., and Austwick, P. K. C.: *Fungal Disease of Domestic Animals II*. Farnham Royal, Commonwealth Argicultural Bureau, 1973.
16. Ajello, L., et al.: The natural history of *Microsporum nanum*. Mycologia 56:873, 1964.
17. Amstutz, H. E.: *Bovine Medicine and Surgery II*. Santa Barbara, CA, American Veterinary Publications, Inc., 1980.
18. Amstutz, H. E.: Bovine skin conditions: A brief review. Mod. Vet. Pract. 60:821, 1979.
19. Andrews, A. H., and Edwardson, J.: Treatment of ringworm in calves using griseofulvin. Vet. Rec. 108:498, 1981.
20. Anonymous: Warning: Sodium hypochlorite can damage metal surfaces. Vet. Med. Small Anim. Clin. 78:1358, 1983.
21. Arora, B. M., et al.: Dermatomycosis in pigs (rubromycosis). Indian Vet. J. 56:791, 1979.
22. Austin, R. J.: Disseminated phycomycosis in a horse. Can. Vet. J. 17:86, 1976.
23. Austwick, P. K. C.: The isolation of *Trichophyton discoides* from cattle. Vet. Rec. 66:224, 1954.
24. Austwick, P. K. C., and Copland, J. W.: Swamp cancer. Nature 250:84, 1974.
25. Awad, F. I.: Studies on epizootic lymphangitis in the Sudan. J. Comp. Pathol. 70:457, 1960.
26. Baker, N. F., and Davis, D. W.: Spray application for the treatment of ringworm in cattle. Vet. Med. 49:275, 1955.
27. Batte, E. G., and Miller, W. S.: Ringworm of horses and its control. JAVMA 123:111, 1953.
28. Baxter, M.: Danger of contact infection from pig ringworm. N.Z. Vet. J. 17:69, 1969.
29. Benbrook, E. A., et al.: A case of blastomycosis in the horse. JAVMA 112:475, 1948.

30. Bennett, S. C. J.: *Cryptococcus* pneumonia in equidae. J. Comp. Pathol. 44:85, 1931.
31. Bennett, S. C. J.: *Cryptococcus* infection in equidae. J. Army Vet. Corps 16:108, 1944.
32. Bese, M., et al.: Ringworm in Angora goats due to *Trichophyton verrucosum*. Vet. Fak. Dergisi. 12:133, 1965.
33. Bibel, D. J., and Le Brun, J. R.: Effect of experimental dermatophyte infection on cutaneous flora. J. Invest. Dermatol. 64:119, 1975.
34. Bibel, D. J., and Smiljanic, R. J.: Interactions of *Trichophyton mentagrophytes* and *micrococci* on skin culture. J. Invest. Dermatol. 72:133, 1979.
35. Biberstein, E. L.: The systemic mycoses. *In*: Howard, J. L.: *Current Veterinary Therapy. Food Animal Practice*. Philadelphia, W. B. Saunders Co., 1981, pp. 753–763.
36. Blackford, J.: Superficial and deep mycoses in horses. Clin. Vet. North Am. Large Anim. Pract. 6:47, 1984.
37. Blank, F.: Ringworm of cattle due to *T. discoides* and its transmission to man. Can. J. Comp. Med. 17:277, 1953.
38. Blank, F., and Craig, C. E.: Family epidemics of ringworm contracted from cattle. Can. Med. Assoc. J. 71:234, 1953.
39. Blank, H., and Rebell, G.: Thiabendazole activity against the fungi of dermatophytosis, mycetomas and chromomycosis. J. Invest. Dermatol. 44:219, 1965.
40. Bliss, E. L.: Tinea versicolor dermatomycosis in the goat. JAVMA 184:1512, 1984.
40a. Blood, D. C., et al.: *Veterinary Medicine V*. Baltimore, Williams & Wilkins Co., 1979.
41. Bohm, K. H., et al.: Mykologische Befunde bei Pferden mit Hautveranderungen in Nordwest-Deutschland-zugleich ein Beitrag zur Frage der Entstehung equiner Dermatomykosen. Berl. Munch. Tierarztl. Wochenschr. 81:397, 1968.
42. Boomker, J., et al.: Black grain mycosis (maduromycosis) in horses. Onderst. J. Vet. Res. 44:249, 1977.
43. Boro, B. R., et al.: Ringworm in animals due to *Epidermophyton floccosum*. Vet. Rec. 107:491, 1980.
44. Brethouwer, A. H.: Ringworm bij runderen. Tijd. Diergeneesk. 107:681, 1982.
45. Bridges, C. H.: Maduromycotic mycetomas in animals. *Curvularia geniculata* as an etiologic agent. Am. J. Pathol. 33:411, 1957.
46. Bridges, C. H., and Beasley, N. N.: Maduromycotic mycetomas in animals—*Brachycladium spiciferum* Bainier as an etiologic agent. JAVMA 137:192, 1960.
47. Bridges, C. H.: Systemic mycoses. *In*: Catcott, E. J., and Smithcors, J. F.: *Equine Medicine and Surgery*. Santa Barbara, CA, American Veterinary Publications, Inc., 1972, p. 119.
48. Bridges, C. H., and Kral, F.: Dermatomycoses. *In*: Catcott, E. J., and Smithcors, J. F.: *Equine Medicine and Surgery II*. Santa Barbara, CA, American Veterinary Publications, Inc., 1972, p. 131.
49. Bridges, C. H.: Dermatological conditions in equidae. Proc. Am. Assoc. Equine Pract. 9:147, 1963.
50. Bridges, C. H., and Emmons, C. W.: Phycomycosis of horses caused by *Hyphomyces destruens*. JAVMA 138:579, 1961.
51. Bridges, C. H., et al.: Phycomycosis of a horse caused by *Entomophthora coronata*. JAVMA 140:673, 1961.
52. Brock, J. M.: *Microsporum nanum*: A cause of tinea capitis. Arch. Dermatol. 84:504, 1961.
53. Brown, G. W., and Donald, G. F.: Equine ringworm due to *Trichophyton mentagrophytes var quinckeanum*. Mycopathol. Mycol. Appl. 23:269, 1964.
54. Brown, R. J., et al.: Equine maduromycosis: A case report. Mod. Vet. Pract. 53:47, 1972.
55. Bubash, G. R., et al.: *Microsporum nanum*: First recorded isolation from animals in the United States. Science 143:366, 1964.
56. Bullen, J. J.: The yeast-like form of *Cryptococcus farciminosus* (Rivolta): (*Histoplasma farciminosum*). J. Pathol. Bacteriol. 61:117, 1949.
57. Bullen, J. J.: Epizootic lymphoangitis: Clinical symptoms, J. R. Army Vet. Corps 22:8, 1951.
58. Cameron, R. D. A.: Porcine dermatoses. University of Sydney Post-Graduate Foundation in Veterinary Science, Veterinary Review No. 15, 1975.
59. Cameron, R. D. A.: Skin diseases of the pig. Proc. Univ. Sydney Post-Grad. Comm. Vet. Sci. 56:445, 1981.
60. Cameron, R. D. A.: *Skin Diseases of the Pig*. Sydney, University of Sydney Post-Graduate Foundation in Veterinary Science, Veterinary Review No. 23, 1984.
61. Carman, M. G., et al.: Dermatophytes isolated from domestic and feral animals. N.Z. Vet. J. 27:136, 1979.
61a. Carmichael, J. W., and Reid, J. F.: *Microsporum nanum* infection in Alberta. Mycopathol. Mycol. Appl. 17:325, 1962.
62. Carter, G. R., et al.: Ringworm of horses caused by an atypical form of *Microsporum canis*. JAVMA 156:1048, 1970.
63. Carter, M. E.: *Microsporum gypseum* isolated from ringworm lesions in a horse. H.Z. Vet. J. 14:92, 1966,
64. Chandler, F. W., et al.: *Histopathology of Mycotic Diseases*. Chicago, Year Book Medical Publishers, Inc., 1980.
65. Chatterjee, A., et al.: Isolation of dermatophytes from dung. Vet. Rec. 107:399, 1980.
66. Chatterjee, A., and Sengupta, D. N.: Ringworm in domestic animals. Indian J. Anim. Health 18:37, 1979.
67. Chauhan, H. V. S., et al.: A fatal cutaneous granuloma due to *E. coronata* in a mare. Vet. Rec. 92:425, 1973.
68. Chineme, C. N., et al.: Ringworm caused by *Trichophyton verrucosum* in young goats. Bull. Anim. Health Prod. 29:75, 1981.
69. Cobb, R. W., et al.: Griseofulvin: Controlled field trials in the treatment of naturally occurring ringworm in calves. Vet. Rec. 75:191, 1963.
70. Coles, B. M., et al.: Equine nodular dermatitis associated with *Alternaria tenuis* infection. Vet. Pathol. 15:779, 1978.
71. Conant, N. F.: A statistical analysis of spore size in the genus *Microsporum*. J. Invest. Dermatol. 4:265, 1941.
72. Connole, M. D.: A review of dermatomycoses of animals in Australia. Aust. Vet. J. 39:130, 1963.
73. Connole, M. D., and Baynes, I. D: Ringworm caused by *Microsporum nanum* in pigs in Queensland. Aust. Vet. J. 42:19, 1966.
74. Connole, M. D., *Microsporum gypseum* ringworm in a horse. Aust. Vet. J. 43:118, 1967.
75. Connole, M. D.: Equine phycomycosis. Aust. Vet. J. 49:214, 1973.
76. Crane, C. S: Equine coccidioidomycosis. Case report. Vet. Med. 57:1073, 1962.
77. Crestian, J., and Luffair, G.: Observation d'une enzootie de teigne du mouton. Rec. Med. Vet. 153:561, 1977.
78. Das, T., et al.: Isolation of *Microsporum nanum* from northeastern region of India. Indian J. Microbiol. 20:326, 1980.
79. Davis, C. L., and Schaefer, W. B.: Cutaneous aspergillosis in a cow. JAVMA 141:1339, 1962.
80. Davis, H. H., and Worthington, W. E.: Equine sporotrichosis. JAVMA 145:692, 1964.
81. Dawson, C. O.: Ringworm in animals. Rev. Med. Vet. Mycol. 6:223, 1963.
82. Dawson, C. O., and Lepper, A. W. D.: *Peyronellaea glomerata* infection of the ear pinna in goats. Sabouraudia 8:145, 1970.
83. Dekeyser, J., et al.: Activité thérapeutique de l'iturine et du chinosol sur la teigne du cheval à *Microsporum equinum*. Bull. Epiz. Dis. Afr. 8:279, 1960.
84. Dodd, D. C., et al.: Infection of swine with *Microsporum nanum*. JAVMA 146:486, 1965.
85. Dunne, H. W., and Leman, A. D.: *Disease of Swine IV*. Ames, Iowa State University Press. 1975.
86. Dvorak, J., and Otcenasek, M.: *Mycological Diagnosis of Animal Dermatophytoses*. The Hague, W. Junk, 1969.
87. Edgson, F. A.: Mass treatment of ringworm in cattle with griseofulvin mycelium. Vet. Rec. 86:58, 1970.
88. Edwardson, J., and Andrews, A. H.: An outbreak of ringworm in a group of young cattle. Vet. Rec. 104:474, 1979.
89. Ek, N.: Ringworm in pigs caused by *Trichophyton verrucosum var. discoides*. Nord. Vet. Med. 17:152, 1965.
90. El-Allawy, T., et al.: An outbreak of ringworm in Oseemy sheep in Egypt. Assiut Vet. Med. J. 7:331, 1980.
91. El-Gundy, M. H., et al.: Histoplasmosis of the eyes of donkeys. II. An electron microscopic study. Assiut Vet. Med. J. 2:235, 1974.
92. Emmons, C. W., and Bridges, C. H.: *Entomophthora coronata*, the etiological agent of a phycomycosis of horses. Mycologia 53:307, 1961.

93. English, M. P.: An outbreak of equine ringworm due to *Trichophyton equinum*. Vet. Rec. 73:578, 1961.

94. Even-Paz, Z., and Raubitschek, F.: Epidemics of tinea capitis due to *T. verrucosum* contracted from cattle or sheep. Dermatologica 120:74, 1960.

95. Fadok, V. A., and Wild, S.: Suspected cutaneous iodism in a horse. JAVMA 183:1104, 1983.

96. Fambach, D.: *Trochosporon equinum*. Ztschr. Infektionskr. 29:124, 1925.

97. Fawi, M. T.: *Histoplasma farciminosum*, the aetiological agent of equine cryptococcal pneumonia. Sabouraudia 9:123, 1971.

98. Fischman, O., and Santiago, M.: *Microsporum canis* infection in a pig. Mycopathol. Mycol. Appl. 30:271, 1966.

99. Fischman, O., et al.: Ringworm infection by *Microsporum canis* in a horse. Mycopathol. Mycol. Appl. 30:273, 1966.

100. Fishburn, F., and Kelley, D. C.: Sporotrichosis in a horse. JAVMA 151:45, 1967.

101. Florian, E., et al.: Active immunization of calves against ringworm. Magy. Allatorv. Lap. 19:529, 1964.

102. Ford, E. J. H.: Ringworm in cattle. An account of an outbreak. Vet. Rec. 68:803, 1956.

103. Fouad, K., et al.: Studies on lachrymal histoplasmosis in donkeys in Egypt. Zbl. Vet. Med. 8:584, 1973.

104. Fowle, L. P., and Georg, L. K.: Suppurative ringworm contracted from cattle. Arch. Dermatol. Syphilol. 56:780, 1947.

105. French, D. D., et al.: Surgical and medical management of rhinophycomycosis (conidiobolomycosis) in a horse. JAVMA 186:1105, 1985.

106. Frey, D., et al.: *Color Atlas of Pathogenic Fungi*. Chicago, Year Book Medical Publishers, Inc., 1979.

107. Gabal, M. A., et al.: The fluorescent antibody technique for diagnosis of equine histoplasmosis (enzootic lymphangitis). Zbl. Vet. Med. B 30:283, 1983.

108. Gabal, M. A., and Khalifa, K.: Study on the immune response and serological diagnosis of equine histoplasmosis (enzootic lymphangitis). Zbl. Vet. Med. B 30:317, 1983.

109. Gabal, M. A.: The effect of amphotericin B, 5-fluorocytosine and nystatin on *Histoplasma farciminosum in vitro*. Zbl. Vet. Med. B 31:46, 1984.

110. Gabal, M. A.: Study on the evaluation of the use of thiabendazole in the treatment and control of bovine dermatophytosis. Mycopathologia 93:163, 1986.

111. Gedek, B.: Mykosen in Rinderbestanden. Zbl. Vet. Med. B 17:234, 1970.

112. Gentles, J. C., and O'Sullivan, J. G.: Correlation of human and animal ringworm in west of Scotland. Br. Med. J. 11:678, 1957.

113. Georg, L. K.: Epidemiology of the dermatophytoses, sources of infection, modes of transmission, and epidemicity. Ann. N.Y. Acad. Sci. 89:69, 1960.

114. Georg, L., et al.: Equine ringworm with specific reference to *Trichophyton equinum*. Am. J. Vet. Res. 18:798, 1957.

115. Georg, L., et al.: *Trichophyton equinum*—a reevaluation of its taxonomic status. J. Invest. Dermatol. 29:27, 1957.

116. Gibbons, W. J.: Sporotrichosis: Case report. Mod. Vet. Pract. 43:92, 1962.

117. Gibbons, W. J.: Aspergillosis. *In:* Gibbons, W. J., et al. (eds.): *Bovine Medicine and Surgery*. Santa Barbara, CA, American Veterinary Publications, Inc., 1970, pp. 247–248.

118. Ginther, O. J.: Clinical aspects of *Microsporum nanum* infection in swine. JAVMA 146:945, 1965.

119. Ginther, O. J., and Bubash, G. R.: Experimental *Microsporum nanum* infection in swine. JAVMA 148:1034, 1966.

120. Ginther, O. J., and Ajello, L.: The prevalence of *Microsporum nanum* infection in swine. JAVMA 146:36, 1965.

121. Goad, M. E. P.: Pulmonary pythiosis in a horse. Vet. Pathol. 21:261, 1984.

122. Gold, T. N., and Jones, B. V.: The use of hexadecamethylene-1:16 bis (isoquinolinium chloride) in the treatment of ringworm in domestic animals. Br. Vet. J. 114:1075, 1958.

123. Gonzalez, H. E., and Ruiz, A.: Espundia equina: Etiologia y pathogenesis de una ficomicosis. Rev. ICA Bogota 10:175, 1975.

124. Gonzalez, H. E., et al.: Tratamiento de la ficomicosis equina

125. subcutanea empleando yoduro de potasio. Rev. ICA Bogota 41:115, 1979.

125. Grunder, H. D., and Muller, U.: Behandlungsversuche mit dem fungiziden Antimykose Natamycin bei der enzootischen Rindertrichophytie. Dtsch. Tierarztl. Wochenschr 86:457, 1979.

125a. Gudding, R., and Ness, B.: Vaccination of cattle against ringworm caused by *Trichophyton verrucosum*. Am. J. Vet. Res. 47:2415, 1986.

126. Gugnani, H. C.: *Trichophyton verrucosum* infection in cattle in India. Mykosen 15:185, 1972.

127. Guha, A. N.: *Aspergillus fumigatus* infection in goats. Indian Vet. J. 36:252, 1959.

128. Guilhon, J., et al.: Teigne du mouton. Bull. Acad. Vet. 28:465, 1955.

129. Guilhon, J., and Obligi, S.: Une nouvelle epizootie de teigne ovine. Bull. Acad. Vet. 29:443, 1956.

130. Gupta, O. P., et al.: Observations on chemotherapy of bovine dermatomycosis (tolnaftate). Indian Vet. Med. J. 5:44, 1981.

131. Gupta, P. K., and Singh, R. P.: Effect of some therapeutics on dermatomycoses (ringworm) in animals. Indian Vet. J. 46:1001, 1969.

132. Gupta, P. K., et al.: A study of dermatomycoses (ringworm) in domestic animals and fowls. Indian J. Anim. Health 9:85, 1970.

133. Gupta, P. K., and Singh, R. P.: A note on the effect of age on the incidence of ringworm in cattle, buffaloes, and horses. Indian J. Anim. Sci. 39:69, 1969.

134. Guss, S. B.: *Management and Diseases of Dairy Goats*. Scottsdale, AZ, Dairy Goat Journal Publishing Corp., 1977.

135. Habbinga, R.: Phycomysosis in an equine. Southwest. Vet. 20:237, 1967.

136. Hagan, W. A., and Bruner, D. W.: *The Infectious Diseases of Domestic Animals III*. Ithaca, Comstock Publishing Associates, 1957.

137. Hajsig, M. S., et al.: Immunoprophylaxis of ringworm (*Trichophyton infection*) in cattle. Praxis Vet. 24:131, 1976.

138. Hajsig, M. S.: *Trichophyton verrucosum* (Bodin 1902) U goveda na podracju nr hrvatske. Vet. Archiv. 27:315, 1957.

139. Hajsig, M. S., and Zukovic, M.: Izolacija *Trichophyton verrucosum* s usi i pausi goveda, te istrazivanje utjecaja dezinsekcije na tok trihofitije. Vet. Archiv. 31:225, 1961.

140. Hajsig, M., and Asaj, A.: Istrazivanja o utjecaju smjestaja goveda na pojavu trihofitije. Vet Archiv. 32:26, 1962.

141. Haley, L. D., and Callaway, C. S.: *Laboratory Manual for Medical Mycology*. PHS Pub. No. 994, Washington, D.C., U.S. Government Printing Office, 1978.

142. Hall, F. R.: Ringworm contracted from cattle in western New York State. Arch. Dermatol. 94:35, 1966.

143. Hall, J. E.: Multiple maduromycotic mycetomas in a colt caused by *Heminthosporium*. Southwest. Vet. 18:233, 1965.

144. Hanselka, D. V.: Equine nasal phycomycosis. Vet. Med. Small Anim. Clin. 72:251, 1977.

145. Harding, R. B.: Treatment of ringworm in the horse with griseofulvin. Vet. Dermatol. News. 6:40, 1981.

146. Hartfield, S. M.: Phycomycosis in a mare. Southwest. Vet. 24:138, 1971.

147. Hasegawa, A., and Usui, K.: Isolation of *Trichophyton equinum* and *Microsporum canis* from equine dermatophytosis. Jpn. J. Med. Mycol. 16:11, 1975.

148. Hiddleston, W. A.: Antifungal activity of penicillium griseofulvin mycelium. Vet. Rec. 86:75, 1970.

149. Hiddleston, W. A.: The use of griseofulvin mycelium in equine animals. Vet. Rec. 87:119, 1970.

150. Hoerlein, A. B.: Studies on animal dermatomycoses. Clinical studies. Cornell Vet. 35:287, 1945.

151. Hoerlein, A. B.: Studies on animal dermatomycoses II. Cultural studies. Cornell Vet. 35:299, 1945.

152. Hoerlein, A. B.: Dermatomycoses. *In:* Gibbons, W. J., et al. (eds.): *Bovine Medicine and Surgery*. Santa Barbara, CA, American Veterinary Publications, Inc., 1970, pp. 231–234.

153. Hopes, R.: Ringworm in the horse—the clinical picture. Vet. Dermatol. News. 6:33, 1981.

154. Hopes, R.: Skin diseases in horses. Vet. Dermatol. News. 1:4, 1976.
155. Horter, R.: Zur Pilzflora hautkranker und-gesunder Schweine. Dtsch. Tierarztl. Wochenschr. 69:717, 1962.
156. Hutchins, D. R.: Skin diseases of cattle and horses in New South Wales. N.Z. Vet. J. 8:85, 1960.
157. Hutchins, D. R., and Johnston, K. G.: Phycomycosis in the horse. Aust. Vet. J. 48:269, 1972.
158. Hutton, R. D., et al.: Scanning electron microscopy of experimental *Trichophyton mentagrophytes* infections in guinea pig skin. Infect. Immun. 21:247, 1978.
159. Ichijo, S., et al.: Equine ringworm by *Trichophyton verrucosum*. Jpn. J. Vet. Sci. 37:407, 1975.
160. Ichijo, S., et al: *Trichophyton equinum* isolated from race horse dermatophytosis. Res. Bull. Obihiro Univ. 10:803, 1978.
161. Ichijo, S., et al.: Dermatomycosis due to *Trichophyton verrucosum* in cows, horses, sheep, and human beings. Jpn. J. Vet. Med. Assoc. 37:506, 1984.
162. Ichijo, S., et al.: Therapeutic effect of BPMC (2-sec-butyl-phenyl-N-methylcarbamate) emulsion for bovine ringworm. Jpn. J. Vet. Med. Assoc. 38:13, 1985.
163. Ichitani, T., and Ameniya, J.: *Pythium gracile* isolated from the foci of granular dermatitis in the horse. Trans. Mycol. Soc. Jpn. 21:263, 1980.
164. Iyer, K. P. R.: An unusual case of epizootic lymphangitis in a mule. Indian J. Vet. Sci. 6:251, 1936.
165. Jocobs, P. H., and Russell, B.: Dermatophyte test medium for systemic fungi. JAMA 224:1649, 1973.
166. Jaksch, W.: Dermatomykosen der Equiden, Karnivoren und einiger Rodentiere in Osterreich, mit einem Beitrag zur normalen Pilzflora der Haut. Wien. Tierarztl. Monatsschr. 50:831, 1963.
167. Jensen, R., and MacKay, D. R.: *Disease of Feedlot Cattle II*. Philadelphia, Lea & Febiger, 1971.
168. Jensen, R., and Swift, B. L.: *Diseases of Sheep II*. Philadelphia, Lea & Febiger, 1982.
169. Jillson, O. F., and Buckley, W. R.: Fungus disease in man acquired from cattle and horses due to *T. faviforme*. N. Engl. J. Med. 246:996, 1952.
170. Johnston, K. G., and Henderson, A. W. K.: Phycomycotic granuloma in horses in the Northern Territory. Aust. Vet. J. 50:105, 1974.
171. Jones, H. E., et al.: Immunologic susceptibility to chronic dermatophytosis. Arch. Dermatol. 110:213, 1974.
172. Jones, T. C., and Maurer, F. D.: Sporotrichosis in horses. Bull. U.S. Army Med. Dept. 74:63, 1944.
173. Joyce, J. R., et al.: The use of amphotericin B in late pregnancy in mares. J. Equine Med. Surg. 1:256, 1977.
174. Jung, H. D.: Die Dermatomykosen und Ihre aktuelle Problematik fur Human und Veterinarmedizin. Monat. Vet. Med. 16:174, 1961.
175. Jungerman, P. F., and Schwartzman, R. M.: *Veterinary Medical Mycology*. Philadelphia, Lea & Febiger, 1972.
176. Kaben, U., and Ritscher, D.: Mikrosporie bei Pferden, unter besonderer Berucksichtigung einer *Microsporum gypseum*—Infektion bei einem Fohlen. Mykosen 11:337, 1968.
176a. Kakepis, E., et al.: Bovine ringworm. An outbreak caused by *Trichophyton mentagrophytes* var. *granulare* in Greece. Intl. J. Dermatol. 25:580, 1986.
177. Kamyszek, F.: Badania nad epizootiologia grzybic skory bydla. Polskie Arch. Wet. 18:69, 1975.
178. Kaplan, W., et al.: The parasitic nature of the soil fungus *Keratinomyces ajelloi*. J. Invest. Dermatol. 32:539, 1959.
179. Kaplan, W., et al.: Equine phaeohyphomycosis caused by *Drechslera spicifera*. Can. Vet. J. 16:205, 1975.
180. Kaplan, W.: Piedra in lower animals. JAVMA 134:113, 1959.
181. Kaplan, W. A., et al.: Isolation of the dermatophyte, *Microsporum gypseum*, from a horse with ringworm. JAVMA 129:381, 1956.
182. Kaplan, W., et al.: Ringworm in horses caused by the dermatophyte *Microsporum gypseum*. JAVMA 131:329, 1957.
183. Kaplan, W., et al.: Public health significance of ringworm in animals. Arch. Dermatol. 96:404, 1967.
184. Khanna, B. M., et al.: Therapeutic effect of thiabendazole on ringworm in calves. Indian Vet. J. 51:562, 1974.
185. Kielstein, P., and Weller, W.: *Trichophyton verrucosum* infection in sheep. Monat. Vet. Med. 20:671, 1965.
186. Kielstein, P.: Zur Immunobiologie der Rindertrichophytie. Monat. Vet. Med. 22:25, 1967.
187. Kielstein, P.: Zur Epidemiologie und Pathologie der Trichophytie unter besonderer Berucksichtigung der veterinar und human medizinischen Literatur. Monat. Vet. Med. 19:174, 1964.
188. Kielstein, P.: *Recent Advances in Human and Animal Mycology*. Bratislava, Czechoslovak Academy of Sciences, 1967.
189. Kielstein, P., and Hubrig, T.: Zur Anwendung von Griseofulvin bei der Behandlung der Rindertrichophytie. Monat. Vet. Med. 22:209, 1967.
190. Kielstein, P., and Gottschalk, C.: Eine *Trichophyton mentagrophytes*: Infektion in einem Schweinezuchtbestund. Monat. Vet. Med. 25:127, 1970.
191. King, D. W.: Systemics of fungi causing entomophthoromycosis. Mycologia 71:731, 1979.
192. King, N. B.: Skin diseases. Univ. Sydney Post-Grad. Comm. Vet. Sci. Proc. 52:199, 1980.
193. Kirkham, W. W., and Moore, R. W.: Sporotrichosis in a horse. Southwest. Vet. 7:354, 1954.
194. Kligman, A. M.: Pathophysiology of ringworm infection in animals with skin infections. J. Invest. Dermatol. 27:171, 1956.
195. Kligman, A. M.: The pathogenesis of tinea capitis due to *Microsporum audouini* and *Microsporum canis*. J. Invest. Dermatol. 81:839, 1952.
196. Knudsen, E. A.: The areal extent of dermatophyte infection. Br. J. Dermatol. 92:413, 1975.
197. Koehne, G.: *Microsporum gypseum* dermatitis in a pig. JAVMA 161:168, 1972.
198. Kral, F.: Classification, symptomatology and recent treatment of animal dermatomycoses (ringworm). JAVMA 127:395, 1955.
199. Kral, F.: Skin diseases. Adv. Vet. Sci. 7:18, 1962.
200. Kral, F., and Schwartzman, R. M.: *Veterinary and Comparative Dermatology*. Philadelphia, J. B. Lippincott Co., 1964.
201. Kral, F.: Ringworm in the horse. Mod. Vet. Pract. 42:32, 1961.
202. Krivanec, K., et al.: Gehauftes Auftreten einer durch *Trichophyton equinum* (Matruchot und Dassonville) hervorgerufenen Dermatophytose bei Rindern. Zbl. Vet. Med. B 25:356, 1978.
203. Kriz, H., et al.: The influence of thiabendazole on trichophytiasis in cattle. Acta Vet. Brno. 40:199, 1971.
204. Kruger, O.: Vergleichende Behandlungsversuche mitdem Antimykotikum Multifungin (Knoll) und anderen Mitteln bei der Trichophytie des Rindes. Diss. Hannover, 1956.
204a. Kubis, A., et al.: Klinische Beuertung des Diethanolamins in der Behandlung der Trichophytose beim jungen Mastrieh. Mykosen 29:85, 1986.
205. Kulkarni, M. P., and Chaudhari, P. G.: A note on the successful treatment of unusual equine ringworm due to *Trichophyton tonsurans var sulfureum*. Indian Vet. J. 46:444, 1969.
206. Kulkarni, V. B., et al.: Equine ringworm caused by *Trichophyton tonsurans var sulfureum*. Indian Vet. J. 46:5, 1969.
207. Kuttin, E. S., et al.: *Trichophyton mentagrophytes* infection in a flock of sheep. Refuah Vet. 31:190, 1974.
208. La Touche, C. J.: Some observations on ringworm in calves due to *T. discoides*. Vet. Rec. 64:841, 1952.
209. La Touche, C. J.: The importance of the animal reservoir of infection in the epidemiology of animal-type ringworm in man. Vet. Rec. 67:666, 1955.
210. Lauder, I. M., and O'Sullivan, J. G.: Ringworm in cattle. Prevention and treatment with griseofulvin. Vet. Rec. 70:949, 1958.
211. Leman, A. D., et al.: *Diseases of Swine V*. Ames, Iowa State University Press, 1981.
212. Lepper, A. W. D.: Experimental bovine *Trichophyton verrucosum* infection. Res. Vet. Sci. 13:105, 1972.
213. Lepper, A. W. D.: Experimental bovine *Trichophyton verrucosum* infection. The cellular responses in primary lesions of the skin resulting from surface or intradermal inoculation. Res. Vet. Sci. 16:287, 1974.

214. Liven, E., and Stenwig, H.: Efficacy of vaccination against ringworm in cattle. Nord. Vet. Med. 37:187, 1985.

215. Lodder, L.: *The Yeasts: A Taxonomic Study*. Amsterdam, North Holland Publishing Co., 1971.

216. Lofstedt, J.: Dermatologic diseases of sheep. Vet. Clin. North Am. Large Anim. Pract. 5:427, 1983.

217. Londero, A. T., and Fischman, O.: *Trichophyton verrucosum* in Brazil. Mycopathol. Mycol. Appl. 28:353, 1966.

218. Londero, A. T., et al.: An epizootic of *Trichophyton equinum* infection in horses in Brazil. Sabouraudia 3:14, 1963.

219. Long, J. R., et al.: *Microsporum nanum*: A cause of porcine ringworm in Ontario. Can. Vet. J. 13:164, 1972.

220. Mahajan, V. M., and Mohapatra, L. N.: Study of human and animal dermatophytes in rural areas. Mykosen 11:793, 1968.

221. Main, P. T.: Ringworm contracted from cattle: A two years' survey in general practice. Practitioner 182:347, 1959.

222. Martin, W. B.: *Diseases of Sheep*. Oxford, Blackwell Scientific Publications, 1983.

223. McClure, J. J., et al.: Immunodeficiency manifested by oral candidiasis and bacterial septicemia in foals. JAVMA 186:1195, 1985.

224. McGinnis, M. R.: *Laboratory Handbook of Medical Mycology*. New York, Academic Press, 1980.

225. McGinnis, M. R., et al.: *Phaeosclera dematioides*, a new etiologic agent of phaeohyphomycosis in cattle. Sabouraudia 23:113, 1985.

226. McKenzie, R. A., and Connole, M. D.: Mycotic nasal granuloma in cattle. Aust. Vet. J. 53:268, 1977.

227. McMullen, W. C.: Equine dermatology. Proc. Am. Assoc. Equine Pract. 22:293, 1976.

228. McMullen, W. C., et al.: Amphotericin B for the treatment of localized subcutaneous phycomycosis in the horse. JAVMA 170:1293, 1977.

229. McMullen, W. C.: The skin. In: Mansmann, R. A., et al. (eds.): *Equine Medicine and Surgery*. Santa Barbara, CA, American Veterinary Publications, Inc., 1982, p. 789.

230. McMullen, W. C.: Phycomycosis. In: Robinson, N. E.: *Current Therapy in Equine Medicine*. Philadelphia, W. B. Saunders Co., 1983, p. 550.

231. McPherson, E. A.: The influence of physiological factors on dermatomycoses in domestic animals. Vet. Rec. 69:1010, 1957.

232. McPherson, E. A.: A survey of the incidence of ringworm in cattle in Northern Britain. Vet. Rec. 69:674, 1957.

233. McPherson, E. A.: *Trichophyton verrucosum* ringworm. A search for control agents. Vet. Rec. 71:425, 1959.

234. McPherson, E. A.: *Trichophyton mentagrophytes*: Natural infection in pigs. Vet. Rec. 68:710, 1956.

235. Meckenstock, E.: Clinical signs and treatment of dermatomycoses in domestic animals. Vet. Med. Rev. 2:79, 1969.

236. Mendoza, L., and Alfaro, A. A.: Equine subcutaneous zygomycosis in Costa Rica. Mykosen 28:545, 1985.

237. Miklausic, B., and Hajsig, M.: Prilog poznavanju dermatomikoza kod domacih zivotinja u nr hrvatskoj. *Trichophyton mentagrophytes* kod konja. Vet. Arch. 30:104, 1960.

238. Miller, R. I., et al.: Black-grained mycetoma in two horses. Aust. Vet. J. 56:347, 1980.

239. Miller, R. I.: Treatment of some equine cutaneous neoplasms. Aust. Vet. Pract. 10:1, 1980.

240. Miller, R. I., and Pott, B.: Phycomycosis of the horse caused by *Basidiobolus haptosporus*. Aust. Vet. J. 56:224, 1980.

241. Miller, R. I., and Campbell, R. S. F.: Clinical observations of phycomycosis. Aust. Vet. J. 58:221, 1982.

242. Miller, R. I.: Investigations into the biology of three phycomycotic fungi pathogenic for horses. Mycopathologia 81:23, 1983.

243. Miller, R. I., and Campbell, R. S. F.: Immunological studies on equine phycomycosis. Aust. Vet. J. 58:227, 1982.

244. Miller, R. I.: Treatment of equine phycomycosis by immunotherapy and surgery. Aust. Vet. J. 57:377, 1981.

245. Miller, R. I.: Equine phycomycosis. Compend. Cont. Educ. 5:S472, 1983.

246. Miller, R. I., and Campbell, R. S. F.: A survey of granulomatous and neoplastic diseases of equine skin in North Queensland. Aust. Vet. J. 59:33, 1982.

247. Miller, R. I., and Campbell, R. S. F.: Haematology of horses with phycomycosis. Aust. Vet. J. 60:28, 1983.

248. Miller, R. I., et al.: Complications associated with immunotherapy of equine phycomycosis. JAVMA 182:1227, 1983.

249. Miller, R. I., and Campbell, R. S. F.: The comparative pathology of equine cutaneous phycomycosis. Vet. Pathol. 21:325, 1984.

250. Miller, R. I., et al.: Cutaneous pythiosis in beef cattle. JAVMA 186:984, 1985.

251. Misra, S. K.: Comparative efficacy of Grisovin, F. P., Ephytol, and Multifungin against *Trichophyton verrucosum* Bodin 1902 infection in cattle. Indian Vet. J. 50:290, 1973.

252. Monga, D. P., et al.: Dermatophytoses due to *Trichophyton mentagrophytes* in adult cattle. Haryana Vet. 13:111, 1974.

253. Monga, D. P., et al.: Use of captan in bovine dermatophytosis. Indian Vet. J. 52:559, 1975.

254. Morganti, L., et al.: First European report of swine infection by *Microsporum nanum*. Mycopathologia 59:179, 1976.

255. Morris, P.: Sporotrichosis. In: Robinson, N. E.: *Current Therapy in Equine Medicine*. Philadelphia W. B. Saunders Co., 1983, p. 555.

256. Mortimer, P. H.: Man, animals, and ringworm. Vet. Rec. 67:670, 1955.

257. Mos, E., et al.: Dermatomycosis caused by *Microsporum nanum* in a herd of swine. Rec. Fac. Med. Vet. Zootec. 15:159, 1978.

258. Muller, G. H., et al.: *Small Animal Dermatology III*. Philadelphia, W. B. Saunders Co., 1983.

259. Mullins, J. F., et al.: *Microsporum nanum*: Review of the literature and a report of two cases. Arch. Dermatol. 94:300, 1966.

260. Mullowney, P. C., and Fadok, V. A.: Dermatologic diseases of horses. Part III. Fungal skin diseases. Compend. Cont. Educ. 6:S324, 1984.

261. Murray, D. R., et al.: Metastatic phycomycosis in a horse. JAVMA 172:834, 1978.

262. Murray, D. R., et al.: Granulomatous and neoplastic diseases of the skin of horses. Aust. Vet. J. 54:338, 1978.

263. Naess, B., and Sandvik, O.: Early vaccination of calves against ringworm caused by *Trichophyton verrucosum*. Vet. Rec. 109:199, 1981.

264. Nazarov, G. S.: Dry-method treatment of ringworm in cattle. Vet. Bull. 26:196, 1954.

265. Neefs, L., and Gillian, L.: Contribution à l'étude de la teigne. Ann. Med. Vet. 76:193, 1931.

266. Negre, L., and Bridre, J.: Un cas de lymphangite épizootique chez l'homme. Bull. Soc. Pathol. Exot. 4:384, 1911.

267. Neuman, M., and Platzner, N.: The treatment of bovine ringworm with thiabendazole. Refuah Vet. 25:46, 1968.

268. Nicolet, J., et al.: *Candida guilliermondii* als wahrscheinliche Ursache einer disseminierten Hautgranulomatose beim Pferd. Schweiz. Arch. Tierheilk. 107:185, 1965.

269. Nierman, M. M., and Lunday, M. E.: *Trichophyton verrucosum* in Indiana. Cutis 26:591, 1980.

270. Nooruddin, M., and Dey, A. S.: Distribution of lesions and clinical severity of dermatophytosis in cattle. Agri-Pract. 6:31, 1985.

271. Noskov, A.: Metody lecenija striguscego lisaja zivotnych. Veterinarija 39:35, 1962.

272. O'Brien, J. D. P., and Sellers, K. C.: A clinical trial of the treatment of cattle ringworm. Vet. Rec. 70:319, 1958.

273. O'Donnell, F. A.: Treatment of leeches in horses. Haver-Lockhart Messenger 41:30, 1961.

274. Oehl, R.: Lymphangitis epizootica beim Schwein. Dtsch. Tierarztl. Wochenschr. 37:39, 1929.

275. Okoshi, S., and Hasegawa, A.: Enzootic of bovine ringworm caused by *T. verrucosum* in Japan. Jpn. J. Vet. Sci. 30:93, 1967.

276. Oldenkamp, E. P.: Natamycin treatment of ringworm in cattle in the United Kingdom. Vet. Rec. 105:554, 1979.

277. Oldenkamp, E. P., and Kommerij, R.: Eeen nieuw therapeuticum op basis van natamycine voor de behandeling van trichophytie bij runderen. Tijdschr. Diergeneeskd. 101:178, 1976.

278. Oldenkamp, E. P., and Spanoghe, L.: De behandeling van trichophytie van het rund met natamycine-S. Tijdschr. Diergeneeskd. 101:1242, 1976

279. Oldenkamp, E. P.: Treatment of ringworm in horses with natamycin. Equine Vet. J. 11:36, 1979.
280. Onizuka, S.: Dermatophyte isolated from horses. Rikugun Jui Dampo 270:1471, 1934.
281. Otcenasek, M., and Komarek, J.: Von einer durch *Trichophyton mentagrophytes* (Robin) Blanchard (1896) hervorgerutenen Dermatophytose des Schweines. Monat. Vet. Med. 25:130, 1970.
282. Otcenasek, M., et al.: Zwei Befunde der *Trichophyton equinum* in menschlichen Lasionen. Dermatol. Wochenschr. 149:438, 1964.
283. Otcenasek, M., et al.: *Microsporum equinum* als Erreger einer Dermatophytose des Pferdes. Zbl. Vet. Med. B 22:833, 1975.
284. Otcenasek, M., et al.: Das gehaufte Auftreten einer Dermatophytose bei der Grofzucht von Pferden. Mykosen 5:131, 1962.
285. Owens, W. R., et al.: Phycomycosis caused by *Basidiobolus haptosporus* in two horses. JAVMA 186:703, 1985.
286. Page, E. H.: Common skin diseases of the horse. Proc. Am. Assoc. Equine Pract. 18:385, 1972.
287. Pal, S., and Gupta, I.: Antifungal activity of "choti dudhi plant" (Euphorbia prostrata AIT and Euphorbia thymifolia LINN) against certain dermatophytes. Indian Vet. J. 56:367, 1979.
288. Pal, M., and Dev, K.: Some observations on the clinical trial of sulfur and calcium lactate in skin disorders. Indian J. Anim. Health 15:173, 1976.
289. Pal, M., and Singh, D. K.: Studies on dermatomycoses in dairy animals. Mykosen 26:317, 1983.
290. Palsson, G.: Geophilic dermatophytes in the soil in Sweden. Studies on their ocurrence and pathogenic properties. Acta Vet. Scand. (Suppl.) 25:1, 1968.
291. Pandey, V. S., and Carbaret, J.: The distribution of ringworm lesions in cattle naturally infected by *Trichophyton verrucosum*. Ann. Rech. Vet. 1:179, 1980.
292. Pandey, V. S.: Some observation on *Trichophyton verrucosum* infection in cattle in Morocco. Ann. Soc. Belge Med. Trop. 59:127, 1979.
293. Pandey, V. S., and Mahin, L.: Observations on ringworm in goats caused by *Trichophyton verrucosum*. Br. Vet. J. 136:198, 1980.
294. Pandey, V. S.: Effect of thiabendazole and tincture of iodine on cattle ringworm caused by *Trichophyton verrucosum*. Trop. Anim. Health Prod 11:175, 1979.
295. Panel Report: Dermatologic problems in cattle. Mod. Vet. Pract. 60:172, 1979.
296. Panel Report: Skin conditions in horses. Mod. Vet. Pract. 56:363, 1975.
297. Pascoe, R. R.: The nature and treatment of skin conditions observed in horses in Queensland. Aust. Vet. J. 49:35, 1973.
298. Pascoe, R. R., and Connole, M. D.: Dermatomycosis due to *Microsporum gypseum* in horses. Aust. Vet. J. 50:380, 1974.
299. Pascoe, R. R.: *Equine Dermatoses*. Sydney, University of Sydney Post-Graduate Foundation in Veterinary Science, Veterinary Review No. 14, 1974.
300. Pascoe, R. R.: Studies on the prevalence of ringworm among horses in racing and breeding stables. Aust. Vet. J. 52:419, 1976.
301. Pascoe, R. R.: The epidemiology of ringworm in race horses caused by *Trichophyton equinum var autotrophicum*. Aust. Vet. J. 55:403, 1979.
302. Pascoe, R. R.: *Equine Dermatoses*. Sydney, University of Sydney Post-Graduate Foundation in Veterinary Science, Veterinary Review No. 22, 1981.
303. Patton, C. S.: *Helminthosporium speciferum* as the cause of dermal and nasal maduromycosis in a cow. Cornell Vet. 67:236, 1977.
304. Pavlovic, R., et al.: Prvi slucajevi trihofitije ovaca u jugoslaviji. Veterinaria (Sarajevo) 32:521, 1983.
305. Pearson, J. K. L., and Rankin, J. E. F.: Griseofulvin in the treatment of bovine ringworm. Vet. Rec. 74:564, 1962.
306. Pepin, G. A., and Austwick, P. K. C.: Skin diseases of domestic animals. II. Skin disease, mycological origin. Vet. Rec. 82:209, 1968.
307. Petrovich, S. V., and Makarchenko, V. A.: Therapeutic efficacy of preparation TF-130 (*Trichophyton faviforme* vaccine). Veterinariya 51:50, 1974.
308. Petrovich, S. V.: Efficacy of the treatment of ringworm in horses. Veterinariya 2:49, 1977.
309. Petzold, K., et al.: Enzootien durch *Trichophyton equinum* bei Pferden. Dtsch. Tierarztl. Wochenschr. 72:302, 1965.
310. Pier, A., and Hughes, J.: *Keratinomyces ajelloi* from skin lesions of a horse. JAVMA 138:484, 1961.
311. Pier, A. C., et al.: Scanning electron microscopy of selected dermatophytes of veterinary importance. Am. J. Vet. Res. 33:607, 1972.
312. Pier, A. C.: Dermatophytosis. In: Howard, J. L.: *Current Veterinary Therapy. Food Animal Practice*. Philadelphia, W. B. Saunders Co., 1981, pp. 1130–1133.
313. Pinello, C. B., et al.: Development of an interpretative system for the identification of yeasts. Species 2:1, 1978.
314. Plambeck, E.: Behandlungsversuche mit Thiabendazol, Monobenzthion und Tego-spray bei der Rindertrichophytie. Diss. Hannover, 1968.
315. Plunkett, J. J.: Epizootic lymphangitis. J. Army Vet. Corps 20:94, 1949.
316. Polonelli, L., and Morace, G.: Antigenic characterization of *Microsporum canis, M. distortum, M. equinum, N. ferrugineum*, and *Trichophyton soudanense* cultures. Mycopathologia 92:7, 1985.
317. Poulain, D., et al.: Experimental study of resistance to infection by *Trichophyton mentagrophytes*: Demonstration of memory skin cells. J. Invest. Dermatol. 74:206, 1980.
318. Powell, F. C., and Muller, S. A.: Kerion of the glabrous skin. J. Am. Acad. Dermatol. 7:490, 1982.
319. Priboth, W.: *Microsporum canis* as cause of ringworm in piglets. Monat. Vet. Med. 17:521, 1962.
320. Pritchard, D., et al.: Eumycotic mycetoma due to *Drechslera rostrata* infection in a cow. Aust. Vet. J. 53:241, 1977.
321. Raab, W. F.: *Natamycin, Its Properties and Possibilities in Medicine*. Stuttgart, Georg Thieme Publishers, 1972.
322. Raper, K. B., and Fennel, D. I.: *The Genus, Aspergillus*. New York, Robert E. Krieger Publishing Co., 1973.
323. Rasulev, S. T.: Immunity to *Trichophyton* infection in cattle. Veterinariya 51:54, 1974.
324. Rebell, G., and Taplin, D.: *Dermatophytes. Their Recognition and Identification*. Coral Gables, University of Miami Press, 1974.
325. Refai, M., and Rieth, H.: Dermatomykose durch *Mikrosporum gypseum* beim Rind. Bull. Pharm. Res. Inst. Takatsuki 65:11, 1965.
326. Refai, M., and Miligy, M.: Ringworm in cattle caused by *Trichophyton verrucosum*. Egypt Vet. Med. Assoc. J. 28:33, 1968.
327. Refai, M., et al.: Uber das Vorkommen von *Trichophyton verrucosum* Infektionen in Agypten mit Hinweis auf die Behandlung mit Griseofulvin. Dtsch. Tierarztl. Wochenschr. 83:62, 1976.
328. Restrepo, L. F., et al.: Rhinophycomycosis from *Entomophthora coronata* in horses. Information on 15 cases. Antioquia Medica 23:13, 1973.
329. Reynolds, I. M., et al.: Cutaneous candidiasis in swine. JAVMA 152:182, 1968.
330. Rieth, H., and El-Fiki, A. V.: Die Rinderflechte-ein aktuelles therapeutisches und hygienisches Problem. Berl. Munch. Tierarztl. Wochenschr. 72:201, 1959.
331. Rieth, H., and El-Fiki, A. V.: Dermatomykose beim Pferd durch *Keratinomyces ajelloi* Vanbreuseghem 1952. Bull. Pharm. Res. Inst. Takatsuki 21:1, 1959.
332. Rinaldi, M. G., et al.: Mycetoma or pseudomycetoma? Mycopathologia 81:41, 1983.
333. Rippon, J. W.: *Medical Mycology. The Pathogenic Fungi and the Pathogenic Actinomycetes*. Philadelphia, W. B. Saunders Co., 1982.
334. Ritscher, D., and Kaben, U.: Hautpilzer-krankungen bei Pferden. Monat. Vet. Med. 26:944, 1971.
335. Roberts, G. A.: Epizootic lymphangitis of solipeds. JAVMA 98:226, 1941.
336. Roberts, J. S., and Keep, J. M.: Infection of the wool of sheep by *Microsporum canis*. Sabouraudia 4:96, 1965.
337. Robinson, H. J., et al.: Thiabendazole: Toxicological, pharmacological, and antifungal properties. Texas Rep. Biol. Med. 27:537, 1969.

338. Robinson, H. J., et al.: Antimycotic properties of thiabendazole. J. Invest. Dermatol. 42:479, 1964.

338a. Roller, J. A., et al.: *Microsporum nanum* infection in hog farmers. J. Am. Acad. Dermatol. 15:935, 1986.

339. Rook, A., and Frain, B. W.: Cattle ringworm. Br. Med. J. 1:1198, 1954.

340. Rook, A.: Animal ringworm. *Trichophyton discoides* and *mentagrophytes* in the Cambridge area. Br. J. Dermatol. 68:11, 1956.

340a. Rotermund, H., et al.: Erste Erfahrungen bei der Anwendung der sowjetischen Trichophytievakzine LTF = 130. Monat. Veterinarmed. 32:576, 1977.

341. Salkin, I. F.: Dermatophyte test medium: Evaluation with nondermatophytic pathogens. Appl. Microbiol. 26:134, 1973.

342. Sanford, S. E., et al.: Submanibular and disseminated zygomycosis (mucormycosis) in feeder pigs. JAVMA 186:171, 1985.

343. Sarkisov, A. K., et al.: Immunization of cattle against trichophytosis. Veterinaria 48:54, 1971.

344. Sarkisov, A. K., and Petrovich, S. V.: Immunity of horses to spontaneous and experimental ringworm. Veterinariya 11:39, 1976.

345. Satija, K. C., and Gautam, O. P.: Ringworm in bovine calves. Indian Vet. J. 49:317, 1972.

346. Saunders, W.: Inflammatory ringworm due to *T. faviforme*. Report of three cases in one family. Arch. Dermatol. 69:365, 1954.

347. Schauffler, A. F.: Maduromycotic mycetoma in an aged mare. JAVMA 160:998, 1972.

348. Schiefer, B., and Mehnert, B.: Maduromykose beim Pferd in Deutschland. Berl. Munch. Tierarztl. Wochenschr 78:230, 1965.

349. Schroder, E., and Bernhard, D.: Thibenzole zur Bekampfung der Trichophytie beim Rind. Prakt. Tierarztl. 60:758, 1979.

350. Schulz, W.: Vergleichende Behandlungsversuche bei der enzootischen Rindertrichophytie mit Mycophyt^R-Gruntex und einem neuen, antimykotisch wirksamen Praparat (Bay-Vet 7294). Dtsch. Tierarztl. Wochenschr. 91:364, 1984.

351. Scott, D. W.: Topical cutaneous medicine, or, "now what should I try." Proc. Am. Anim. Hosp. Assoc. 46:89, 1979.

352. Scott, D. W., et al.: Caprine dermatology. I. Normal skin, bacterial and fungal disorders. Compend. Cont. Educ. 6:S190, 1984.

353. Scott, D. W., and Manning, T. O.: Equine folliculitis and furunculosis. Equine Pract. 2:20, 1980.

354. Scott, D. W.: Folliculitis and furunculosis. *In*: Robinson, N. E.: *Current Therapy in Equine Medicine*. Philadelphia, W. B. Saunders Co., 1983, p. 542.

355. Scott, D. B.: An outbreak of ringworm in Karakul sheep caused by a physiological variant of *Trichophyton verrucosum* Bodin. Onderstepoort J. Vet. Res. 42:49, 1975.

356. Sellers, K. C., et al.: Preliminary observations on natural and experimental ringworm in cattle. Vet. Rec. 68:729, 1956.

357. Shipton, W. A., et al.: Cell wall, zoospore, and morphological characteristics of Australian isolates of *Pythium* causing equine phycomycosis. Trans. Br. Mycol. Soc. 79:15, 1982.

358. Simpson, J. G., et al.: A case of chromoblastomycosis in a horse. Vet. Med. Small Anim. Clin. 61:1207, 1966.

359. Singh, S.: Equine cryptococcosis (epizootic lymphangitis). Indian Vet. J. 32:260, 1956.

360. Singh, T.: Studies on epizootic lymphangitis. I. Modes of infection and transmission of equine histoplasmosis (epizootic lymphangitis). Indian J. Vet. Sci. 35:102, 1965.

361. Singh, T.: Studies on epizootic lymphangitis. Indian J. Vet. Sci. 36:45, 1966.

362. Singh, T., et al.: Studies on epizootic lymphangitis. II. Pathogenesis and histopathology of equine histoplasmosis. Indian J. Vet. Sci. 35:111, 1965.

363. Singh, T., and Varmani, B. M. L.: Some observations on experimental infection with *Histoplasma farciminosum* (Rivolta) and the morphology of the organism. Indian J. Vet. Sci. 37:471, 1967.

364. Slagsvold, L.: Favus in the skin of goats and sheep. Norsk. Vet. Tidsskr. 45:361, 1933.

365. Smallwood, J. E.: A case of phycomycosis in the equine. Southwest. Vet. 22:150, 1969.

366. Smith, J. M. B., et al.: *Trichophyton equinum var autotrophicum*: Its characteristics and geographic distribution. Sabouraudia 6:296, 1968.

367. Smith, J. M. B., et al.: Animals as a reservoir of human ringworm in New Zealand. Aust. J. Dermatol. 10:169, 1969.

368. Smith, J. M. B.: An unusual dermatophyte from horses in New Zealand. Sabouraudia 5:124, 1966.

369. Smith, J. M. B., and Steffert, I. J.: *Microsporum nanum* in New Zealand pigs. N.Z. Vet. J. 14:97, 1966.

370. Spanoghe, L., and Oldenkamp, E. P.: Mycological and clinical observations on ringworm in cattle after treatment with natamycin. Vet. Rec. 101:135, 1977.

371. Stannard, A. A.: Equine dermatology. Proc. Am. Assoc. Equine Pract. 22:273, 1976.

372. Stannard, A. A.: Diagnostic aids in dermatology. Mod. Vet. Pract. 60:548, 1979.

373. Stenwig, H.: Isolation of dermatophytes from domestic animals in Norway. Nord. Vet. Med. 37:161, 1985.

374. Sweatman, J. C.: Clinical manifestations and treatment of bovine ringworm. Cornell Vet. 37:3, 1947.

375. Tabuchi, K., et al.: Papular dermatitis in pigs. Therapeutic trials against *Aspergillus*. Bull. Azabu Vet. Coll. 11:67, 1963.

376. Takatori, K., et al.: Occurrence of equine dermatophytosis in Hokkaido. Jpn. J. Vet. Sci. 43:307, 1981.

377. Takatori, K., and Hasegawa, A.: Mating experiment of *Microsporum canis* and *M. equinum* isolated from animals with *Nannizzia otae*. Mycopathologia 90:59, 1985.

378. Takatori, K., and Ichijo, S.: Human dermatophytosis caused by *Trichophyton equinum*. Mycopathologia 90:15, 1985.

379. Tanner, A. C., and Quaife, R. A.: *Microsporum gypseum* as the cause of ringworm in a horse. Vet. Rec. 111:396, 1982.

380. Thakur, D. K., et al.: Dermatomycosis in goats in India. Mykosen 25:442, 1981.

381. Thakur, D. K., and Verma, B. B.: A report on *Trichophyton rubrum* infection in a calf. Indian Vet. J. 61:163, 1984.

382. Thomas, S.: Einsatz von Schwetel (sulf. dep) zur Bekampfung der Trichopytie des Rindes. Monat. Vet. Med. 37:451, 1982.

383. Thomsett, L. R.: Laboratory procedures in the diagnosis of equine ringworm. Vet. Dermatol. News. 6:35, 1981.

384. Thomsett, L. R.: Skin diseases of the horse. In Pract. 1:15, 1979.

385. Thorold, P. W.: Equine dermatomycosis in Kenya caused by *Microsporum gypseum*. Vet. Rec. 65:280, 1953.

386. Thorold, P. W.: Equine sporotrichosis. J. S. Afr. Vet. Med. Assoc. 22:81, 1951

386a. Tornquist, M., et al.: Vaccination against ringworm in specialized beef production. Acta Vet. Scand. 26:21, 1985.

387. Tsuji, S., and Kuchii, T.: Ringworm in military horses. Rikugun Jui Dampo 417:138, 1944.

388. Uvarov, O.: Recent advances in the treatment of skin diseases with special reference to griseofulvin. Vet. Rec. 73:258, 1961.

389. Kane, J., et al.: *Microsporium equinum* in North America. J. Clin. Microbiol. 16:943, 1982.

390. Vanbreuseghem, R., et al.: Signification de l'isolement d'une souche de *Keratinomyces ajelloi*, Vanbreuseghem 1952, à partir de l'homme. Arch. Belg. Dermatol. Syphiligr. 12:130, 1956.

391. Viola, C., and Stefanon, G.: Treatment of ringworm of beef calves with trichlorfon (Neguvon). Vet. Bull. 698, 1968.

392. Wawrzkiewicz, K., and Chrol, M.: Treatment and prevention of ringworm in cattle with "Bovitrichovac" vaccine. Med. Weter. 33:337, 1977.

393. Wawrzkiewicz, K., and Zielkowska, G.: Immunological response in guinea pigs and calves infected experimentally with *Trichophyton verrucosum*. Mykosen 22:314, 1979.

394. Wegmann, E.: Trichlorfon treatment of ringworm in horses. Mod. Vet. Pract. 67:636, 1986.

395. Weidman, F. O.: Cutaneous torulosis. Arch. Dermatol. Syphilol. 31:58, 1935.

395a. Weksberg, F., et al.: Unusual tinea corporis caused by *Trichophyton verrucosum*. Intl. J. Dermatol. 25:653, 1986.

396. Woloszyn, S., et al.: Studies on occurrence and control of dermatomycosis in horses. Med. Weter. 32:14, 1976.

CHAPTER 8

PROTOZOAL DISEASES

Protozoa are unicellular animals in whom activities such as metabolism and locomotion are carried out by organelles of the cell.[7, 30, 46] Parasitic protozoa are an important cause of livestock disease in many areas of the world. Some of these protozoal diseases have an associated dermatosis (Table 8–1), but the cutaneous disorders are of minimal importance compared with disorders that involve other organ systems. In this chapter, the cutaneous changes associated with various protozoal diseases of livestock will be characterized. For detailed information on other clinicopathologic, diagnostic, and therapeutic aspects of these diseases, the reader is referred to specific articles in the references.

TRYPANOSOMIASIS

Members of the genus *Trypanosoma* are found in livestock, principally in the blood and tissue fluids, although a few invade tissue cells.[7, 46] They are transmitted by blood-sucking arthropods and insects. Diagnosis is based on demonstrating the trypanosomes (elongated, central or terminal kinetoplast, flagellum, tapered ends, 12 to 35 μm in length and 1 to 3 μm in diameter) in blood or tissue fluids.

T. brucei (*T. pecaudi*) has been reported to cause urticarial plaques over the neck, chest, and flanks of cattle in Africa. Direct smears revealed numerous trypanosomes, and skin biopsy revealed perivascular to diffuse dermatitis, with numerous lymphocytes, histiocytes, and extravascular trypanosomes.[32] *T. congolense* (*T. pecorum, T. nanum*) causes edema of the distal extremities and genitals in horses in Africa.[46] *T. equinum* causes Mal de Caderas in horses in Central and South America, which is characterized by urticarial plaques that become crusted and alopecic over the neck and flanks.[35, 46] *T. evansi* (*T. annamense, T. soudanense*) causes surra (Indian for "rotten")

in horses in Asia and Africa, which is characterized by urticarial lesions over the neck and flanks.[35, 46] *T. vivax* (*T. caprae, T. angolense*) infection of horses in Africa and Central and South America has been associated with urticaria.[46]

T. equiperdum is the cause of dourine (Arabic for "unclean") in horses in Africa, Asia, Southeastern Europe, and Central and South America.[7, 35, 46] The disease is transmitted mainly by coitus. Initial cutaneous changes include edema of the vulva in mares and the prepuce in stallions as well as occasional papules that may ulcerate. Depigmentation may be a striking sequela in these areas. Later, an urticarial eruption appears, which is especially prominent over the neck, chest, flanks, and back. Urticarial plaques are 2 to 10 cm in diameter, wax and wane, and usually have a depressed center. When the urticarial lesions resolve, focal areas of hypo- or hyperhidrosis may persist.

LEISHMANIASIS

Members of the genus *Leishmania* rarely cause disease in livestock.[35, 46] The amastigote

TABLE 8–1. Protozoan Parasites Associated with Skin Lesions in Large Animals

Class: Zoomastigophorea
Order: Kinetoplastida
Family: Trypanosomatidae
Genera: *Trypanosoma*
Leishmania
Class: Sporozoea
Order: Eucoccidiida
Family: Sarcocystidae
Subfamily: Toxoplasmatinae
Genus: *Besnoitia*
Subfamily: Sarcocystinae
Genus: *Sarcocystis*
Order: Piroplasmida
Family: Theileriidae
Genus: *Theileria*

stages (Leishman-Donovan bodies) are found in endothelial cells and cells of the mononuclear phagocytic system. They are circular or oval in shape and 2 to 4 μm in diameter. When the organism is stained with Romanowsky's stains, the cytoplasm is blue, and the oval nucleus is red and lies to one side. At right angles to the nucleus is a kinetoplast that stains red to purple. *Phlebotomus* spp. sandflies are the chief vectors.

Cutaneous leishmaniasis, characterized by nonhealing ulcers with raised edges and depressed granulating centers, has been reported in the horse.[4, 35] Smears revealed numerous Leishman-Donovan bodies.

SARCOCYSTOSIS

Members of the genus *Sarcocystis* are being increasingly recognized as an important cause of disease in cattle.[7, 10, 28, 40, 44, 46] Carnivores (especially dogs and cats) eat beef containing bradyzoites and pass oocysts or sporocysts in their feces. Cattle eat feedstuffs contaminated with carnivore feces, from which sporozoites are released in the intestinal tract and invade many tissues. Schizogony occurs in the endothelial cells of blood vessels in most organs.[18–22, 27] At various times, the cattle parasites have been referred to as *S. blanchardi*, *S. cruzi*, and *S. fusiformis*, but intermediate-to-definitive host names are least confusing and are gaining popularity: *S. bovicanis* (ox to dog) and *S. bovifelis* (ox to cat). At present, only mild or no clinical signs are attributed to *S. bovifelis* infection.

Sarcocystosis (sarcosporidiosis, Dalmeny disease) is believed to affect from 75 to 98 percent of the cattle in the United States[7, 10, 16, 28, 44] and 80 percent of the cattle in Norway,[7, 9, 36] and has been reported in Germany.[8] After an incubation period of about 7 to 28 days, cattle may develop fever, anorexia, lameness, and anemia and may lose weight.* Affected cattle may lose the tail switch (rat-tail) (Fig. 8–1) and develop alopecia of the pinnae and distal extremities. Sarcocystosis may be a cause of poor hair coat and patchy alopecia in goats.[15, 16, 20]

In tissues, basophilic parasitic cysts (few to several millimeters in size) are round, oval, or elongated and are filled with variable numbers of metrocytes and bradyzoites.[19, 27, 28, 33, 46] Me-

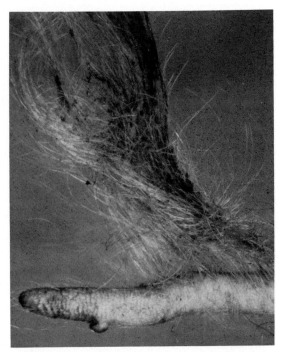

FIGURE 8–1. *Bovine sarcocystosis. "Rat-tailed" appearance is due to loss of switch (Courtesy J. M. King).*

trocytes are densely arranged, round to oval basophilic bodies at the periphery of the cysts, whereas bradyzoites are centrally located and crescentic or banana-shaped. The cysts may be surrounded by degeneration, necrosis, and an infiltration of lymphocytes, histiocytes, and plasma cells.

Experimental studies have suggested that amprolium and salinomycin may have a prophylactic benefit in sarcocystosis in cattle and sheep (Fig. 8–2).[22, 24, 37, 38]

BESNOITIOSIS

Members of the genus *Besnoitia* cause significant disease in cattle, goats, and horses.[7, 46, 51] Infection is acquired by ingesting feedstuffs contaminated with cat feces (*B. besnoiti*), by bites from blood-sucking insects, and by the parenteral injection of blood during the acute stage of infection. The definitive host of *B. bennetti* in the horse is not known.

Besnoitiosis (globidiosis) is reported to affect cattle in Africa, Asia, Southern Europe, and South America.[1, 5–7, 25, 31, 43] After an incubation period of 6 to 10 days, affected cattle develop pyrexia, anorexia, photophobia, generalized lymphadenopathy, and warm, painful swellings on the distal extremities and ven-

---

*References 7, 10, 16, 23, 26, 28, 41, 44, 47

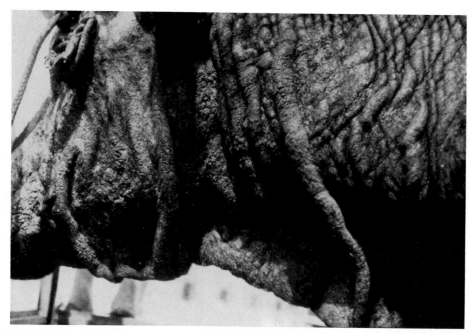

FIGURE 8–2. *Bovine besnoitiosis. Marked alopecia, lichenification, and crusting of face and neck (Courtesy P. Bland).*

trum. The skin then becomes markedly thickened, lichenified, and alopecic and may fissure and ooze (Fig. 8–2). In chronic cases, the skin is markedly scaly and crusty. In goats, besnoitiosis (*B. besnoitii*) ("dimple") is characterized by thickening, lichenification, alopecia, fissuring, and oozing of the skin on the legs, ventrum, and scrotum.[11–13, 34] In addition, subcutaneous papules (about 1 mm in diameter) may be present over the hindquarters. In horses, besnoitiosis (*B. bennetti*) is characterized by generalized thickening, lichenification, alopecia, and scaling.[2, 3, 46, 48] In addition, multiple papules (0.5 to 5 mm in diameter) may be present in the subcutis of the perineal, genital, and abdominal areas.

Skin biopsy reveals parasitic cysts, which appear to develop within fibroblasts.[3, 11, 13, 42, 46] The cysts may be up to 600 μm in diameter and contain numerous crescentic or banana-shaped bradyzoites (2 to 7 μm long). The cysts may be surrounded by degeneration, necrosis, fibrosis, and a mixed inflammatory cell infiltrate.

THEILERIASIS

Members of the genus *Theileria* are an important cause of disease in cattle.[7, 46] The piroplasm stage occurs in erythrocytes and is characterized by forms that are shaped like rods, ovals, commas, and rings and that are 1.5 to 2 μm by 0.5 to 1.0 μm. With Romanowsky's stains, they have a blue cytoplasm with a red chromatin granule at one end. The actively multiplying forms of the parasite that occur chiefly in the cytoplasm of lymphocytes and occasionally in endothelial cells are schizonts (Koch's blue bodies). They are circular or irregularly shaped and are 2 to 12 μm in diameter. With Romanowsky's stains, the schizonts have a blue cytoplasm and a variable number of red chromatin granules. Transmission occurs via ticks. Diagnosis is based on demonstrating the parasites in blood, lymph nodes, and tissue fluids.

T. parva is the cause of East Coast fever or bovine theileriasis in cattle in Africa.[7, 46] The disease may be associated with the development of papules and nodules containing numerous theilerial schizonts over the neck and trunk as well as demodicosis.[50] *T. annulata* is a cause of bovine theileriasis in Asia, Southern Europe, and Northern Africa.[46] Cutaneous lesions may be seen and include wheals or papules (0.1 to 0.5 cm in diameter), which begin on the face, neck, and shoulders and then become generalized.[17, 29, 39, 45, 49] The lesions are very firm, and pruritus may be intense. Numerous schizonts are found in smears from the lesions, and skin biopsy reveals a diffuse neutrophilic dermatitis with central necrosis and hemorrhage.

REFERENCES

1. Basson, P. A., et al.: Observations on the pathogenesis of bovine and antelope stains of *Besnoitia besnoitti* (Marotel, 1912) infection in cattle and rabbits. Onderstepoort J. Vet. Res. 37:105, 1970.
2. Bennett, S. C. J.: A peculiar equine sarcosporidium in the Anglo-Egyptian Sudan. Vet. J. 83:297, 1927.
3. Bennett, S. C. J.: *Globidium* infections in the Sudan. J. Comp. Pathol. Ther. 46:1, 1933.
4. Bennett, S. C. J.: Equine cutaneous leishmaniasis: Treatment with berberine sulphate. J. Comp. Pathol. Ther. 48:241, 1935.
5. Besnoit, C., and Robin, V.: Sarcosporidiose cutanée chez une vache. Rec. Med. Vet 90:327, 1913.
6. Bigalke, R. D., et al.: Studies in cattle on the development of a live vaccine against bovine besnoitiosis. J. S. Afr. Vet. Med. Assoc. 45:207, 1974.
7. Blood, D. C., et al.: *Veterinary Medicine VI*. London, Baillière Tindall, 1983.
8. Boch, J. K. E., et al.: Drei Sarkosporidienarten bei Schlachtrindern in Suddeutschland. Berl. Munch. Tierarztl. Wochenschr. 91:426, 1978.
9. Bratberg, B., and Landverk, T.: Sarcocystis infection and myocardial pathological changes in cattle from south-eastern Norway. Acta Vet. Scand. 21:395, 1980.
10. Briggs, M., and Foreyt, W.: Sarcocystosis in cattle. Compend. Cont. Educ. 7:S396, 1985.
11. Bwangamoi, O.: A preliminary report on the finding of *Besnoitia besnoitii* in goat skins affected with dimple in Kenya. Bull. Epizoot. Dis. Afr. 15:263, 1967.
12. Bwangamoi, O.: Besnoitiosis and other skin diseases of cattle (*Bos indicus*) in Uganda. Am. J. Vet. Res. 29:737, 1968.
13. Cheema, A. H., and Toofanian, F.: Besnoitiosis in wild and domestic goats in Iran. Cornell Vet. 69:159, 1979.
14. Collins, G. H., and Crawford, S. J. S.: Sarcocystosis in goats: Prevalence and transmission. N.Z. Vet. J. 26:288, 1970.
15. Collins, G. H., and Charleston, W. A. G.: Studies on *Sarcocystis* species. IV. A species infecting dogs and goats: Development in goats. N.Z. Vet. J. 27:260, 1979.
16. Corner, A. H., et al.: Dalmeny disease. An infection of cattle presumed to be caused by an unidentified protozoan. Can. Vet. J. 4:252, 1963.
17. Deore, P. A., et al.: A case of cutaneous theileriasis in a graded calf. Indian Vet. J. 56:794, 1979.
18. Dubey, J. P.: A review of *Sarcocystis* of domestic animals and of other coccidia of cats and dogs. JAVMA 169:1061, 1976.
19. Dubey, J. P., et al.: Sarcocystosis in newborn calves fed *Sarcocystis cruzi* sporocysts from coyotes. Am. J. Vet. Res. 43:2147, 1982.
20. Dubey, J. P., et al.: Sarcocytosis in goats: Clinical signs and pathologic and hematologic findings. JAVMA 178:683, 1981.
21. Fayer, R., and Johnson, A. J.: Development of *Sarcocystis fusiformis* in calves infected with sporocysts from dogs. J. Parasitol. 59:1135, 1973.
22. Fayer, R., and Johnson, A. J.: Effect of amprolium on acute sarcocystosis in experimentally infected calves. J. Parasitol. 61:932, 1975.
23. Fayer, R., et al.: Abortion and other signs of disease in cows experimentally infected with *Sarcocystis fusiformis* from dogs. J. Infect. Dis. 134:624, 1976.
24. Foreyt, W.: Evaluation of decoquinate, lasalocid, and monensin against experimentally induced sarcocystosis in calves. Am. J. Vet. Res. 47:1674, 1986.
25. Frank, M., et al.: Prevalence of antibodies against *Besnoitia besnoiti* in beef and dairy cattle in Israel. Refuah Vet. 34:83, 1977.
26. Frelier, P. I. G., et al.: Sarcocystosis: A clinical outbreak in dairy calves. Science 195:1341, 1977.
27. Frelier, P. I. G., et al.: Bovine sarcocystosis: Pathological features of naturally occurring infection. Am. J. Vet. Res. 40:651, 1979.
28. Giles, R. C., et al.: Sarcocystosis in cattle in Kentucky. JAVMA 176:543, 1980.
29. Grimpet, J.: Symptômes cutanés de la theileriose bovine. Bull. Acad. Vet. Fr. 26:535, 1953.
30. Howard, J. L.: *Current Veterinary Therapy. Food Animal Practice II*. Philadelphia, W. B. Saunders Co., 1986.
31. Hussein, M. F., and Haroun, E. M.: Bovine besnoitiosis in the Sudan: A case report. Br. Vet. J. 131:85, 1975.
32. Ikede, B. O., and Losos, G. T.: Pathological changes in cattle infected with *Trypanosoma brucei*. Vet. Pathol. 9:272, 1972.
33. Johnson, A. J., et al.: Experimentally induced sarcocystis infection in calves: Pathology. Am. J. Vet. Res. 36:995, 1975.
34. Kaliner, G.: Vorkommen von Besnoitien zysten in Ziegenlunge. Berl. Munch. Tierarztl. Wochenschr. 86:229, 1973.
35. Kral, F., and Schwartzman, R. M.: *Veterinary and Comparative Dermatology*. Philadelphia, J. B. Lippincott Co., 1964.
36. Landsverk, T.: An outbreak of sarcocystosis in a cattle herd. Acta Vet. Scand. 20:238, 1979.
37. Leek, R. G., and Fayer, R.: Amprolium for prophylaxis of ovine sarcocystosis. J. Parasitol. 66:100, 1980.
38. Leek, R. G., and Fayer, R.: Experimental *Sarcocystis ovicanis* infection in lambs: Salinomycin chemoprophylaxis and protective immunity. J. Parasitol. 69:271, 1983.
39. Manickam, R., et al.: Histopathology of cutaneous lesions in *Theileria annulata* infection of calves. Indian Vet. J. 61:13, 1984.
40. Markus, M. B.: *Sarcocystis* and sarcocystosis in domestic animals and man. Adv. Vet. Sci. 22:159, 1978.
41. Meads, E. B.: Dalmeny disease—another outbreak—probably sarcocystosis. Can. Vet. J. 17:271, 1976.
42. Neuman, M., and Nobel, T. A.: Observations on the pathology of besnoitiosis in experimental animals. Zbl. Vet. Med. B28:345, 1981.
43. Pols, J. W.: Studies on bovine besnoitiosis with special reference to the aetiology. Onderstepoort J. Vet. Res. 28:265, 1960.
44. Sanders, D. E.: Sarcocystosis in cattle: An emerging disease. Mod. Vet. Pract. 66:599, 1985.
45. Shastri, U. V., et al.: Cutaneous lesions and some other unusual findings in cases of theileriosis in graded calves. Indian Vet. J. 59:188, 1982.
46. Soulsby, E. J. L.: *Helminths, Arthropods and Protozoa of Domesticated Animals VII*. London, Baillière Tindall, 1982.
47. Stalheim, O. H. V.: Update of bovine toxoplasmosis and sarcocystosis with emphasis on their role in bovine abortion. JAVMA 176:299, 1980.
48. Terrell, T. G., and Stookey, J. L.: *Besnoitia besnoiti* in two Mexican burros. Vet. Pathol. 10:177, 1973.
49. Tsur-Tchernomoretz, I., et al.: Two cases in bovine theileriasis (*Th. annulata*) with cutaneous lesions. Refuah Vet. 17:100, 1960.
50. Uilenberg, G., and Zwart, D.: Skin nodules in East Coast fever. Res. Vet. Sci. 26:243, 1979.
51. Wallace, G. D., and Frenkel, J. K.: *Besnoitia* species (Protozoa, Sporozoa, Toxoplasmatidae): Recognition of cyclic transmission by cats. Science 188:369, 1975.

CHAPTER 9

PARASITIC DISEASES

Dermatoses caused by ectoparasites are the most common skin disorders of large animals.* Animal suffering—through annoyance, irritability, pruritus, disfigurement, secondary infections, and myiasis—is often great. Decreased food intake, resulting in decreased weight gains or in weight loss; decreased milk production; hide damage; wool loss; difficulties in estrus detection; death; and the financial burdens of diagnostic, therapeutic, or preventive programs can lead to astronomic economic losses. In addition, many of the ectoparasites are important in the transmission of various viral, protozoal, helminthic, fungal, and bacterial diseases. The important arachnids, insects, and helminths associated with skin disease in large animals are listed in Tables 9–1 through 9–3.

The treatment of ectoparasitism is a complex topic.[348, 396, 440] Significant differences exist in the regional availability of, and regulations governing, parasiticidal agents. Species and age differences (e.g., most organophosphates are not recommended for animals younger than three to four months of age) must be considered. In addition, the veterinarian must be knowledgeable about the restrictions on the use of such agents regarding (1) meat and milk withdrawal times, (2) use in pregnant animals, (3) use in lactating animals, and (4) use in breeding animals. Some general guidelines for the treatment of ectoparasitisms are presented in Tables 9–4 through 9–7.

MITES

Psoroptic Mange

Psoroptic mange (common scab, body mange) is a devastating pruritic dermatitis of cattle and sheep in many areas of the world and a rather frequent cause of otitis externa in goats and horses.

Cause and Pathogenesis

Psoroptes spp. mites (0.4 to 0.8 mm long) are nonburrowing and feed on tissue fluids.* Their life cycle on the host is completed in 10 to 12 days. The mites are capable of surviving off the host for up to two weeks under many environmental conditions. It has been recommended that infected premises be evacuated for at least two weeks when appropriate decontamination procedures cannot be instituted.[459, 774, 849] *P. ovis* and *P. cuniculi* were maintained under various environmental conditions, off animals, for up to 48 and 84 days, respectively.[429] The researchers suggested stable quarantine periods of 7 and 12 weeks, respectively. Transmission is by direct and indirect contact. The incubation period varies from two to eight weeks. In experimentally infested cattle, specific serum antibody against *P. ovis* was detected when skin lesions became visible, and levels increased as mite numbers and lesion severity grew.[264, 265]

The classification of *Psoroptes* spp. mites is apparently in a state of disarray. Most authors agree that (1) *P. ovis* is the cause of body mange in cattle and sheep, (2) *P. equi* is the cause of body mange in the horse, (3) *P. cuniculi* is an ear mite in the horse, goat, sheep, and rabbit, and (4) *P. natalensis* affects cattle in South Africa and South America.[63, 478, 644, 734, 771] Others espouse the controversial opinion that *P. caprae* (ears and body of goats) and *P. hippotis* (ears of horses) are separate species.[406, 434, 517, 734] Another area of controversy is the long-held host specificity of these mites.[459, 734] Workers in the United States and

---

*References 14, 80, 112–114, 118, 120, 123, 134, 221, 282, 299–301, 343, 347, 360, 420, 437, 455, 459, 464, 469, 575–578, 584

---

*References 14, 63, 80, 184, 211, 259, 260, 360, 437, 459, 478–481, 497, 715, 734, 771, 774, 849, 858–862

TABLE 9–1. Arachnids Associated with Skin Disease in Large Animals

Class: Arachnida
  Order: Acarina
    Suborder: Sarcoptiformes
      Family: Sarcoptidae
        Sarcoptes scabiei var. *bovis*
        S. scabiei var. *caprae*
        S. scabiei var. *equi*
        S. scabiei var. *ovis*
        S. scabiei var. *suis*

      Family: Psoroptidae
        Psoroptes cuniculi (horse, goat, sheep)
        P. caprae (goat)
        P. equi (horse)
        P. hippotis (horse)
        P. natalensis (cow)
        P. ovis (cow, sheep)
        Chorioptes bovis (cow)
        C. caprae (goat)
        C. equi (horse)
        C. ovis (sheep)
        C. texanus (goat)

      Family: Acaridae
        Acarus farinae
        Caloglyphus berlesei

    Suborder: Trombidiformes
      Family: Trombiculidae
        Euschoengastia latchmani
        Neoschoengastia americana
        Trombicula alfreddugési
        T. autumnalis
        T. sarcina

      Family: Pediculoididae
        Pediculoides ventricosus

      Family: Demodicidae
        Demodex bovis (cow)
        D. caballi
        D. caprae (goat)
        D. equi (horse)
        D. ghanensis (cow)
        D. ovis (sheep)
        D. phylloides (pig)
        Demodex sp. (cow)

      Family: Cheyletidae
        Psorergates bos (cow)
        P. ovis (sheep)

    Suborder: Mesostigmata
      Family: Dermanyssidae
        Dermanyssus gallinae

      Family: Gamasidae
        Raillietia auris (cow)
        R. caprae (goat)
        R. manfredi (goat)

    Suborder: Ixodoidea
      Family: Argasidae
        *Otobius megnini** (North and South America, Africa)
        *Ornithodorus coriaceus** (North America)
        O. lahorensis (Asia)
        O. moubata (Africa)
        O. porcinus (Africa)
        O. savignyi (Africa, Near East)
      Family: Ixodidae
        Ixodes ricinus (Europe, Africa, Asia)
        I. persulcatus (Europe, Asia)
        I. canisuga (Britain)
        I. pilosus (Africa)
        I. rubicundus (Africa)
        *I. scapularis** (North America)
        *I. cookei** (North America)
        *I. pacificus** (North America)
        I. holocyclus (Australia)
        Boophilus annulatus (Central America, Africa)
        B. microplus (Central and South America, Australia, Africa, Asia)
        B. calcaratus (Africa)
        B. decoloratus (Africa)

        Margaropus winthemi (Europe, Asia, Africa)

        Hyalomma plumbeum (Europe, Asia, Africa)
        H. excavatum (Europe, Asia, Africa)

        Rhipicephalus appendiculatus (Africa)
        R. capensis (Africa)
        R. neavei (Africa)
        R. jeanelli (Africa)
        R. ayrei (Africa)
        R. pulchellus (Africa)
        *R. sanguineus** (cosmopolitan)
        R. evertsi (Africa)
        R. bursa (Europe)

        Haemaphysalis leachi (Africa, Asia, Australia)
        H. cinnabarina (Africa, Asia, Europe)
        H. longicornis (Asia, Australia, New Zealand)
        H. bancrofti (Australia)

        Dermacentor reticulatus (Europe)
        D. marginatus (Africa, Asia)
        *D. andersoni** (North America)
        *D. variabilis** (North America)
        *D. nitens** (North, Central, and South America)
        *D. albipictus** (North America)
        *D. occidentalis** (North America)
        D. nigrolineatus (North America)

        Amblyomma hebraeum (Africa)
        A. gemma (Africa)
        A. variegatum (Africa)
        *A. americanum** (North America)
        *A. cajennense** (North, Central, and South America)
        *A. maculatum** (North America)
  Order: Araneidea
  Spiders

*Ticks recovered from large animals in the United States

TABLE 9–2. Insects Associated with Skin Disease in Large Animals

Class: Insecta
  Subclass: Pterygota
    Division: Exopterygota
      Order: Mallophaga
          Damalinia bovis (cow)
          D. caprae (goat)
          D. crassipes (goat)
          D. equi (horse)
          D. limbata (goat)
          Bovicola painei (goat)
      Order: Siphunculata
        Family: Haematopinidae
          Haematopinus asini (horse)
          H. eurysternus (cow)
          H. quadripertusus (cow)
          H. suis (pig)
        Family: Linognathidae
          Linognathus africanus (sheep, goat)
          L. ovillus (sheep)
          L. pedalis (sheep)
          L. stenopsis (goat)
          L. vituli (cow)
          Solenopotes capillatus (cow)
    Division: Endopterygota
      Order: Siphonaptera
          Ctenocephalides canis
          C. felis
          Echidnophaga gallinacea
          Pulex irritans
          Tunga penetrans
          Vermipsylla spp.
      Order: Diptera
        Suborder: Nematocera
          Family: Culicidae
          Aedes spp.
          Anopheles spp.
          Culex spp.
          Culicoides spp.

          Family: Simuliidae
          Simulium spp.
        Suborder: Brachycera
          Family: Tabanidae
          Tabanus spp.
          Haematopota spp.
          Chrysops spp.
        Suborder: Cyclorrhapha
          Family: Gasterophilidae
          Gasterophilus spp.
          Family: Muscidae
          Musca spp.
          Stomoxys calcitrans
          Hydrotaea spp.
          Haematobia spp.
          Family: Calliphoridae
          Subfamily: Calliphorinae
          Calliphora spp.
          Chrysomyia spp.
          Phormia spp.
          Callitroga spp.
          Booponus intonsus
          Auchmeromyia luteola
          Subfamily: Sarcophaginae
          Sarcophaga spp.
          Wohlfahrtia spp.
          Family: Oestridae
          Hypoderma bovis (cow, horse)
          H. lineatum (cow, horse)
          Przhevalskiana silenus (goat, sheep)
          Family: Cuterebridae
          Dermatobia hominis
          Cuterebra spp.
          Family: Hippoboscidae
          Hippobosca spp.
          Melophagus ovinus
      Order: Hymenoptera
      Bees and Wasps

TABLE 9–3. Helminths Associated with Skin Disease in Large Animals

Class: Nematoda
  Order: Ascaridida
    Superfamily: Oxyuroidea
      Family: Oxyuridae
         Oxyuris equi (horse)
  Order: Rhabditida
    Superfamily: Rhabditoidea
      Family: Rhabditidae
         Pelodera strongyloides (horse, cow, sheep)
         Rhabditis bovis (cow)
  Order: Strongylida
    Superfamily: Strongyloidea
      Family: Strongyloididae
         Strongyloides papillosus (sheep, goat)
         S. westeri (horse)
    Superfamily: Ancylostomatoidea
      Family: Ancylostomatidae
         Bunostomum trigonocephalum (sheep)
         B. phlebotomum (cow)
    Superfamily: Metastrongyloidea
      Family: Protostrongylidae
         Parelaphostrongylus tenuis (goat)
  Order: Spirurida
    Superfamily: Spiruroidea
      Family: Spiruridae

         Habronema muscae (horse)
         H. majus (horse)
         Draschia megastoma (horse)
    Superfamily: Filarioidea
      Family: Filariidae
         Suifilaria suis (pig)
         Parafilaria bovicola (cow)
         P. multipapillosa (horse)
         Elaeophora schneideri (sheep)
      Family: Setariidae
         Stephanofilaria assamensis (cow, goat)
         S. dedoesi (cow, goat)
         S. kaeli (cow, goat)
         S. okinawaensis (cow)
         S. stilesi (cow)
      Family: Onchocercidae
         Onchocerca cervicalis (horse)
         O. gibsoni (cow, horse)
         O. gutturosa (cow, horse)
         O. ochengi (cow)
         O. reticulata (horse)
    Superfamily: Dracunculoidea
      Family: Dracunculidae
         Dracunculus insignis (cow, horse)
         D. medinensis (horse, cow)

TABLE 9–4. Guidelines for Treatment of External Parasites of Horses*

Chemical	Concentration/Form	Parasites Affected†
Coumaphos	0.06% spray; 1% dust	F, L, T
Dioxathion	0.15% spray	F, L, M, T
Ivermectin	200–300 µg/kg PO‡	H, O
Lime sulfur	2–5% spray/dip	L, M
Lindane	0.03% spray/dip	L, M, T
Malathion	0.5% spray/dip; 5% dust	F, L, M, T
Methoxychlor	0.5% spray/dip	F, L, M, T
Stirofos	1% spray	F, L, M, T

*Read all product labels closely for appropriate use of product and safety precautions.
†F, flies; H, habronemiasis; L, lice; M, mites; O, onchocerciasis; T, ticks
‡PO, orally

TABLE 9–5. Guidelines for Treatment of External Parasites of Cattle*

Chemical	Concentration/Form	Parasites Affected†
Coumaphos	0.125–0.3% spray/dip	F, L, M, T, W
Crotoxyphos	0.25–1% spray; 3% dust	F, L, W
Dioxathion	0.15% spray/dip	F, L, T
Famphur	1% dust	F, L, W
Fenthion	20% pour-on	F, L, W
Fenvalerate	0.05% spray; 8% ear tag	F, L, T
Flucythrinate	7.5% ear tag	F, T
Ivermectin	200–300 µg/kg PO or SCI‡	M, P, W
Lime sulfur	2–5% spray/dip	M
Lindane	0.03–0.06% spray/dip	L, M, T
Malathion	0.5% spray; 5% dust	F, L, M, T
Methoxychlor	0.5% spray; 10% dust; 0.2–0.25% dip	F, L, M, T
Permethrin	0.015% spray; 0.25% dust; 10% ear tag	F, T
Phosmet	20% pour-on	F, L, M, T, W
Stirofos	0.35% spray; 3% dust	F, L, T
Trichlorfon	0.2% spray/dip	L, M, T, W

*Read all product labels closely for appropriate use of product and safety precautions.
†F, flies; L, lice; M, mites; P, parafilariasis; T, ticks; W, warbles
‡PO, orally; SCI, subcutaneous injection

TABLE 9–6. Guidelines for Treatment of External Parasites of Swine*

Chemical	Concentration/Form	Parasites Affected†
Amitraz	0.05–0.1% spray/dip	L, M, T
Ciodrin	0.25% spray	L
Coumaphos	0.06–0.12% spray; 1% dust	L, M, T
Diazinon	0.05% spray	L, M
Dioxathion	0.15% spray/dip	L, T
Fenchlorphos	0.0014% spray	L, M
Ivermectin	300 µg/kg SCI or PO‡	L, M
Lime sulfur	2–5% spray/dip	M
Lindane	0.06% spray/dip	L, M, T
Malathion	0.5% spray	L, M, T
Phosmet	20% pour-on	M
Trichlorfon	0.125% spray	L, M

*Read all product labels closely for appropriate use of product and safety precautions.
†L, lice; M, mites; T, ticks
‡SCI, subcutaneous injection; PO, orally

TABLE 9–7. Guidelines for Treatment of External Parasites of Sheep and Goats*

Chemical	Concentration/Form	Parasites Affected†
Amitraz	250 ppm dip	M
Chlorfenvinphos	0.05–0.1% spray	K, L, T
Chlorpyrifos	0.05–0.25% spray	K, L, T
Coumaphos	0.05–0.3% spray/dip; 0.5–1% dust	K, L, T
Crotoxyphos	0.1–0.25% spray/dip; 3% dust	K, L, M, T
Diazinon	0.03–0.1% spray/dip	K, L, M
Dioxathion	0.15% spray/dip	K, L
Fenvalerate	0.025% spray; 10% water-dispersible liquid	K, L
Lime sulfur	2–5% dip	K, L, M
Lindane	0.03–0.05% spray; 0.03% dip	K, L, M, T
Malathion	0.5% spray; 5% dust	K, L, M, T
Methoxychlor	0.5% spray/dip; 5% dust	K, L, M, T
Phosmet	0.15–0.25% spray/dip	K, L, M
Trichlorfon	0.2% spray/dip	K, L, M

*Read all product labels closely for appropriate use of product and safety precautions.
†K, keds; L, lice; M, mites; T, ticks

West Germany have shown that *P. ovis* isolated from cattle or sheep can easily produce lasting infestations when applied to either species.[63, 432, 476, 478, 644, 849] In addition, psoroptic mites isolated from cattle were used to produce skin disease in rabbits,[476] and psoroptic mites were transmitted from rabbits and goats to sheep.[771] Psoroptic mites do not affect humans.

In cattle and sheep, *P. ovis* populations are usually much smaller in spring and summer.* In spring and summer, smaller mite populations reside in body folds, especially in the perineum, inguinal region, and interdigital areas. Thus, clinical signs are most severe in fall and winter. Interestingly, it has been shown that cattle that are restrained from grooming develop high mite populations and clinical signs in summer.[304]

CLINICAL FEATURES

In cattle, psoroptic mange is worldwide in occurrence.† In the United States, it is especially common in the western and central states. There are no apparent age, breed, or sex predilections. The primary clinical sign is intense pruritus, which often begins on the shoulders and rump. Nonfollicular papules and pustules, crusts, excoriations, alopecia, and lichenification are seen. Generalized skin involvement and secondary infections are common. Severely infested cattle develop a mild anemia and lymphopenia, marked neutro-

penia, variable eosinophilia, and increased fibrinogen and gamma globulin levels.[760a]

In sheep, psoroptic mange occurs in many parts of the world.* In the United States, ovine psoroptic mange was thought to have been eradicated in the early 1970s. However, anecdotal reports suggest that it still occurs.[578] There are no apparent age, breed, or sex predilections. The chief clinical sign is intense pruritus, which usually begins over the trunk and rump. Yellowish, nonfollicular pustules develop into yellow crusts, and the fleece becomes characteristically moist and matted over the crusts. The crusts then darken and lift away from the skin with any wool that has not already been rubbed off. Affected sheep are often hyperesthetic and "mouth" characteristically when touched, and some will roll on the ground. *P. cuniculi* is an occasional cause of ear mites in sheep.[866]

In goats in North America, Australia, New Zealand, Europe, India, and Africa, *P. cuniculi* (and possibly *P. caprae*) is very commonly found in the ears.† There are no apparent age, breed, or sex predilections. Many affected goats appear to be clinically normal, whereas others show head shaking, ear scratching, and variable degrees of excessive cerumen accumulation or crusts and alopecia on the pinnae. Severe infestations may result in otitis media or otitis interna and yellowish-brown crusts (Fig. 9–1) over the poll, face, pasterns, and interdigital areas.

*References 14, 211, 261, 306, 437, 459, 478, 497, 643, 735, 774
†References 14, 80, 240, 353, 406, 428, 432, 478, 497, 604

*References 21, 26, 80, 95, 211, 212, 267, 360, 406, 437. 459, 597, 620, 659, 660, 735, 774, 851
†References 98, 164, 434, 455, 498, 517, 730, 731, 771. 782, 810, 847, 866

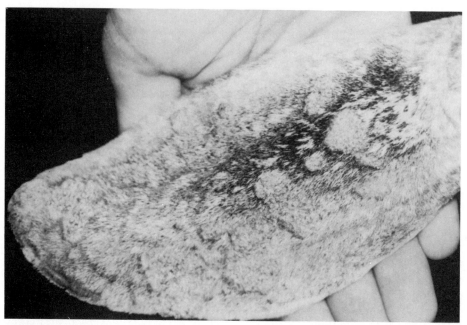

FIGURE 9–1. Marked crusting and alopecia on the pinna of a goat with psoroptic mange.

In horses in North America, Great Britain, and Australia, *P. cuniculi* (and possibly *P. hippotis*) are commonly found in the ears.* *P. equi* causes body mange in horses.[244, 245a, 353, 406, 469, 586, 734] There are no apparent age, breed, or sex predilections. Horses infested with *P. cuniculi (hippotis)* may be clinically normal or may show variable degrees of head shaking and ear scratching and rubbing and may have a lop-eared appearance. Horses infested with *P. equi* manifest intense pruritus, nonfollicular papules, crusts, scales, excoriations, and alopecia, especially affecting the ears, mane, and tail.

DIAGNOSIS

The differential diagnosis includes sarcoptic mange, chorioptic mange, psorergatic mange, lice, keds, and fly-bite dermatitis. Definitive diagnosis is based on history, physical examination, skin scrapings, and otoscopic examination. Body mites are usually easily demonstrated in skin scrapings (Figs. 9–2 and 9–3). Ear mites can be very difficult to demonstrate without a thorough otoscopic examination (usually requires chemical restraint) and microscopic examination of material gathered from deep within the ear canal. Skin biopsy

reveals varying degrees of superficial perivascular dermatitis with numerous eosinophils.[760] Eosinophilic microabscesses and focal areas of epidermal edema, leukocytic exocytosis, and necrosis (epidermal "nibbles") may be found. Mites are rarely seen.

CLINICAL MANAGEMENT

Psoroptic mange in cattle and sheep is often a devastating disease. Intense, unremitting pruritus results in annoyance, irritability, decreased food intake, decreased weight gains or weight loss, decreased milk production, hide damage, wool loss, difficulties in estrus detection, secondary infections and myiasis, increased susceptibility to other diseases, and even death.* In the United States, bovine and ovine psoroptic mange are reportable diseases.

The factors that complicate the detection and control of psoroptic mange in cattle and sheep are complex and include (1) complacency in detecting and reporting the disease, (2) infested animals' moving undetected through market channels, (3) changes in the intensity and complexity of the cattle-feeding industry, (4) inadequate treatment (increased use of systemic organophosphates, which are not as effective as lindane and toxaphene), (5)

*References 23, 245, 344, 364, 442, 493, 582–584, 639, 700, 734

*References 14, 62, 80, 146, 346, 360, 394, 437, 459, 478, 497, 748, 774, 792

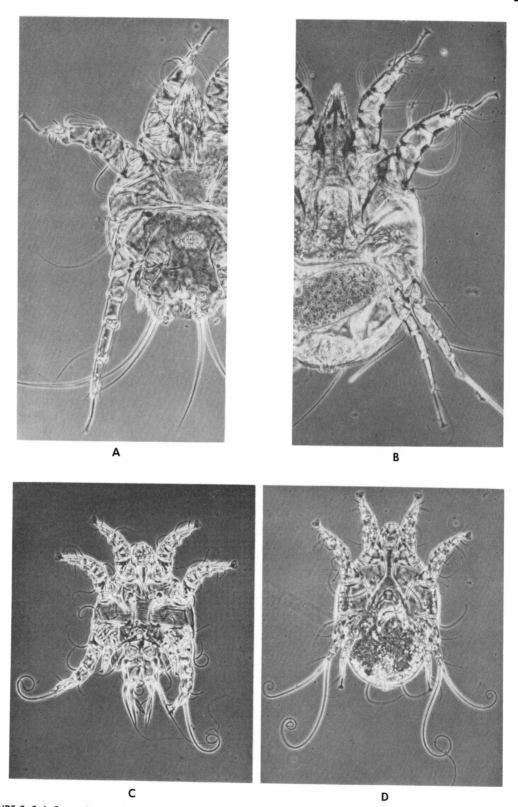

A

B

C

D

FIGURE 9–2. A, Psoroptes, *male* (× *100*). B, Psoroptes, *female* (× *100*). C, Chorioptes, *male* (× *100*). D, Chorioptes, *female* (× *100*). (With permission from Georgi, J. R.: Parasitology for Veterinarians, 3rd ed. Philadelphia, W. B. Saunders Co., 1980, p. 59.)

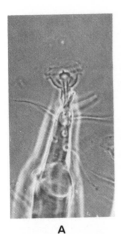 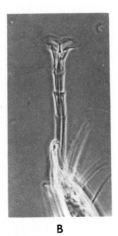

A   **B**

FIGURE 9–3. Sarcoptiform pretarsi (pedicle plus caruncle equals pretarsus). A, Otodectes, pretarsus with short pedicle (Chorioptes pretarsi also have short pedicles). B, Psoroptes, pretarsus with long jointed pedicle. (With permission from Georgi, J. R.: Parasitology for Veterinarians, 3rd ed. Philadephia, W. B. Saunders Co., 1980, p. 57.)

the addition to the list of USDA-permitted dips of acaricides that are known not to eradicate mites on a single dipping, (6) misinterpretation of summertime remissions as cures, (7) the influence of substandard, partially effective, off-season, and unauthorized treatments, and (8) the developing resistance of some mite populations to various acaricides.* All animals that have come into contact with infected animals and all exposed animals should be treated.

In cattle in the United States, one recognized method of treatment for psoroptic mange is spray-dipping or vat-dipping. Vat-dipping is essentially impossible in the Northeast. Only three approved dips are listed by the USDA: (1) 0.3 percent coumaphos (two dippings essential; no withholding period prior to slaughter), (2) 0.20 to 0.25 percent phosmet (two dippings essential), and (3) 2.0 percent hot lime sulfur (essentially reserved for use on lactating dairy cattle; no milk residue; three times at ten-day intervals). The state regulatory agency and the manufacturer's label for the treatment product should be consulted to learn precise directions for use, precautions, intervals between dippings and slaughter, and so forth.[345, 346, 497, 520]

Ivermectin has been shown to be very effective in the treatment of bovine psoroptic mange and has been approved by the U.S. Department of Agriculture for use in the national eradication program.* A single subcutaneous injection of 200 μg/kg has been shown to result in a rapid decrease in live mites and egg counts and a complete absence of all mites and eggs 20 days after treatment.[416, 480, 481, 861, 862] However, surviving mites on ivermectin-treated cattle are infectious for at least fourteen days after treatment.[305, 481, 759a, 862] Ivermectin is generally a safe drug in cattle, having no teratogenic effects and no effect on breeding performance or semen quality in bulls. Rare toxicities include acute esophagitis and posterior paresis, resulting from the death of the first instar of *Hypoderma lineatum* in the esophagus and *H. bovis* in the spinal canal, respectively. There is a 35-day withholding period before slaughter. Withdrawal times in milk have not been established; therefore, the drug should not be used in female dairy cattle of breeding age. Amitraz has been reported to be effective in bovine psoroptic mange[192] but is not approved in the United States.

In sheep, the only recognized method of treatment for psoroptic mange is vat-dipping (one-minute immersion). State-approved acaricides and quarantine procedures should be employed. Dipping is most effective if done within two weeks after shearing and must be repeated in 10 to 14 days.† Acaricides reported to be effective include 0.3 percent coumaphos, 0.15 to 0.25 percent phosmet, 0.03 to 0.1 percent diazinon, 2.0 percent hot lime sulfur, and 125 ppm propetamphos.

For years, lindane was the preferred dip for ovine psoroptic mange, but environmental considerations have curtailed its use in many parts of the world.[212, 360, 437, 459] In addition, the use of lindane in some countries has been accompanied by the development of resistant strains of *P. ovis*.[26, 412, 413, 459, 659, 660] *P. ovis* strains resistant to organophosphates have also been reported.[95, 660] Amitraz has been reported to be effective where organochlorine or organophosphate resistance was seen.[95, 459]

An investigative approach to the therapy for ovine psoroptic mange has involved the use of

---

*References 297, 346, 437, 459, 477, 478, 497, 520, 647, 735, 812

*References 51, 240, 305, 432, 480, 481, 604, 759a, 861, 862

†References 80, 90, 267, 360, 393, 395, 437, 459, 578, 597, 646, 660, 757, 758

drying agents.[314, 459] Mixtures of zinc and aluminum oxides applied topically reduce the moisture content of fleece by 30 percent for 10 to 12 weeks. In addition, such applications have been shown to reduce significantly the incidence of fleece rot and blowfly strike. This approach also has the advantage of not creating resistant strains of mites.

Considering the efficacy of ivermectin in bovine psoroptic mange (see earlier), it would appear that an evaluation of this drug in ovine psoroptic mange is also warranted.

In goats, psoroptic ear mites have been successfully treated with commercial otic preparations used in the treatment of ear mites in dogs and cats.[455, 730, 731] Examples include one part rotenone (Canex) in three parts mineral oil and thiabendazole (Tresaderm). Ears should be thoroughly cleaned, if possible, and treated twice weekly for three weeks with the otic acaricide. When cutaneous lesions are present as well, total body dips or sprays (at least twice, at a 14-day interval) with 0.25 percent crotoxyphos, 0.25 percent coumaphos, 0.2 percent trichlorfon, 0.5 percent malathion, and 2 percent lime sulfur are effective. Based on the efficacy of ivermectin in bovine psoroptic mange (see preceding), this drug may also prove to be useful in caprine psoroptic mange.

In horses, psoroptic ear mites have been successfully treated with numerous organochlorine and organophosphate otic preparations.[406, 442, 584, 700] Rotenone (Canex) in mineral oil is also effective. Ears should be thoroughly cleaned, if possible, and treated twice weekly for three weeks with the otic acaricide. When psoroptic body mange is present, total body dips or high-powered sprays (80 to 100 pounds per square inch) with 0.5 percent malathion, 0.06 percent coumaphos, 0.5 percent methoxychlor, and 0.03 percent lindane are effective when applied at least twice, at 14-day intervals.[244, 406, 440, 469, 584, 586] Lime sulfur (2 percent) is also effective but may require weekly application for three to four weeks. Based on the efficacy of ivermectin in bovine psoroptic mange (see preceding), this drug may also prove to be effective in equine psoroptic mange. In fact, ivermectin (200 μg/kg given subcutaneously) was reported to cure psoroptic mange in donkeys (*P. equi* infestation).[2a]

Amitraz appears to be an unacceptable acaricide for use in horses. Horses sprayed with 0.025 percent amitraz developed somnolence, depression, ataxia, muscular weakness, and progressive large intestinal impaction

beginning within 24 to 48 hours of treatment.[25, 584, 652, 652a]

Sarcoptic Mange

Sarcoptic mange (barn itch, scabies, head mange) is a common cause of pruritic dermatitis in swine, cattle, goats, and, rarely, sheep and horses.

CAUSE AND PATHOGENESIS

Sarcoptes spp. mites (0.25 to 0.6 mm in diameter) tunnel through the epidermis and feed on tissue fluids and possibly epidermal cells.* The life cycle on the host is completed in two to three weeks. The mites are quite susceptible to drying and survive only a few days off the host. Transmission is by direct and indirect contact. The incubation period varies from a few hours to several weeks, depending on the method and severity of exposure and on prior sensitization of the host.

Sarcoptes scabiei may infest a variety of hosts. Similar-looking mites found in different species are regarded by some as different mite species. However, the dominant view is that *S. scabiei* in various species are varieties of the same organism that have undergone evolution and adaptation to a particular host.[459a, 562, 734] Although the mite tends to be species-specific, cross-infestations among animals and between animals and humans are not uncommon.†

In humans, scabies of animal origin is characterized by pruritic erythematous papules, especially on the forearms, chest, abdomen, and thighs.[266, 562, 658] Burrows are not commonly produced, and mites are not usually demonstrated in skin scrapings. The infestation is usually self-limited and generally clears spontaneously within four to six weeks if the patient is not re-exposed to the animal source.

The primary constant clinical sign in sarcoptic mange of any species is pruritus, and much of this is associated with a hypersensitivity reaction to mite product(s).‡ In swine, experimental infestation with *S. scabiei* var. *suis* results in crusts on the ears within one to ten weeks.§ These aural crusts disappear in 7 to

---

*References 80, 122, 123, 320, 360, 406, 420, 437, 455, 562, 734

†References 14, 137, 303, 353, 406, 562, 579, 734

‡References 122, 123, 343, 406, 420, 437, 441, 455, 459a, 459b, 497, 562, 854, 855

§References 74, 127, 343, 420, 459a, 459b, 536, 703, 704

18 weeks and are followed by a widespread pruritic, erythematous papular eruption. During this hypersensitivity state, tissue and blood eosinophilia are present, intradermal skin tests using mite antigen are positive (immediate and delayed-type hypersensitivity reactions), and mites are difficult or impossible to find in skin scrapings.

Severe, chronic sarcoptic mange is more common in animals when feeding, management, and hygiene procedures are poor.[80, 123, 420, 459a, 459b, 497] Studies in swine have demonstrated that diets deficient in protein and iron result in reduced hypersensitivity responses and a greater tendency to develop chronic scabies.[127, 343, 420, 703, 704]

CLINICAL FEATURES

In swine, sarcoptic mange is the most important ectoparasitic disease throughout the world.* Few swine herds, other than specific pathogen–free herds, are free of the disease. There are no apparent age, breed, or sex predilections. The only constant clinical sign of infestation is pruritus. Clinical signs of rubbing and scratching in the absence of lice must be assumed to be scabies until proved otherwise. Initial infection is characterized by crusts and excoriations in and on the ears. In healthy pigs, these lesions tend to regress after 7 to 18 weeks, and a widespread erythematous, nonfollicular, maculopapular eruption appears, especially over the rump, flanks, and abdomen (see Plate 5). Without effective therapy, lesions progress to lichenification and crusting. Lesions characteristic of chronic sarcoptic mange (thick, asbestos-like crusts in the ears, and crusts on the head and neck) develop in only a few animals, especially those that are debilitated for other reasons. The mites favor the ears, and this site is often the only source of lesions and mites.

In cattle, sarcoptic mange occurs throughout the world.† In the United States, it is a reportable disease. There are no apparent age, breed, or sex predilections. The primary clinical sign is intense pruritus, especially over the face, neck, shoulders, and rump (Figs. 9–4 and 9–5). Nonfollicular papules, crusts, excoriations, alopecia, and lichenification are usually

seen, and generalized skin involvement can occur.

In goats, sarcoptic mange occurs throughout the world.* There are no apparent age, sex, or breed predilections. The chief clinical sign is intense pruritus, especially over the face, ears, neck, and limbs (Figs. 9–6 and 9–7). Skin lesions are as previously described for cattle. Peripheral lymphadenopathy is usually prominent.

In sheep, sarcoptic mange is generally considered to be rare throughout the world.† In the United States, sarcoptic mange has supposedly never been recognized in sheep and is thus a reportable disease. However, anecdotal reports suggest that it does occur.[578] There are no apparent age, breed, or sex predilections. The primary clinical sign is pruritus, which tends to involve the face, ears, and limbs and rarely spreads to wooled areas. Excoriations, crusts, alopecia, lichenification, and hyperpigmentation are often present.

In horses, sarcoptic mange is generally considered to be rare throughout the world.‡ In the United States, equine sarcoptic mange has been officially eradicated and is thus reportable. However, recent anecdotal reports suggest that it is the most common form of mange in horses in the United States.[469] There are no apparent age, breed, or sex predilections. The chief clinical sign is pruritus, which usually begins on the head and neck and spreads caudally. Nonfollicular papules, crusts, excoriations, alopecia, and lichenification are usually seen.

DIAGNOSIS

The differential diagnosis includes psoroptic mange, chorioptic mange, psorergatic mange, lice, keds, and fly-bite dermatoses. Definitive diagnosis is based on history, physical examination, skin scrapings (Figs. 9–8 through 9–10), skin biopsy, and response to therapy. Mites are often very difficult to find in scrapings.§ In swine, crusts and cerumen gathered from the ear canal and pinna are the most consistent sources of mites.[122, 123, 127, 420, 704, 706]

---

*References 2, 141, 185, 235, 236, 277, 310, 369, 387, 408, 449, 455, 459a, 579, 585, 716–718, 816, 853
†References 80, 353, 360, 406, 411, 437, 459, 520, 774, 853
‡References 80, 97, 227, 230, 245, 344, 353, 362, 406, 421, 631, 756
§References 14, 122, 123, 221, 360, 420, 437, 455, 459, 547

---

*References 80, 82, 88, 103, 123, 129, 178, 221, 245, 274, 292a, 321, 343, 370, 374, 420, 459a, 473, 596, 667, 701, 827
†References 14, 80, 111, 353, 406, 414, 428, 497, 577

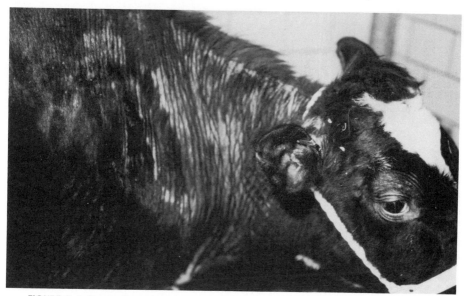

FIGURE 9–4. Sarcoptic mange in a cow. Alopecia and crusts on face, ears, and neck.

FIGURE 9–5. Sarcoptic mange in a cow. Alopecia and lichenification over neck.

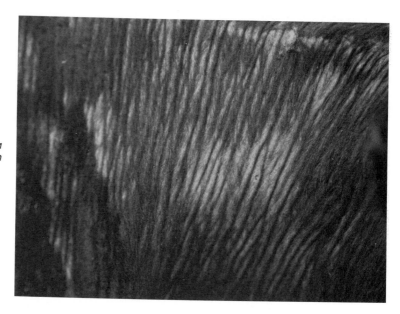

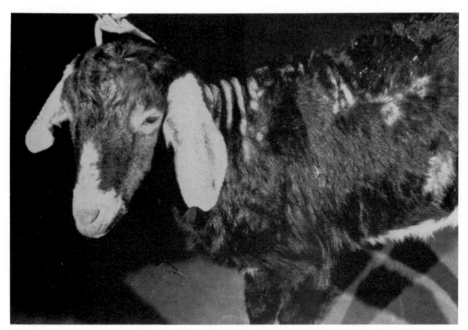

FIGURE 9–6. Sarcoptic mange in a goat. Alopecia and crusts on face, ears, neck, and trunk.

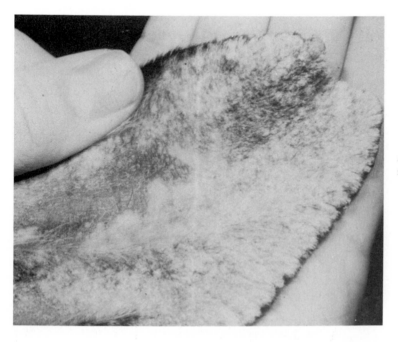

FIGURE 9–7. Sarcoptic mange in a goat. Extensive crusting of pinna.

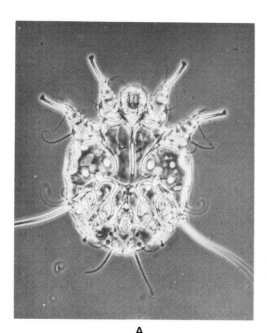 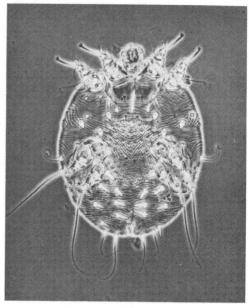

A   B

FIGURE 9–8. A, Sarcoptes, *male (× 100).* B, Sarcoptes, *female (× 100). (With permission from Georgi, J. R.:* Parasitology for Veterinarians, *3rd ed. Philadelphia, W. B. Saunders Co., 1980, p. 57.)*

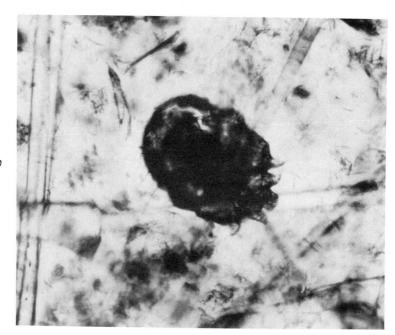

FIGURE 9–9. Sarcoptes *mite in skin scraping from a pig.*

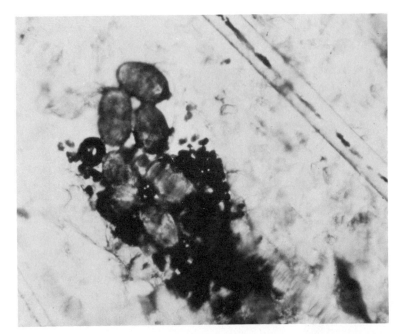

FIGURE 9–10. Sarcoptes *eggs and fecal pellets in skin scraping from a pig.*

Skin biopsy reveals varying degrees of superficial perivascular dermatitis with numerous eosinophils.[74, 185, 406, 455, 459b, 668, 704] Eosinophilic microabscesses and focal areas of epidermal edema, leukocytic exocytosis, and necrosis (epidermal nibbles) may be seen. Mites may be seen within parakeratotic scale crusts and in subcorneal "tunnels," but this is uncommon (Fig. 9–11). Occasionally, deep perivascular dermatitis with lymphoid nodules may be seen.

Because of the frequently negative results of skin scrapings and skin biopsy, response to therapy is often employed in determining a presumptive diagnosis.* This is especially practical for small groups of animals and for individual animals (show animals, working animals, pets).

CLINICAL MANAGEMENT

Sarcoptic mange is often a severe disease. Intense, constant pruritus results in annoyance, irritability, decreased food intake, anemia, decreased weight gains or weight loss, decreased milk production, difficulties in estrus detection, lowered conception as well as reproductive problems, hide damage, wool loss, secondary infections and myiasis, increased susceptibility to other diseases, and even death.† Factors that complicate the detection and control of sarcoptic mange are complex and include many of the items considered for psoroptic mange (see prior discussion on psoroptic mange.[80, 346, 478, 547]). All animals that have come into contact with infected animals and all exposed animals should be treated.

In cattle in the United States, the only recognized methods of treatment of sarcoptic mange are spray-dipping and vat-dipping. Vat-dipping is essentially impossible in the Northeast. Only three approved dips are listed by the USDA: (1) 0.3 percent coumaphos (two dippings, no withholding period), (2) 0.20 to 0.25 percent phosmet (two dippings), and (3) 2.0 percent hot lime sulfur (essentially reserved for use on lactating diary cattle; no milk residue; three times at ten-day intervals). In addition, some states use 0.06 percent lindane (two dippings; use on beef cattle; not within 30 days prior to calving; 30-day withdrawal period). Ivermectin has been shown to be effective in the treatment of bovine sarcoptic mange.[414, 690] A single subcutaneous injection approximating 200 μg/kg was curative.

In sheep, the only recognized method of treatment for sarcoptic mange is vat-dipping (one-minute immersion). State-approved acaricides and quarantine procedures should be employed. Dipping is most effective if done within two weeks after shearing and must be repeated in 10 to 14 days.[80, 360, 437, 459] Acaricides reported to be effective include 0.3 percent coumaphos, 0.15 to 0.25 percent phosmet, 0.03 to 0.1 percent diazinon, and 2.0 percent hot

---

*References 14, 122, 123, 245, 414, 420, 455, 547, 731
†References 14, 80, 128, 221, 310, 329, 343, 406, 420, 437, 455, 459, 473, 497, 702, 816

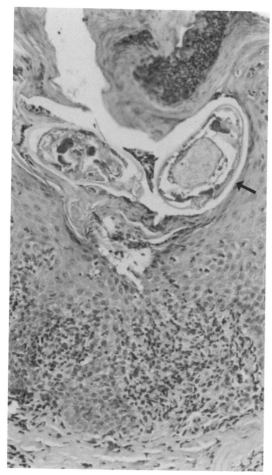

FIGURE 9–11. Porcine sarcoptic mange. Mites (arrow) in subcorneal tunnels.

lime sulfur. In light of the efficacy of ivermectin in bovine psoroptic and sarcoptic mange (see previous sections) and porcine sarcoptic mange (see later), this drug may prove to be effective in ovine sarcoptic mange.

In goats, sarcoptic mange may be treated with 0.25 percent crotoxyphos, 0.25 percent coumaphos, 0.2 percent trichlorfon, 0.5 to 2.0 percent malathion, or 2 percent lime sulfur sprays or dips.* Weekly therapy for four to six weeks is often necessary. Ivermectin (200 μg/ kg given subcutaneously) is also effective.

In horses, sarcoptic mange may be treated with spray or dip applications of 0.5 percent malathion, 0.03 percent lindane, 0.06 percent coumaphos, 0.5 percent methoxychlor, or 2 percent lime sulfur.[80, 244, 406, 440] At least two treatments at a 14-day interval should be administered. In light of the efficacy of ivermec-

tin in bovine psoroptic and sarcoptic mange and porcine sarcoptic mange, this drug may prove to be useful in equine sarcoptic mange. Amitraz does not appear to be an acceptable acaricide in the horse (see discussion on psoroptic mange).

In swine, although effective insecticides have been available for years, sarcoptic mange continues to be an increasingly serious problem, especially in intensive production units.* This problem is related to pork producers' lack of appreciation of the economic losses caused by sarcoptic mange, (2) hit or miss treatments that do not take into account the short life cycle of the mite, (3) the failure of many currently available acaricides to kill mite eggs, (4) the lack of treatment rooms or pens in a majority of intensive swine units, and (5) the inaccurate perception that rubbing and scratching are normal behaviors for swine.

Since young nursing piglets are infected by mites from sows, any successful treatment and control programs must begin with the breeding herd.† All replacement animals added to the herd should be kept in isolation, if possible, until they have received two treatments at a ten-day interval. Gestating gilts and sows should receive three treatments at seven-day intervals, beginning 21 days before farrowing. Boars should receive similar therapy. Weaned pigs should be treated twice at a ten-day interval, at six to eight weeks of age.

Lindane 0.06 percent spray has long been the acaricide of choice.‡ Inappropriate use of lindane has produced abortions in pregnant sows and toxicity in newborn piglets. Other acaricides reported to be effective as sprays for porcine sarcoptic mange include 0.5 percent malathion, 0.12 percent coumaphos, 0.05 percent diazinon, 0.125 percent trichlorfon, and 0.1 percent amitraz.§ Acaricidal sprays should be applied to the entire body, with special attention given to the ears. Proper treatment and hygiene regimens for the housing areas are vital. Animals showing chronic mange lesions should be culled.

Ivermectin has been shown to be very effective in the treatment of porcine sarcoptic mange.[10, 11, 152, 417, 459c, 581, 691] Single subcutaneous (300 μg/kg) or oral (300 to 500 μg/kg) doses

---

*References 141, 236, 277, 455, 718, 719, 730, 731, 767

*References 123, 129, 221, 274, 343, 374, 420, 441
†References 123, 127, 129, 221, 343, 420, 441, 596
‡References 122, 123, 129, 221, 343, 420, 441, 773
§References 123, 129, 221, 274, 343, 374, 420, 441, 462, 696, 863.

of ivermectin were found to be curative and nontoxic. Treatment 8 to 37 days before farrowing prevented transmission to offspring.

A 20 percent phosmet pour-on was reported to be effective for porcine sarcoptic mange.[329] A dose of 20 mg/kg was poured on the back line. This procedure not only cured active infestations but also prevented transmission of infestations from sows to their piglets when administered three days prior to farrowing. No toxicities were reported.

Chorioptic Mange

Chorioptic mange (leg mange, tail mange, symbiotic scab, foot mange) is a common cause of dermatitis in cattle, goats, sheep, and occasionally horses.

CAUSE AND PATHOGENESIS

Chorioptic mites (0.3 to 0.5 mm long) are surface-inhabiting parasites that feed on epidermal debris.[80, 734, 770] The life cycle takes about two to three weeks and is completed on the host. It is generally stated that the mites live only a few days off the host. However, recent studies of *Chorioptes bovis* under various environmental conditions, off the animal, showed that the mites could survive up to 69 days.[429] The researchers recommended a stable quarantine period of ten weeks. Transmission is by direct and indirect contact.

Sweatman felt that *Chorioptes bovis, C. ovis,* and *C. equi* were all one species, *C. bovis.*[770] He recognized only one other species, *C. texanus,* from the ears of goats in Texas. However, because of the apparent lack of interspecies transmission of chorioptic mange, most authors currently recognize four species: *C. bovis* (cattle), *C. caprae* (goats), *C. equi* (horses), and *C. ovis* (sheep).* *Chorioptes* spp. mites do *not* affect humans.

Mite populations are usually much larger during cold weather.† Thus, clinical signs are usually seen, or are more severe, in winter. This seasonality of mite populations and clinical signs is thought to be under the influence of temperature, humidity, and wetting of the host. The disease often spontaneously regresses during summer as mite numbers become very small. During this clinically inapparent stage of infestation, mites are more

easily demonstrated around the coronet and interdigital areas.

Because the mites can be demonstrated on normal sheep and cattle,* it has been theorized that a hypersensitivity to mite products is present in animals manifesting dermatitis.

CLINICAL FEATURES

Chorioptic mange occurs in cattle, goats, sheep, and horses in most parts of the world.† In general, there are no apparent age, breed, or sex predilections.

In goats, infestation with *C. caprae* is fairly common, especially in stabled goats during the winter in the northeastern United States.‡ Lesions consist of nonfollicular papules, crusts, alopecia, erythema, oozing, and ulceration. Pruritus is usually marked. Lesions are most commonly seen on the feet, hind legs (Fig. 9–12), udder, scrotum, tail, and perineal area but may also be seen on the neck and flank.

In cattle, *C. bovis* infestation is common, especially in stabled dairy cattle during the winter in the northeastern United States.§ Clinical signs are as previously described for goats (Fig. 9–13; see Plate 6). In addition, a syndrome characterized by coronitis, footrot–like lesions, muzzle lesions, weight loss, and a drop in milk production has been described.[460, 492, 497]

In sheep, *C. ovis* is most commonly seen in Europe, New Zealand, and Australia during the winter.‖ In the United States, ovine chorioptic mange has been eradicated and is a reportable disease. Clinical signs are as described for goats and cattle. Some authors believe that chorioptic mite infestations may predispose to ovine foot-rot in some instances.[460] Rams can become temporarily infertile as a result of scrotal dermatitis.[322, 333, 336, 626, 627] Yellowish exudate and crusts up to several centimeters in thickness may literally encase the scrotum and testicles. The average testicular temperature in such animals is 0.6 to 3.1°C higher than that in normal rams. Testicular atrophy and spermatogenic arrest may

---

*References 80, 244, 406, 459, 469, 497, 731, 734
†References 80, 244, 459, 497, 769, 770, 772

*References 80, 322, 460, 497, 769, 770, 772
†References 80, 244, 245, 437, 455, 459, 469, 497, 731
‡References 85, 220, 310, 337, 387, 389, 406, 455, 731, 853
§References 13, 14, 22, 36, 37, 80, 202, 406, 414, 418, 428, 497, 614, 853
‖References 21, 80, 104, 135, 155, 228, 237, 322, 333, 360, 437, 459, 467, 489, 613, 640, 774

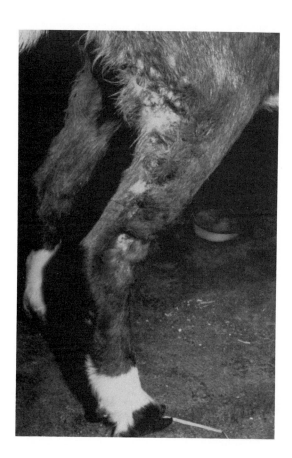

FIGURE 9–12. Chorioptic mange in a goat. Alopecia and crusts on hind leg.

FIGURE 9–13. Chorioptic mange in a cow. Alopecia, papules, and crusts in perineal area.

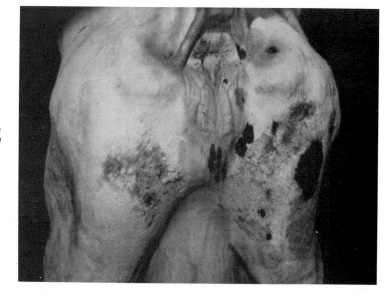

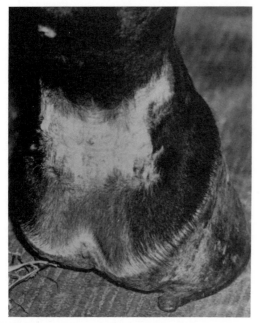

FIGURE 9–14. Chorioptic mange in a horse. Alopecia and crusting on caudal pastern area.

occur but are reversible if the chorioptic mange is successfully treated.

In horses, *C. equi* infestations are most commonly seen in draft horses and other horses with feathered fetlocks, especially during winter.* Clinical signs are as described for

---

*References 23, 80, 134, 244, 245a, 344, 406, 469, 475, 583, 584, 786, 853

goats, cattle, and sheep, with the fetlocks, pasterns, and tail being particularly affected (Fig. 9–14). Horses with widespread lesions have been seen.[81, 406, 469, 490, 639]

DIAGNOSIS

The differential diagnosis includes sarcoptic and psoroptic mange (ruminants) and tail rubbing (insect hypersensitivity, food allergy, lice, oxyuriasis, or stable vice) and grease heel (see Chapter 15, discussion on equine pastern dermatitis) in horses. Definitive diagnosis is based on history, physical examination, and examination of skin scrapings (Fig. 9–2, 9–3, and 9–15). *Chorioptes* spp. mites are usually easy to demonstrate. These mites are frequently quite active and fast-moving. The author recommends using a mixture of one part rotenone to three parts of mineral oil for the skin-scraping solution. Skin biopsy reveals variable degrees of superficial perivascular dermatitis with numerous eosinophils. Eosinophilic epidermal microabscesses and focal epidermal necrosis, leukocytic exocytosis, and edema (epidermal nibbles) may be seen. Mites are rarely found (Fig. 9–16).

CLINICAL MANAGEMENT

All animals that have come into contact with infected animals should be treated simultaneously. In cattle, total body applications of 0.03

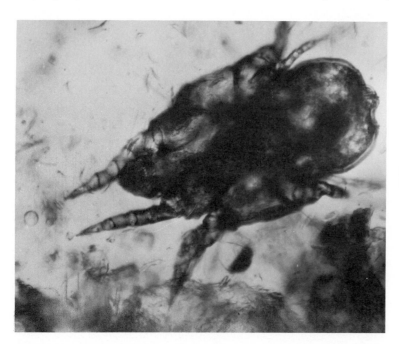

FIGURE 9–15. Chorioptes caprae in skin scraping from a goat.

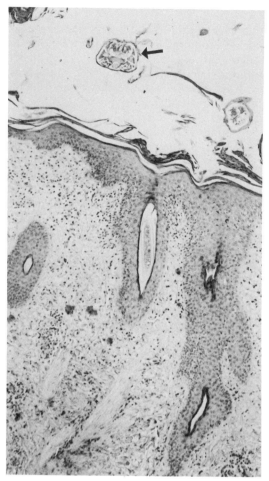

FIGURE 9–16. Bovine chorioptic mange. Superficial perivascular dermatitis with mite segments (arrow) in surface keratin.

percent coumaphos or 0.25 percent crotoxyphos (twice, at a 10- to 14-day interval) or 2 percent lime sulfur (weekly for four weeks) have been effective.*

In goats, 0.25 percent crotoxyphos, 0.25 percent coumaphos, and 0.2 percent trichlorfon have been effective when applied as total body dips or sprays at least twice at a 10- to 14-day interval.[455, 730, 731] Lime sulfur (2 percent applied as a spray or dip, weekly for four weeks) is also effective and safe in lactating dairy goats.

In sheep, chorioptic mange is a reportable disease in many parts of the world (including the United States). State-approved acaricidal treatments and quarantine procedures should be employed. The dipping-vat (one-minute im-mersion) is the only recognized way of treating sheep.[360, 520] Dipping is most effective if done within two weeks after shearing and repeated in 10 to 14 days. Coumaphos (0.2 percent), 0.15 to 0.25 percent phosmet, and 2 percent lime sulfur have been reported to be effective.[80, 360, 437, 459]

In horses, 0.25 percent crotoxyphos, applied to the total body on a weekly basis for three to four treatments, is effective.[23, 244, 584] In addition, 0.5 percent malathion, 0.5 percent methoxychlor, and 0.06 percent coumaphos are effective when applied at least twice, at a 14-day interval.[440] The author has used 2 percent lime sulfur weekly with success. In vivo and in vitro resistance of *C. equi* to coumaphos has been reported,[81] after which weekly treatments with 0.03 percent lindane were effective. Ivermectin (200 μg/kg given orally, repeat in two weeks) has recently been reported to be effective.[245a]

Psorergatic Mange

Psorergatic mange (itch mite, Australian itch) is a common skin disorder of sheep in many parts of the world and an occasional cause of skin disease in cattle.

Cause and Pathogenesis

Psorergatic mites are small (0.1 to 0.2 mm in diameter), host-specific parasites that burrow in the epidermis of sheep (*Psorergates ovis*) and cattle (*P. bos*).* The life cycle is completed on the host and takes about 35 days. Mite populations are highest and clinical signs more severe in winter and spring.† Transmission is by direct and indirect contact, but mites cannot survive for more than a few days off the host. Psorergatic mites do not affect humans.

Clinical Features

In sheep, psorergatic mange has been reported in the United States, Australia, New Zealand, Africa, and South America.‡ Psorergatic mange has been eradicated from sheep in the United States and is a reportable disease. There are no apparent age, breed, or sex

---

*References 14, 80, 282, 461, 497, 577, 724

*References 71, 80, 360, 437, 459, 510, 553, 734
†References 295, 360, 437, 448, 452, 459, 712, 714
‡References 42, 65, 80, 131, 174, 245, 296, 360, 406, 437, 459, 508, 510, 642, 712, 714, 720, 837

predilections. Affected sheep develop intense pruritus and variable degrees of fleece derangement, characterized by matted, chewed, broken, and absent wool in regions accessible to the sheep's mouth—the lateral thorax, flanks, and thighs. The affected skin is often quite scaly.

In cattle, psorergatic mange has been reported in the United States, Canada, and South Africa.[71, 414, 553, 641, 734] There are no apparent age, breed, or sex predilections. Affected cattle usually show subtle degrees of patchy alopecia and scaling, with little or no pruritus. Occasionally, cattle will develop severe dorsally distributed alopecia, scaling, and pruritus. *P. bos* can also be recovered from cattle with normal skins and hair coats.

DIAGNOSIS

In sheep, the differential diagnosis includes lice, keds, and psoroptic and sarcoptic mange. Psorergatic mange usually lacks the papular dermatitis, marked crusting, and excoriations seen with psoroptic and sarcoptic mange. In cattle, the major differential diagnoses are lice and shedding. Definitive diagnosis is based on history, physical examination, and skin scrapings (Fig. 9–17). The mites may be difficult to find, requiring several skin scrapings. Skin biopsy reveals varying degrees of superficial perivascular dermatitis with eosinophils. Mite segments may be seen in the stratum corneum.

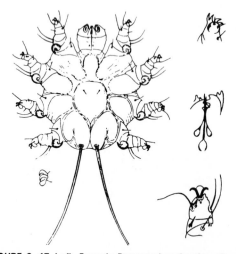

FIGURE 9–17. Left, *Female Psorergates simplex (Tyrell).* Right, *Palps, chelicera and tarsus I of* Psorergates ovis. *(With permission from Baker, W. E., et al.:* A Manual of the Mites of Medical or Economic Importance. *New York, National Pest Control Association, 1956, p. 170.)*

CLINICAL MANAGEMENT

In sheep, psorergatic mange can cause significant economic losses through wool damage and weight loss. Mite populations are highest in the spring, and therapeutic dips and sprays are least effective (slower in working) at this time.* Thus, if husbandry practices allow, it is best to treat the disease in summer. Topical applications (dip or spray) of 2 to 3 percent lime sulfur, 0.2 percent malathion, 0.3 percent coumaphos, and 0.03 to 0.3 percent diazinon are effective when administered at least twice, at a 14-day interval.

In cattle, psorergatic mange usually causes no apparent economic losses. Thus, although 2 to 3 percent lime sulfur dips or sprays are effective in eliminating the parasites,[71] treatment is not usually rendered. Recently, the subcutaneous administration of ivermectin was reported to be curative.[553]

Demodectic Mange

Demodectic mange (follicular mange, demodicosis) is a follicular dermatosis of cattle, goats, swine, and, rarely, sheep and horses.

CAUSE AND PATHOGENESIS

Demodectic mites are normal residents of the skin in all large animals.† The mites live in hair follicles and sebaceous glands, are host-specific, and complete their entire life cycle on the host. The life cycle of most demodicids has not been carefully studied but is assumed to be completed in 20 to 35 days.

Under most environmental conditions, demodicids can survive only several minutes to a couple of days off the host.[549] Studies in cattle[241, 257, 262, 834] and dogs[496] have shown that (1) demodectic mites are acquired during the first two to three days of life by direct contact with the dam, (2) animals delivered by cesarean section and raised away from other animals did not harbor demodectic mites, and (3) confining normal adult animals with severely infested and diseased animals for several months did not produce disease in the normal animals. In addition, attempts to transmit clinical de-

---

*References 210, 295–297, 437, 459, 508, 510, 710–714, 720
†References 40, 44, 68, 122, 123, 241, 256, 258, 340, 360, 405, 406, 420, 441, 527, 529, 530, 548, 549, 608, 610, 721, 734

modicosis to sheep, horses, and swine by direct contact and by applying mites to the skin were unsuccessful.[68, 122, 223] Thus, demodectic mange is not thought to be a contagious disease in most instances.

Because demodectic mites are normal residents of the skin, it is likely that animals manifesting clinical disease resulting from this parasite are, in some manner, immunocompromised. Demodicosis in dogs is known to occur as a result of immunosuppression (drugs or diseases) and genetic predilection (selective immunodeficiency?).[496] In large animals, many authors have suggested that clinical demodicosis probably occurs only in animals that are immunocompromised (debilitation, concurrent disease, poor nutrition, or stress).* In horses, demodicosis has been reported in association with chronic treatment with systemic glucocorticoids.[693] Thus, in herd outbreaks of demodicosis, one must consider genetic predilection and endogenous and exogenous causes of immunosuppression as playing significant roles.

CLINICAL FEATURES

Bovine demodectic mange is worldwide in occurrence and has no apparent age or sex predilections.† In the United States, Holsteins are commonly affected, perhaps suggesting genetic predilection. Three species of demodicids have been isolated from cattle: *Demodex bovis* (eyelids and body skin; 200 to 240 μm long),[549, 721, 734] *D. ghanensis* (eyelids; 400 μm long),[44, 721] and an unclassified *Demodex* sp. (eyelids and body skin; 195 ± 6 μm long).[721] Clinical signs consist of usually asymptomatic follicular papules and nodules, especially over the withers, neck, back, and flanks (Fig. 9–18). Generalized skin involvement can occur. The lesions are usually attached to the overlying skin, and the overlying skin is usually normal in appearance. Occasionally, ulceration, fistulae, abscesses, and crusts may be seen, especially if follicular rupture or secondary bacterial infections, or both, have occurred.

Caprine demodectic mange is caused by *D. caprae* (224 to 315 μm long), is worldwide in occurrence, and has no apparent age, breed, or sex predilections.‡ Clinical signs consist of usually asymptomatic follicular papules and nodules, especially over the face, neck, shoulders, and sides (Fig. 9–19). Other findings were previously described for bovine demodectic mange.

Porcine demodectic mange is caused by *D. phylloides* (230 to 265 μm long), is worldwide in occurrence, and has no apparent age, breed, or sex predilections.* Clinical signs consist of usually asymptomatic, skin-colored or erythematous follicular papules and, occasionally, pustules and nodules, especially on the snout, eyelids, ventral neck, ventral thorax, ventral abdomen, and medial thighs. Secondary staphylococcal pyoderma may occur.

Ovine demodectic mange is caused by *D. ovis* (240 to 280 μm long), is worldwide but uncommon to rare in occurrence, and has no apparent age, breed, or sex predilections.† Clinical signs include usually asymptomatic alopecia, erythema, and scaling of the face, neck, shoulders, and back. Crusts, pustules, and abscesses may be seen, and the pinnae, limbs, and coronets may occasionally be affected.

Equine demodectic mange is worldwide but very rare in occurrence and has no apparent age, breed, or sex predilections.‡ Horses possess two species of demodicid mites: *D. caballi* (264 to 453 μm in length; eyelids and muzzle) and *D. equi* (179 to 236 μm in length; body). Clinical signs consist of usually asymptomatic alopecia and scaling, especially over the face, neck, shoulders, and forelimbs (Fig. 9–20). Papules and pustules may be seen.

DIAGNOSIS

The differential diagnosis includes other follicular dermatoses: staphylococcal folliculitis, dermatophytosis, and dermatophilosis. Definitive diagnosis is based on history, physical examination, skin scrapings, and skin biopsy. Alopecic, erythematous, scaling areas of skin should be squeezed firmly and scraped deeply until blood is drawn. Papular or nodular lesions should be incised on the surface and evacuated manually, revealing a thick, caseous, whitish to yellowish exudate, which is literally loaded with demodectic mites (Fig. 9–21).

---

*References 80, 123, 360, 406, 441, 529, 530, 693, 721, 727, 731, 819
†References 13, 14, 44, 80, 119, 241, 256, 258, 404, 406, 511, 527, 528, 601, 726, 727, 777, 791, 834, 853
‡References 49, 79, 80, 87, 154, 166, 222, 239, 252, 302, 310, 316, 406, 454, 455, 656, 725, 730, 731, 736, 766, 846

---

*References 80, 120, 122, 123, 221, 317, 343, 368, 400, 405, 420, 529, 606, 827
†References 12, 28, 39, 80, 102, 132, 223, 398, 405, 406, 509, 530, 665, 692
‡References 68, 70, 72, 344, 353, 405, 406, 433, 469, 666, 693, 693a, 786, 848

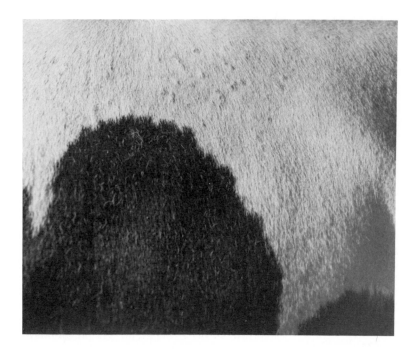

FIGURE 9–18. Bovine demodectic mange. Multiple papules on lateral thorax.

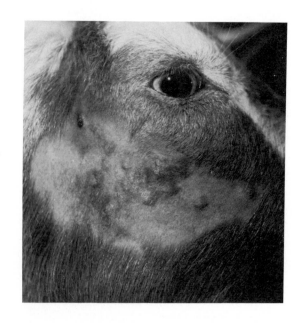

FIGURE 9–19. Caprine demodectic mange. Multiple papules on cheek (area has been clipped).

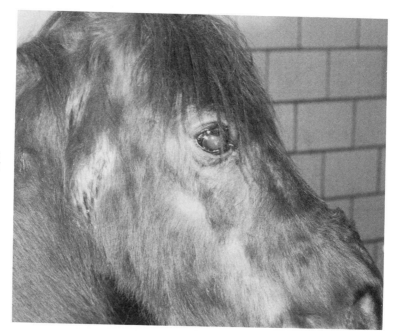

FIGURE 9–20. Equine demodectic mange. Patchy alopecia and scaling on face.

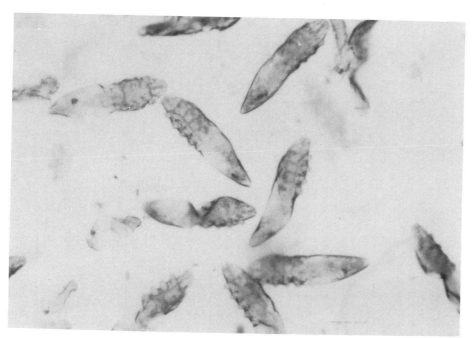

FIGURE 9–21. Demodex caprae *in skin scraping from a goat.*

Skin biopsy reveals hair follicles distended to varying degrees with demodectic mites.* Often, the degree of follicular distention results in very large follicular cysts (Fig. 9–22). In many cases, there is minimal inflammatory response. Alternatively, varying degrees of perifolliculitis, folliculitis, furunculosis, and foreign body granuloma formation (Fig. 9–23) may be seen. The granulomatous inflammation may contain numerous eosinophils, and the mites may be coated with Hoeppli-Splendore material.[278]

CLINICAL MANAGEMENT

Because demodectic mange (1) is usually asymptomatic, (2) may spontaneously regress, and (3) has been refractory to most therapeutic agents and regimens, treatment is not usually attempted.† Severe infestations may result in significant economic losses through hide damage and wool loss.‡ It has been reported that 2 percent trichlorfon (Neguvon) applied as a total-body dip, every other day for three treatments (after clipping, if needed), is curative

---

*References 28, 102, 119, 223, 298, 455, 527, 529, 530, 555, 693

†References 13, 14, 80, 122, 123, 221, 244, 278, 343, 360, 405, 420, 497, 511, 693, 727, 730, 731, 853

‡References 12, 14, 80, 123, 221, 406, 420, 455, 511, 527, 529, 530, 721, 728

for demodectic mange in sheep, swine, and cattle.[529, 530, 787] In goats, localized lesions may be incised, expressed manually, and infused with either Lugol's iodine or rotenone in alcohol (1:3).[730, 731, 777] For generalized lesions in goats, two therapeutic regimens have been reported to be curative: (1) ronnel in propylene glycol (180 ml of 33 percent ronnel in 1000 ml of propylene glycol; apply to one third of the body surface daily until cured; clip if needed),[455, 730] and (2) rotenone in alcohol (1:3) applied to one quarter of the body surface daily until the entire body has been treated (four days).[787]

Considering the difficulties associated with treatment and the probable importance of genetic predilection in disease susceptibility, it may be best to cull severely affected animals and not use affected animals for breeding stock.

Trombiculidiasis

Trombiculidiasis (trombidiosis, chiggers, harvest mite, scrub itch mite, leg itch, heel bug) is a fairly common dermatosis of horses and sheep in many parts of the world.

CAUSE AND PATHOGENESIS

Trombiculid adults and nymphs are free-living and feed on invertebrate hosts or

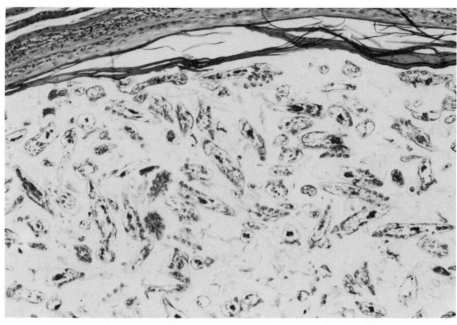

FIGURE 9–22. Caprine demodectic mange. Follicular cyst filled with mites.

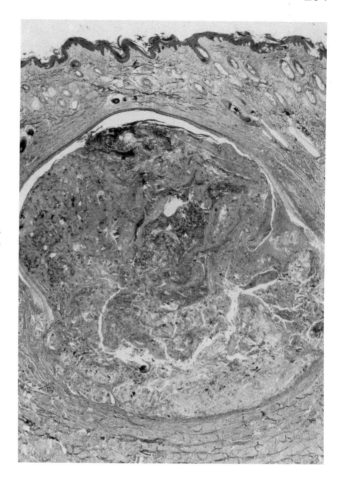

FIGURE 9–23. Bovine demodectic mange. Dermal granuloma arising from ruptured hair follicle.

plants.[244, 245, 734] The larvae normally feed (suck tissue fluids) on small rodents but may also attack large animals and humans. Skin lesions produced by feeding larvae consist of papules and wheals. Because some animals manifest extreme pruritus, and other animals none, it is theorized that the pruritic animals may have developed a hypersensitivity reaction to larval salivary antigen(s).

Trombiculid larvae measure 0.2 to 0.4 mm in length and vary in color from red to orange to yellow. In North and South America, *Trombicula (Eutrombicula) alfreddugèsi, Euschoengastia latchmani,* and *Neoschoengastia americana* are important trombiculids that inhabit forested and swampy areas. *T. (Neotrombicula) autumnalis*, the harvest mite, or heel bug, of Europe and Australia, inhabits chalky soils, grasslands, and cornfields. *T. sarcina* is the blacksoil itch, or leg itch, mite of Australia.

Trombiculid larvae are usually active in summer and fall. After feeding (seven to ten days), the larvae drop off the host to molt.

CLINICAL FEATURES

Trombiculidiasis generally occurs in the late summer and fall, when larvae are active. Trombiculids may attack any large animal; humans, horses, and sheep are most commonly affected.* The infestation is seen primarily in pastured animals, horses in infested paddocks, or horses taken on trail rides through infested fields and woods. There are no apparent age, breed, or sex predilections.

Skin lesions consist of papules and wheals, especially on the distal limbs, muzzle, face, neck, and ventral thorax and abdomen. Close examination of early lesions reveals brightly colored trombiculids, singly or in clusters. Pruritus may be intense or absent. Cutaneous edema, exudation, crusting, and ulceration may be prominent, especially in sheep. Affected sheep may show decreased feed con-

---

*References 23, 80, 93, 157, 244, 245a, 270, 284, 344, 360, 406, 459, 469, 583, 584, 632, 786, 853

sumption, may lose weight, and may suffer significant wool damage.

DIAGNOSIS

The differential diagnosis includes chorioptic mange, psoroptic mange, sarcoptic mange, contact dermatitis, forage mites, biting flies, staphylococcal folliculitis, and dermatophilosis. Definitive diagnosis is based on history, physical examination, and demonstrating the trombiculids grossly or microscopically, or both, in skin scrapings. Because the larvae only feed on the animal for a few days, demonstrating the trombiculids may be impossible in chronic cases. Presumptive diagnosis is then based on the time of year, exposure to trombiculid-infested areas, physical findings, and response to therapy. Skin biopsy reveals varying degrees of superficial perivascular dermatitis with numerous eosinophils.

CLINICAL MANAGEMENT

Treatment of trombiculidiasis may not be necessary, since the disease is self-limiting if further contact with the trombiculids is avoided. In severe cases, a single application (dip or spray) of a topical parasiticidal agent such as 2 percent lime sulfur, 0.25 to 0.5 percent malathion, 0.06 to 0.3 percent coumaphos, 0.03 to 0.1 percent diazinon, or 0.25 percent chlorpyrifos may be helpful.* Severely pruritic animals may benefit from a few days' treatment with systemic glucocorticoids.

Forage Mites

Mites from the families Acaridae (Tyroglyphidae) and Pediculoididae (Pyemotidae) may cause dermatitis in animals and humans.[244, 395, 410, 658, 734] Because these free-living mites normally feed on organic matter (Acaridae) or insects in straw and grain (Pediculoididae), the dermatoses they produce are often called grain itch, straw itch, cheese itch, copra itch, and so on.

These so-called forage mites have been reported to cause pruritic or nonpruritic papulocrustous dermatoses in horses (*Pediculoides ventricosus* or *Pyemotes tritici; Acarus farinae*), sheep (*Caloglyphus berlesei, Acarus* sp.), and swine (*Acarus* sp.) in areas of skin that contact the contaminated foodstuff (muzzle, head, neck, limbs, ventral thorax, and abdomen).* In humans, forage mites produce a pruritic papular to urticarial dermatosis in contact areas within 12 to 16 hours after attacking.[266, 658]

The differential diagnosis includes sarcoptic mange, psoroptic mange, chorioptic mange, contact dermatitis, trombiculidiasis, and fly bites. Definitive diagnosis is based on history, physical examination, and microscopic demonstration of the mites (0.3 to 0.6 mm long) in skin scrapings and forage samples. Skin biopsy reveals varying degrees of superficial perivascular dermatitis with numerous eosinophils.

Therapy consists of eliminating the contaminated forage. The dermatosis resolves spontaneously within a few days.[266, 410, 658]

Poultry Mite

The poultry mite, *Dermanyssus gallinae*, is known to occasionally attack horses, cattle, and humans.[406, 584, 734] Adult mites live and lay eggs in cracks and crevices in the walls of poultry houses or in bird nests. Adult mites suck blood and are 0.6 to 1 mm in length. Lesions consist of pruritic papules and crusts in contact areas (especially limbs, muzzle, and ventrum).

Diagnosis is based on history, physical examination, and demonstrating the mites in skin scrapings or the environment. Therapy consists of elimination or treatment of infested premises with miticidal sprays such as 0.5 percent malathion, 0.5 percent methoxychlor, 0.3 percent coumaphos, 0.1 percent diazinon, or 2 percent lime sulfur.

Ear Mites

In addition to *Psoroptes* spp. mites, *Raillietia* spp. mites are known to parasitize the ear canals of large animals.[734] In cattle, *R. auris* has been reported from Africa and South America.[254, 558] Infested cattle showed no signs of disease. In goats, *R. caprae* has been reported from the United States,[415] Brazil,[268] and Mexico.[609] *R. manfredi* has been reported in Australian goats.[150] Again, infested goats showed no signs of disease.

---

*References 244, 360, 440, 459, 469, 583, 584

*References 80, 334, 410, 431, 546, 583, 584

TICK INFESTATION

Ticks are an important ectoparasite of large animals all around the world (Table 9–1).*

CAUSE AND PATHOGENESIS

Ticks may harm their hosts by (1) injuries done by bites, which may predispose to secondary infections and myiasis, (2) sucking blood (a single adult female tick may remove 0.5 to 2.0 ml blood), (3) transmitting various viral, protozoal, rickettsial, and bacterial diseases, and (4) causing tick paralysis. In addition, economic losses through hide damage and diagnostic, therapeutic, or control programs may be sizable. Together, these effects may vary from a situation in which it is impossible to raise livestock to one in which great expenses are incurred. In tropical and temperate areas, ticks are responsible for the loss of hundreds of millions of dollars annually.

Argasid (soft) ticks, such as *Otobius megnini* and *Ornithodorus coriaceus*, lay their eggs in sheltered spots, such as cracks in poles, under boxes or stones, and in crevices in walls.[734] Larvae and nymphs suck blood and lymph and drop off the host to become adults.

Ixodid (hard) ticks, such as *Dermacentor albipictus* and *Amblyomma americanum*, lay their eggs in sheltered areas, such as wall crevices, cracks in wood near the ground, and under stones and clods of soil.[734] Larvae (seed ticks) climb onto grass and shrubbery and wait for a suitable host to pass by.

According to the number of hosts required during their life cycle, ticks can be classified into three groups: (1) one-host ticks (all three instars engorge on the same animal; two ecdyses take place on the host), (2) two-host ticks (larva engorges and molts on host, and nymph drops off after engorging; nymph molts on the ground, and the imago seeks a new host), and (3) three-host ticks (require a different host for every instar, drop off host each time after engorging, and molt on the ground). Each species of tick is adapted to certain ranges of temperature and moisture. In general, ticks are not especially host-specific. Local reactions to tick bites are variable, depending on the properties of the tick in question and on the host-parasite relationship.[843] Differences in animal susceptibility to tick infestation have been recognized clinically, pathologically, and immunologically.* The ability of animals to resist tick infestations is dependent on immune mechanisms, including: (1) humoral immunity, (2) cell-mediated immunity, (3) delayed-type hypersensitivity, (4) immediate hypersensitivity, and (5) cutaneous basophil hypersensitivity. Because of the importance of tick-borne diseases, research into mechanisms of immunity to ticks is currently active.

CLINICAL FEATURES

Ticks are important ectoparasites of goats,[45, 46, 678, 740] sheep,† cattle,[14, 80, 282, 308, 406, 518] and horses.‡ They are not usually a problem in swine.[221, 420] Tick-related dermatoses are most commonly seen in spring and summer. Although ticks may attack any portion of the body surface, favorite areas include the ears, face, neck, axillae, groin, distal limbs, and tail. Initial skin lesions consist of papules, pustules, wheals, and, occasionally, nodules centered around a tick. These primary lesions develop crusts, erosions, ulcers, and alopecia. Pain and pruritus are variable.

Otobius megnini (the spinose ear tick) attacks all large animal species. Otitis externa, characterized by considerable irritation, inflammation, and a waxy discharge, is the result. Secondary bacterial infection is common. Affected animals may exhibit head tilting, head shaking, and ear rubbing and appear lop-eared.

In Australia, a hypersensitivity syndrome in horses is associated with the larvae of *Boophilus microplus*.[406, 469, 584, 633] Most cases occur in late summer or early fall, and only sensitized horses are affected. The onset of clinical signs is rapid and may be evident within 30 minutes of infestation. Affected horses exhibit multiple papules and wheals, which are most numerous on the lower legs and muzzle. Close examination reveals larval ticks embedded in a serous exudate in the center of the lesions. Pruritus is intense.

---

*References 38, 60, 62, 80, 308, 607, 734, 748, 783, 853

*References 3a, 7–9, 24, 30, 67, 75, 91, 99–101, 177, 197, 327, 328, 364a, 374a, 403, 514, 556, 636, 637, 648–651, 685, 761, 765, 778, 796, 808a, 824–826, 838, 840, 841a, 843

†References 21, 80, 290, 360, 406, 459, 678

‡References 80, 134, 245a, 406, 469, 583, 584, 759, 797

DIAGNOSIS

A definitive diagnosis of tick infestation is simply based on demonstrating the ticks. Specific identification of the ticks is of value in determining the control measures required.

Skin biopsy findings vary with the duration of the lesion and the host-parasite relationship.* Reactions in primary infestations are characterized by varying degrees of focal epidermal necrosis and edema, with the subjacent dermis showing edema and infiltration with neutrophils, eosinophils, and mononuclear cells. Reactions in previously infested hosts are characterized by marked intraepidermal vesicopustular dermatitis (marked spongiosis, microabscesses containing eosinophils and basophils), marked subepidermal edema, and marked dermal infiltration with basophils, eosinophils, and mononuclear cells. Persistent nodular reactions are distinguished by diffuse dermatitis in which lymphohistiocytic cells predominate, with lesser numbers of eosinophils and plasma cells and frequent lymphoid nodules or follicles (pseudolymphomatous reaction). In all histopathologic forms of tick-bite reactions, tick mouthparts (chelicerae and hypostomes) may be found penetrating the epidermis or embedded in the dermis or both.

CLINICAL MANAGEMENT

Therapy is usually directed at temporarily reducing the tick population.† Total eradication is usually very difficult and is generally reserved for vectors of economically important infectious diseases. Suitable insecticides are applied to the entire body surface every two to three weeks. One-host ticks may require only two to three applications, whereas multiple-host ticks often require periodic applications throughout tick season. Knowledge of the insecticidal resistance of the local tick population is extremely important.‡

Sprays or dips with 0.06 percent lindane or 0.5 percent toxaphene used to be very effective and popular. However, with increasing concern over residues in animals and the environment and the development of resistant *Boophilus* spp. strains, organophosphates and pyrethroids have become increasingly popular. However, organophosphate- and pyrethroid-resistant strains are now emerging, as well. Commonly espoused tickicides include 0.025 percent amitraz, 0.05 to 0.1 percent chlorfenvinphos, 0.05 percent chlorpyrifos, 0.05 percent coumaphos, 0.05 percent diazinon, 0.1 percent dioxathion, 0.25 to 0.5 percent malathion, 0.1 to 0.2 percent trichlorfon, 150 ppm cypermethrin, 150 ppm cypothrin, 200 ppm propetamphos, 25 ppm decamethrin, and 30 to 75 ppm flumethrin.* Slow-release insecticide devices (e.g., ear tags) have shown promise for tick control.† Recently, it has been reported that certain ixodid ticks were prevented from engorging on cattle and reproducing by daily and oral doses (greater than 50 μg/kg) of ivermectin[214] and that tick control could be achieved with subcutaneous injections (200 μg/kg) of ivermectin every two to four weeks during tick season.[541, 542, 592]

Treatment of *O. megnini* ear infestations is relatively simple.[14, 377, 469, 584, 734, 776] As many ticks as possible should be mechanically removed and the ear cleared of exudate. Lindane (one part), xylol (two parts), and pine oil (17 parts) has been a popular, effective otic tickicide and repellent when applied every three to four weeks. In addition, many commercial otic miticides and tickicides are effective, such as rotenone (one part) in mineral oil (three parts).

Other methods of tick control having variable application and efficacy include (1) burning of pasture, (2) land cultivation, (3) repellents, and (4) sterile hybrids.[440, 734]

SPIDERS

Spiders have poison glands in their cephalothorax that open through pores on the tips of the chelicerae.[734] They apparently attack large animals rarely.

In Australia, *Ixeuticus robustus* (black house spider, window spider) has been known to bite horses.[583, 584] The spider (5 to 10 mm in diameter) is commonly found in unused buildings and older stables, in characteristic funnel-like webs. It is nocturnal, often being found on stable walls and floors at night. Edematous plaques are produced by spider bites, usually on the neck and body of affected horses. The

---

*References 8, 30, 290, 514, 637, 685, 778, 843
†References 14, 80, 221, 360, 420, 440, 459
‡References 62, 232, 341, 440, 543, 621, 734, 748, 835

*References 14, 62, 80, 90, 173, 214–217, 232, 343, 420, 440, 455, 459, 466, 469, 497, 540, 543, 584, 645, 734, 852
†References 4, 58, 172, 177, 427, 780, 781

condition occurs overnight. Diagnosis is based on history, physical examination, presence of spiders, and elimination of other causes. Treatment consists of local cold packs and systemic glucocorticoids and antihistamines for two to three days. Control consists of avoiding infested premises or having a commercial exterminator power-spray the premises.

LICE INFESTATION

Infestation with lice (pediculosis) is a common cause of skin disease in large animals throughout the world.

CAUSE AND PATHOGENESIS

Lice are highly host-specific, obligate parasites that spend their complete life cycle (20 to 40 days) on the host.* Biting lice feed on exfoliated epithelium and cutaneous debris. Sucking lice feed on blood and tissue fluid. Nits 1 to 2 mm long are attached to hairs by a clear adhesive secretion by female lice (3 to 6 mm in length). Under favorable environmental conditions, lice can live two to three weeks off the host, but less than seven days is more typical. Transmission is by direct and indirect contact.

Lice populations are much larger and, therefore, clinical signs most obvious in winter.† This seasonality of pediculosis is related to lower skin and hair or wool temperatures, longer winter coats, overcrowding, poor nutrition, and possibly other stresses associated with cold weather. In cattle, ambient temperatures of over 78°F produce skin temperatures of 100 to 125°F.[14, 282] At 100°F, biting lice do not progagate, and at 125°F, biting lice are killed after one hour of exposure. Similarly, in sheep, the mean temperature of wool 3 cm long in summer is 178 ± 70°F at the tips, and 109 ± 1°F at the skin.[447, 502–507] Lice are killed in one hour at 118°F, in 30 minutes at 122°F, and in five minutes at 131°F. Thus, in summer, only small populations of lice generally survive in protected areas such as inside the ears, between the legs, and in the brush of the tail.

CLINICAL FEATURES

Lice are common ectoparasites of cattle throughout the world.* There are no particular age, breed, or sex predilections. Light louse infestation may cause no clinical signs. Heavy infestations cause pruritus and restlessness. Sucking lice (*Haematopinus eurysternus*, *Linognathus vituli*, and *Solenopotes capillatus* in the United States) are commonly found around the poll, nose, eyes, neck, brisket, withers, tail, axillae, and groin. Biting lice (*Damalinia bovis*) prefer the neck, withers, and tailhead. Rubbing, scratching, and excessive grooming lead to a rough and dishevelled coat, patchy alopecia and excoriations, and hairballs in calves. Patchy to generalized scaling is common (Fig. 9–24). Heavy sucking louse infestations may produce varying degrees of anemia.

Pediculosis is a cosmopolitan disease of sheep.† There are no apparent age, breed, or sex predilections. Biting lice (*D. ovis* in the United States) are commonly found on the neck and back (see Plate 6). Sucking lice prefer the face (*L. ovillus*) and lower legs (*L. pedalis*). Clinical signs are as previously described for cattle. Additionally, *L. pedalis* may cause lameness.

In goats, lice are the most common ectoparasites in most areas of the world.‡ There are no apparent age, breed, or sex predilections. Pediculosis is an especially devastating disease, economically, in Angora goats. Biting lice (*D. caprae* in the United States) and sucking lice (*L. stenopsis*) are most commonly found on the neck, trunk, and groin. *D. ovis* can be transferred between goats and sheep.[315] Clinical signs are as described for cattle.

In horses, lice are common ectoparasites in most parts of the world.§ There are no apparent age, breed, or sex predilections. Biting lice (*D. equi*) prefer the dorsolateral trunk (see Plate 6), whereas sucking lice (*H. asini*) favor the mane, tail, and fetlocks. Clinical signs are as described for cattle.

Pediculosis is the second most common ec-

---

*References 80, 244, 420, 437, 455, 457, 459, 497, 734
†References 14, 80, 221, 234, 244, 282, 360, 437, 455, 459, 469, 497, 500–507, 584, 680, 694, 808

---

*References 13, 14, 80, 156, 282, 381, 406, 497, 513, 519, 561, 577, 734
†References 21, 80, 111a, 111b, 360, 406, 437, 459, 500, 578
‡References 59, 200, 220, 310, 387, 406, 455, 513, 678, 683, 730, 731
§References 23, 80, 134, 244, 245a, 344, 469, 575, 576, 584, 786, 853

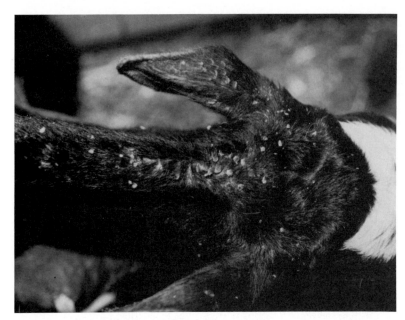

FIGURE 9–24. Bovine pediculosis. Crusts and scaling over head, ears, and neck.

toparasitism of swine throughout the world.* There are no apparent age, breed, or sex predilections. The sucking louse, *H. suis*, is the only louse of swine. It prefers the ears, neck, axillae, and groin. Clinical signs are as described for cattle. Hog lice are important in the transmission of swinepoxvirus and play a role in conditions of complex etiology, such as ear and tail biting. Hog lice also may temporarily feed on humans.

DIAGNOSIS

The differential diagnosis of pediculosis includes sarcoptic mange, psoroptic mange, chorioptic mange, psorergatic mange, keds, fly-bite dermatoses, trombiculidiasis, forage mites, seborrheic skin disease, and shedding. Definitive diagnosis is based on history, physical examination, and demonstration of lice or nits, or both (Fig. 9–25). Skin biopsy reveals varying degrees of superficial perivascular dermatitis with numerous eosinophils. Focal areas of epidermal necrosis, edema, and leukocytic exocytosis (epidermal nibbles) as well as eosinophilic intraepidermal microabscesses may be seen.

CLINICAL MANAGEMENT

Louse infestation may produce substantial economic losses through decreased weight

gains or weight losses, decreased milk production, hide and wool damage, secondary infections and myiasis, anemia, and increased susceptibility to other diseases.*

Treatment of pediculosis is usually easy and effective. Sprays are effective in horses, cattle, goats, and swine, and treatment should be repeated in two weeks.† Special attention should be given to the ears. Recommended insecticidal sprays include 0.06 percent lindane, 0.05 to 0.1 percent chlorfenvinphos, 0.05 to 0.2 percent coumaphos, 0.25 percent chlorpyrifos, 0.03 to 0.05 percent diazinon, 0.5 percent malathion, 0.1 to 1.0 percent crotoxyphos, 0.2 percent trichlorfon, 200 ppm propetamphos, and 0.15 percent dioxathion. In sheep, sprays or, preferably, dips are most effective when employed after shearing.

Pour-ons are simple and effective and are preferred in inclement weather.‡ Recommended insecticidal pour-ons include famphur, fenthion, phosmet, trichlorfon, and cypermethrin. In sheep, pour-ons are easier, quicker, and less stressful than dipping.[323] Fenthion pour-on, as marketed for cattle, has occasionally caused severe urticarial reactions

---

*References 50, 80, 123, 221, 335, 343, 406, 420, 513, 779, 827, 853

*References 14, 80, 121, 123, 147, 159, 160, 221, 234, 244, 344, 360, 379, 420, 437, 455, 459, 469, 497, 519, 563, 584, 595, 680, 731, 779, 786, 808
†References 14, 29, 76, 80, 90, 123, 165, 183, 221, 244, 297, 310, 360, 378, 420, 437, 455, 459, 474, 497, 519, 560, 577, 578, 584, 678, 731, 740, 786
‡References 123, 323, 343, 380, 381, 497, 519, 563, 584, 645

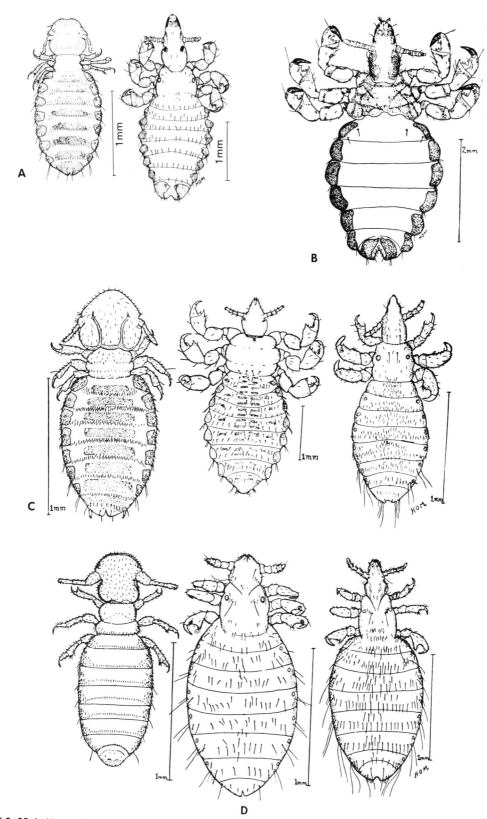

FIGURE 9–25. A, *Lice of the horse*. Left, Damalinia equi. Right, Haematopinus asini. B, *Female* Haematopinus suis. C, *Cattle lice*. Left, Damalinia bovis. Center, Haematopinus eurysternus. Right, Linognathus vituli. D, *Sheep lice*. Left, Damalinia ovis. Center, Linognathus pedalis. Right, L. africanus. *(With permission from Soulsby, E. J. L.: Helminths, Arthropods and Protozoa of Domesticated Animals, 7th ed. London, Baillière Tindall, 1982, pp. 370, 372, 373.)*

237

in horses.[584] Widespread wheals occur within 12 hours of application and usually resolve in 24 to 36 hours with symptomatic therapy. Even licensed pour-on products can cause primary irritant contact dermatitis.[96]

Powders or dusts are effective and are often used during inclement weather.* Recommended chemicals include 0.5 to 1.0 percent coumaphos, 4 to 6 percent malathion, 1.0 percent chlorpyrifos, 3 percent crotoxyphos, and 1 percent rotenone. In addition, commercial flea powders licensed for use in cats have been used safely and effectively in goats.[455, 730, 731] Powders should be applied weekly for three to four treatments.

It has been reported that ivermectin is effective against sucking lice in swine,[50, 752] cattle,[51, 52, 416, 690] and goats.[731] Single subcutaneous injections of 200 to 300 µg/kg were curative. Results in the treatment of biting lice have been erratic.[11a, 416, 480, 690]

Resistance to lindane has been reported for lice in sheep (*D. ovis*)[853] and swine (*H. suis*).[488] Resistance to organophosphate compounds has been reported for lice in goats.[43, 474, 494, 740, 790]

Improved hygiene, nutrition, and cleansing of the environment (e.g., bedding, blankets, and tack) are important control measures.

KED INFESTATION

Keds (sheep ticks) cause a pruritic skin disorder in sheep and goats in most parts of the world.

CAUSE AND PATHOGENESIS

The ked, *Melophagus ovinus*, is a blood-sucking, wingless, hairy, leathery insect 4 to 7 mm long.[360, 437, 459, 526, 734] Keds spend their entire life on the host. The female ked attaches her larvae to hair and wool by means of a sticky substance. The life cycle is about five to six weeks. Engorged female keds can live up to eight days off the host. Transmission is by direct and indirect contact.

Ked populations are highest in fall and winter.† Spring shearing and summer ambient temperatures reduce ked numbers dramatically. Poorly fed or debilitated animals appear to be more susceptible.

CLINICAL FEATURES

Keds are fairly common ectoparasites of sheep and goats in many parts of the world.* There are no apparent age, breed, or sex predilections. Ked populations are highest, and clinical signs most severe, in winter. The chief clinical sign is intense pruritus. The most commonly affected areas are the neck, sides, rump, and abdomen. Rubbing, chewing, and scratching produces broken wool, alopecia, and excoriations. Ked excrement stains the wool. Heavy infestations can cause anemia. Keds transmit the blue-tongue virus.

DIAGNOSIS

The differential diagnosis includes sarcoptic mange, psoroptic mange, chorioptic mange, psorergatic mange, lice, trombiculidiasis, and forage mites. Definitive diagnosis is based on history, physical examination, and demonstration of keds (Fig. 9–26).

CLINICAL MANAGEMENT

Ked infestations can cause significant economic losses through hide damage, wool damage, weight loss, decreased milk production, secondary infections, and anemia.†

Treatment is usually easy and effective. Sprays, dips, and dusts may be utilized as described for the treatment of lice (see prior section). In the United States, the two approved insecticides are coumaphos (0.125 percent spray or dip, or 0.5 percent dust) and malathion (0.5 percent spray or dip, or 4 percent dust).[435] For keds, three treatments are given at 10- to 14-day intervals. Resistance to organochlorines has been reported for sheep keds.[853]

Considering the efficacy of injectable ivermectin in sucking lice infestations of cattle and swine (see previous discussion), this compound may prove to be useful for ked control.

FLEAS

Fleas occasionally parasitize goats and pigs and, rarely, sheep, cattle, and horses. Adult

---

*References 343, 420, 437, 455, 459, 519, 730, 731
†References 279, 360, 437, 459, 523, 526, 734

*References 21, 80, 279, 280, 310, 360, 406, 435, 437, 455, 459, 578, 730, 734
†References 80, 279, 280, 360, 435, 437, 455, 459, 523, 730, 731, 853

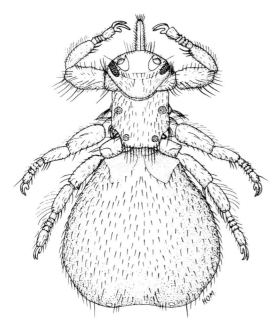

FIGURE 9–26. Adult *Melophagus ovinus. (With permission from Soulsby, E. J. L.: Helminths, Arthropods and Protozoa of Domesticated Animals, 7th ed. London, Baillière Tindall, 1982, p. 440.)*

fleas are blood-sucking, wingless, laterally compressed insects 2 to 4 mm long. Eggs (about 0.5 mm long) are deposited in dust and dirt or on the host. Fleas are much less permanent parasites than, for example, lice and frequently leave their hosts. Longevity and life cycle vary with different species of fleas, according to whether they are fed or not, and according to ambient temperature and humidity.[734] Flea populations are largest in summer and fall.

Fleas are not markedly host-specific and have been reported to infest swine (*Ctenocephalides felis, C. canis, Echidnophaga gallinacea, Pulex irritans, Tunga penetrans*),* goats (*Ctenocephalides* spp.),[250, 455, 513, 550, 683] sheep (*Ctenocephalides* spp.),[161, 250, 550, 683, 806] cattle (*C. felis*),[78, 171] and horses (*T. penetrans, E. gallinacea*).[406, 734] Clinical signs include varying degrees of rubbing, scratching, and chewing as well as broken wool, alopecia, excoriations, nonfollicular papules, and crusts, especially over the trunk. In swine, *T. penetrans* infestations tend to localize around the snout, feet, scrotum, and teats.[151, 817] Sows with teat lesions may suffer from agalactia, with resultant piglet deaths. Heavy infestations in goats and

sheep, especially on kids and lambs or debilitated animals, may result in anemia, poor feeding behavior and weight losses, and even death.[250] In swine, fleas may transmit swinepoxvirus.[123, 221, 420]

Successful treatment and control regimens must focus on the animals *and* the environment.[123, 221, 420, 734] Numerous organophosphates may be used as sprays or dips on the animals, as described for lice (see preceding section). In addition, dusts such as 4 to 6 percent malathion, 1 percent rotenone, and commercial flea powders licensed for use in cats may be used. Similarly, insecticidal sprays and dusts should be used on the premises.

FLIES

Domestic livestock are liable to almost perpetual attack from a variety of flies. Animal and production losses are enormous.* Estimated costs to producers for livestock insect control and losses resulting from these ectoparasites in the United States exceed 3 billion dollars annually.[729]

Biting Flies

Mosquitoes

Mosquitoes (*Aedes* spp., *Anopheles* spp., *Culex* spp.) are important nuisances and vectors of numerous viral and protozoal diseases to large animals throughout the world.† Substantial economic losses occur via decreased weight gains, decreased milk production, hide damage, and disease transmission.

Mosquito eggs are laid on water or on floating vegetable matter, and each species has its special requirements. Mosquito populations are largest during warm weather and after rainfall. Adults may fly distances up to several kilometers and tend to feed (suck blood) at night.

Mosquito bites produce wheals and papules that are variably pruritic or painful.‡ Unlike the papules and wheals caused by the bites of many other insects, close examination of mos-

---

*References 122, 123, 151, 221, 343, 420, 806, 817

---

*References 23, 62, 80, 221, 297, 420, 437, 459, 469, 497, 584, 734, 748, 755
†References 23, 80, 206, 221, 406, 420, 455, 469, 472, 584, 734, 746–748
‡References 206, 221, 420, 469, 472, 583, 584

quito bites reveals no central crust. Individual lesions resolve spontaneously in one to two days. Large swarms of mosquitoes cause animals to be very restless at night and may cause death.

Control measures are usually directed against both the larval and the adult stages.[440, 734] Antilarval methods include the use of larvicidal compounds (e.g., pyrethrins and organophosphates) and the reduction or removal of breeding sites. Antiadult methods include residual environmental sprays or aerosols (e.g., organophosphates and pyrethroids) and mosquito screens. Repellent sprays for animals have a short duration of action (a few hours) and are not practical for grazing animals.

Culicoides Gnats

Culicoides spp. (biting midges, gnats, "punkies," sandflies, "no-see-ums") are important nuisances and vectors of various diseases to large animals throughout the world.[80, 406, 729, 734, 748]

Culicoides spp. eggs are laid in water. Gnat populations are largest during warm weather and most active when there is little or no breeze. Adult gnats are blood-suckers, and the different species vary in their preferred feeding times (morning versus evening) and sites (dorsum versus ventrum) (Fig. 9–27).

Culicoides spp. bites produce immediate pain and pruritus followed by papules and wheals. Individual lesions and associated symptoms may persist for several days. In the horse, *Culicoides* gnats are a cause of insect hypersensitivity and ventral midline dermatitis.

Control of these gnats is difficult.[440, 469, 584, 729, 734] Adult gnats are of such minute size (1 to 3 mm long) that they can pass through conventional 14- to 16-mesh mosquito screens. Combinations of stabling (dusk, dawn, or constantly), special screens (32-mesh), and residual environmental sprays and time-operated spray-mist insecticide systems are usually employed.

Black Flies

Simulium spp. (black flies, buffalo gnats, sandflies) are severe nuisances and vectors of various viral, protozoal, and filariid diseases to large animals throughout the world.*

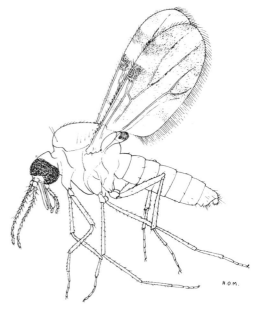

FIGURE 9–27. Culicoides. *(With permission from Soulsby, E. J. L.: Helminths, Arthropods and Protozoa of Domesticated Animals, 7th ed. London, Baillière Tindall, 1982, p. 393.)*

Simulid eggs are laid on stones or plants just below the surface of the water in running streams. Black fly populations are largest and most active in spring and early summer, especially in the morning and evening. Adult black flies (1 to 5 mm long) are blood-suckers and vicious biters (Fig. 9–28).

Black flies cause great annoyance and irritation and even deaths in all large animal species.* Simulid bites (*S. pecuarum* and *S. venustum* in the United States) cause painful papules and wheals, which often become vesicular, hemorrhagic, and necrotic. Favorite biting sites are the ears, head, neck, and ventrum. Localization of lesions to the intermandibular skin of horses may be seen. Simulid bites have been incriminated in the pathogenesis of equine aural plaques (see Chapter 17, discussion on papillomatosis). Black flies may also be an important cause of insect hypersensitivity in horses (see Chapter 10, discussion on insect hypersensitivity). In addition to painful, damaging bites, a heat-stable, alcohol- and ether-soluble toxin secreted by simulids causes cardiorespiratory dysfunction.[293, 294, 469, 584, 734] The toxin causes increased capillary permeability, with consequent major loss of circulatory fluids

---

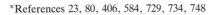

*References 23, 80, 406, 584, 729, 734, 748

---

*References 14, 23, 110, 134, 245a, 273, 282, 406, 420, 469, 471, 729, 734, 748, 755

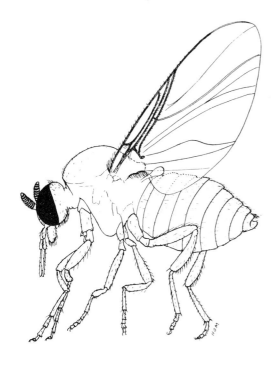

FIGURE 9–28. Simulium *imago. (With permission from Soulsby, E. J. L.: Helminths, Arthropods and Protozoa of Domesticated Animals, 7th ed. London, Baillière Tindall, 1982, p. 394.)*

into extravascular spaces. Systemic signs produced include depression, weakness, staggering, tachypnea, tachycardia, weak pulse, and potential shock and death.

Skin biopsy reveals varying degrees of superficial perivascular dermatitis with numerous eosinophils (Fig. 9–29).[110, 273] Focal areas of epidermal necrosis (nibbles), purpura, and subepidermal hemorrhagic bullae may be seen.

Control of simulids is difficult because the adults can fly 3 to 5 km or more.[440, 469, 584, 729, 734] Stabling during the day, residual environmental sprays or aerosols, and frequent applications of repellents to animals are all helpful, when possible or practical. Treatment of severe cutaneous reactions in animals is accomplished with systemic glucocorticoids as needed.

Horseflies

Tabanids (*Tabanus* spp., *Chrysops* spp., and *Haematopota* spp.), commonly called horseflies, deerflies, or breeze flies, cause great economic losses worldwide through their disturbing effects as nuisances and through trans-

mission of various viral, protozoal, bacterial, and filariid diseases.*

Tabanid eggs are laid in the vicinity of water, usually on the leaves of plants. Fly populations are largest in summer and most active on hot, sultry days. Adult tabanids (10 to 20 mm long) are blood-suckers and vicious biters (Fig. 9–30).

Horseflies cause great annoyance and irritation.† Tabanid bites produce painful, pruritic papules and wheals with a central ulcer and hemorrhagic crust. Favorite biting sites are the ventrum, legs, neck, and withers.

Control of tabanids is difficult.[440, 729, 734, 748] Stabling during the day, residual environmental sprays or aerosols, and frequent applications of repellents to animals are all helpful, when possible or practical. Recently, ear tags impregnated with permethrin and cypermethrin were reported to be effective.[430]

Stable Flies

Stomoxys calcitrans, the stable fly, is a cosmopolitan cause of annoyance and disease transmission (viral, protozoal, and helminthic).‡

Stable fly eggs are laid in manure and moist, decaying vegetable matter. Fly populations are largest in summer and fall. Adult flies (6 to 7 mm long) are blood-suckers and prefer fairly strong light (Fig. 9–31).

Stable flies cause great annoyance and irritation.§ Stable fly bites cause pruritic and painful papules and wheals with a central crust. Favorite biting sites are the neck, back, chest, groin, and legs. In horses, *Stomoyxs calcitrans* may be one cause of insect hypersensitivity (see Chapter 10, discussion on insect hypersensitivity).

Control measures are directed at destroying breeding places and the use of residual environmental sprays and aerosols.‖ Ear tags impregnated with cypermethrin are also reported to be effective.[593] Regular (at least twice weekly) removal of moist bedding, hay, and manure along with preventing the accumulation of weed heaps, grass cuttings, and vege-

---

*References 80, 221, 420, 440, 469, 471, 729, 734, 748
†References 80, 221, 245a, 406, 420, 455, 469, 471, 584, 729, 734, 748, 867
‡References 80, 221, 420, 455, 469, 584, 729, 734, 748
§References 14, 23, 80, 143, 245a, 387, 388, 406, 455, 469, 584, 729, 734, 748, 755
‖References 124, 125, 440, 469, 686, 729, 734

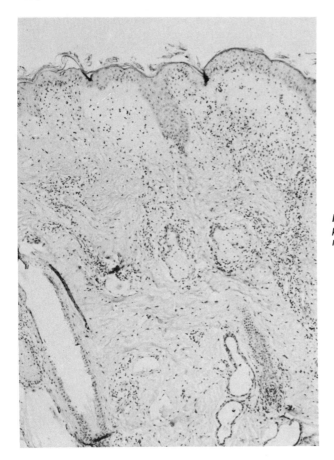

FIGURE 9–29. Blackfly bite in a cow. Superficial perivascular dermatitis with marked subepidermal edema.

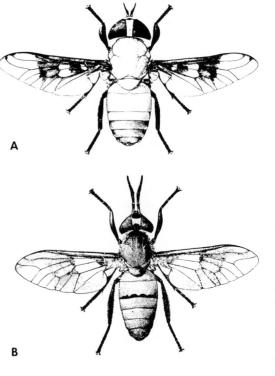

FIGURE 9–30. A, Tabanus latipes. B, Chrysops fixissimus. (With permission from Smart, J.: Cychorrhapha. In: Edwards, F. W., et al.: British Blood Sucking Flies. London, British Museum, 1939.)

A

B

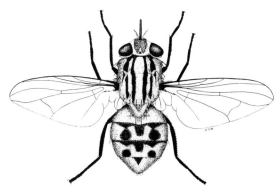

FIGURE 9–31. Female Stomoxys calcitrans. (With permission from Soulsby, E. J. L.: Helminths, Arthropods and Protozoa of Domesticated Animals, 7th ed. London, Baillière Tindall, 1982, p. 409.)

table refuse is very helpful. Other areas of research in stable fly control include (1) attractant toxicant devices (ultraviolet light attracts flies to pyrethroid-containing fiberglass panels,[469] (2) fly predator systems,[469] and (3) sterile-male release techniques.[469]

Horn Flies

Haematobia (Lyperosia) spp. flies, the horn flies, are a ubiquitous cause of annoyance and disease transmission (protozoal and helminthic)* among cattle and horses.

Horn fly eggs are laid in the fresh dung of cattle. Fly populations are largest in summer. Adult horn flies (3 to 4 mm long) are blood-suckers and spend most of their lives on the host, tending to congregrate around the base of the horns, shoulders, and back when ambient temperature is less than 70°F and on the ventrum when it is hot or rainy, or both.

Horn flies cause great annoyance and irritation in cattle and horses.† Bites produce pruritic to painful papules and wheals with a central crust, which occur over the dorsum or ventrum. In horses, *H. irritans* is a cause of ventral midline dermatitis in the United States.

Control of horn flies is relatively easy, as adult flies spend most of their life on the host.[14, 440, 729, 734, 748, 755] Regular spraying with various organophosphates or self-application of organophosphates with the use of back-rubbers or dust bags achieves good control. In general, there are five categories of horn fly control: (1) direct applications of insecticides (sprays, dusts, dips, or pour-ons), (2) free-choice and forced-used self-application devices (back-rubbers, dust bags, or treadle sprayers), (3) ultra–low-volume applications of insecticides from aerial or ground units, (4) feeding of insecticides, and (5) ear tags.*

Musca spp. and *Hydrotaea* spp. Flies

Musca spp. and *Hydrotaea* spp. flies are cosmopolitan causes of annoyance.[14, 80, 459, 584, 657, 734] In general, these flies do not pierce the skin but feed from wounds and add to the inflammatory response.

M. autumnalis is the face fly of North America.[14, 657, 734] Fly eggs are deposited in fresh manure. Adult flies (6 to 8 mm long) are active in summer and fall and gather around the eyes and nostrils to feed on ocular and nasal discharges. Economic losses through annoyance, disruption of grazing, reduced weight gains, and decreased milk production are great.[14, 80, 188, 208, 657, 734] *M. vetustissima* is the bush fly, or face fly, of Australia.[23, 271, 388, 455, 584]

Hydrotaea irritans is the head fly or forest fly of sheep and cattle in Europe and Australia.[21, 351, 459, 734, 755, 828] Although these flies do not possess piercing or biting mouthparts, their rasping labellae prevent healing of minor wounds and lead to rapid expansion of the lesions. Fly eggs are deposited on manure and decaying vegetation, and fly populations are largest in summer and most active at the edges of woods in which the flies find shelter. Adult flies (4 to 7 mm long) are attracted to animal movement and wounds, particularly those that appear to arise spontaneously at the skin-horn junction in young sheep and cattle and in fighting rams. Affected animals shake and rub their heads. Horned breeds of sheep and those with haired faces appear to be more susceptible. While the head flies are active, wounds do not heal. Secondary infections, myiasis, weight loss due to interruption of feeding, and permanent disfigurement are possible sequelae.

Control methods for *M. autumnalis* are effective and generally include the five categories described for horn fly control. However, there are no totally effective, practical control meas-

---

*References 14, 23, 80, 126, 245a, 282, 319, 406, 729, 734, 748
†References 14, 23, 80, 187, 282, 406, 469, 584, 729, 734, 748

---

*References 31, 77, 124, 179, 208, 338, 371, 390, 391, 430, 440, 593, 686, 729, 734, 748, 857

ures for use against *H. irritans*.[459] Avoiding the grazing of pasture with extensive tree cover would be helpful. Protective canvas head caps give good to complete protection but are expensive and time-consuming to use.[272, 459] Repellents, except for 0.05 percent crotoxyphos in pine tar oil, are ineffective.[272, 459] The spray application of 0.1 percent permethrin, 500 ppm cyhalothrin, or 1000 ppm cypermethrin significantly decreases the incidence and severity of disease, if applied every two weeks throughout fly season.[19, 857] In addition, ear tags containing 8.5 percent cypermethrin or 10 percent permethrin were reported to be effective.[20, 21, 338, 430, 593, 857]

Equine Ventral Midline Dermatitis

Ventral midline dermatitis is a distinctive, common, fly-related dermatosis of horses.[244, 245a, 469, 471, 576, 584, 741] The condition is caused by the bites of *Haematobia (Lyperosia) irritans* (the horn fly) and *Culicoides* spp. gnats. Thus, the dermatosis is quite seasonal, corresponding to fly season (spring to fall). Ventral midline dermatitis occurs most commonly in horses over four years of age, with no apparent breed or sex predilections.

Clinical signs consist of one to several sharply demarcated areas of punctate ulcers, hemorrhagic crusts, thickening, and alopecia on the ventral midline (see Plate 6). The umbilical area is most commonly affected, but lesions may occur anywhere on the ventral midline, thorax to abdomen. Leukoderma is commonly seen. The majority of horses on the premises are usually affected. Pruritus varies from intense to minimal, possibly reflecting the presence or absence of a hypersensitivity reaction to fly salivary antigen(s) in a given horse.

Diagnosis is based on history, physical examination, and the presence of the flies. Skin biopsy reveals varying degrees of superficial perivascular dermatitis with numerous eosinophils.[244, 741] Intraepidermal eosinophilic microabscesses, focal areas of epidermal necrosis (nibbles), and hypomelanosis may be seen.

Treatment consists of gentle cleansing and topical applications of antibiotic-glucocorticoid creams or ointments until healed. Severely pruritic animals may require systemic glucocorticoids for two to three days. Control is achieved by the frequent topical application (two to three times daily) of fly repellents or a thick layer of petrolatum.

Louse Flies

Louse flies, including *Hippobosca equina* (cosmopolitan), *H. maculata* (Africa and South America), and *H. rufipes* (Africa), parasitize horses and cattle in many parts of the world.[80, 406, 734] These flies are often called forest flies or keds. Female flies (about 1 cm long) deposit larvae in sheltered spots where there is dry soil or humus (Fig. 9–32). The flies are most numerous in sunny weather.

Adult louse flies suck blood and tend to cluster in the perineal and inguinal regions. They remain for long periods on their hosts and are not easily disturbed. Louse flies are a source of irritation and fly-worry.

Louse flies are readily killed by numerous organophosphate and organochlorine sprays.

Bees and Wasps

Bees and wasps have been reported to attack large animals.[80, 406, 584, 844] The honeybee, *Apis mellifera*, has been reported to attack horses in the summer, producing single to multiple edematous wheals and plaques anywhere on the body (apisination).[584] The barbed stinger with attached venom sac may be observed in the center of skin lesions. Severe attacks may produce angioedema of the head, eyelids, nostrils, and lips. Treatment includes the careful removal of stingers (avoid compressing the venom sac) and systemic glucocorticoids.

Yellow jacket attacks were reported to cause vesicles, wheals, and crusts on the ears, snout, eyelids, anus, vulva, scrotum, axillae, and flank of swine.[824] Affected swine were nervous, unthrifty, and polydipsic. Gastric ulcers and sudden deaths were seen. Skin biopsies revealed varying degrees of superficial perivascular dermatitis with numerous eosinophils. Separating the swine from the yellow jackets resulted in complete recovery.

Gasterophiliasis

Gasterophiliasis (bots) is a rare cause of skin disease in the horse.[406, 469, 734] Adult flies (botflies) are active in summer, and the females glue their eggs to the hairs of horses on the distal legs and shoulders (*G. intestinalis*), intermandibular area (*G. nasalis*), and face (*G. haemorrhoidalis, G. pecorum,* and *G. inermis*). Eggs apparently hatch in response to temperature increases and licking. Larvae pen-

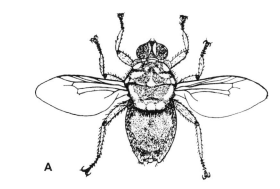

FIGURE 9–32. A, Hippobosca rufipes. B, *Wing of Hippobosca rufipes. (With permission from Soulsby, E. J. L.: Helminths, Arthropods and Protozoa of Domesticated Animals, 7th ed. London, Bailliere Tindall, 1982, p. 439.)*

A

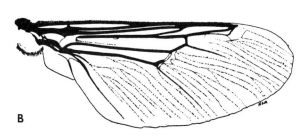

B

etrate skin or mucosa, develop in the stomach, pass with the feces, and pupate in the ground.

Gasterophilus spp. larvae that penetrate facial skin and oral mucosa, including *G. haemorrhoidalis* (global), *G. pecorum* (Europe, Asia, and Africa), and *G. inermis* (northern hemisphere), have been reported to rarely cause dermatitis and stomatitis.[406, 734] Cutaneous gasterophiliasis (gasterophilosis cutis, dermatitis aestivalis buccarum) is characterized by 1- to 2-mm wide grayish-white, crooked streaks in the skin of the cheeks, neck, and shoulders (Fig. 9–33). These streaks may extend by 1.5 to 3 cm in 24 hours. The hair over these palpable, twinelike tracts may become rough and fall out, revealing a scaling skin surface. Depigmentation may be seen, but pruritus is mild or absent. Rarely, similar lesions have also been described in humans, especially on the arms.[406, 658, 734]

Diagnosis is based on history, physical examination, and demonstration of the migrating larvae. Skin biopsy reveals larvae in an apparently normal or mildly inflamed dermis.[406]

Therapy for cutaneous gasterophiliasis is not necessary, as the disease is self-limiting and, rarely, symptomatic. For external treatment of bot eggs, a warm water wash that contains an insecticide (0.06 percent coumaphos, 0.15 percent dioxathion, 0.5 percent malathion, or 0.5 percent stirofos) will stimulate hatching and kill the larvae.[440, 734] Therapy for stomach bots

consists of the administration of oral products such as carbon disulfide, trichlorfon, thiabendazole, or ivermectin.[16, 80, 734] Treatment is usually administered twice yearly, approximately one month after the first frost and again in late winter.

Myiasis

Hypodermiasis

Hypodermiasis (warbles, grubs) is a common disorder of cattle, goats, and, occasionally, horses and sheep in many parts of the world.

CAUSE AND PATHOGENESIS

The larval stages of *Hypoderma bovis* and *H. lineatum*, the ox warbles, are common parasites of cattle, and occasionally horses and humans, in many countries in the northern hemisphere.* Adult flies (13 to 15 mm long) occur in summer and fix their eggs (1 mm long) to the hairs of cattle and horses, especially on the legs. *H. bovis* lays its eggs singly, while *H. lineatum* deposits a row of six or more on a hair. Larvae hatch in about four days and

---

*References 14, 80, 276, 282, 311, 406, 497, 521, 658, 734

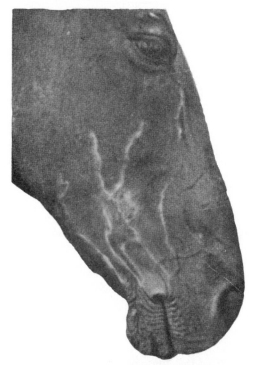

FIGURE 9–33. Gasterophilus myiasis (Courtesy F. Chládek). (With permission from Kral, F., and Schwartzman, R. M.: Veterinary and Comparative Dermatology. Philadelphia, J. B. Lippincott Co., 1964, p. 398.)

crawl down the hair to the skin, which they penetrate. The larvae wander in the subcutaneous tissue, apparently via the elaboration of proteolytic enzymes,[17, 61, 521, 525, 709] up the leg and toward the diaphragm, and they gradually increase in size. The winter resting sites of first-stage larvae are the submucosal connective tissue of the esophagus for *H. lineatum* and the region of the spinal canal and epidural fat for *H. bovis*. Larvae reach these sites weeks or months after hatching and remain in them for fall and winter, growing to 12 to 16 mm in length. During January and February, the now second-stage larvae migrate toward the dorsum of the host's body and reach the subcutaneous tissue of the back (the spring resting site), where they mature to third-stage larvae. When the parasites arrive under the skin of the back, swellings begin to form. The skin over each swelling becomes perforated (breathing pore). This is the "warble" stage of infestation, and it lasts about 30 days. In spring, the mature larvae (25 to 28 mm long) wriggle out of their cysts and fall to the ground to pupate.

In horses, goats, sheep, and humans, *Hypoderma* larvae usually do not mature and complete the life cycle.[244, 406, 521, 734, 741, 742] In addition, aberrant migrations may cause serious effects, such as neurologic disorders.

Hypersensitivity or toxic reactions associated with the accidental or deliberate rupture of third-stage larvae and the therapeutic destruction of second-stage larvae have been recorded in cattle.[243, 289, 313, 497, 521, 734] Anaphylaxis-like reactions may be mediated by Type I (reaginic) and Type III (Arthus) hypersensitivity reactions to larva-associated allergen(s).[83, 84] Reactions similar to toxic reactions have been recognized clinically[15, 383, 385, 497, 521, 681] and have been produced experimentally with intravenous and intradermal injections of soluble larval toxin.[243]

Przhevalskiana silenus (synonyms: *Hypoderma silenus, H. crossi, P. crossi,* and *P. aegagi*) parasitizes goats, sheep, and, occasionally, horses in Europe and Asia.* Adult flies are active from April to June and fix their eggs to hairs on the legs and chest. Larvae hatch out and crawl down to the skin, which they penetrate. The larvae migrate in the subcutaneous connective tissue up the legs to the back. *All* larval stages are found in the subcutaneous tissues of the back. Third-stage larvae produce subcutaneous nodules and cysts in spring, cut breathing pores, and drop on the ground to pupate.

In Central and South America, larvae of *Dermatobia hominis* are known to attack cattle, sheep, goats, swine, and humans.[406, 658, 734, 748] Adult female flies (12 mm long) capture mosquitoes or other blood-sucking flies and glue a batch of eggs to the abdomen of the captive fly. When the transport fly alights on a warm-blooded host, the larvae of *D. hominis* hatch and penetrate the skin. The larvae develop subcutaneously and produce a painful swelling with a central pore. Mature larvae (25 mm long) drop to the ground and pupate.

The larvae of *Cuterebra* spp. flies have been reported rarely to parasitize swine.[163, 221, 420] Adult flies (20 mm or more in length) oviposit near rodent and rabbit burrows.[734] Larvae hatch at intervals and penetrate the skin of hosts in spring and summer. The larvae develop subcutaneously, especially in the neck, and produce cysts with a central pore. Larvae mature in about 30 days and drop to the ground to pupate.

---

*References 1, 27, 162, 291, 422, 512, 673–675, 707, 733, 798, 811

CLINICAL FEATURES

Hypodermiasis is a common disorder of cattle in many parts of the northern hemisphere.* There are no apparent breed or sex predilections. Calves and younger cattle are more frequently and more severely affected than older cattle, suggesting the development of some degree of acquired immunity. Indeed, acquired immunity to *H. lineatum* has been demonstrated in cattle by in vitro and in vivo immunologic techniques,[48, 285, 286, 451, 605] suggesting that vaccination may be a future means of controlling this disease.

Swarms of adult *Hypoderma* flies (heel flies, gadflies) cause annoyance and fright, and cattle may be seen running (gadding), apparently trying to avoid the flies. Larva-associated cutaneous lesions appear in the spring as numerous subcutaneous nodules and cysts over the back. These lesions develop a central hole, or breathing pore, in which the third-stage larvae may be seen. Accidental or deliberate rupture of third-stage larvae may produce anaphylactic reactions, characterized by depression, salivation, lacrimation, defecation, edema of the head and anus, dyspnea, and death.†

In horses, *Hypoderma* larvae infestations are occasionally seen.‡ Affected horses are often in close proximity to cattle, and younger horses or those in poor condition seem to be more susceptible. Subcutaneous nodules and cysts are most commonly seen over the withers in spring and are usually few in number. Most lesions develop a breathing pore. Many lesions are painful. Rupture of the third-stage larvae may produce anaphylactoid reactions.[244, 344] Intracranial migration of first-stage *Hypoderma* larvae with resultant neurologic disorders have been reported.[312, 557]

Hypoderma larvae rarely affect humans.[406, 658, 734] Abdominal pain, subcutaneous migratory tracts, and local warble formation (cyst, furuncle, abscess) have been reported.

Hypodermiasis caused by *P. silenus* is common in goats and sheep in Asia and Europe.§ There are no apparent age, breed, or sex predilections. Larva-associated cutaneous lesions appear in spring as numerous subcutaneous nodules and cysts over the back. The lesions develop a central pore in which the third-stage larvae may be seen. Goats frequently have numerous lesions, whereas sheep often have only a few.

DIAGNOSIS

The differential diagnosis includes infectious granulomas, parafilariasis (cattle and horses), epidermoid and dermoid cysts, neoplasms, and equine eosinophilic granuloma. Definitive diagnosis is based on history, physical examination, and demonstration of the larvae. Dermatohistopathologic findings vary from a larva confined in a subcutaneous and dermal cyst (the walls of which are formed by dense connective tissue, which is often infiltrated by neutrophils and eosinophils) to severe suppurative, pyogranulomatous, or granulomatous reactions containing numerous eosinophils and larval segments (Fig. 9–34).[142, 709]

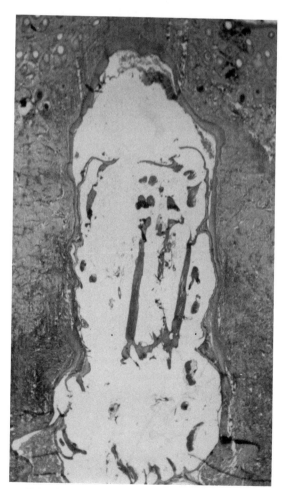

FIGURE 9–34. Equine hypodermiasis. Warble surrounded by fibrosis and pyogranulomatous dermatitis.

*References 14, 282, 406, 497, 521, 734, 748
†References 14, 15, 80, 282, 289, 313, 497, 521
‡References 41, 244, 245, 287, 344, 406, 469, 575, 576, 602, 682, 742, 786
§References 1, 27, 162, 291, 422, 512, 673, 707, 733, 798, 811

CLINICAL MANAGEMENT

In cattle and goats, hypodermiasis causes major economic losses resulting from annoyance, reduced weight gains or weight losses, decreased milk production, carcass and hide depreciation, and control programs.*

In cattle, hypodermiasis is usually controlled with systemic organophosphate compounds administered as feed additives, drenches, boluses, subcutaneous injections, dips, sprays, or pour-on or spot-on solutions.† Safe and effective treatment dates differ from region to region and year to year, depending on such factors as (1) which *Hypoderma* sp. is involved, (2) environmental temperature, and (3) anatomic location of migrating or resting larvae. Obviously, therapy is safest when larvae are not in a vital anatomic position (e.g., esophagus and spinal canal) and is most effective soon after fly season is over. Ivermectin, at a dosage of 200 µg/kg, has been reported to be 99 percent effective against all parasitic stages of *H. bovis* and *H. lineatum*. Recently, topical ivermectin (0.5 percent solution poured down the back at a dosage of 500 µg/kg) was reported to be highly effective against *H. bovis* and *H. lineatum*.[11a]

A variety of side effects may follow treatment of cattle for hypodermiasis.‡ Organophosphate toxicity is usually seen in less than 10 percent of the cattle treated and is characterized by varying combinations of lacrimation, pollakiuria, diarrhea, muscle fasciculation, ptyalism, hyperperistalsis of the gut, and bloat. Signs of toxicity usually peak in severity at 24 to 48 hours after treatment. Antidotal therapy, if needed, involves the administration of atropine. Death of *H. lineatum* larvae in the wall of the esophagus may result in esophagitis and bloat. Death of *H. bovis* larvae in the spinal canal may result in meningitis, periostitis, osteomyelitis, and posterior paralysis. Therapy includes the administration of glucocorticoids, phenylbutazone, and antibiotics. Animals that recover usually do so within about three to five days.

In horses, *Hypoderma* infestations are usually treated by *gently* enlarging the breathing pore with a scalpel and extracting the grub.[244, 469, 575, 576, 742, 786] Routine wound care is rendered as needed. Alternatively, the entire nodule may be surgically excised, or the larvae may be allowed to drop out by themselves.[344] In areas of high incidence, pour-on insecticides (such as 13.4 percent cruformate, 30 ml/45 kg) are effective preventives.[469, 682] Such treatments should be done at the time of year recommended for treatment of cattle.

For goats with hypodermiasis due to *P. silenus*, trichlorfon was found to be an effective drug for control.[672, 677] Goats were given a single backwash with 2 percent trichlorfon in December or January, resulting in a 92 and 98 percent reduction in the number of grubs, respectively. A single oral dose of trichlorfon (7 mg/kg) was not as effective.

Calliphorine Myiasis

Calliphorine myiasis (blowfly strike) is a common disorder of all large animals, especially sheep, in most areas of the world.

CAUSE AND PATHOGENESIS

Calliphorine myiasis is caused by flies from the genera *Lucilia*, *Calliphora*, *Phormia*, and *Chrysomyia*.* *L. cuprina* and *L. sericata* are the chief cause of calliphorine myiasis in Australia and Great Britain, respectively, while *L. caesar* and *L. illustris* are cosmopolitan in distribution. *Calliphora erythrocephala* and *C. vomitoria* strike sheep in Great Britain, while *C. stygia*, *C. australis*, *C. augur*, *C. fallax*, *C. nociva*, and *Microcalliphora varipes* strike sheep in Australia. *Chrysomyia chloropyga* and *C. albiceps* are sheep blowflies in Africa; *C. rufifacies* and *C. micropogon* are sheep blowflies in Australia. In North America, the most important blowflies are *Phormia regina* and *P. terrae-novae*.

Adult blowflies (6 to 12 mm long) lay clusters of light-yellow eggs (up to 3000 altogether) in wounds, soiled wool, or carcasses, being attracted by the odor of decomposing matter. Larvae hatch from eggs in 8 to 72 hours and reach full size in 2 to 19 days, depending on the temperature, amount and suitability of food, and competition with other larvae. Full-grown larvae (10 to 14 mm long) are grayish white or pale yellow and hairy or smooth.

---

*References 14, 17, 62, 64, 80, 282, 497, 521, 630, 673, 734, 748, 755

†References 14, 17, 80, 219, 276, 282, 383, 384, 439, 457, 458, 497, 521, 628–630, 655, 661, 676, 679, 684, 788, 789

‡References 14, 15, 80, 153, 243, 383, 385, 497, 521, 628, 681, 850

---

*References 14, 23, 80, 221, 282, 309, 324, 360, 387, 388, 420, 437, 455, 459, 497, 584, 734, 828, 868

Larvae pupate in the ground, in dry parts of a carcass, or even in the wool of live animals.

The factors that influence the occurrence of calliphorine myiasis can be classified into two groups: those controlling the number of flies and those determining the susceptibility of the host.

The proliferation of flies is seasonal because the adults are adapted to definite ranges of temperature and humidity. They are most abundant in late spring, early summer, and early fall. The abundance and suitability of food for the adults and larvae are of great importance.

The flies can be classified as (1) *primary flies*, which initiate a strike by laying eggs on living animals, (2) *secondary flies*, which usually lay their eggs on animals already struck, the larvae extending the injury done by the larvae of the primary flies, and (3) *tertiary flies*, which come last of all, the larvae of which do little further damage. The most important primary blowflies are *Phormia regina* (North America), *L. cuprina* (Australia), and *L. sericata* (Great Britain and New Zealand). Important secondary flies include *Chrysomyia* spp. and *Sarcophaga* spp. The ubiquitous *Musca domestica* is a common tertiary fly.

The susceptibility of the host depends on inherent factors, which can be influenced by selective breeding, and on temporary factors, which can be otherwise controlled. For instance, sheep are struck most commonly in the breech or crutch and around the tail, where wool is soiled and skin macerated by diarrheic feces and by urine. Major predisposing factors in this area are conformational, especially narrowness of the breech and wrinkling of the skin. Rams and wethers soil the wool of the sheath with urine. Rams with deep head folds or with horns lying close to the head may develop intertrigo, which attracts blowflies. Any other part of the body may be struck if undressed wounds are present. Myiasis over the dorsum is usually the result of prolonged wet weather and bacterial activity (fleece rot), and breeds of sheep with short or coarse wool, which dries faster, are less commonly affected than breeds with longer or finer wool.

Unless a wound is present to attract the flies and provide a suitable substrate for the larvae, bacterial activity appears to be important in preparing favorable conditions (see Chapter 4, discussion on ovine fleece rot). In wool that is kept moist, wool and skin scales become pasty and form a suitable medium for bacteria. Bacterial activity produces an odor that attracts flies and, probably, an exudative skin reaction that provides food for the larvae until they are able to pierce the skin. The larvae of primary blowflies initiate the strike and create favorable conditions for secondary flies. Primary blowfly larvae secrete proteolytic enzymes that digest and liquefy host tissues, which prepares the site for secondary blowfly larvae.

Recent studies of *Lucilia cuprina* strike in sheep[551, 552, 671] have demonstrated antibody responses, including reaginic antibody, and have suggested a genetic basis for resistance to fly-strike and the possibility of vaccination against fly-strike.

CLINICAL FEATURES

Calliphorine myiasis is an important disorder of all large animals, especially sheep, in most parts of the world.* Although any age, breed, or sex of animal may be struck, Merino sheep appear to be particularly susceptible because of the presence of highly developed skin folds. The disorder is most severe in spring, early summer, and early fall.

Clinically, blowfly strike is frequently classified in terms of the anatomic site attacked. Wound strike may occur on any wounded part of the body, such as results from fighting, accidents, surgical procedures (castration, docking, or dehorning), and other forms of trauma (ear marking, branding, or shearing). Breech, crutch, and tail strike follow soiling of these areas from diarrhea and urine scald. Pizzle strike follows soiling of the sheath of rams and wethers with urine. Poll strike follows fight wounds or intertrigo (deep head skin folds, close-lying horns). Body strike affects the dorsum, especially the withers, and usually follows prolonged wet weather and resultant fleece rot. Strike also complicates virtually any dermatosis.

Affected animals often stand with their heads down, do not feed properly, and are restless. The lesions are usually pruritic and painful, and animals shake, rub, scratch, and chew affected areas. Lesions consist of foul-smelling ulcers, often with scalloped margins. The ulcers often have a "honeycombed" appearance and are filled with larvae (maggots). Affected animals may die of toxemia and septicemia.

---

*References 14, 21, 80, 134, 221, 282, 309, 360, 387, 388, 420, 437, 455, 459, 497, 591, 695, 762, 793, 828

DIAGNOSIS

Definitive diagnosis is based on history, physical examination, and identification of the larvae. The different larvae may be identified by means of the structure of their spiracles and the cephalopharyngeal skeleton[734, 868] and must be differentiated from screw-worm larvae.

CLINICAL MANAGEMENT

The financial losses arising from calliphorine myiasis result from wool and hide damage, decreased weight gains or weight losses, decreased milk production, death, and treatment or control programs.*

Control programs are based on management practices that decrease the susceptibility of animals and on the use of insecticides to kill flies and larvae. Selected breeding has been used in attempts to produce sheep with flatter or plainer breeches.[734, 828] Surgical removal of breech folds (Mule's operation) is an older surgical technique that has helped to reduce the incidence of breech strike.[360, 437, 459, 734, 828] Crutching (clipping the wool from around the tail and in the breech) is very effective in reducing breech and tail strike.[360, 459, 734, 828] Ringing (clipping the wool from around the belly and sheath of rams) is very useful for reducing the incidence of pizzle strike.[828] Surgical procedures should be avoided during fly season, when possible.

Routine spraying or dipping with organophosphates (0.04 percent diazinon, 0.0125 percent chlorpyrifos, 0.05 percent chlorfenvinphos, or 0.05 percent coumaphos) and pyrethroids (e.g., permethrin, cypermethrin, and cypothrin) is helpful for controlling adult flies and larvae.† In Australia, *Lucilia cuprina* has developed resistance to many insecticides.[828] A strain of blowfly in which females are blind and cannot survive in the field and males are partially sterile offers the possibility that control of blowflies could be accomplished by genetic manipulation.[269]

Treatment of individual animals includes (1) a thorough cleansing and débriding of the wound, (2) application of topical insecticide (e.g., malathion or coumaphos) in *ointment* form (persists long enough to prevent reinfestation), and (3) other symptomatic therapy (e.g., antibiotics) as needed.‡

---

*References 309, 360, 437, 459, 497, 734, 748
†References 14, 21, 80, 360, 437, 459, 497, 697, 734, 748, 828, 865
‡References 14, 80, 282, 309, 360, 437, 459, 497, 734, 828

Screw-Worm Myiasis

Screw-worm myiasis is a serious disease of livestock in many parts of the world.

CAUSE AND PATHOGENESIS

The name screw-worm is given to the larvae of *Callitroga hominivorax* and *C. macellaria*, both of which occur in North, Central, and South America, and *Chrysomyia bezziana*, which occurs in Africa and Asia.[23, 734, 748, 868]

Adult flies (10 to 15 mm long) deposit clusters of eggs at the edge of a wound and near natural body openings on the host. These species have become so adapted to parasitic life that they breed only in wounds and sores on their hosts and not in carcasses. Larvae hatch in 10 to 12 hours and mature in three to six days, after which they leave to pupate in the ground. Mature larvae are about 15 mm long.

Wounds, accidental or surgical, rainy weather, and virtually any dermatosis predispose to screw-worm attack. The larvae (maggots) penetrate into the tissues, which they liquefy, and extend the lesion considerably.

CLINICAL FEATURES

Screw-worm myiasis is a serious disease of all large animals, especially cattle, swine, sheep, and horses, and humans may also be attacked.* The disease is most severe in spring, early summer, and early fall. There are generally no age, breed, or sex predilections.

Predisposing factors for screw-worm, and thus the areas of the body often affected, generally parallel those previously discussed for calliphorine myiasis. Common sites are wounds from shearing, dehorning, castration, docking, fighting, wire cuts, ear marking, and branding; the navel of newborn animals; cancer eye in cattle; severe pinkeye in cattle; and tick-bite lesions. In addition, larvae are often found in the mouth, feeding on the gums or lips of newborn calves, kids, and lambs. Lesions are as described for calliphorine myiasis, but screw-worm lesions tend to be more severe and more painful and pruritic and to have a fouler smell. Severe infections are common, and death (toxemia, septicemia) from screw-worm myiasis is common.

Cattle experimentally infested with *Chrysomyia bezziana* developed intermittent pyrexia,

---

*References 14, 23, 80, 221, 282, 309, 360, 387, 388, 406, 420, 437, 455, 459, 497, 545, 584, 685, 734, 868

neutrophilia, anemia, decreased total serum protein levels, and a progressive rise in serum globulin concentrations.[350]

DIAGNOSIS

Definitive diagnosis is based on history, physical examination, and identification of the larvae. Screw-worm myiasis is a reportable disease in the United States, and if the disease is suspected, larvae should be collected, preserved in 70 percent alcohol, and forwarded to an appropriate laboratory for identification.

The histopathology of experimental infestation of cattle with *C. bezziana* has been reported.[350] Two distinct phases were evident: (1) an initial phase of necrosis, neutrophil infiltration, and hemorrhage associated with tissue invasion and growth of larvae and (2) a fibroplastic healing phase in which eosinophils and mast cells were prominent.

CLINICAL MANAGEMENT

The financial losses from screw-worm myiasis can be astronomic and result from wool and hide damage, decreased weight gains or weight losses, decreased milk production, and death.*

Treatment of individual animals includes (1) a thorough cleansing and débriding of the wound, (2) application of a topical insecticide (e.g., malathion or coumaphos) in ointment form, and (3) other symptomatic therapy (e.g., antibiotics) as needed.

Prophylactic measures include those previously described for calliphorine myiasis. The most dramatic campaign against screw-worm flies and their larvae was the one carried out for the eradication of *Callitroga hominivorax* from the United States by the release of male flies sterilized by irradiation.[54, 55, 297, 734] Occasional screw-worm attacks are still recorded in the extreme southern United States, especially south Texas, as the flies are still present in Mexico and other parts of Central and South America.

HELMINTHS

Habronemiasis

Habronemiasis is a common cause of ulcerative cutaneous granulomas in horses around the world.

---

*References 14, 80, 134, 221, 282, 309, 360, 420, 437, 459, 497, 734, 748, 755, 868

CAUSE AND PATHOGENESIS

Three nematodes are involved in producing cutaneous habronemiasis in horses: *Habronema muscae*, *H. majus (H. microstoma)*, and *Draschia megastoma (H. megastoma)*.* The adults of all three nematodes inhabit the horse's stomach, *D. megastoma* residing in nodules. Eggs and larvae are passed with the feces and are ingested by the maggots of intermediate hosts: *Musca domestica*, the housefly (for *H. muscae* and *D. megastoma*), and *Stomoxys calcitrans*, the stable fly (for *H. majus*). Infectious larvae are deposited on the horse, especially in moist areas or open wounds, while the flies are feeding. Larvae are also capable of penetrating intact skin.[539, 734] Larvae deposited near the mouth are swallowed and complete the parasitic life cycle in the horse's stomach. Larvae deposited on the nose migrate to the lungs, and those on other areas of the body migrate locally within the skin.

There is reason to believe that habronemiasis is, at least in part, a hypersensitivity (allergic) disorder.† First, the disease is seasonal, with spontaneous remission occurring in winter and with larvae *not* overwintering in tissues. Second, the disease is sporadic, often affecting a single horse in a herd. Third, the disease often recurs in the same horse every summer. Fourth, systemic glucocorticoids, as the sole form of treatment, may be curative.

CLINICAL FEATURES

Habronemiasis (summer sores, bursautee, bursatti, swamp cancer, "kunkurs," "esponja", granular dermatitis) has been reported in horses from most parts of the world.‡ There are no apparent age, breed, or sex predilections. The disease usually begins in spring and summer when fly populations are active and often regresses partially or totally during the winter.

Lesions are most commonly seen on the legs, ventrum, prepuce, urethral process of the penis, and medial canthus of the eyes (Figs. 9–35 and 9–36; see Plate 6). Often, chronic wetting or wounds are predisposing factors. The onset of cutaneous habronemiasis is often characterized by the rapid development of papules or the failure of a wound to heal and

---

*References 245, 365, 392, 539, 662, 663, 734, 814
†References 244, 392, 469–471, 584, 744, 814
‡References 80, 170, 175, 181, 182, 349, 365, 392, 426, 469–471, 486, 584, 594, 602, 616, 722, 813, 814

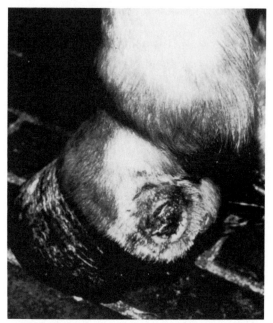

FIGURE 9–35. Equine habronemiasis. Ulcerated nodule on pastern.

the development of exuberant granulation tissue. Lesions may be solitary or multiple and are characterized by the rapid development of granulomatous inflammation, ulceration, intermittent hemorrhage, a serosanguineous exudate, and exuberant granulation. Pruritus varies from mild to severe. Small (1 mm in diameter) yellowish granules may be seen within the diseased tissue. The granules do not branch as do those (leeches) seen with py-

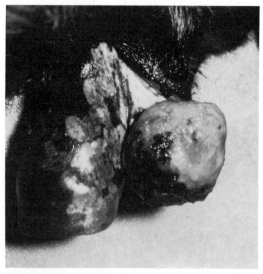

FIGURE 9–36. Equine habronemiasis. Large ulcerative granuloma on prepuce.

thiosis and zygomycosis (see Chapter 7, discussion on pythiosis and zygomycosis). These granules represent necrotic, caseous to calcified foci surrounding nematode larvae. Habronemiasis involving the urethral process may result in dysuria and pollakiuria.[255, 708, 753]

Conjunctival habronemiasis is common and usually characterized by yellowish, gritty plaques on the palpebral and bulbar conjunctivae.[367, 426, 469–471, 622, 814] Eyelid granulomas and blepharitis may be seen in some cases.

Pulmonary habronemiasis is apparently uncommon and is usually asymptomatic.[*] Multiple granulomas with central caseous necrosis are found at necropsy in the interstitial and peribronchial areas of the lungs.

Gastric habronemiasis is usually asymptomatic,[80, 469–471, 584, 814] although a fatal gastric abscess attributed to *D. megastoma* has been reported.[794]

Habronema and *Draschia* larvae have been suspected of facilitating tissue invasion by *Corynebacterium pseudotuberculosis* (cutaneous abscesses, see Chapter 6, discussion on *Corynebacterium pseudotuberculosis* abscesses) and *Rhodococcus equi* (lung abscess).[32, 471, 624]

DIAGNOSIS

The differential diagnosis includes bacterial and fungal granulomas, equine sarcoid, squamous cell carcinoma, and exuberant granulation tissue. Definitive diagnosis is based on history, physical examination, direct smears, and biopsy. Deep scrapings or smears from lesions, especially if the yellowish granules are retrieved, may reveal nematode larvae (40 to 50 μm long and 2 to 3 μm wide) in association with numerous eosinophils and mast cells. However, caution is warranted for two reasons: (1) such scrapings and smears are frequently negative and (2) *Habronema* and *Draschia* larvae may invade other ulcerative dermatoses, such as equine sarcoid, squamous cell carcinoma, and infectious granulomas.

Biopsy reveals varying degrees of nodular to diffuse dermatitis (Fig. 9–37).[†] The inflammatory reaction contains numerous eosinophils and mast cells. A characteristic feature of habronemiasis is multifocal areas of discrete coagulation necrosis, which consume all cutaneous structures in the area. Nematode larvae, few to many, may be found in these necrotic

*References 32, 392, 469–471, 594, 745, 795, 814
†References 109, 189, 193, 244, 392, 469–471, 499, 584, 622, 623, 723, 823

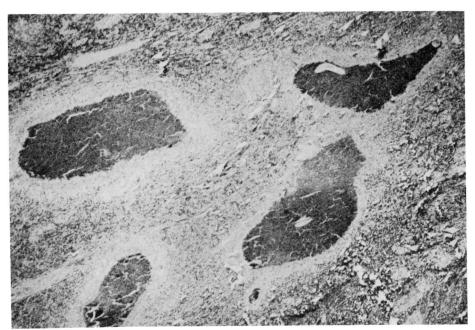

FIGURE 9–37. Equine habronemiasis. Multifocal areas of discrete dermal necrosis with palisading granuloma formation.

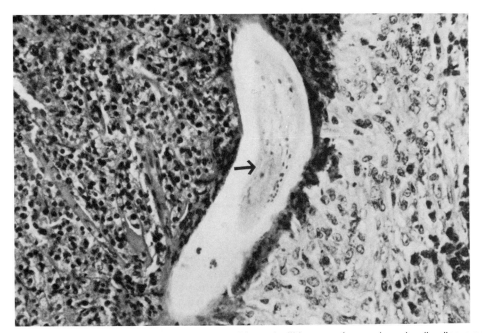

FIGURE 9–38. Equine habronemiasis. Nematode segment (arrow) within area of necrosis and palisading granuloma.

foci in about 50 percent of the specimens examined (Fig. 9–38). Palisading granulomas may develop around the necrotic foci.

CLINICAL MANAGEMENT

Habronemiasis has been managed with a plethora of therapeutic regimens.* However, there is little to suggest that an optimal therapeutic protocol for equine habronemiasis exists. Any therapeutic regimen will need to be individualized, with factors such as site of lesion, size of lesion, number of lesions, economics, and practicality receiving appropriate consideration.

In general, a combination of local and systemic therapy is most effective. Massive or medically refractory lesions may be eliminated surgically or, at least, debulked prior to vigorous topical and systemic therapy.† Lesions of a thickness within the capability of a cryotherapy unit have been treated successfully using a double freeze-thaw cycle.[255, 470, 487, 584, 708, 814]

Systemic therapy most commonly involves the use of organophosphates, ivermectin, or glucocorticoids.‡ One of the most commonly used systemic organophosphate compounds is trichlorfon.[86, 470, 584, 814] Trichlorfon is administered intravenously, at a dose of 22 mg/kg, in 1 L of 5 percent dextrose or saline by means of a 5-cm, 16-gauge needle, with attention given to avoiding perivascular injection. The solution is preferably autoclaved before use. Treatment may be repeated in two weeks, if necessary. The animal should not have been dewormed or sprayed with organophosphates within the last two weeks.[469] Some horses may exhibit mild side effects, such as restlessness and pawing. Pretreatment with atropine is unnecessary and may cause ileus and flatulent colic. Healing usually occurs within about 30 days, although some individuals fail to respond to trichlorfon.[392] A fatal case of acute hemolytic anemia in a horse with cutaneous and pulmonary habronemiasis was thought to be precipitated by systemic organophosphate therapy.[745]

Ivermectin has been reported to be very effective for the treatment of equine habronemiasis.[16, 325] A single intramuscular injection of 200 μg/kg ivermectin was reported to be curative in 84 percent of the horses treated, with the rest of the animals requiring a second or third injection at ten-day intervals. Because of the toxicities (predominantly clostridial infection and toxicosis),[16, 373, 386] associated with injectable ivermectin, this product is no longer available in the United States. It is presumed that the ivermectin oral product (Eqvalan paste) that is available will be equally as effective as the intramuscular product, while avoiding the problems of clostridial infection and toxicosis and, possibly, decreasing the risk of anaphylaxis.[94, 271, 373] The most common side effect of any ivermectin therapy in the horse is post-treatment cutaneous edema and pruritus, especially along the ventral midline, less so around the face. This occurs in 10 to 25 percent of horses treated and is presumed to be associated with massive destruction of *Onchocerca cervicalis* microfilariae in these areas.[16, 373]

Systemic glucocorticoids have been found to be very effective as the sole systemic agent in equine habronemiasis.[244, 245, 392, 470, 744, 814] Prednisone or prednisolone given orally at 1 mg/kg, once daily, results in a marked resolution of most lesions within 7 to 14 days. Such therapeutic observations emphasize the probable role of hypersensitivity in this disease.

A myriad of concoctions have been used for topical therapy of habronemiasis.* Commonly, these topical potions contain ingredients that are larvacidal, antimicrobial, anti-inflammatory, penetrating, and protective (Table 9–4). It is interesting to note that most of these topical concoctions contain a glucocorticoid! Such topical preparations are usually applied daily and bandaged. One of the older topical agents used in the treatment of cutaneous habronemiasis is glycerin.† A typical formulation is 50 ml glycerin, 20 ml formalin, and 1000 ml distilled water. The mixture is applied daily until the lesion(s) sloughs off!

Conjunctival habronemiasis has been successfully treated topically with 0.03 percent echothiophate (Phospholine Iodide) drops, twice daily, in combination with ophthalmic ointment (Maxitrol) containing neomycin, polymyxin B, and dexamethasone three times daily until healed.[622] Other similar topical protocols have also been recommended.[367, 469, 471]

---

*References 80, 182, 406, 469–471, 571, 584, 622, 670, 734, 814
†References 469–471, 571, 584, 753, 754, 814
‡References 80, 86, 325, 406, 469–471, 571, 584, 624, 814, 836

---

*References 80, 182, 406, 469–471, 584, 622, 814
†References 182, 325, 406, 469–471, 584, 622

Fly control, though difficult, will reduce the incidence of habronemiasis.[440, 470, 814] Prompt and proper removal and disposal of manure and soiled bedding are vital. Residual sprays on the walls, barn or stall mister systems, repellents applied to the horses, and cattle insecticide ear tags affixed to the mane and tail are all helpful.[440, 469, 470, 814]

Elimination of adult *Habronema* and *Draschia* nematodes from the stomach is another logical point of attack.[80, 470, 814] Recommended products include dichlorvos and carbon disulfide.

Onchocerciasis

Onchocerciasis is an important cause of skin disease in horses and cattle throughout the world.

CAUSE AND PATHOGENESIS

Five species from the genus *Onchocerca* are associated with cutaneous lesions in horses and cattle in different parts of the world.[35, 115, 116, 566, 567, 734] The prevalence of infection for all five *Onchocerca* species is very high, ranging from 20 to 100 percent of a given population of animals.

O. gibsoni infests cattle in Africa, Asia, and Australia.* Adult worms (up to 20 cm long) live in connective tissue nodules in the brisket and lateral stifle areas and produce microfilariae (240 to 280 μm long), which are most plentiful in the dermis of the brisket. *Culicoides* spp. gnats serve as intermediate hosts.

O. gutturosa infests cattle and horses in North America, Africa, Australia, and Europe.† Adult worms (up to 60 cm long) inhabit the ligamentum nuchae in horses and cattle and the connective tissue of the scapula, stifle, and hip areas in cattle. Microfilariae (200 to 230 μm long) are most numerous in the dermis of the face, neck, back, and ventral midline. Numerous *Simulium* spp. and *Culicoides* spp. gnats serve as intermediate hosts.

O. reticulata infests horses in Europe and Asia.[35, 570, 734, 750, 764] Adult worms (up to 50 cm long) live in the connective tissue of the flexor tendons and the suspensory ligament of the fetlock, especially in the frontlegs. Microfilariae (310 to 395 μm long) are most numerous

in the dermis of the legs and ventral midline. *Culicoides* spp. gnats serve as intermediate hosts.

O. ochengi infests cattle in Africa.[115, 116, 559] Adult worms (up to 25 cm long) inhabit the dermis of the udder and scrotum, and occasionally the flanks, sides, and head. Microfilariae (156 to 207 μm long) are most numerous in the dermis of the scrotum, udder, and ventral midline. *Simulium* spp. gnats serve as intermediate hosts.

O. cervicalis infests horses throughout the world.* Adult worms (up to 30 cm long) inhabit the funicular portion of the ligamentum nuchae. They are usually encased in a necrotizing, pyogranulomatous to granulomatous reaction with marked fibrosis and dystrophic mineralization. Microfilariae (200 to 240 μm long) are most numerous on the ventral midline (especially at the umbilicus), then the face and neck. Microfilariae are not evenly distributed in the skin and tend to be present in nests or pockets. Additionally, microfilariae tend to be situated more deeply in the dermis in winter. *Culicoides* spp. gnats and, possibly, mosquitoes serve as intermediate hosts.

Onchocerca sp. microfilariae were found in the skin of a pig with a generalized crusting dermatosis.[618] Further details were not available.

In infestations with *O. gibsoni*, *O. gutturosa*, *O. ochengi*, and *O. reticulata*, cutaneous nodules are produced by a granulomatous and fibrous reaction to adult worms. The exception would be *O. gutturosa* infestations in the horse, which may be nonpathogenic.[568]

In equine *O. cervicalis* infestations, the cutaneous lesions are associated with the microfilariae.† A unique clinical syndrome, distinctive dermatohistopathologic findings, and response to microfilaricidal chemotherapy define equine cutaneous onchocerciasis. Because most horses are infested with *O. cervicalis*, but only certain horses develop clinical signs, cutaneous onchocerciasis is thought to represent a hypersensitivity reaction to microfilarial antigen(s).‡ In humans, cutaneous reactions to *O. volvulus* microfilariae are thought to represent Type I and Type III hypersensitivity reactions.[732] Both in horses and humans, dead and dying microfilariae provoke the most in-

---

*References 73, 92, 107, 358, 565, 567, 638
†References 33, 34, 89, 92, 140, 225, 229, 231, 233, 253a, 352, 401, 515, 516, 567–569, 749, 750, 763

*References 6, 35, 66, 80, 158, 244, 419, 456, 468, 482, 484, 566, 568, 584, 611, 688, 741–743, 784, 786, 807, 830
†References 244, 267a, 468, 469, 471, 584, 741–743
‡References 244, 245, 468, 469, 471, 741–743

tense inflammatory reactions.* In fact, an exacerbation of cutaneous signs in association with microfilaricidal therapy is well-known, important to anticipate, and called the Mazzotti reaction.† Microfilariae are more numerous in skin with lesions than in clinically normal skin.[468, 471] *O. cervicalis* microfilariae may also invade ocular tissues, where they may be associated with keratitis, uveitis, peripapillary choroidal sclerosis, and vitiligo of the bulbar conjunctiva of the lateral limbus.‡ Here, again, the sudden killing of numerous microfilariae with chemotherapy may produce a severe exacerbation in ocular disease. It has been reported that horses with ocular onchocerciasis usually have more microfilariae in their skin than do horses without ocular involvement.[136, 483, 743]

In the past, *O. cervicalis* adult worms were incriminated as a cause of fistulous withers and poll evil in horses.§ However, necropsy examinations in large numbers of normal horses and those with fistulous withers have failed to support this belief.[80, 483, 635, 688]

It is not known how long the adults and microfilariae of the various *Onchocerca* spp. survive in the host. In humans, *O. volvulus* adults are believed to live up to 16 years, and the microfilariae up to five years.[522, 732]

CLINICAL FEATURES

Equine cutaneous onchocerciasis associated with *O. cervicalis* infestation is worldwide.‖ In the United States, the incidence of *O. cervicalis* infestation in clinically normal horse populations varies from 25 to 100 percent.¶

There are no apparent breed or sex predilections. Affected horses are usually four years of age or older, with horses younger than two years rarely showing clinical signs.

The clinical signs of equine cutaneous onchocerciasis are nonseasonal in nature, although they may be more severe during warm weather. This warm weather exacerbation of clinical signs is probably attributable to the additive effects of the insect vectors, *Culicoides* spp. gnats. Lesions may be seen exclusively on the face and neck (especially close to the mane) (Figs. 9–39 and 9–40), on the ventral chest and abdomen (see Plate 7), or in all these areas. Lesions vary in appearance from focal annular areas of alopecia, scaling, crusting, and inflammatory plaques to widespread areas of alopecia, erythema, ulceration, oozing, crusting, and lichenification. Pruritus varies from mild to severe. An annular lesion in the center of the forehead is thought to be highly suggestive of cutaneous onchocerciasis.[244, 419, 741, 744] Leukoderma may be seen in combination with the lesions just described or alone and is usually irreversible. Alopecia from permanent scarring may be a sequela. Seborrhea sicca (heavy scaling) may be seen in some horses.

Ocular signs may be seen in conjunction with cutaneous onchocerciasis and include variable combinations of (1) sclerosing keratitis (originating at the temporal limbus and growing toward the center), (2) vitiligo of the bulbar conjunctiva bordering the temporal limbus, (3) white nodules (0.5 to 1 mm in diameter) in the pigmented conjunctiva around the temporal limbus, (4) a round or crescent-shaped patch of depigmentation bordering the optic disc (peripapillary choroidal sclerosis), and (5) uveitis.*

O. reticulata adult worms cause subcutaneous nodules in the area of the flexor tendons and suspensory ligament of the fetlock, especially in the frontlegs, in horses in Europe and Asia.[35, 80, 570, 734, 750, 764] Severely affected horses may have extensive swelling and lameness in association with the infestation.

In cattle, three *Onchocerca* spp. are known to produce skin lesions. In North America, Europe, Africa, and Australia, adult *O. gutturosa* produce asymptomatic firm subcutaneous nodules over the shoulder, hip, and stifle regions.† In Africa, Asia, and Australia, adult *O. gibsoni* produce asymptomatic firm subcutaneous nodules over the brisket, hip, and stifle areas.‡ In Africa, adult *O. ochengi* produce asymptomatic firm subcutaneous and dermal papules and nodules of the scrotum, udder, flanks, sides, and head.[115, 116]

---

*References 244, 468, 469, 471, 522, 732, 741–743
†References 16, 244, 326, 373, 419, 468, 469, 471, 522, 732, 741–743
‡References 136, 436, 468, 469, 471, 531, 653, 687, 741–743
§References 3, 117, 339, 599, 600, 654, 751
‖References 66, 201, 244, 267a, 326, 419, 456, 463, 468, 469, 471, 575, 576, 584, 741, 742, 764, 784, 786, 807
¶References 133, 148, 226, 436, 445, 446, 465, 468, 611, 612, 688, 743

---

*References 136, 468, 469, 471, 653, 687, 741, 742
†References 33, 34, 225, 233, 401, 619, 689, 749, 763, 830
‡References 92, 107, 116, 358, 565, 567, 638, 750

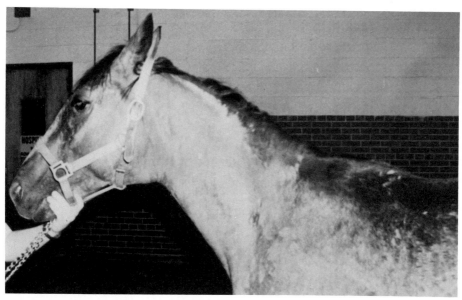

FIGURE 9–39. Equine cutaneous onchocerciasis. Alopecia, scaling, and crusting of face, neck, and withers.

DIAGNOSIS

The differential diagnosis for equine cutaneous onchocerciasis includes dermatophytosis, fly-bite dermatoses (seasonal), sarcoptic mange, psoroptic mange, *Pelodera* dermatitis, trombiculidiasis, and food hypersensitivity. The differential diagnosis for bovine onchocerciasis includes bacterial and fungal granulomas, demodicosis, parafilariasis, viral nodules, and neoplasia. Definitive diagnosis is based on history, physical examination, and skin biopsy.

Skin scrapings and direct smears are unreliable for the demonstration of microfilariae. *Onchocerca* spp. microfilariae are rarely found in the peripheral blood. An excellent technique for demonstrating *Onchocerca* spp. microfilariae in skin involves taking a punch biopsy (4 to 6 mm in diameter), mincing the specimen with a razor or scalpel blade, and

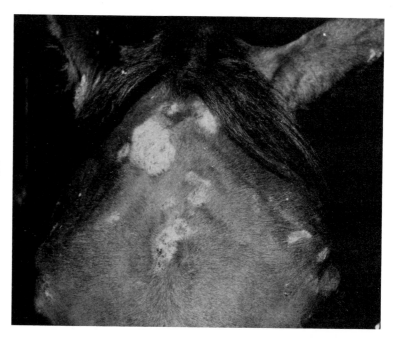

FIGURE 9–40. Equine cutaneous onchocerciasis. Alopecic, crusted plaques on forehead.

placing the minced skin on a glass slide or in a Petri dish and covering it with room temperature physiologic saline.[244, 468, 469, 471, 741, 742] After allowing this preparation to incubate at room temperature for 30 minutes, the specimen is examined under a microscope for the rapid motion of microfilariae in the saline. Saline containing preservatives (e.g., alcohol) should not be used, as such solutions may kill the microfilariae, not allowing their migration out of the minced skin. In addition, it must be remembered that this technique only confirms the presence of *Onchocerca* spp. microfilariae and does *not*, by itself, justify a diagnosis of cutaneous onchocerciasis.

In equine cutaneous onchocerciasis, skin biopsy reveals varying degrees of superficial and deep perivascular dermatitis, to diffuse dermatitis with numerous eosinophils (Fig. 9–41). Numerous microfilariae are usually seen in the superficial dermis, often surrounded by degranulating eosinophils (Fig. 9–42). Fibrosis tends to be prominent in older lesions. Occasional histopathologic findings include (1) necrosis of hair follicle epithelium, (2) focal areas of collagenolysis in the superficial dermis, where microfilariae may often be found, and (3) lymphoid nodules in the deep dermis or subcutis. Again, it must be emphasized that *Onchocerca* microfilariae may be found in the skin of normal horses as well as in lesions from potentially *any* equine dermatosis. Thus, the mere finding of microfilariae in a biopsy is *not* diagnostic of cutaneous onchocerciasis. Typical historical and physical findings must be accompanied by the indicated histopathologic changes.

In bovine cutaneous onchocerciasis, adult worms are the nidus for necrosis, abscess formation, mineralization, and granulomatous to pyogranulomatous inflammation.* Eosinophils may be prominent, and Hoeppli-Splendore material may be seen on the worm cuticle. Microfilariae are found in the surrounding connective tissue and lymphatics.

CLINICAL MANAGEMENT

Equine cutaneous onchocerciasis is a cause of discomfort, irritability, and disfigurement. Permanent leukoderma and scarring alopecia are potentially devastating sequelae for valuable show horses. Bovine cutaneous onchocerciasis causes economic losses as a result of hide damage and carcass trimming.[116, 567]

---

*References 33, 34, 116, 358, 567, 689, 830

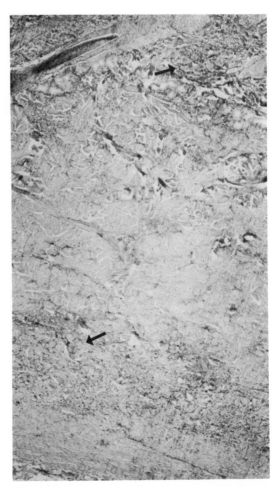

FIGURE 9–41. Equine cutaneous onchocerciasis. Superficial (arrow) and deep (arrow) perivascular dermatitis.

The treatment of choice for equine cutaneous onchocerciasis would appear to be ivermectin.[16, 267a, 326, 373, 397, 602a, 744] A single intramuscular injection of 200 µg/kg produced clinical remission within two to three weeks in most horses treated, which correlated with the disappearance of microfilariae from minced skin preparations and skin biopsies. Occasional horses require a second or third treatment at one-month intervals.[16] Ivermectin paste may be given orally at the same dosage with equal efficacy and without the severe side effects of clostridial infection and toxemia occasionally seen with the injectable preparation.[16, 267a, 373, 602a, 744] The paste may be given to pregnant mares, breeding stallions, and performance horses.

Levamisole is also effective for the treatment of equine cutaneous onchocerciasis.[244, 245, 267a, 419, 576, 744] The drug is given orally at 11 mg/kg once daily for seven days. Levamisole is un-

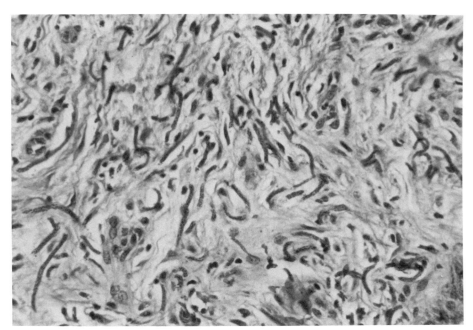

FIGURE 9–42. Equine cutaneous onchocerciasis. Numerous microfilariae associated with eosinophils and lymphocytes.

palatable to many horses and should be coated and administered with molasses, Karo syrup, or peanut butter.

In the past, diethylcarbamazine was also used to treat equine cutaneous onchocerciasis.* The drug was given orally at 5 mg/kg once daily for 21 days. However, this regimen was laborious and not totally satisfactory in many areas of North America.[244, 267a, 419, 468, 469, 471, 744]

In Australia, it has been reported that fenbendazole (60 mg/kg orally, daily for five days) and mebendazole (50 mg/kg orally, daily for five days) are effective for the treatment of equine cutaneous onchocerciasis.[584] In the United States, oral thiabendazole was found to be ineffective.[744]

Regardless of which microfilaricide is used, certain ancillary procedures should be followed: (1) a thorough ocular examination prior to therapy and (2) concurrent systemic glucocorticoid administration for the first five days of microfilaricidal treatment. Massive destruction of microfilariae may exacerbate both the cutaneous and ocular inflammation for the first three to four days of therapy.† Similar reactions are known to occur in humans as well.[522, 658, 732] Additional side effects attributable to levamisole include hyperhidrosis, head pressing, mild colic, and hyperesthesia to sounds, which last for one to five days.[244, 245, 744] The oral administration of prednisone or prednisolone, 1 mg/kg daily for five days, obviates or greatly reduces the severity of these side effects.

None of the microfilaricides presently in use are known to kill adult Onchocerca worms. Thus, periodic retreatments are to be expected. Pending the reproductive activity of the adult worms, retreatment for microfilariae and associated clinical signs may be necessary every 2 to 12 months. In humans, suramin (a urea-derivative) is known to kill adults and microfilariae of O. volvulus.[732] This drug is administered intravenously (weekly for five weeks), produces numerous side effects (including nephrotoxicity), and has apparently not been evaluated in horses.

Successful treatment for bovine cutaneous onchocerciasis has not been reported.

Stephanofilariasis

Stephanofilariasis is a common cause of skin disease in cattle and is occasionally seen in goats in many parts of the world.

CAUSE AND PATHOGENESIS

Many species of the genus Stephanofilaria are associated with skin disease in cattle. In

*References 468, 469, 471, 575, 584, 741, 742
†References 16, 136, 244, 326, 373, 468, 469, 471, 687, 741, 742, 744

the United States, Canada, the Soviet Union, and Australia, *S. stilesi* produces an often ventrally oriented dermatitis.* In Indonesia, *S. dedoesi* produces a dermatitis of the face, neck, forequarters, and dewlap (cascado).[105, 354, 495] *S. kaeli* produces a dermatitis on the lower extremities (filarial sore, Krian sore) in Malaysia.[106, 246–249, 438] In India and the Soviet Union, *S. assamensis* produces a dermatitis of the shoulders (hump sore).† In Japan, *S. okinawaensis* produces lesions on the muzzle and teats.[402, 802–805]

Adult worms (3 to 8 mm in length) are usually found in small cystlike structures at the base of hair follicles. Microfilariae are found in the surrounding dermal tissue and lymphatics. The microfilariae are ingested by various flies that serve as intermediate hosts: *Haematobia (Lyperosia) irritans* and *L. titillans (S. stilesi)* and *Musca conducens (S. okinawaensis, S. kaeli, S. assamensis)*.[246, 248, 587, 590, 803] Infective larvae are then transmitted through cutaneous wounds to cattle and goat hosts.

Clinical Features

In the United States, stephanofilariasis occurs most commonly in the west and southwest.‡ There are no apparent age or sex predilections, and range (beef) cattle are more commonly affected than dairy cattle.[80, 497, 729] The incidence of infection in a herd varies from 25 to 90 percent. In all countries, stephanofilariasis is a nonseasonal dermatitis, although the condition is often worse in warm weather and improves when the weather turns cold. This exacerbation of disease severity in warm weather is presumably the result of the activity of fly intermediate hosts at this time of year.

Clinically, stephanofilariasis is characterized by papules, crusts, ulcers, alopecia, hyperkeratosis, and thickening of the skin (see Plate 7). Pruritus is variable. Leukoderma may be prominent. In North America, *S. stilesi* produces lesions on the ventral chest and abdomen, flank, udder, teats, and, occasionally, the face and neck.§ Teat lesions may predispose to mastitis.

In other parts of the world, stephanofilariasis may present as a dermatitis on the shoulders, neck, pinnae, and feet (hump sore; *S. assamensis*),* over the face, neck, forequarters, and dewlap (cascado; *S. dedoesi*),[105, 354, 495] over the distal extremities and pinnae (filarial or Krian sore; *S. kaeli*),[106, 246–249, 438] and over the muzzle and teats (*S. okinawaensis*).[402, 802–805] Unidentified *Stephanofilaria* spp. have been reported to cause dermatitis in cattle in Africa[554] and Germany.[203–205]

Stephanofilariasis has been reported rarely in goats. *S. kaeli* was reported to cause a crusting dermatitis on the feet of goats in Malaysia,[249] and *S. assamensis* and *S. dedoesi* were isolated from crusting dermatoses of goats in India and Indonesia.[249, 588]

In general, stephanofilariasis is of minor economic importance. Financial losses are associated with hide damage and secondary flystrike.

Diagnosis

The differential diagnosis includes dermatophytosis, *Pelodera* dermatitis, chorioptic mange, fly-bite dermatitis (especially horn flies), contact dermatitis, and zinc-responsive dermatitis. Definitive diagnosis is based on history, physical examination, skin scrapings, and skin biopsy techniques. Deep skin scrapings may reveal *Stephanofilaria* spp. larvae but are often negative.

Skin biopsies should be taken for maceration in saline (see discussion on onchocerciasis) and for histologic examination. Histopathologic findings include varying degrees of folliculitis, nodular dermatitis, and superficial and deep perivascular dermatitis.† Eosinophils are usually the predominant inflammatory cell. Adult nematodes are seen coiled within cystlike structures at the base of hair follicles (Fig. 9–43). Microfilariae are found in the dermal connective tissue and lymphatics and are often surrounded by leukocytes, especially eosinophils (Fig. 9–44).

Clinical Management

Because stephanofilariasis is often economically unimportant and successful treatment may be economically or logistically impracti-

---

*References 13, 14, 18, 144, 198–200, 245, 330, 331, 363, 363a, 366, 424, 450, 729
†References 47, 168, 194, 356, 453, 544, 587–589, 615, 737
‡References 14, 80, 199–201, 245, 366, 424, 497, 729
§References 13, 14, 144, 199–201, 366, 424, 450, 729

---

*References 138, 139, 169, 186, 356, 357, 544, 572–574, 580, 664, 698, 699, 738
†References 168, 195, 204, 363, 438, 554, 818

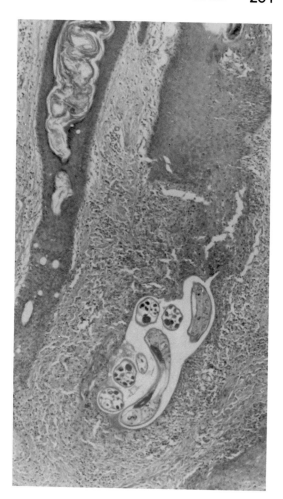

FIGURE 9–43. Bovine stephanofilariasis. Adult nematode segments in cyst at base of inflamed hair follicle.

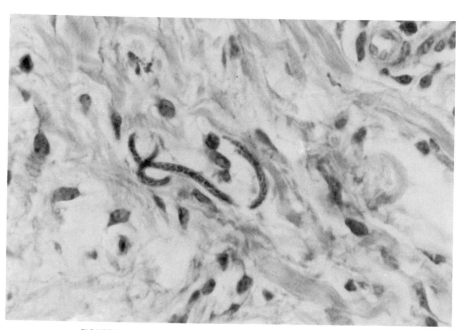

FIGURE 9–44. Bovine stephanofilariasis. Microfilariae in dermis.

cal, therapy is often not undertaken. In addition, *S. stilesi* infections may spontaneously regress within two to three years.[497, 729]

Where treatment has been tried, topical or systemic organophosphates have given the best results.[224] Daily topical applications of 6 to 10 percent trichlorfon ointment,* 2 percent coumaphos ointment,[495] or 4 percent chlorfenvinphos (Supona)[167] for one to two weeks have been recommended. Systemic treatment with trichlorfon (60 mg/kg given orally, repeated in four weeks) was also reported to be effective.[203, 205]

Stibophen (0.63 gm/50 kg, given subcutaneously, repeated weekly for three treatments) was reported to be curative in most cases.[203, 205] In Japan, levamisole was used to treat *S. okinawaensis* infections.[805] Levamisole hydrochloride (7.5 gm/100 kg, given orally) or levamisole phosphate (364 mg active ingredient/45 kg, given subcutaneously) produced a rapid reduction in microfilaria numbers in association with clinical improvement. However, all microfilariae were not killed. In both groups of cattle treated with levamisole, many animals developed salivation and tachypnea within 10 to 20 minutes after treatment. These side effects disappeared in 60 to 90 minutes. Levamisole hydrochloride administered intramuscularly[491] or levamisole ointment applied twice daily for five days was reported to be curative for bovine stephanofilariasis in India.[372]

Parafilariasis

Parafilariasis is a common cause of seasonal hemorrhagic nodules in cattle and horses in many parts of the world.

CAUSE AND PATHOGENESIS

Parafilariasis (hemorrhagic filariasis, dermatorrhagie parasitaire, summer bleeding) is caused by *Parafilaria multipapillosa* in horses and *P. bovicola* in cattle.[56, 734] Adult worms (30 to 70 mm in length) live in the subcutaneous and intermuscular connective tissues, coiled within nodules. The subcutaneous nodules open to the surface and discharge a bloody exudate, in which embryonated eggs and larvae are found. Various flies serve as vectors or intermediate hosts: *Haematobia atripalpis* (for *P. multipapillosa*) and several *Musca* spp.

(for *P. bovicola* and *P. multipapillosa*).* Experimental inoculation of infectious *P. bovicola* larvae into cattle produced typical skin lesions when given intraconjunctivally but *not* when given subcutaneously.[56] The prepatent period is about seven to ten months.[56, 533, 534, 820]

Suifilaria suis has been reported as a cause of skin disease in South African pigs.[734] Details on the life cycle of this parasite are apparently not known.

CLINICAL FEATURES

Equine parafilariasis (*P. multipapillosa*) has been reported in Eastern Europe and Great Britain.† The disease appears in the spring and summer. Papules and nodules arise suddenly, especially over the neck, shoulders, and trunk. The lesions, which are not usually painful or pruritic, proceed to open to the surface, discharge a bloody exudate, develop reddish-black crusts, and then heal. New lesions continue to develop as old ones heal. The disease regresses spontaneously during fall and winter. Affected horses are usually healthy otherwise.

Bovine parafilariasis (*P. bovicola*) has been reported in the Philippines, Africa, Asia, Europe, and Canada.‡ The disease occurs seasonally in spring and summer, with nodules appearing suddenly, especially over the neck, shoulders, and trunk (Fig. 9–45). The lesions follow the same course as described for equine parafilariasis. Affected cattle are usually otherwise healthy. Bovine parafilariasis can cause economic losses through downgrading of meat quality and slaughter condemnation.[57, 58, 832]

In South Africa, *Suifilaria suis* has been reported to cause a vesicular and ulcerative dermatitis in swine.[734]

DIAGNOSIS

The differential diagnosis includes bacterial, fungal, and parasitic granulomas, hypodermiasis, and angiomatosis (cattle). Definitive diagnosis is based on history, physical examination, direct smears, and skin biopsy. Direct smears from hemorrhagic exudate contain larvae (about 0.2 mm in length), rectangular embryonated eggs (25 μm by 50 μm), and

---

*References 47, 167, 203, 205, 247, 589, 615

*References 53, 56, 283, 288, 444, 532, 533, 734
†References 53, 149, 283, 288, 342, 344, 406, 599, 617, 785, 845
‡References 56–58, 130, 180, 251, 355, 382, 409, 444, 485, 532, 534, 535, 537, 538, 598, 799, 809, 829, 832, 839

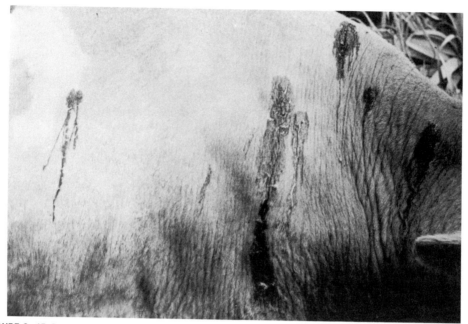

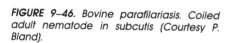
FIGURE 9–45. Bovine parafilariasis. Multiple bleeding ulcers over neck and shoulder (Courtesy P. Bland).

numerous eosinophils. Skin biopsy reveals nodular to diffuse dermatitis.[355, 598] The centers of the lesions contain coiled adult nematodes surrounded by necrotic debris and an inflammatory infiltrate containing numerous eosinophils (Fig. 9–46). Necrotic tracts lead from the central core of the lesions to the epidermal surface.

CLINICAL MANAGEMENT

Many cases of parafilariasis will recur annually for three to four years and then apparently resolve.[53, 80, 406, 534, 734] Only in cattle have extensive therapeutic trials on parafilariasis been attempted. Thiacetarsamide sodium (intravenously), suramin (intravenously), dieth-

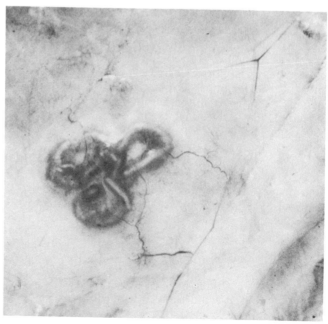
FIGURE 9–46. Bovine parafilariasis. Coiled adult nematode in subcutis (Courtesy P. Bland).

ylcarbamazine (orally), fenchlorphos (orally), trichlorfon (intramuscularly), phosmet (pour-on), and mebendazole (orally) were found to be ineffective.[820, 821] Although early noncontrolled studies reported that antimony compounds (intramuscularly) were effective,[307, 382, 669, 739] recent studies have failed to confirm these findings.[821]

Recent studies have shown that four drugs have a very favorable therapeutic effect in bovine parafilariasis: (1) nitroxynil, given subcutaneously at 20 mg/kg, repeated in three days,[821, 831–833] (2) levamisole, given intramuscularly at 12 mg/kg/day for four days,[820, 821] (3) fenbendazole, given orally at 20 mg/kg/day for five days,[820] and (4) ivermectin, given once subcutaneously at 200 to 400 µg/kg.[767] A period of nine weeks after treatment should be allowed prior to slaughter to permit lesions to resolve.

Elaeophoriasis

Elaeophoriasis (filarial dermatitis, sore head) is an uncommon cause of dermatitis, stomatitis, rhinitis, and keratitis in sheep in the western and southwestern United States.

Cause and Pathogenesis

Elaeophora schneideri normally parasitizes mule deer.[145, 332, 359, 360, 437, 734] Sheep become infected when grazing mountain ranges (most above an altitude of 2000 m) with infected deer during fly season. Horseflies of the genus *Hybomitra* and *Tabanus* serve as intermediate hosts. Adult worms (60 to 100 mm in length) occupy the lumina of the common carotid and internal maxillary arteries as well as the brachial, celiac, anterior mesenteric, tibial, and common digital arteries. Microfilariae (about 250 µm in length) accumulate in the capillaries and connective tissue of the dermis and submucosa, especially in the head and limbs. The prepatent period is about five to six months, and adult worms live three to four years. Skin and mucosal lesions are produced by (1) inflammatory reaction against microfilariae and (2) ischemia from vessel occlusion.

Clinical Features

Clinical signs of elaeophoriasis are first seen in adult sheep in winter, after the sheep have grazed mountain ranges in the west and south-western United States the previous summer.* There are no breed or sex predilections, and most affected sheep are older than one year. Morbidity is low, usually less than 0.5 percent of the flock.

Lesions are usually unilateral.[176, 209, 359, 360, 375] Skin lesions are most commonly seen on the poll, forehead, and face, less commonly on the limbs, abdomen, and feet. Affected skin becomes inflamed, alopecic, ulcerated, and crusted. There is often extensive hemorrhaging from the lesions, and pruritus is usually intense. Coronet involvement may result in deformed hooves. In addition to cutaneous lesions, affected sheep may have ipsilateral stomatitis (multiple ulcers, 1 to 5 mm in diameter, of the buccal mucosa and the hard and soft palates), keratoconjunctivitis, and rhinitis (multiple yellowish papules in the mucosa of the anterior and posterior nares, turbinates, ethmoturbinates, and frontal sinuses). Occasionally, neurologic signs and sudden death may be seen.

Diagnosis

The differential diagnosis includes photodermatitis, ulcerative dermatosis, and staphylococcal dermatitis. Definitive diagnosis is based on history, physical examination, and skin biopsy techniques. Skin biopsies should be taken for maceration in saline (see prior discussion on onchocerciasis) and for histologic examination. Histopathologic findings include variable degrees of nodular to diffuse dermatitis.[175, 359, 360] Eosinophils are the predominant inflammatory cell, and microfilarial segments are seen intra- and extravascularly.

Clinical Management

Elaeophoriasis often spontaneously regresses, after periods of intermittent and incomplete healing, within three to four years.[245, 359, 360, 437] The disease has little economic importance, as the incidence is low, and few sheep die. For all these reasons, elaeophoriasis is rarely treated.

Successful therapy has been reported with (1) piperazine, 50 mg/kg given orally for three days,[176, 437, 734] (2) diethylcarbamazine, 100 mg/kg given orally,[176, 734] and (3) antimony compounds, given intramuscularly.[176, 376, 437] The death of adult worms in heavily infested

---

*References 80, 176, 209, 245, 359, 360, 375, 437

sheep may cause death of the host resulting from occlusion of major arteries. Prevention is centered around avoiding the grazing of mountain ranges known to harbor infected deer and flies.

Oxyuriasis

Oxyuriasis (pin worms, thread worms) affects horses in most areas of the world.[23, 80, 244, 245, 734] The overall economic importance of the disease is not great. *Oxyuris equi* infests the cecum and colon, and adult female worms crawl out of the anus and lay their eggs in clusters on the perineal skin. Eggs eventually fall off onto the ground, and infection takes place by ingestion. The activity of the female worms and, possibly, irritating substances in the material that cements the eggs to the perineal skin cause variable degrees of pruritus.

Oxyuriasis is primarily a disease of stabled horses.[23, 80, 244, 584, 734] Pruritus ani results in constant rubbing of the tail base, which produces varying degrees of broken hairs and excoriation (rat-tail). Affected horses are often restless and irritable and may have a poor appetite.

The differential diagnosis includes insect hypersensitivity, pediculosis, chorioptic mange, food hypersensitivity, drug eruption, and stable vice. Definitive diagnosis is based on history, physical examination, and demonstration of eggs on the perineal skin. The eggs are encased in a cream-colored, gelatinous material. Clear acetate tape applied to the area will remove the eggs. The tape is then placed on a glass slide and examined microscopically for the presence of the characteristic operculated eggs.

Therapy consists of routine worming with thiabendazole, mebendazole, cambendazole, fenbendazole, ivermectin, or pyrantel pamoate[23, 80, 244, 584, 734, 864] and improving stable management and hygiene.

Strongyloidosis

Strongyloidosis has been reported in most countries throughout the world.[80, 734] The overall economic importance of the disease is not usually very great. *Strongyloides* spp. infect the small intestine of sheep, cattle, and goats (*S. papillosus*)[80, 734] and horses (*S. westeri*).[80, 734] Infection is acquired by ingestion or percutaneous penetration of infectious larvae.

In sheep and goats, repeated percutaneous penetration by infectious larvae may produce a pruritic, erythematous, pustular dermatitis in areas of skin that contact the contaminated environment (feet, legs, ventral abdomen, and chest).* The larvae are suspected of being important in the introduction of the microorganisms involved in foot-rot. In horses, it is thought that the disruption of the skin's integrity by penetrating *S. westeri* larvae may predispose to *Rhodococcus equi* lymphangitis.[80, 196, 238]

The differential diagnosis includes contact dermatitis, *Pelodera* dermatitis, trombiculidiasis, hookworm dermatitis, chorioptic mange, and dermatophytosis. Definitive diagnosis is based on history, physical examination, and fecal flotation. Skin biopsy reveals varying degrees of superficial and deep perivascular dermatitis with numerous eosinophils.[801] Fortuitous sections may reveal necrotic tracts and nematode larvae surrounded by inflammatory cells.

Therapy consists of routine worming with thiabendazole, cambendazole, fenbendazole, levamisole, or ivermectin and improving sanitation (eliminating warm, moist areas).[80, 437, 443, 459, 734]

Pelodera Dermatitis

Pelodera dermatitis (rhabditic dermatitis) is an uncommon skin condition associated with infection by the nematode *Pelodera strongyloides.*

CAUSE AND PATHOGENESIS

Pelodera (Rhabditis) strongyloides is a facultative nematode parasite, 1 to 1.5 mm in length.[14, 80, 437, 497, 734] It usually leads a free-living existence in damp soil and decaying organic matter. Under moist, filthy environmental circumstances, the larvae can invade the skin of domestic animals, producing a parasitic folliculitis. Affected skin is that in contact with the contaminated environment. The infection is self-limited if the environmental source of the nematode is eliminated.

CLINICAL FEATURES

Pelodera dermatitis has been reported in cattle,[14, 200, 201, 425, 625] horses,[213, 253] and sheep[69,

---

*References 80, 292, 437, 459, 730, 731, 800, 801

[437] in North America. No age, breed, or sex predilections are apparent. The disease occurs in association with moist, filthy environmental conditions.

Skin lesions are seen in areas of skin that are in close, frequent contact with the contaminated environment. The dermatitis is characterized by papules, pustules, ulcers, crusts, alopecia, scales, and erythema on the limbs, ventral thorax and abdomen, and, occasionally, the flank and neck. Pruritus is usually moderate to marked.

In East Africa, *Rhabditis bovis* has been reported to cause an otitis externa in cattle.[361, 407] Affected animals have a putrid-smelling otorrhea that is frequently complicated by myiasis. Large numbers of rhabditid larvae are found in the aural exudate, and therapy with various otic insecticides is effective.

DIAGNOSIS

The differential diagnosis includes stephanofilariasis, onchocerciasis, fly bites, contact dermatitis, trombiculidiasis, dermatophytosis, and various types of mange. Definitive diagnosis is based on history, physical examination, skin scrapings, and skin biopsy.

Deep skin scrapings usually reveal numerous small (about 600 μm in length), motile nematode larvae. The adult and larval nematodes may also be detected in samples of the bedding and soil. Skin biopsy reveals varying degrees of perifolliculitis, folliculitis, and furunculosis. Nematode segments are present within hair follicles and dermal pyogranulomas (Fig. 9–47). Eosinophils are numerous.

CLINICAL MANAGEMENT

Treatment is simple and effective. Complete removal and destruction of contaminated bedding and other environmental fomites is mandatory. The infected premises may be washed and sprayed with an insecticide such as malathion.

Pelodera dermatitis is a self-limited infection as long as the environmental source of the parasite is eliminated. Clinical signs regress spontaneously in one to four weeks. Severely affected animals may be treated with medicated shampoos to remove crusts and exudative debris. Secondary pyodermas may require topical antimicrobial agents (povidone-iodine or chlorhexidine) or systemic antibiotics. If pruritus is severe, systemic glucocorticoids may

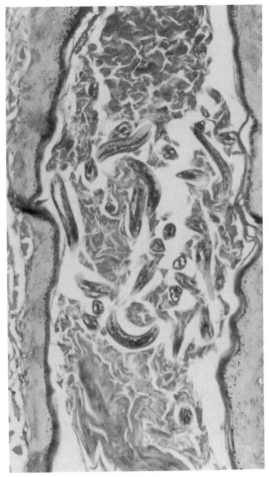

FIGURE 9–47. Bovine pelodera dermatitis. Nematode segments in hair follicle.

be administered for a few days. In severe infections, recovery may be hastened by the use of topical insecticides, especially organophosphate compounds such as malathion.

Hookworm Dermatitis

Hookworm dermatitis has been reported in cattle and sheep throughout the world.[80, 734] Hookworm disease may result in severe economic losses from blood loss, diarrhea, and poor growth. *Bunostomum* species infect the small intestine of cattle (*B. phlebotomum*) and sheep (*B. trigonocephalum*). Nematode eggs are passed in the feces, and infection occurs by ingestion or percutaneous penetration of infectious larvae.

Repeated percutaneous penetration by infectious larvae may produce a pruritic, erythematous dermatitis in areas of skin that contact the contaminated environment (especially feet and legs).[80, 406, 734] Affected animals are irritable and are seen to stomp, kick, and lick their feet.

The differential diagnosis includes contact dermatitis, *Pelodera* dermatitis, trombiculidiasis, strongyloidosis, and chorioptic mange. Definitive diagnosis is based on history, physical examination, and fecal flotation.

Therapy consists of routine worming with thiabendazole, fenbendazole, or levamisole and improving sanitation.[80, 734]

Dracunculiasis

There are a few anecdotal reports of dracunculiasis (dracunculosis, dracontiasis) in horses and cattle in the veterinary literature.[406, 734] *Dracunculus medinensis* (guinea worm, dragon worm) occurs in Asia and Africa, and *D. insignis* in North America. Adult female worms (up to 100 cm in length) live in subcutaneous nodules, which ulcerate. When the lesions contact water, the uterus of the worm prolapses through its anterior end and discharges a mass of larvae (500 to 750 μm in length). Aquatic crustaceans (*Cyclops* spp.) serve as intermediate hosts, and infection occurs when contaminated water is ingested.

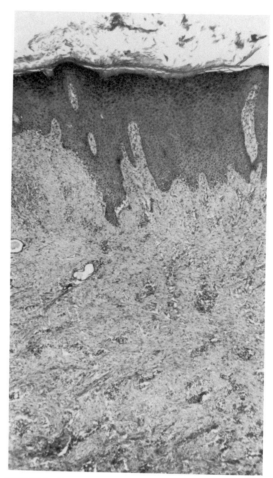

FIGURE 9–49. Caprine parelaphostrongylosis. Fibrosing dermatitis.

Lesions are usually solitary and occur most commonly on the limbs and abdomen. The subcutaneous nodules may be pruritic or painful, and just before the nodules open to the surface, the host may show urticaria, pruritus, and pyrexia.

Diagnosis is based on history, physical examination, observation of the female worm within the draining nodule, and direct smears of the exudate (larvae). Treatment classically is to gently remove the adult worm by carefully winding it up on a stick over a period of several days. Alternatively, the nodule may be surgically excised.

Control measures depend on improving contaminated water supplies.

Parelaphostrongylosis

Parelaphostrongylus tenuis is a common parasite of white-tailed deer in North America.[734] Adult nematodes inhabit the cranial venous sinuses and subdural spaces. Larvae are passed

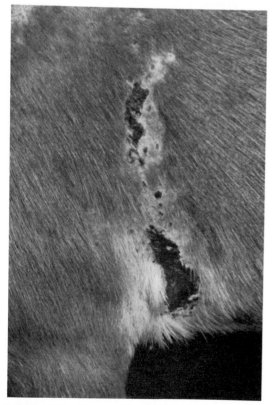

FIGURE 9–48. Caprine parelaphostrongylosis. Linear, vertical area of alopecia, crusting, and ulceration.

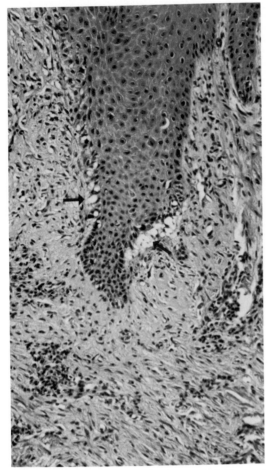

FIGURE 9–50. Caprine parelaphostrongylosis. Hydropic degeneration of epidermal basal cells (arrows).

and deep perivascular accumulations of mononuclear cells (Fig. 9–49).[455] Focal areas of hydropic degeneration of epidermal basal cells have been a consistent finding (Fig. 9–50).

Therapy is difficult to evaluate because of the variable course of this disease.[455, 730, 731] Levamisole, thiabendazole, and systemic glucocorticoids have been recommended for therapeutic trials.

in deer feces, and terrestrial snails and slugs serve as intermediate hosts. Infection occurs via ingestion of intermediate hosts.

In goats, *P. tenuis* infection produces neurologic disorders as larvae migrate through the spinal canal.[730, 734] A unique dermatosis has been observed in some paretic and nonparetic goats with *P. tenuis* infection.[455, 730, 731] Focal, linear, vertically oriented skin lesions are seen on the shoulder, thorax, or flank (Fig. 9–48). The lesions are usually unilateral and characterized by alopecia, ulceration, crusting, and scarring. It has been theorized that migrating *P. tenuis* larvae irritate dorsal nerve roots, resulting in pruritus and excoriation along dermatomes.

Diagnosis is based on history, physical examination, cerebrospinal fluid analysis (eosinophils, increased protein), and skin biopsy. Histopathologic findings include varying degrees of fibrosing dermatitis with superficial

REFERENCES

1. Abul-Hab, J., and Al-S'adi, H.: Seasonal occurrence of Przhevalskiana silenus Brauer (Diptera:Oestridae) warble flies on goats and sheep in the Baghdad area, Iraq. Beitr. Trop. Landwirtsch. Veterinarmed. 12:153, 1974.
2. Abu-Samra, M. T., et al.: Mange in domestic animals in the Sudan. Ann. Trop. Med. Parasitol. 75:627, 1981.
2a. Abu-Samra, M. T., et al.: Five cases of psoroptic mange in the domestic donkey (*Equus asinus asinus*) and treatment with ivermectin. Equine Vet. J. 19:143, 1987.
3. Ackert, J. E., and O'Neal, W. S.: Parasitism and fistulous withers. JAVMA 77:28, 1930.
3a. Agbede, R. I. S., et al.: Immunization of cattle against *Boophilus microplus* using extracts derived from adult female ticks: Histopathology of ticks feeding on vaccinated cattle. Intl. J. Parasitol. 16:35, 1986.
4. Ahrens, E. H., and Cocke, J.: Comparative test with insecticide-impregnated ear tags against the Gulf Coast tick. J. Econ. Entomol. 71:764, 1978.
5. Ahrens, E. H., et al.: Prevention of screw-worm infestation in cattle by controlling Gulf Coast ticks with slow-release insecticide devices. J. Econ. Entomol. 70:581, 1977.
6. Alicata, J. E.: Microfilarial infestation in the skin of a horse. North Am. Vet. 17:39, 1936.
7. Allen, J. R., and Humphreys, S. J.: Immunization of guinea pigs and cattle against ticks. Nature 280:491, 1979.
8. Allen, J. R., et al.: Histology of bovine skin reaction to *Ixodes holocyclus* Neumann. Can. J. Comp. Med. 41:26, 1977.
9. Allen, J. R., et al.: Langerhans cells trap tick salivary gland antigens in tick-resistant guinea pigs. J. Immunol. 122:563, 1979.
10. Alva-Valdes, R., et al.: Efficacy of ivermectin against the mange mite *Sarcoptes scabiei var suis* in pigs. Am. J. Vet. Res. 45:2113, 1984.
11. Alva-Valdes, R., et al.: The effects of sarcoptic mange on the productivity of confined pigs. Vet. Med. 82:258, 1986.
11a. Alva-Valdes, R., et al.: Efficacy of ivermectin in a topical formulation against induced gastrointestinal and pulmonary nematode infections, and naturally occurring grubs and lice in cattle. Am. J. Vet. Res. 47:2389, 1986.
12. Amiel, J. P.: Alterations des cuirs dans la Demodecie des petits ruminants. Rec. Med. Vet. 105:331, 1929.
13. Amstutz, H. E.: Bovine skin conditions: A brief review. Mod. Vet. Pract. 60:821, 1979.
14. Amstutz, H. E.: *Bovine Medicine and Surgery II.* Santa Barbara, CA, American Veterinary Publications, Inc., 1980.
15. Anderson, P. H., and Kirkwood, A. C.: A reaction in cattle to toxins of *Hypoderma bovis* (warble fly) larvae. Br. Vet. J. 124:569, 1968.
16. Anderson, R. R.: The use of ivermectin in horses: Research and clinical observations. Compend. Cont. Educ. 6:S516, 1984.
17. Andrews, A. H.: Warble fly: The life cycle, distribution, economic losses, and control. Vet. Rec. 103:348, 1978.
18. Anonymous: Filarial dermatitis in cattle caused by the nematode *Stephanofilaria stilesi*. Vet. Scope 5:8, 1955.
19. Appleyard, W. T.: Field assessment of permethrin in the control of sheep head fly disease. Vet. Rec. 110:7, 1982.

20. Appleyard, W. T., et al.: Use of pyrethroid-impregnated tags in the control of sheep headfly disease. Vet. Rec. 115:463, 1984.

21. Appleyard, B., and Bailie, H.: Parasitic skin diseases of sheep. In Pract. 6:4, 1984.

22. Arnold, R. M.: Deaths of calves following dipping in chlordane. JAVMA 115:462, 1949.

23. Arundell, J. H.: Parasites of the Horse. Sydney, University of Sydney Post-Graduate Foundation in Veterinary Science, Veterinary Review No. 18, 1978.

24. Askenase, P. W., and Worms, M. J.: Immune cutaneous basophil resistance to parasite ticks. Fed. Proc. 38:1220, 1979.

25. Auer, D. E., et al.: Illness in horses following spraying with amitraz. Aust. Vet. J. 61:257, 1984.

26. Ault, C. N., et al.: Resistencia del Psoroptes communis var ovis Frente al hexachlorociclohexano. Rev. Med. Vet. 13:357, 1962.

27. Austen, E. E.: A new species of warble fly which attacks goats in Cyprus. Bull. Entomol. Res. 22:423, 1931.

28. Aynaud, M.: Kystes a Demodex, Kystes sebaces et absces du mouton. Ann. Inst. Pasteur 46:306, 1931.

29. Babcock, O. G.: DDT for the control of goat lice. J. Econ. Entomol. 37:138, 1944.

30. Bagnall, B. G.: The Australian paralysis tick, Ixodes holocyclus. Aust. Vet. J. 51:159, 1975.

31. Bailie, H. D., and Morgan, D. W. T.: Field trials to assess the efficacy of permethrin for the control of flies on cattle. Vet. Rec. 106:124, 1980.

32. Bain, A. M., et al.: Habronema megastoma larvae associated with pulmonary abscesses in a foal. Aust. Vet. J. 45:101, 1969.

33. Bain, O., et al.: Validité des deux espèces Onchocerca lienalis et O. gutturosa chez les bovines. Ann. Parasitol. Hum. Comp. 53:421, 1978.

34. Bain, O.: Transmission de l'onchocerque bovine, Onchocerca gutturosa, par Culicoides. Ann. Parasitol. Hum. Comp. 54:483, 1979.

35. Bain, O.: Redescription de cinq espèces d'onchocerques. Ann. Parasitol. Hum. Comp. 50:763, 1975.

36. Baker, D. W.: Cattle mange and scabies. Vet. Med. 42:57, 1947.

37. Baker, D. W., and Howe, I. G.: Cattle mange in New York State. JAVMA 116:280, 1950.

38. Baker, D. W.: Ticks found in New York State. Cornell Vet. 36:84, 1946.

39. Baker, D. W., and Nutting, W. B.: Demodectic mange in New York State sheep. Cornell Vet. 40:140, 1950.

40. Baker, D. W., and Fisher, W. F.: The incidence of demodectic mites in the eyelids of various mammalian hosts. J. Econ. Entomol. 62:942, 1969.

41. Baker, D. W., and Monlux, W. S.: Hypoderma myiasis in the horse. J. Parasitol. 25:15, 1939.

42. Baker, J. A. F.: Some clinical aspects of itch mite (Psorergates ovis) infestation of Merino sheep in South Africa. J. S. Afr. Vet. Med. Assoc. 39:53, 1968.

43. Baker, J. A. F.: Resistance to certain organophosphorus compounds by Linognathus africanus on Angora goats in South Africa. J. S. Afr. Vet. Med. Assoc. 40:411, 1969.

44. Baker, K. P.: Demodex spp. in the meibomian gland of Irish cattle. Vet. Rec. 92:699, 1973.

45. Baker, M. K., and Ducasse, F. B. W.: Tick infestation of livestock in Natal. J. S. Afr. Vet. Med. Assoc. 38:447, 1967.

46. Baker, M. K., and Ducasse, F. B. W.: Tick infestation of livestock in Natal. J. S. Afr. Vet. Med. Assoc. 39:55, 1968.

47. Baki, M. A., and Dewan, M. L.: Evaluation of treatment of stephanofilariasis (humpsore) with Neguvon (Bayer) by clinical pathological studies. Bangladesh Vet. J. 9:1, 1975.

48. Baron, R. W., and Weintraub, J.: Immunization of Cattle Against Warbles. Research Highlights, Research Station, Alberta, Canada, 1981, p. 24.

49. Barrett, S.: Skin lesions of demodectic mange in the goat. Trans. R. Soc. Trop. Med. Hyg. 52:301, 1958.

50. Barth, D., and Brakken, E. S.: The activity of 22,23-dihydroavermectin B₁ against the pig louse, Haematopinus suis. Vet. Rec. 106:388, 1980.

51. Barth, D.: Untersuchungen uber die wiksamkeit von ivermectin Gegenuber Ektoparasiten des Rindes. Prakt. Tierarztl. 4:328, 1980.

52. Barth, D., and Preston, J. M.: Efficacy of ivermectin against the sucking louse Solenopotes capillatus. Vet. Rec. 116:267, 1985.

53. Baumann, R.: Beobachtungen beim parasitaren sommerbluten der Pferde. Wien. Tierarztl. Monatsschr. 33:52, 1946.

54. Baumhover, A. H., et al.: Screw-worm control through release of sterilized flies. J. Econ. Entomol. 48:462, 1955.

55. Baumhover, A. H., et al.: Field observations on the effects of releasing sterile screw-worms in Florida. J. Econ. Entomol. 52:1202, 1959.

56. Bech-Nielsen, S., et al.: Parafilaria bovicola (Tubangui 1934) in cattle: Epizootiology—vector studies and experimental transmission of Parafilaria bovicola to cattle. Am. J. Vet. Res. 43:948, 1982.

57. Bech-Nielsen, S., et al.: Parafilaria bovicola (Tubangui 1934) in cattle: Epizootiology—disease occurrence. Am. J. Vet. Res. 43:945, 1982.

58. Bech-Nielsen, S., et al.: Benefit/cost-studier for alternativa bekampningsmetoder for Parafilaria bovicola. Svensk. Vet. 33:435, 1981.

59. Becklund, W. W.: The long-nosed cattle louse, Linognathus vituli, collected from a goat. J. Parasitol. 43:637, 1957.

60. Becklund, W. W.: Ticks of veterinary significance found on imports in the United States. J. Parasitol. 54:622, 1968.

61. Beesley, W. N.: Observations on the biology of the ox warble-fly. III. Dermolytic properties of larval extracts. Ann. Trop. Med. Parasitol. 63:159, 1969.

62. Beesley, W. N.: Control of arthropods of medical and veterinary importance. Adv. Parasitol. 11:115, 1973.

63. Beesley, W. N.: Sheep scab = cattle scab? Vet. Rec. 114:388, 1984.

64. Beesley, W. N.: Economics and progress of warble fly eradication in Britain. Vet. Med. Rev. 4:334, 1974.

65. Bell, D. S., et al.: Psorergates ovis—a cause of itchiness in sheep. JAVMA 120:117, 1952.

66. Bellocq, P., and Guilhem, P.: Guérison spectaculaire d'un cas de Dermite estivale des Equidés. Rec. Med. Vet. 136:663, 1960.

67. Bennett, G. F.: Boophilus microplus (Acarina-Ixodoidea) experimental infestations on cattle restrained from grooming. Exper. Parasitol. 26:323, 1969.

68. Bennison, J. C.: Demodicosis of horses with particular reference to equine members of the genus Demodex. J. R. Army Vet. Corps 14:34, 1943.

69. Bergeland, M. E., et al.: Dermatitis in sheep caused by Pelodera strongyloides. Proc. Helminthol. Soc. Wash. 43:230, 1976.

70. Berger, D.: Acariasis in the horse. Vet. J. 67:383, 1911.

71. Bergstrom, R. C., and Etherton, S. L.: Psorergatid mites from cattle in Wyoming. Vet. Med. Small Anim. Clin. 78:1761, 1983.

72. Besch, E. D., and Griffiths, H. J.: Demonstration of Demodex equi (Railliet, 1895) from a horse in Minnesota. JAVMA 155:82, 1956.

73. Beveridge, I., et al.: An investigation of biting midges in relation to their potential as vectors of bovine onchocerciasis in north Queensland. J. Aust. Entomol. Soc. 20:349, 1981.

74. Bindseil, E.: Histopathologiske undersogelser af Sarcoptesskab hos svin med specielt henblik pa forandringernes immunologiske natur. Danske Dyrl. Med. 57:470, 1974.

75. Binta, M. G., and Cunningham, M. R.: Cutaneous responses of cattle to extracts from Rhipicephalus appendiculatus larvae. Vet. Parasitol. 15:67, 1984.

76. Biswal, G.: Hazards of gammexane with reference to treatment of pediculosis in goats. Indian Vet. J. 31:426, 1955.

77. Blackman, G. G., Hodson, M. J.: Further evaluation of permethrin for biting-fly control. Pestic. Sci. 8:270, 1977.

78. Blackman, D. M., and Nolan, M. P.: Ctenocephalides felis infestation in Holstein calves. Agri-Pract. 5:6, 1984.

79. Blandford, T. B., and Beesley, W. N.: Pustular demodectic mange in a goat. Vet. Rec. 77:693, 1965.

80. Blood, D. C., et al.: Veterinary Medicine VI. London, Baillière Tindall, 1983.

81. Boersema, J. H.: De effectiviteit van coumaphos tegen *Chorioptes bovis* bij een paard met beenschurft. Tijdschr. Diergeneeskd. 103:377, 1978.

82. Bogatko, W.: Studies on the occurrence of *Sarcoptes scabiei* in clinically healthy pigs. Med. Weter. 30:38, 1974.

83. Boulard, C.: Evolution des anticorps circulants chez les bovins traités contre l'hypodermose. Ann. Rech. Vet. 6:143, 1975.

84. Boulard, C.: Circulating antibodies and blood histamine in cattle after treatment against hypodermosis. Vet. Parasitol. 5:379, 1979.

85. Bouvier, G.: Premier cas de gale chorioptique chez le chamois. Schweiz. Arch. Tierheilkd. 103:36, 1961.

86. Boyd, C. L., and Bullard, T. L.: Organophosphate treatment of cutaneous habronemiasis in horses. JAVMA 153:324, 1968.

87. Boyle, J. A.: Demodectic mange on goats. Vet. Rec. 85:478, 1969.

88. Brackenridge, D. T.: Mange in pigs: A survey. N.Z. Vet. J. 6:166, 1958.

89. Braide, E. I., et al.: Bovine onchocerciasis in Tompkins County, New York. Cornell Vet. 71:332, 1981.

90. Bramley, P. S., and Henderson, D.: Control of sheep scab and other ectoparasites with propetamphos. Vet. Rec. 115:460, 1984.

91. Branagan, D.: The feeding performance of the ixodid *Rhipicephalus appendiculatus* Neum. on rabbits, cattle, and other hosts. Bull. Entomol. Res. 64:387, 1974.

92. Bremner, K. C.: Morphologic studies on the microfilariae of *Onchocerca gibsoni* and *Onchocerca gutturosa*. Aust. J. Zool. 3:324, 1955.

93. Brennan, J. M., and Yunker, C. E.: A new species of *Euschoengastia* of potential veterinary importance. J. Parasitol. 50:311, 1964.

94. Bridges, E. R.: The use of ivermectin to treat genital cutaneous habronemiasis in a stallion. Comp. Cont. Educ. 7:S94, 1985.

95. Bridi, A. A., et al.: Controle de um surto de sarna psoroptica ovina com suposta resistencia a organoclorados e organofosforados, usando-se amitraz 12.5% CE. Arq. Fac. Vet. UFRGS 4–5:135, 1976–1977.

96. Britt, A. G., et al.: Effects of a pour-on insecticidal formulation on sheep skin. Aust. Vet. J. 61:329, 1984.

97. Brizard, A.: Le benzoate de benzyle dans le traitement des gales du cheval. Rev. Med. Vet. 94:267, 1943.

98. Brizard, A.: Nouveau cas d'otacariase de la chevre. Rev. Med. Vet. 91:93, 1939.

99. Brossard, M.: Relations immunologiques entre bovins et tiques, plus particulièrement entre bovins et *Boophilus microplus*. Acta Trop. 33:15, 1976.

100. Brown, S. J., and Askenase, P. W.: Immune rejection of ectoparasites (ticks) by T cell and IgG1 antibody recruitment of basophils and eosinophils. Fed. Proc. 42:1744, 1983.

101. Brown, S. J., et al.: Bovine resistance to *Amblyomma americanum* ticks: An acquired immune response characterized by cutaneous basophil infiltrates. Vet. Parasitol. 16:147, 1984.

102. Brownlee, A. A.: *Demodex* found in sheep in Britain. J. Comp. Pathol. 48:68, 1935.

103. Brownlee, W. M., and Harrison, J. R.: Sarcoptic mange in pigs. Vet. Rec. 72:1022, 1960.

104. Bruere, A. N.: Some clinical aspects of hypo-orchidism (small testes) in the ram. N.Z. Vet. J. 18:189, 1970.

105. Bubberman, C., and Kraneveld, F. C.: Over een dermatitis squamosa et crustosa circumscript bij het rund in Nederlandsch-Indie, genamd cascado. III. Het voorkommen van cascado bij de geit. Ned. Ind. Diergeneeskd. 46:67, 1933.

106. Buckley, J. J. C.: On a new species of *Stephanofilaria* causing lesions on the legs of cattle in the Malay Peninsula. J. Helminthol. 15:233, 1937.

107. Buckley, J. J. C.: On *Culicoides* as a vector of *Onchocerca gibsoni*. J. Helminthol. 16:21, 1938.

108. Buhlmann, V.: Untersuchungen uber Sarcoptes suis-Milbenbefall beim Schwein. Schweiz. Arch. Tierheilkd. 122:253, 1980.

109. Bull, L. B.: A granulomatous affection of the horse—habronemic granulomata (cutaneous habronemiasis of Railliet). J. Comp. Pathol. Ther. 29:187, 1916.

110. Burghardt, H. F., et al.: Dermatitis in cattle due to *Simulium* (black flies). Cornell Vet. 41:311, 1951.

111. Burrichter, D.: Sarcoptic mange in a calf. Iowa State Univ. Vet. 28:121, 1966.

111a. Butler, A. R.: Effects of closantel on face lice (*Linognathus ovillus*) of sheep. Aust. Vet. J. 63:89, 1986.

111b. Butler, A. R.: Observations on the control of ovine face lice (*Linognathus ovillus*) with closantel. Aust. Vet. J. 63:371, 1986.

112. Bwangamoi, O.: The incidence of skin diseases of cattle in Uganda. Bull. Epizoot. Dis. Afr. 16:115, 1968.

113. Bwangamoi, O.: A survey of skin diseases and defects which downgrade hides and skins in East Africa. I. Cattle. Bull. Epizoot. Dis. Afr. 17:185, 1969.

114. Bwangamoi, O.: A survey of skin diseases and defects which downgrade hides and skins in East Africa. II. Goats. Bull. Epizoot. Dis. Afr. 17:197, 1969.

115. Bwangamoi, O.: *Onchocerca ochengi* new species, an intradermal parasite of cattle in East Africa. Bull. Epizoot. Dis. Afr. 17:321, 1969.

116. Bwangamoi, O.: Dermatitis in cattle caused by *Onchocerca ochengi* Bwandamoi, 1969, and the effect of the adult filaria on the finished leather. Bull. Epizoot. Dis. Afr. 17:435, 1969.

117. Chambers, F.: The parasitic origin of poll evil and fistulous withers. Vet. Rec. 45:759, 1932.

118. Bwangamoi, O., and DeMartini, J.: A survey of skin diseases and defects which downgrade hides and skins in East Africa. III. Sheep. Bull. Epizoot. Dis. Afr. 18:243, 1970.

119. Bwangamoi, O.: The pathogenesis of demodicosis in cattle in East Africa. Br. Vet. J. 127:30, 1970.

120. Bwangamoi, O.: A survey of skin diseases of pigs in Kenya. Bull. Epizoot. Dis. Afr. 20:19, 1972.

121. Callinan, A. P. L.: Effects of artificially induced infestations of the cattle louse, *Linognathus vituli*. Aust. Vet. J. 56:484, 1980.

122. Cameron, R. D. A.: Skin diseases of the pig. Proc. Univ. Sydney Post-Grad. Comm. Vet. Sci. 56:445, 1981.

123. Cameron, R. D. A.: *Skin Diseases of the Pig.* Sydney, University of Sydney Post-Graduate Foundation in Veterinary Science, Veterinary Review No. 23, 1984.

124. Campbell, J. B., and Raun, E. S.: Aerial ULV and LV applications of insecticides for control of the stable fly and horn fly. J. Econ. Entomol. 64:1170, 1971.

125. Campbell, J. B., and Hermanussen, J. F.: Efficacy of insecticides and methods of insecticidal application for control of stable flies in Nebraska. J. Econ. Entomol. 64:1188, 1971.

126. Campbell, J. B.: Effect of horn fly control on cows as expressed by increased weaning weights of calves. J. Econ. Entomol. 69:711, 1976.

127. Cargill, C. F., and Dobson, K. J.: Experimental *Sarcoptes scabiei* infestation in pigs. I. Pathogenesis. Vet. Rec. 104:11, 1979.

128. Cargill, C. F., and Dobson, K. J.: Experimental *Sarcoptes scabiei* infestation in pigs. II. Effects on production. Vet. Rec. 104:33, 1979.

129. Cargill, C. F.: The treatment and control of sarcoptic mange. Proc. Univ. Sydney Post-Grad. Comm. Vet. Sci. 56:87, 1981.

130. Carmichael, I. H., and Koster, S.: Bovine parafilariosis in southern Africa: A preliminary report. Onderstepoort J. Vet. Res. 45:213, 1978.

131. Carter, H. B.: A skin disease of sheep due to an ectoparasitic mite, *Psorergates ovis* Womersley 1941. Aust. Vet. J. 17:193, 1941.

132. Carter, H. B.: Follicle mite (*Demodex*) in Australian sheep. Aust. Vet. J. 18:120, 1942.

133. Caslick, E.: Further study of a parasite found in the ligamentum nuchae of equines. Rep. N.Y. State Vet. 32:162, 1922.

134. Catcott, E. J., and Smithcors. J. F.: *Equine Medicine and Surgery II.* Santa Barbara, CA, American Veterinary Publications, Inc., 1972.

135. Cave, T. W.: The foot-scab mite of sheep (*Symbiotes communis var ovis*, Railliet). J. Comp. Pathol. Ther. 22:50, 1909.

136. Cello, R. M.: Ocular onchocerciasis in the horse. Equine Vet. J. 3:148, 1971.

137. Chakraverty, A. N., et al.: Case notes of scabies in a family transmitted from goats. Indian Med. Gazette 99:153, 1953.

138. Chatterjee, A., et al.: Parasitic dermatitis of the muzzle of a cow with clinical signs of leukoderma. Indian J. Anim. Health 21:97, 1982.

139. Chatterjee, A., and Chakrabarti, A.: Some uncommon lesions of stephanofilarial dermatitis in cattle of West Bengal (India). Indian J. Anim. Health 22:69, 1983.

140. Chauhan, P. P. S., and Pande, B. P.: Morphological variations within the species *Onchocerca armillata* and *O. gutturosa* in buffaloes and cattle in India, with special reference to the male tail and cuticular ornamentation. J. Helminthol. 52:343, 1978.

141. Chauhan, P. P. S., and Bhatia, B. B.: Scabies in sheep and goats. Indian Farming 30:31, 1980.

142. Cheema, A. H.: Observations on the histopathology of warble infestation in goats by the larvae of *Przhevalskiana silenus*. Zbl. Vet. Med. B 24:648, 1977.

143. Cheng, T. H.: The effect of biting fly control on weight gain in beef cattle. J. Econ. Entomol. 51:275, 1958.

144. Chitwood, B. G.: A nematode, *Stephanofilaria stilesi*, new species from the skin of cattle in the United States. North Am. Vet. 15:25, 1934.

145. Clark, G. C., and Hibler, C. P.: Horse flies and *Elaeophora schneideri*. J. Wildl. Dis. 9:21, 1973.

146. Clymer, B. C.: Cattle scabies cut feedlot profits. Feedlot Manage. 20:27, 1978.

147. Collins, R. C., and Dewirst, L. W.: Some effects of the suckling louse, *Haematopinus eurysternus*, on cattle on unsupplemented range. JAVMA 146:129, 1965.

148. Collins, R. C.: Onchocerciasis of horses in southeastern Louisiana. J. Parsitol. 59:1016, 1973.

149. Condamine, M., and Drouilly, M.: Description de la filaire femelle (cause determinate des boutons hemorrhagiques). Rec. Med. Vet. 55:1145, 1878.

150. Cook, R. W.: Ear mites, *Raillietia manfredi* and *Psoroptes cuniculi* in goats in New South Wales. Aust. Vet. J. 57:72, 1981.

151. Cooper, J. E.: An outbreak of *Tunga penetrans* in a pig herd. Vet. Rec. 80:365, 1967.

152. Courtney, C. H., et al.: Ivermectin for the control of swine scabies: Relative values of prefarrowing treatment of sows and weaning treatment of pigs. Am. J. Vet. Res. 44:1220, 1983.

153. Cox, D. D., et al.: Posterior paralysis in a calf caused by cattle grubs (*Hypoderma bovis*) after treatment with a systemic insecticide for grub control. JAVMA 157:1088, 1970.

154. Cram, E. B.: Demodectic mange of the goat in the United States. JAVMA 66:475, 1925.

155. Crawford, R., et al.: Chorioptic mange of the scrotum of rams. N.Z. Vet. J. 18:209, 1970.

156. Creighton, J. T., and Dennis, D. M.: The tail louse in Florida. J. Econ. Entomol. 40:911, 1948.

157. Crogan, W. E.: Trombidiosis of sheep. Aust. Vet. J. 25:103, 1949.

158. Cummings, E., and James, E. R.: Prevalence of equine onchocerciasis in the southeastern and midwestern United States. JAVMA 186:1202, 1985.

159. Cummins, L. J., and Tweedle, N. E.: The influence of light infestations of *Linognathus vituli* on the growth of young cattle. Aust. Vet. J. 53:591, 1977.

160. Cummins, L. J., and Graham, J. F.: The effect of lice infestation on the growth of Hereford calves. Aust. Vet. J. 58:194, 1982.

161. Curasson, G.: *Ctenocephalides canis* parasite du mouton. Bull. Soc. Pathol. Exot. 18:755, 1925.

162. Cwilich, R., and Shimshoni, A.: The identification of larvae of the fly *Przhevalskiana aegagri* on goats in Israel. Refuah Vet. 22:258, 1965.

163. Dalmat, H. L.: A contribution to the knowledge of the rodent warble flies (Cuterebridae). J. Parasitol. 29:311, 1943.

164. DaMassa, A. J.: Prevalence of mycoplasmas and mites in the external auditory meatus of goats. Calif. Vet. 37:10, 1985.

165. Darrow, D. I.: Biting lice of goats: Control with dichlorvos-impregnated resin neck collars. J. Econ. Entomol. 66:133, 1973.

166. Das, D. N., and Misra, S. C.: Studies on caprine demodectic mange with institution of effective therapeutic measures. Indian Vet. J. 49:96, 1972.

167. Das, P. K., et al.: Study on the efficacy of some organophosphate compounds in the treatment of stephanofilarial dermatitis in cattle. Orissa Vet. J. 11:110, 1977.

168. Das, P. K., et al.: Studies on the pathoanatomy of the skin in *Stephanofilaria assamensis* Pande, 1936, infection in cattle. Indian J. Anim. Sci. 45:543, 1975.

169. Das, P. K., et al.: Incidence of stephanofilarial dermatitis in cattle. Orissa Vet. J. 10:69, 1975.

170. Datta, S. C. A.: The etiology of Bursati. Indian J. Vet. Sci. Anim. Husb. 3:217, 1933.

171. Daubney, R., and Hudson, J. R.: Preliminary note on the transmission of haemorrhagic septicemia by the flea *Ctenocephalides felis* Bouche. J. Comp. Pathol. 47:211, 1934.

172. Davey, R. B., et al.: Control of the southern cattle tick with insecticide-impregnated ear tags. J. Econ. Entomol. 73:651, 1980.

173. Davey, R. B., and Ahrens, E. H.: Control of *Boophilus* ticks in heifers with two pyrethroids applied as sprays. Am. J. Vet. Res. 45:1008, 1984.

174. Davis, J. W.: Studies of the sheep mite, *Psorergates ovis*. Am. J. Vet. Res. 15:255, 1954.

175. Davis, C. L., and Kemper, H. E.: Histological diagnosis of filarial dermatitis in sheep. JAVMA 118:103, 1951.

176. Davis, J. W., and Anderson, R. C.: *Parasitic Diseases of Wild Mammals*. Ames, Iowa State Univ. Press, 1971.

177. de Castro, J. J., et al.: Effects on cattle of artificial infestations with the tick *Rhipicephalus appendiculatus*. Parasitology 90:21, 1985.

178. deChaneet, G.: Porcine sarcoptic mange in Western Australia. Aust. Vet. J. 48:581, 1972.

179. Defoliart, G. R.: Dusting for horn fly control on beef herds. J. Econ. Entomol. 49:393, 1956.

180. deJesus, Z.: Haemorrhagic filariasis in cattle caused by a new species of *Parafilaria*. Philippine J. Sci. 55:125, 1934.

181. deJesus, Z.: Habronemiasis seriously affecting improved types of horses in Thailand. J. Thai. Vet. Med. Assoc. 10:61, 1959.

182. deJesus, Z.: Observations on habronemiasis in horses. Philippine J. Vet. Med. 2:133, 1963.

183. deLeon, D. D., et al.: Control of *Haematopinus suis* and *Ascaris lumbricoides* of swine with certain organic phosphorus compounds. JAVMA 138:179, 1961.

184. DeLoach, J. R.: *In vitro* feeding of *Psoroptes ovis* (*Acari:Psoroptidae*). Vet. Parasitol. 16:117, 1984.

185. Deorani, V. P. S., and Chaudhuri, R. P.: On the histopathology of the skin lesions of goats affected by sarcoptic mange. Indian J. Vet. Sci. 35:150, 1965.

186. Deorani, V. P. S.: Studies on the pathogenicity in stephanofilarial hump sore among cattle in India. Indian J. Vet. Sci. 37:87, 1967.

187. DePaasch, P. A., and dePaasch, L. H.: Haematobia irritans (mosca del cuerno) en un hato de vacas de ordena en la costa de vera cruz. Veterinaria (Mex. City) 15:113, 1984.

188. Depner, K. R.: Distribution of the face fly *Musca autumnalis* in western Canada and the relation between its environment and population density. Can. Entomol. 101:97, 1969.

189. Descazeaux, M., and Morel, R.: Relations entre les habronemoses cutanées et gastriques du cheval. Bull. Acad. Vet. Fr. 6:364, 1933.

190. Descazeaux, M., and Morel, R.: Diagnostic bioloque des habronemoses gastriques du cheval. Bull. Soc. Pathol. Exot. 26:1010, 1933.

191. Desch, C. E., and Nutting, W. B.: Redescription of *Demodex caballi* (= *D. folliculorum var. equi* Railliet, 1895) from the horse, *Equus caballas*. Acarologia 20:235, 1978.

192. Detry, M.: Essai d'un nouvel agent antiparasitaire dans la

lutte contre la gale bovine: l'amitraz (taktic N.D.). Ann. Med. Vet. 129:173, 1985.

193. Devakula, S., et al.: The biopsy technic as an aid in the diagnosis of equine cutaneous habronemiasis. J. Thai. Vet. Med. Assoc. 13:7, 1962.

194. Dewan, M. L., and Rahman, M. M.: Isolation of microorganisms from stephanofilariasis (humpsore) and their roles in the initiation of the disease. Bangladesh Vet. J. 4:25, 1970.

195. Dewan, M. L.: Histopathology of stephanofilariasis (hump sore) at different stages of its development. Bangladesh J. Agri. Sci. 2:49, 1975.

196. Dewes, H. F.: *Strongyloides westeri* and *Corynebacterium equi* in foals. N.Z. Vet. J. 20:82, 1972.

197. Dickinson, R. G., et al.: Prostaglandin in the saliva of the cattle tick *Boophilus microplus*. Aust. J. Exper. Biol. Med. Sci. 54:475, 1976.

198. Dies, K. H., and Pritchard, J.: Bovine stephanofilarial dermatitis in Alberta. Can. Vet. J. 26:361, 1985.

199. Dikmans, G.: Observations on stephanofilariasis in cattle. Proc. Helminthol. Soc. Wash. 1:42, 1934.

200. Dikmans, G.: Nematodes as the cause of a recently discovered skin disease of cattle in the United States. North Am. Vet. 15:22, 1934.

201. Dikmans, G.: Skin lesions of domestic animals in the United States due to nematode infestation. Cornell Vet. 38:3, 1948.

202. Diplock, P. T., and Hyre, R. H. J.: Chorioptic mange in cattle associated with a severe fall in milk production. N. S. Wales Vet. Pract. 10:100, 1976.

203. Dirksen, G., and Radermacher, F.: Erste Ergebrisse der Allgemeinbehandlung der Stephanofilariose ("Sommerwunden") des Rindes mit Antiomosan und Neguvon. Dtsch. Tierarztl. Wochenschr. 67:70, 1960.

204. Dirksen, G.: Stephanofilarien als Ursache der "Sommerwunden" des Rindes in den nordwestdeutschen Weidegebieten. Dtsch. Tierarztl. Wochenschr. 66:85, 1959.

205. Dirksen, G., and Radermacher, F.: Weitere Erfahrungen mit der Allgemeinbehandlung der Stephalofilariose ("Summerwunden") des Rindes mit Antimosan[R] and Neguvon.[R] Vet. Med. Nach. 60:227, 1960.

206. Dobson, K. J.: External parasites of pigs. Mosquitoes. Proc. Univ. Sydney Post-Grad. Comm. Vet. Sci. 19:349, 1973.

207. Dorsey, C. K.: Face-fly control experiments on quarter horses. J. Econ. Entomol. 59:86, 1966.

208. Dorsey, C. K., et al.: Face fly and hornfly control on cattle—1962–1964. J. Econ. Entomol. 59:726, 1966.

209. Douglas, J. R., et al.: *Elaeophora schneideri* Wehr and Dikmans, 1935 (Nematoda, Filarioidea) in California sheep. Cornell Vet. 44:252, 1954.

210. Downing, W., and Mort, P.: Experiments in the control of the itch mite, *Psorergates ovis*, Womersley, 1941. Aust. Vet. J. 38:269, 1962.

211. Downing, W.: The life-history of *Psoroptes communis var ovis* with particular reference to latent or suppressed scab. J. Comp. Pathol. Ther. 49:163, 1936.

212. Downing, W.: The control of psoroptic scab on sheep by benzene hexachloride and DDT. Vet. Rec. 59:581, 1947.

213. Dozsa, L.: Dermatitis in large animals . . . selected case histories. Mod. Vet. Pract. 47:45, 1966.

214. Drummond, R. O., et al.: Control of ticks systemically with Merck MK-933, an avermectin. J. Econ. Entomol. 74:432, 1981.

215. Drummond, R. O., and Whetstone, T. M.: Lone star tick: Laboratory tests of acaricides. J. Econ. Entomol. 66:1274, 1973.

216. Drummond, R. O., et al.: *Boophilus annulatus* and *B. microplus*: Sprays and dips of insecticides for control on cattle. J. Econ. Entomol. 65:1354, 1972.

217. Drummond, R. O., and Gladney, W. J.: Acaricides applied to cattle for control of the lone star tick. Southwest. Entomol. 3:96, 1978.

218. Drummond, R. O.: Cattle–*Hypoderma lineatum* animal systemic insecticide test. Proc. Entomol. Soc. Am. 5:216, 1980.

219. Drummond, R. O., et al.: Small-scale field tests with dermally applied animal systemic insecticides for control of the common cattle grub. J. Econ. Entomol. 63:1233, 1970.

220. Dunn, P.: Diseases of dairy goats. In Pract. 2:21, 1980.

221. Dunne, H. W., and Leman, A. D.: *Diseases of the Swine IV*. Ames, Iowa State Univ. Press, 1975.

222. Durant, A. J.: Demodectic mange of the milk goat. Vet. Med. 39:268, 1944.

223. duToit, R., and Fiedler, O. G. H.: Demodicosis in sheep in South Africa. J. S. Afr. Vet. Med. Assoc. 38:281, 1967.

224. Dutta, P. A., and Hazarika, R. N.: Chemotherapy of stephanofilarial dermatitis in bovines. Indian Vet. J. 53:221, 1976.

225. Eberhard, M. L.: Studies on the *Onchocerca* found in cattle in the United States. I. Systematics of *O. gutturosa* and *O. lienalis* with a description of *O. stilesi* sp. n. J. Parasitol. 65:379, 1979.

226. Eberhard, M. L., and Winkler, W. G.: Onchocerciasis among ungulate animals in Georgia. J. Parasitol. 60:971, 1974.

227. Eberhard, T.: Erfahrungen bei der Gasbehundlung der Pferderaude mit Schwefeldioxyd. Monat. Prakt. Tierheilkd. 32:81, 1921.

228. Edgar, D. G.: Examination of rams for fertility. N.Z. Vet. J. 7:61, 1959.

229. Eichler, D. A., and Nelson, G. S.: Studies on *Onchocerca gutturosa* and its development in *Simulium ornatum*. J. Helminthol. 65:245, 1971.

230. Eisenblatter, K.: Beitrag zur Behandlung der Pferderaude. Berl. Tierarztl. Wochenschr. 32:185, 1916.

231. Elbihari, S., and Hussein, H. S.: *Onchocerca gutturosa* in Sudanese cattle. Rev. Elev. Med. Vet. Pays Trop. 31:179, 1978.

232. Elliot, M., et al.: The future of pyrethroids in insect control. Ann. Rev. Entomol. 23:443, 1978.

233. El Sinnary, K., and Hussein, H. S.: *Culicoides kingi*, Austen: A vector of *Onchocerca gutturosa* (Neumann, 1910) in the Sudan. Ann. Trop. Med. Parasitol. 74:655, 1980.

234. Ely, D. G., and Harvey, T. L.: Relation of ration to shortnosed cattle louse infestations. J. Econ. Entomol. 62:431, 1969.

235. Endrejat, E.: Ueber die Schaf-und Ziegenraude. Tierarztl. Rundsch. 45:637, 1939.

236. Endrejat, E.: Die Behandlung der *Sarcoptes raude* der Ziegen mit Neguvon. Tierarztl. Umsch. 14:313, 1959.

237. Endrejat, E.: Uber den derzeitigen Stand der Schfraudebekampfung. Berl. Munch. Tierarztl. Wochenschr. 1:7, 1950.

238. Etherington, W. G., and Prescott, J. F.: *Corynebacterium equi* cellulitis associated with *Strongyloides* penetration in a foal. JAVMA 177:1025, 1980.

239. Euzeby, J., et al.: La demodecie de la chevre en France. Bull. Acad. Vet. Fr. 49:423, 1976.

240. Euzeby, J., et al.: Les avermectines dans la therapeutique des gales des bovins. Bull. Acad. Vet. Fr. 54:273, 1981.

241. Everett, A. L., et al.: Effects of some important ectoparasites on the grain quality of cattle-hide leather. J. Am. Leather Chem. Assoc. 72:6, 1977.

242. Eyre, P., et al.: Reaginic (type I, anaphylactic) antibodies produced in calves in response to *Hypoderma* larvae. Vet. Rec. 107:280, 1980.

243. Eyre, P., et al.: Local and systemic reactions in cattle to *Hypoderma lineatum* larval toxin: Protection by phenylbutazone. Am. J. Vet. Res. 42:25, 1981.

244. Fadok, V. A., and Mullowney, P. C.: Dermatologic diseases of horses part I. Parasitic dermatoses of the horse. Compend. Cont. Educ. 5:S615, 1983.

245. Fadok, V. A.: Parasitic skin diseases of large animals. Vet. Clin. North Am. Large Anim. Pract. 6:3, 1984.

245a. Fadok, V. A.: Ectoparasites. In: Robinson, N. E.: Current Therapy in Equine Medicine II. Philadelphia, W. B. Saunders Co., 1987, p. 622.

246. Fadzil, M.: *Musca conducens* Walker, 1859—its prevalence and potential as a vector of *Stephanofilaria kaeli* in Peninsular Malaysia. Kajian Vet. 5:27, 1973.

247. Fadzil, M.: *Stephanofilaria kaeli* infection in cattle in Peninsular Malaysia—prevalence and treatment. Vet. Med. Rev. 1:44, 1977.

248. Fadzil, M.: The development of *Stephanofilaria kaeli* Buck-

ley, 1937, in *Musca conducens*, Walker, 1859. Kajian Vet. 7:1, 1975.

249. Fadzil, M., et al.: *Stephanofilaria kaeli* Buckley, 1937, as the cause of chronic dermatitis on the foot of a goat and on the ears and teats of cattle in West Malaysia. Vet. Rec. 92:316, 1973.

250. Fagbemi, B. O.: Effect of *Ctenocephalides felis strongylus* infestation on the performance of West African dwarf sheep and goats. Vet. Q. 4:92, 1982.

251. Fain, A., and Herin, V.: *Parafilaria bovicola* Tubangui (1934) au Ruanda-Urandi. Description du male. Ann. Parasitol. Hum. Comp. 25:167, 1950.

252. Farjoun, E., et al.: Infestation of Saanen goats in Israel with *Demodex caprae*. Refauh Vet. 38:114, 1981.

253. Farrington, D. O., et al.: *Pelodera strongyloides* dermatitis in a horse in Iowa. Vet. Med. Small Anim. Clin 71:1199, 1976.

253a. Ferenc, S. A., et al.: *Onchocerca gutturosa* and *Onchocerca lienalis* in cattle: Effect of age, sex, and origin on prevalence of onchocerciasis in subtropical and temperate regions of Florida and Georgia. Am. J. Vet. Res. 47:2266, 1986.

254. Ferguson, W., and Lavoipierre, M. M. J.: The occurrence of *Raillietia auris* in Zebu cattle in Nigeria. Vet. Rec. 74:678, 1962.

255. Finocchio, E. J., and Meriam, J. C.: Surgical correction of myiasitic urethritis granulosa. Vet. Med. Small Anim. Clin. 71:1629, 1976.

256. Fisher, W. F.: Incidence of demodectic mange in beef cattle and limed cattle hides. J. Am. Leather Chem. Assoc. 65:547, 1970.

257. Fisher, W. F.: Natural transmission of *Demodex bovis stilesi* in cattle. J. Parasitol. 59:223, 1973.

258. Fisher, W. F.: Incidence of demodicosis in commercially pickled steer hides. J. Am. Leather Chem. Assoc. 69:5, 1974.

259. Fisher, W. F., and Wilson, G. I.: Precipitating antibodies in cattle infested by *Psoroptes ovis* (Acarina:Psoroptidae). J. Med. Entomol. 14:146, 1977.

260. Fisher, W. F., and Wright, F. C.: Susceptibility of scabies-naive Hereford and Brahman calves to *Psoroptes ovis* infestations. Southwest. Entomol. 6:57, 1981.

261. Fisher, W. F.: Recent advances in psoroptic acariasis and demodectic mange of domestic animals and sarcoptic scabies of humans. Intl. J. Dermatol. 20:585, 1981.

262. Fisher, W. F., et al.: Natural transmission of *Demodex bovis stilesi* to dairy calves. Vet. Parasitol. 7:233, 1980.

263. Fisher, W. F., and Wright, F. C.: Effects of the sheep scab mite on cumulative weight gains in cattle. J. Econ. Entomol. 74:234, 1981.

264. Fisher, W. F., and Crookshank, H. R.: Effects of *Psoroptes ovis* (Acarina-Psoroptidae) on certain biochemical constituents of cattle serum. Vet. Parasitol. 11:241, 1982.

265. Fisher, W. F.: Development of serum antibody activity as determined by enzyme-linked immunosorbent assay to *Psoroptes ovis* (Acarina:Psoroptidae) antigens in cattle infected with *P. ovis*. Vet. Parasitol. 13:363, 1983.

266. Fitzpatrick, T. B., et al.: *Dermatology in General Medicine II*. New York, McGraw-Hill Book Co., 1979.

267. Flower, P. J.: A new outbreak of sheep scab (*Psoroptes ovis*) in Lesotho and the measures taken to control it. Trop. Anim. Health Prod. 10:207, 1978.

267a. Foil, C. S.: Cutaneous onchocerciasis. *In*: Robinson, N. E.: Current Therapy in Equine Medicine II. Philadelphia, W. B. Saunders Co., 1987, p. 627.

268. Fonseca, A. H., et al.: *Raillietia caprae* (Acari:Mesostigmata) em caprinos e ovinos no Brasil. Pesq. Vet. Bras. 3:29, 1983.

269. Foster, G. G., et al.: Genetic manipulation of sheep blow fly populations. Aust. Adv. Vet. Sci. 1978:86, 1978.

270. Fraser, A. C.: Heel-bug in the Thoroughbred horse. Vet. Rec. 50:1455, 1938.

271. French, D. D., et al.: Comparison of the anti-strongyle activity of a micellar formulation of ivermectin given parentally and per os. Vet. Med. Small Anim. Clin. 78:1778, 1983.

272. French, N., et al.: Control of headfly on sheep. Vet. Rec. 100:40, 1977.

273. Frese, K., and Thiel, W.: Zur Pathologie der Hautveranderungen beim Kriebelmuckenbefall des Rindes. Zbl. Vet. Med. B 21:618, 1974.

274. Frick, W., et al.: Ergebnisse der Ektoparasitenbekumpfung bei Schweinen in einem Kreis. Monat. Vet. Med. 29:612, 1974.

275. Funk, K.: Cutaneous nematodiasis. Southwest. Vet. 17:68, 1963.

276. Gansser, A.: Zur Biologie der Dasselfliege und zur Bekampfung der Dasselplage durch Abfangen der Dasselfliegen. Schweiz. Arch. Tierheilkd. 99:17, 1957.

277. Garg, R. K.: Efficacy of some insecticides against sarcoptic mange in goats. Vet. Bull. 45:352, 1975.

278. Gearhart, M. S., et al.: Bilateral lower palpebral demodicosis in a dairy cow. Cornell Vet. 71:305, 1981.

279. Gecheva, G.: Seasonal dynamics of *Melophagus ovinus* in sheep. Vet. Med. Nauki 8:67, 1971.

280. Gecheva, G.: Pathogenic role of *M. ovinus* in sheep: Hematological aspects. Vet. Med. Nauki 9:89, 1972.

281. Gibbons, W. J.: Summer sores. Mod. Vet. Pract. 49:76, 1968.

282. Gibbons, W. J., et al.: *Bovine Medicine and Surgery II*. Santa Barbara, CA, American Veterinary Publications, Inc., 1970.

283. Gibson, T. E., et al.: *Parafilaria multipapillosa* in the horse. Vet. Rec. 76:774, 1964.

284. Gill, D. A., et al.: Trombidiosis of sheep. Aust. Vet. J. 21:22, 1945.

285. Gingrich, R. E.: Differentiation of resistance in cattle to larvae *Hypoderma lineatum*. Vet. Parasitol. 7:243, 1980.

286. Gingrich, R. E.: Acquired resistance to *Hypoderma lineatum*: Comparative immune response of resistant and susceptible cattle. Vet. Parasitol. 9:233, 1982.

287. Girard, R.: Un cas d'evolution d'*Hypoderma bovis* de Geer sur le cheval. C. R. Acad. Sci. 208:306, 1939.

288. Gnedina, M. A., and Osipov, A. N.: Contribution to the biology of the nematode *Parafilaria multipapillosa* parasite in the horse. Helminthologia 2:13, 1960.

289. Goetze, R.: Verluste und Erkrankungen bei der Abdasselung durch Dasselanaphylaxie. Dtsch. Tierarztl. Wochenschr. 42:258, 1934.

290. Goksu, K., and Ozgencil, B.: Kuzu ve koyunda *Rhipicephalus sanguineus* Latreille, 1806 (Acarina:Ixodoidea) dan ileri gelen dis kulak derisi lezyonlari. Vet. Fak. Derg. Ank. Univ. 17:7, 1970.

291. Goksu, K., and Dincer, S.: Koyunlarda hypodermoisis durumu. Vet. Fak. Derg. Ank. Univ. 20:234, 1973.

292. Gordon, H. M.: *Strongyloides papillosus* in goats. Proc. Univ. Sydney Post-Grad. Comm. Vet. Sci.—Control and Therapy, No. 1758, May, 1984.

292a. Gourreau, J. M.: Principales dermatoses parasitaires chez le porc en France. Point Vet. 14:55, 1982.

293. Grafner, G., et al.: Occurrence and harmful effects of the blackflies in the Schwerin district of East Germany. Angew. Parasitol. 17:2, 1976.

294. Grafner, G., and Hiepe, T.: Beitrag zum Krankheitsbild und zur Pathogenese des Kriebelmuckenbefalles bei Weidetieren. Monat. Vet. Med. 34:538, 1979.

295. Graham, N. P. H.: Some observations on the bionomics of the itch mite (*Psorergates ovis*) of sheep and its control with lime sulfur dips. J. Coun. Scient. Ind. Res. Aust. 16:206, 1943.

296. Graham, N. P. H.: The control of itch mite (*Psorergates ovis*) in sheep. Aust. Vet. J. 35:153, 1959.

297. Graham, O. H., and Hourrigan, J. L.: Eradication programs for the arthropod parasites of livestock. J. Med. Entomol. 13:629, 1977.

298. Graubman, H. D., and Schulz, W.: Ein Beitrag zur Histopathologie der Demodikose beim Rind. Arch. Exp. Vet. Med. 22:831, 1968.

299. Green, H. F.: A survey of skin diseases in goats in Kenya and their effect on the finished leather. J. Soc. Leather Trades Chem. 40:259, 1956.

300. Green, H. F.: A survey of skin diseases of cattle in Kenya

and their effect on the finished leather. J. Soc. Leather Trades Chem. 41:418, 1957.

301. Green, H. F.: A survey of skin diseases of hair sheep in Kenya and their effect on the finished leather. J. Soc. Leather Trades Chem. 43:85, 1959.

302. Griffin, C. A., and Dean, D. J.: Demodectic mange in goats. Cornell Vet. 34:308, 1944.

303. Griffiths, R. B., et al.: Some parasitic diseases of zoonotic interest recorded by the regional veterinary diagnostic laboratory, Selangor, during 1965–1968. Kajian Vet. 2:13, 1969.

304. Guillot, F. S.: Population increase of Psoroptes ovis (Acari:Psoroptidae) on stanchioned cattle during summer. J. Med. Entomol. 18:44, 1981.

305. Guillot, F. S., and Meleney, W. P.: The infectivity of surviving Psoroptes ovis (Hering) in cattle treated with ivermectin. Vet. Parasitol. 10:73, 1982.

306. Guillot, F. S., and Cole, N. A.: Development and transmission of psoroptic mange of cattle in feed lots in endemic and nonendemic regions. Vet. Parasitol. 16:127, 1984.

307. Gulati, R. L.: Filaria haemorrhagica in cattle and its treatment. Indian Vet. J. 11:32, 1934.

308. Gunn, F. L.: Ticks. In Howard, J. L.: Current Veterinary Therapy. Food Animal Practice. Philadelphia, W. B. Saunders Co., 1981, p. 1137.

309. Gunn, F. L.: Myiasis. In: Howard, J. L.: Current Veterinary Therapy. Food Animal Practice. Philadelphia, W. B. Saunders Co., 1981, p. 1139.

310. Guss, S. B.: Management of Diseases of Dairy Goats. Scottsdale, AZ, Dairy Goat Journal Publishing Corp., 1977.

311. Haberman, W. O., et al.: The occurrence of Hypoderma larvae in the spinal canal of cattle. Aust. J. Agric. Res. 78:637, 1949.

312. Hadlow, W. J., et al.: Intracranial myiasis by Hypoderma bovis (Linnaeus) in a horse. Cornell Vet. 67:272, 1977.

313. Hadwen, S., and Bruce, E. A.: Anaphylaxis in cattle and sheep, produced by the larvae of Hypoderma bovis, H. lineatum, and Oestrus ovis. JAVMA 51:15, 1917.

314. Hall, C. A., et al.: The effect of a drying agent (B26) on wool moisture and blowfly strike. Res. Vet. Sci. 29:186, 1980.

315. Hallam, G. J.: Transmission of Damalinia ovis and Damalinia caprae between sheep and goats. Aust. Vet. J. 62:344, 1985.

316. Hardenbergh, J. G., and Schlotthauer, C. F.: Demodectic mange of the goat and its treatment. JAVMA 67:486, 1925.

317. Harland, E. C., et al.: Demodectic mange of swine. JAVMA 159:1752, 1971.

318. Harvey, T. L., and Brethour, J. R.: Treatment of one beef animal per herd with permethrin for horn fly control. J. Econ. Entomol. 72:532, 1979.

319. Harvey, T. L., and Brethour, J. R.: Effect of horn flies on weight gains of beef cattle. J. Econ. Entomol. 72:516, 1979.

320. Haupt, W., and Siebert, W.: Untersuchungen zur Lebensdauer von Grabmilben und deren Entwicklungsstadien in Hautgeschabseln von Schweinen unter verschiedenen um veltbedingungen. Arch. Exp. Vet. Med. 37:613, 1983.

321. Heard, T. W.: Sarcoptes scabiei infestation in pigs. Vet. Rec. 104:61, 1979.

322. Heath, A. C. G.: The scrotal mange mite, Chorioptes bovis (Hering, 1845) on sheep: Seasonality, pathogenicity, and intra-flock transfer. N.Z. Vet. J. 26:307, 1978.

323. Henderson, D., and McPhee, I.: Cypermethrin pour-on for control of the sheep body louse (Damalinia ovis). Vet. Rec. 113:258, 1983.

324. Hepburn, G. A.: Sheep blowfly research. Onderstepoort J. Vet. Sci. Anim. Ind. 18:13, 1943.

325. Herd, R. P., and Donham, J. C.: Efficacy of ivermectin against cutaneous Draschia and habronema infection (summer sores) in horses. Am. J. Vet. Res. 42:1953, 1981.

326. Herd, R. P., and Donham, J. C.: Efficacy of ivermectin against Onchocerca cervicalis microfilarial dermatitis in horses. Am. J. Vet. Res. 44:1102, 1983.

327. Hewetson, R. W., and Nolan, J.: Resistance of cattle to cattle tick, Boophilus microplus. I. The development of

328. Hewetson, R. W.: Resistance by cattle to the cattle tick, Boophilus microplus. III. The development of resistance to experimental infestations by purebred Sahiwal and Australian Illawarra Shorthorn cattle. Aust. J. Agric. Res. 22:331, 1971.

329. Hewett, G. R., and Heard, T. W.: Phosmet for the systemic control of pig mange. Vet. Rec. 111:558, 1982.

330. Hibler, C. P.: The life history of Stephanofilaria stilesi Chitwood, 1934. J. Parasitol. 50:34, 1964.

331. Hibler, C. P.: Development of Stephanofilaria stilesi in the horn fly. J. Parasitol. 52:890, 1966.

332. Hibler, C. P., et al.: Experimental infection of sheep and deer with Elaeophora schneideri. J. Wildl. Dis. 6:110, 1970.

333. Hiepe, T., and Splisteser, H.: Untersuchungen uber Vorkommen, Diagnostik der durch Chorioptes ovis bedingten FuBraude in Schafherden. Monat. Vet. Med. 17:776, 1962.

334. Hiepe, T., et al.: Enzootisches Auftreten von Hautveranderungen mit Wollausfall in Schafbestanden infolge Caloglyphus-berlesei-Befalls. Monat. Vet. Med. 33:901, 1978.

335. Hiepe, T., and Ribbeck, R.: The pig louse (Haematopinus suis). Angew. Parasitol. 16:233, 1975.

336. Hiepe, T., et al.: Untersuchungen zum Krankheitsbild der durch Chorioptes ovis bedingten FuBraude des Schafes. Monat. Vet. Med. 23:578, 1968.

337. Hightower, B. G.: Ectoparasites taken from Texas goats. J. Econ. Entomol. 44:287, 1951.

338. Hillerton, J. E., et al.: Control of flies (Diptera:Muscidae) on dairy heifers by Flectron ear-tags. Br. Vet. J. 141:160, 1985.

339. Hilmy, N., et al.: The role of Onchocerca reticulata as the cause of fistulous withers and ulcerative wounds of the back in solipeds, and its treatment. Cairo Fac. Vet. Med. J. 14:149, 1967.

340. Himonas, C. A., et al.: Demodectic mites in eyelids of domestic animals in Greece. J. Parasitol. 61:767, 1975.

341. Hitchcock, L. F.: Resistance of the cattle tick B. microplus to benzene hexachloride. Aust. J. Agric. Res. 4:360, 1953.

342. Hobday, F.: Some uncommon parasites. J. Comp. Pathol. Ther. 11:266, 1898.

343. Hogg, A., and Swieczkowski, T.: External parasites of swine. Vet. Clin. North Am. Large Anim. Pract. 4:343, 1982.

344. Hopes, R.: Skin diseases in horses. Vet. Dermatol. News. 1:4, 1976.

345. Hourrigan, J. L.: Safe use of pesticides on livestock. JAVMA 157:1818, 1970.

346. Hourrigan, J. L.: Spread and detection of psoroptic scabies of cattle in the United States. JAVMA 175:1278, 1979.

347. Howard, J. L., et al.: Current Veterinary Therapy. Food Animal Practice. Philadelphia, W. B. Saunders Co., 1981.

348. Howard, J. L., et al.: Current Veterinary Therapy. Food Animal Practice II. Philadelphia, W. B. Saunders Co., 1986.

349. Howell, C. E., and Hart, G. H.: An apparent hereditary epithelial defect factor, the possible etiology of Bursattee in horses. JAVMA 71:347, 1927.

350. Humphrey, J. D., et al.: Chrysomyia bezziana: Pathology of old world screw-worm fly infestations in cattle. Exp. Parasitol. 49:381, 1980.

351. Hunter, A. R.: Sheep headfly disease in Britain. Vet. Rec. 97:95, 1975.

352. Hussein, M. F., et al.: Onchocerca gutturosa infection in Sudanese cattle. Br. Vet. J. 131:76, 1975.

353. Hutyra, F., et al.: Special Pathology and Therapeutics of the Diseases of Domestic Animals III. Chicago, Eger, 1926.

354. Ihle, J. E. W., and Ihle-Landenberg, M. E.: Over een dermatitis squamosa et crustosa circumscripta bij het rund in Nederlandsch-Indie, genaamd cascado. II. Stephanofilaria dedoesi een nematode uit de huid van het rund. Ned. Ind. Diergeneeskd. 45:279, 1933.

355. Ishihara, K., et al.: Occurrence of cutaneous hemorrhagic parafilariasis in cattle. Jpn. J. Vet. Sci. 44:669, 1982.

356. Islam, A. W. M. S.: Biology of Stephanofilaria assamensis and epizootiology of stephanofilariasis in cattle of Bangladesh. Veterinariya (Moscow) 15:112, 1971.

357. Islam, A. W. M. S.: Stephanofilariasis (hump sore) in cattle

of Bangladesh. I. Incidence of hump sore in different districts and geographical areas of Bangladesh. Bangladesh J. Agri. Sci. 4:127, 1977.

358. Isshiki, O.: Studies on bovine onchocerciasis in Korea. Jpn. J. Vet. Sci. 25:375, 1963.

359. Jensen, R., and Seghetti, L.: Elaeophoriasis in sheep. JAVMA 127:499, 1955.

360. Jensen, R., and Swift, B. I.: *Diseases of Sheep II*. Philadelphia, Lea & Febiger, 1982.

361. Jibbo, J. M. C.: Bovine parasitic otitis. Bull. Epizoot. Dis. Afr. 14:59, 1966.

362. Johnk, M.: Arsenik in der Behandlung der Raude. Berl. Tierarztl. Wochenschr. 35:3, 1919.

363. Johnson, S. J., et al.: Stephanofilariasis in cattle. Aust. Vet. J. 57:411, 1981.

363a. Johnson, S. J., et al.: The distribution and prevalence of Stephanofilariasis in cattle in Queensland. Aust. Vet. J. 63:121, 1986.

364. Johnston, L. A. Y.: A note on psoroptic otoacariasis in a horse in North Queensland. Aust. Vet. J. 39:208, 1963.

364a. Johnston, L. A. Y., et al.: Immunization of cattle against *Boophilus microplus* using extracts derived from adult females: Effects of induced immunity on tick populations. Intl. J. Parasitol. 16:27, 1986.

365. Johnston, T. H., and Bancroft, M. J.: The life history of *Habronema* in relation to *Musca domestica* and native flies in Queensland. Proc. R. Soc. 32:61, 1920.

366. Jones, C. K., et al.: Occurrence of *Stephanofilaria stilesi* in Texas. Southwest. Vet. 21:139, 1968.

367. Joyce, J. R., et al.: Treatment of habronemiasis of the adnexa of the equine eye. Vet. Med. Small Anim. Clin. 67:1008, 1972.

368. Kadlec, V.: *Demodex suis*. Vet. Med. (Prague) 20:441, 1975.

369. Kale, S. M., and Panchegaonkar, M. R.: Treatment of sarcoptic mange in goats with oil of Karanj. Indian Vet. J. 46:622, 1969.

370. Kamyszek, F.: Sarcoptic mange in pigs. A problem in large herds. Wiad. Parazytol. 21:281, 1975.

371. Kantack, B. H., et al.: Hornfly and face fly control on range cattle with ultra-low-volume malathion sprays. J. Econ. Entomol. 60:1766, 1967.

372. Karim, R.: A report on the dermatitis around the eyes of cattle due to stephanofilaria and its chemotherapy. Indian Vet. J. 61:419, 1984.

373. Karns, P. A., and Luther, D. G.: A survey of adverse effects associated with ivermectin use in Louisiana horses. JAVMA 185:782, 1984.

374. Keller, H., et al.: Zur tilgung der *Sarcoptes*—raude beim schwein. Schweiz. Arch. Tierheilkd. 114:573, 1972.

374a. Kemp, D. H., et al.: Immunization of cattle against *Boophilus microplus* using extracts derived from adult female ticks: Feeding and survival of the parasite on vaccinated cattle. Intl. J. Parasitol. 16:115, 1986.

375. Kemper, H. E.: Filarial dermatosis in sheep. North Am. Vet. 19:36, 1938.

376. Kemper, H. E., and Roberts, I. H.: Treatment of filarial dermatosis of sheep. Am. J. Vet. Res. 7:350, 1946.

377. Kemper, H. E., et al.: Hexachlorocyclohexane as an acaricide for the control of the spinose ear tick in cattle. North Am. Vet. 28:665, 1947.

378. Kemper, H., et al.: DDT emulsions for the destruction of lice on cattle, sheep, and goats. Am. J. Vet. Res. 9:373, 1948.

379. Kettle, P. R.: The influence of cattle lice (*Damalinia bovis* and *Linognathus vituli*) on weight gain in beef animals. N.Z. Vet. J. 22:10, 1974.

380. Kettle, P. R., and Pearce, D. M.: Pour-on insecticides for the control of cattle lice (*Linognathus vituli* and *Damalinia bovis*). N.Z. Vet. J. 22:76, 1974.

381. Kettle, P. R.: Pour-on insecticides for the control of *Linognathus vituli*. N.Z. Vet. J. 20:167, 1972.

382. Khajuria, R. R.: Incidence and control of parafilariasis in bovines in Jammu province. Indian Vet. J. 43:749, 1966.

383. Khan, M. A.: Toxicity of systemic insecticides: Efficacy of dermal and parenteral applications of cruformate for systemic control of *Hypoderma* spp. in cattle. Vet. Rec. 93:525, 1973.

384. Khan, M. A.: Extermination of cattle grubs *Hypoderma* spp. on a regional basis. Vet. Rec. 83:97, 1968.

385. Khan, M. A.: Some factors involved in systemic insecticide toxicosis: Esophageal lesions in heifers treated with coumaphos, cruformate, and trichlorfon. Can. J. Anim. Sci. 51:411, 1971.

386. Kilgore, R. L., et al.: Response of horses to repeated intramuscular injections of ivermectin. Vet. Med. Small Anim. Clin. 78:1894, 1983.

387. King, N. B.: External parasites. Proc. Univ. Sydney Post-Grad. Comm. Vet. Sci. 52:215, 1980.

388. King, N. B.: Goat practice summer management problems. Proc. Univ. Sydney Post-Grad. Comm. Vet. Sci. 52:39, 1980.

389. King, N. B.: Skin diseases. Proc. Univ. Sydney Post-Grad. Comm. Vet. Sci. 52:199, 1980.

390. Kinzer, H. G.: Aerial application of ultra-low-volume insecticides to control the horn fly on unrestrained range cattle. J. Econ. Entomol. 62:1515, 1969.

391. Kinzer, H. G.: Ground application of ultra-low-volume malathion and fenthion for horn fly control in New Mexico. J. Econ. Entomol. 63:736, 1970.

392. Kirkland, K. C., et al.: Habronemiasis in an Arabian stallion. Equine Pract. 3:34, 1981.

393. Kirkwood, A. C., et al.: The efficacy of showers for control of ectoparasites of sheep. Vet. Rec. 102:50, 1978.

394. Kirkwood, A. C.: Effect of *Psoroptes ovis* on the weight of sheep. Vet. Rec. 107:469, 1980.

395. Kirkwood, A. C., and Quick, M. P.: Diazinon for the control of sheep scab. Vet. Rec. 108:279, 1981.

396. Kirkwood, A.: Insecticides and dips for farm animals. In Pract. 5:198, 1983.

397. Klei, T. R., et al.: Efficacy of ivermectin (22,23-dihydroavermectin B_1) against adult *Setaria equina* and microfilaria of *Onchocerca cervicalis* in ponies. J. Parasitol. 66:859, 1980.

398. Klein, W.: Schwere Raude bei Schafen durch die Akarusmilbe (*Demodex folliculorum*). Dtsch. Tierarztl. Wochenschr. 29:105, 1921.

399. Knese, K.: Die Sarkoptesraude der Pferde und ihre Behandlung. Berl. Tierarztl. Wochenschr. 32:185, 1916.

400. Koch, F.: Demodicosis in the pig. Vet. Med. Rev. 1:67, 1979.

401. Kolstrup, N.: *Onchocerca gutturosa* in Danish cattle: Prevalence, geographic distribution, and host vector relationships. Acta Vet. Scand. 16:1, 1975.

402. Kono, I., and Fukuyoski, S.: Leucoderma of the muzzle of cattle induced by a new species of *Stephanofilaria*. Jpn. J. Vet. Sci. 29:312, 1967.

403. Koudstaal, D., et al.: *Boophilus microplus*: Rejection of larvae from British breed cattle. Parasitology 76:379, 1978.

404. Koutz, F. R.: *Demodex folliculorum* studies. V. Demodectic mange in cattle. Vet. Med. 50:305, 1955.

405. Koutz, F. R.: *Demodex folliculorum* studies. IX. The prevalence of demodectic mange in various animals. Speculum 17:19, 1963.

406. Kral, F., and Schwartzman, R. M.: *Veterinary and Comparative Dermatology*. Philadelphia, J. B. Lippincott Co., 1964.

407. Kreis, H. A.: Ein neuer Nematode aus dem ausseren Gehorgang von Zeburindern in Ostafrika, *Rhabditis bovis* n. sp. Schweiz. Arch. Tierheilkd. 106:372, 1964.

408. Kress, F., and Stockl, W.: Uber den Kalzium-, Phosphor-, Kupfer-und Eisengehalt im Serum gesunder und an Sarkoptesraude (*Sarcoptes rupicaprae*) erkrankter Ziegen. Wien. Tierarztl. Monatsschr. 51:260, 1964.

409. Kretzmann, P. M., et al.: Manifestations of bovine parafilariasis. J. S. Afr. Vet. Assoc. 55:127, 1984.

410. Kunkle, G. A., and Greiner, E. C.: Dermatitis in horses and man caused by the straw itch mite. JAVMA 181:467, 1982.

411. Lal, J., et al.: Studies on the comparative efficacy of Cedrus deodara oil, benzyl benzoate and tetraethylthiuram monosulphide against sarcoptic mange in sheep. Indian Vet. J. 53:543, 1976.

412. Laranja, R. J.: Organochlorine and organophosphorus resistance in a strain of *Psoroptes ovis*. Biol. Inst. Pesq. Vet. 5:5, 1978.

413. Lastra, H. C.: Brief review of acaricides for sheep in use in Argentina. Gaceta Vet. 34:531, 1972.

414. Lavigne, C., and Smith, H. J.: Treatment of sarcoptic mange in Canadian cattle with ivermectin. Can. Vet. J. 24:389, 1983.

415. Lavoipierre, M. M. J., and Larsen, P. H.: A note on a new ear mite discovered in the auditory canal of California feral goats. Calif. Vet. 35:23, 1981.

416. Leaning, W. H. D.: Ivermectin as an antiparasitic agent in cattle. Mod. Vet. Pract. 65:669, 1984.

417. Lee, R. P., et al.: Efficacy of ivermectin against sarcoptic scab in pigs. Vet. Rec. 107:503, 1980.

418. Leeman, W.: Die Chorioptes—oder FuBraude beim. Pferd. Schweiz. Arch. Tierheilkd. 96:588, 1954.

419. Lees, M. J., et al.: Cutaneous onchocerciasis in the horse: Five cases in Southwestern British Columbia. Can. Vet. J. 24:3, 1983.

420. Leman, A. D., et al.: Diseases of Swine V. Ames, Iowa State Univ. Press, 1981.

421. Lepinay, R.: Les essais pratiques de traitement de la gale des chevaux par les gaz sulfureaux. Rec. Med. Vet. 93:653, 1917.

422. LeRiche, P. D. R., et al.: Notes on the goat warble-fly Przhevalskiana aegagri Brauer 1863, in Cyprus. J. Natl. Hist. 7:615, 1973.

423. Lewis, J. C.: Equine granuloma in the Northern Territory of Australia. J. Comp. Pathol. Ther. 27:1, 1914.

424. Levine, N. D., and Morrill, C. C.: Bovine stephanofilarial dermatitis in Illinois. JAVMA 127:528, 1955.

425. Levine, N. D., et al.: Nematode dermatitis in cattle associated with Rhabditis. JAVMA 116:294, 1950.

426. Lewis, J. C., and Seddon, H. R.: Habronemic conjunctivitis. J. Comp. Pathol. Ther. 31:87, 1918.

427. Liddel, J. S., and Clayton, R.: Long duration Fly control on cattle using cypermethrin-impregnated ear tags. Vet. Rec. 110:502, 1982.

428. Liebisch, A., and Petrich, J.: Zur gegenwartigen Verbreitung und Bekampfung dier Rinderraude in Norddeutschland. Dtsch. Tierarztl. Wochenschr. 84:424, 1977.

429. Liebisch, A., et al.: Untersuchungen zur Uberle bensdauer von Milben der Arten Psoroptes ovis, Psoroptes cuniculi und Chorioptes bovis abseits des belebten Wirtes. Dtsch. Tierarztl. Wochenschr. 92:181, 1985.

430. Liebisch, A.: Untersuchungen uber die Langzeltwirkung insektizidhaltiger Ohrmarken (Permethrin und Cypermethrin) zur Berkampfung von Fliegen und Bremsen bei Weiderind in Norddeutschland. Dtsch. Tierarztl. Wochenschr. 92:186, 1985.

431. Linklater, K. A., and Rogerson, T.: Alopecia in housed ewes. Vet. Rec. 110:565, 1982.

432. Linklater, K. A., and Gillespie, I. D.: Outbreak of psoroptic mange in cattle. Vet. Rec. 115:211, 1984.

433. Linton, R. C.: The presence of Demodex folliculorum in the horse. Vet. J. 72:79, 1916.

434. Littlejohn, A. I.: Psoroptic mange in the goat. Vet. Rec. 82:148, 1968.

435. Livingston, C. W.: The sheep ked (Melophagus ovinus). In: Howard, J. L.: Current Veterinary Therapy. Food Animal Practice. Philadelphia, W. B. Saunders Co., 1981, p. 1157.

436. Lloyd, S., and Soulsby, E. J. L.: Survey for infection with Onchocerca cervicalis in horses in Eastern United States. Am. J. Vet. Res. 39:1962, 1979.

437. Lofstedt, J.: Dermatologic diseases of sheep. Vet. Clin. North Am. Large Anim. Pract. 5:427, 1983.

438. Loke, Y. W., and Ramachandran, C. P.: The pathology of lesions in cattle caused by Stephanofilaria kaeli Buckley, 1937. J. Helminthol. 41:161, 1967.

439. Loomis, E. C., et al.: Control of Hypoderma lineatum and H. bovis in California, 1970–1972, using crufomate, fenthion, and imidan in new low-volume and usual pour-on formulations. J. Econ. Entomol. 66:439, 1973.

440. Loomis, E. C.: Common ectoparasites and their control. In: Robinson, N. E.: Current Therapy in Equine Medicine. Philadelphia, W. B. Saunders Co., 1983, p. 529.

441. Love, R. J.: Skin diseases. Proc. Univ. Sydney Post-Grad. Comm. Vet. Sci. 56:111, 1981.

442. Lucas, K. M.: Psoroptic otoacariasis of the horse. Aust. Vet. J. 22:186, 1946.

443. Ludwig, K. G., et al.: Efficacy of ivermectin in controlling Strongyloides westeri infections in foals. Am. J. Vet. Res. 44:314, 1983.

444. Lundquist, H.: Parafilaria Bovicola (Tubangui, 1934) established in Swedish cattle. Nord. Vet. Med. 35:57, 1983.

445. Lyons, E. J., et al.: Prevalence of microfilariae (Onchocerca spp.) in skin of Kentucky horses at necropsy. JAVMA 179:899, 1981.

446. Lyons, E. T., et al.: Onchocerca spp. frequency in Thoroughbreds at necropsy in Kentucky. Am. J. Vet. Res. 47:880, 1986.

447. MacFarlane, W. V., et al.: Heat and water in tropical Merino sheep. Aust. J. Agric. Res. 9:217, 1958.

448. MacHardy, W. M.: A literature review with some comments on the sheep itch mite (Psorergates ovis Womersley). J. S. Afr. Vet. Med. Assoc. 36:237, 1965.

449. MacKenzie, D.: Goat Husbandry. London, Faber and Faber, 1957.

450. Maddy, K. T.: Stephanofilarial dermatitis of cattle. North Am. Vet. 36:275, 1955.

451. Magat, A., and Boulard, C.: Essaisde vaccination contre l'hyperdermose bovine avec un vaccin contenant une collagenase brute extraite des larves de ler stade d'Hypoderma lineatum. C. R. Acad. Sci. 270:728, 1970.

452. Malan, F. S., and Roper, N. A.: The seasonal incidence of the sheep itch mite, Psorergates ovis Womersley under subtropical conditions. J. S. Afr. Vet. Assoc. 53:171, 1982.

453. Malviya, H. C.: Stephanofilarial infections in cattle and buffalo in Andaman Islands. Indian J. Helminthol. 24:68, 1972.

454. Manley, F. H.: Note on caprine demodectic mange. Vet. Rec. 47:118, 1935.

455. Manning, T. O., et al.: Caprine dermatology. Part III. Parasitic, allergic, hormonal, and neoplastic disorders. Compend. Cont. Educ. 7:S437, 1985.

456. Marcoux, M., et al.: Infection par Onchocerca cervicalis au Québec: Signes cliniques et méthode de diagnostic. Can. Vet. J. 18:108, 1977.

457. Marquardt, W. C., and Fritts, D. H.: Control of cattle grubs by an orally administered organic phosphorus compound. JAVMA 131:562, 1957.

458. Marquardt, W. C., et al.: Control of cattle grubs and lice in Montana. JAVMA 137:589, 1960.

459. Martin, W. B.: Diseases of Sheep. Oxford, Blackwell Scientific Publications, 1983.

459a. Martineau, G. P., et al.: Pathophysiology of sarcoptic mange in swine—part I. Compend. Cont. Educ. 9:F51, 1987.

459b. Martineau, G. P., et al.: Pathophysiology of sarcoptic mange in swine—part II. Compend. Cont. Educ. 9:F93, 1987.

459c. Martineau, G. P., et al.: Control of Sarcoptes scabiei infection with ivermectin in a large intensive piggery. Can. Vet. J. 25:235, 1984.

460. Matthysse, J. G., and Marshall, J.: The importance, relationship to footrot, and control of Chorioptes bovis on cattle and sheep. Adv. Acarol. 1:39, 1963.

461. Matthysse, J. G., et al.: Controlling lice and chorioptic mange mites on dairy cattle. J. Econ. Entomol. 60:1615, 1967.

462. Mauck, C., and Mickwitz, G.: Kombinierte Raude-und Spulwurmtherapie mit Neguvon im Absatzferkelalter. Dtsch. Tierarztl. Wochenschr. 72:521, 1965.

463. Maurer, N. D., and Bell, P. R.: Evaluation of injectable trichlorfon as a treatment for onchocerciasis in horses. Southwest. Vet. 30:176, 1977.

464. McCulloch, B., and Tungaraza, R.: Skin diseases in cattle hides and goat skins in Northwestern Tanzania. E. Afr. Agric. For. J. 32:240, 1967.

465. McCullough, C., et al.: Onchocerciasis among ungulate animals in Maryland. J. Parasitol. 63:1065, 1977.

466. McDougall, K. W., and Lewis, I. J.: Behavior of amitraz in cattle dipping baths. Aust. Vet. J. 61:137, 1984.

467. McKenna, C. T., and Pulsford, M. F.: A note on the occurrence of Chorioptes communis var ovis on sheep in South Australia. Aust. Vet. J. 23:146, 1947.

468. McMullen, W. C.: Onchocercal filariasis. Southwest. Vet. 25:1979, 1972.

469. McMullen, W. C.: The skin. *In*: Mansmann, R. A., et al.: *Equine Medicine and Surgery III*. Santa Barbara, CA, American Veterinary Publications, Inc., 1982.

470. McMullen, W. C.: Habronemiasis. *In*: Robinson, N. E.: *Current Therapy in Equine Medicine*. Philadelphia, W. B. Saunders Co., 1983, p. 551.

471. McMullen, W. C.: Equine dermatology. Proc. Am. Assoc. Equine Pract. 22:293, 1976.

472. McMullen, W. C.: Mosquitoes. *In*: Howard, J. L.: *Current Veterinary Therapy. Food Animal Practice*. Philadelphia, W. B. Saunders Co., 1981, p. 1156.

473. McPherson, E. A.: Sarcoptic mange in pigs. Vet. Rec. 72:869, 1960.

474. Medley, J. G., and Drummond, R. O.: Tests with insecticides for control of lice on goats and sheep. J. Econ. Entomol. 56:658, 1963.

475. Mehls, H. J.: Eine seltene Form der *Chorioptes*—Raude beim Pferd. Berl. Munch. Tierarztl. Wochenschr. 1:9, 1952.

476. Meleney, W. P.: Experimentally induced bovine psoroptic acariasis in a rabbit. Am. J. Vet. Res. 28:892, 1967.

477. Meleney, W. P., and Roberts, I. H.: Evaluation of acaricidal dips for control of *Psoroptes ovis* on sheep. JAVMA 151:725, 1967.

478. Meleney, W. P., and Christy, J. E.: Factors complicating the control of psoroptic scabies of cattle. JAVMA 173:1473, 1978.

479. Meleney, W. P., and Fisher, W. F.: The effect of exposure to mites, *Psoroptes ovis*, on calves of varying susceptibility to common scabies. Proc. Ann. Meet. U.S. Anim. Health Assoc. 83:340, 1979.

480. Meleney, W. P.: Control of psoroptic scabies on calves with ivermectin. Am. J. Vet. Res. 43:329, 1982.

481. Meleney, W. P., et al.: Residual protection against cattle scabies afforded by ivermectin. Am. J. Vet. Res. 43:1767, 1982.

482. Mellor, P. S.: Studies on *Onchocerca cervicalis* Railliet and Henry, 1910. I. *Onchocerca cervicalis* in British horses. J. Helminthol. 47:97, 1973.

483. Mellor, P. S.: Studies on *Onchocerca cervicalis* Railliet and Henry, 1910: II. Pathology in the horse. J. Helminthol. 47:111, 1973.

484. Mellor, P. S.: Studies on *Onchocerca cervicalis* Railliet and Henry, 1910. III. Morphologic and taxonomic studies on *Onchocerca cervicalis* from British horses. J. Helminthol. 48:145, 1974.

485. Metianu, T.: Considerations sur la Parafilariose haemorrhagique des bovins. *Parafilaria bovicola* en Roumanie. Ann. Parasitol. Hum. Comp. 24:54, 1949.

486. Meyrick, J. J.: Bursattee. Vet. J. 7:318, 1878.

487. Migiola, S.: Cryosurgical treatment of equine cutaneous habronemiasis. Vet. Med. Small Anim. Clin. 73:1073, 1978.

488. Miller, R. B., and Olson, L. D.: Epizootic of concurrent cutaneous streptococcal abscesses and swinepox in a herd of swine. JAVMA 172:676, 1978.

489. Miller, S. J., and Moule, G. R.: Clinical observations on the reproductive organs of Merino rams in pastoral Queensland. Aust. Vet. J. 30:353, 1954.

490. Mirck, M. H.: Een geval van uitebreide Chorioptes schurft bij een paard. Tijdschr. Diergeneeskd. 98:580, 1973.

491. Mitra, K., et al.: Stephanofilarial dermatitis at the base of the horn and at the poll region of cattle in the saluc belt of West Bengal (India) and its treatment. Indian J. Anim. Health 23:22, 1984.

492. Monlux, W. S., et al.: Foot rot and a mucosal-type disease caused by *Chorioptes bovis*. JAVMA 138:379, 1961.

493. Montali, R. J.: Ear mites in a horse. JAVMA 169:630, 1976.

494. Moore, B., et al.: Tests of insecticides for the control of goat lice in 1957 and 1958. J. Econ. Entomol. 52:980, 1959.

495. Muchlis, A., and Soetijono, P.: A short report on the use of Asuntal ointment in the treatment of Cascado and hoof myiasis. Vet. Med. Rev. 2:134, 1973.

496. Muller, G. H., et al.: *Small Animal Dermatology III*. Philadelphia, W. B. Saunders Co., 1983.

497. Mullowney, P. C.: Dermatologic diseases of cattle part I. Parasitic diseases. Compend. Cont. Educ. 3:S334, 1981.

498. Munro, R., and Munro, H. M.: Psoroptic mange in goats in Fiji. Trop. Anim. Health Prod. 12:1, 1980.

499. Murray, D. R., et al.: Granulomatous and neoplastic diseases of the skin of horses. Aust. Vet. J. 54:338, 1978.

500. Murray, M. D.: Infestation of sheep with the face louse. Aust. Vet. J. 31:22, 1955.

501. Murray, M. D.: Distribution of eggs of *Damalinia ovis* on sheep. Aust. J. Zool. 5:173, 1957.

502. Murray, M. D.: Influence of skin temperature on populations of *Linognathus pedalis*. Aust. J. Zool. 8:349, 1960.

503. Murray, M. D.: Influence of temperature and humidity on development of eggs of *Damalinia ovis*. Aust. J. Zool. 8:357, 1960.

504. Murray, M. D.: Biologies of *L. pedalis* and *L. ovillus*. Aust. J. Zool. 11:153, 1963.

505. Murray, M. D.: Populations of *L. ovillus*. Aust. J. Zool. 11:157, 1963.

506. Murray, M. D.: Influence of shearing and solar energy on populations of *D. ovis*. Aust. J. Zool. 16:725, 1968.

507. Murray, M. D., and Gordon, G.: Population dynamics of *D. ovis*. Aust. J. Zool. 17:179, 1969.

508. Murray, M. D.: A preliminary note on the efficacy of some of the new insecticides against *Psorergates ovis* the itch mite of sheep. Aust. Vet. J. 33:122, 1957.

509. Murray, M. D.: Demodectic mange in sheep. Aust. Vet. J. 35:93, 1959.

510. Murray, M. D.: The life cycle of *Psorergates ovis* Womersley, the itch mite of sheep. Aust. J. Agric. Res. 12:965, 1961.

511. Murray, M. D., et al.: Demodectic mange of cattle. Aust. Vet. J. 52:49, 1976.

512. Mustafeyev, A. S.: Infestation of sheep warble flies. Veterinariya (Moscow) 38:68, 1961.

513. Mustaffa-Babjee, A.: Lice and fleas of animals in Malaysia. Kajian Vet. 2:37, 1969.

514. Musatov, V. A.: The reaction of animal skin to the repeated attachment and feeding of ixodid ticks. Parazitologiya 4:66, 1970.

515. Mwaiko, G. L.: The development of *Onchocerca gutturosa* Neumann to infective stage in *Simulium vorax* Pomeroy. Tropenmed. Parasitol. 32:276, 1981.

516. Mwaiko, G. L.: *Onchocerca gutturosa* in Tanzanian cattle. Tanz. Vet. Bull. 1:8, 1979.

517. Naik, R. N.: Existence of otoacariasis (ear mange) in goats in India. Vet. J. 45:43, 1939.

518. Neitz, W. O.: Sweating sickness: The present state of our knowledge. Onderstepoort J. Vet. Res. 28:3, 1959.

519. Nelson, D. L.: Lice (pediculosis). *In*: Howard, J. L.: *Current Veterinary Therapy. Food Animal Practice*. Philadelphia, W. B. Saunders Co., 1981, p. 1141.

520. Nelson, D. L.: Mites (mange). *In*: Howard, J. L.: *Current Veterinary Therapy. Food Animal Practice*. Philadelphia, W. B. Saunders Co., 1981, p. 1143.

521. Nelson, D. L.: Cattle grubs (Hypoderma myiasis). *In*: Howard, J. L.: *Current Veterinary Therapy. Food Animal Practice*. Philadelphia, W. B. Saunders Co., 1981, p. 1145.

522. Nelson, G. S.: Onchocerciasis. Adv. Parasitol. 8:173, 1970.

523. Nelson, W. A., and Qually, M. C.: Annual cycles in numbers of sheep ked. Can. J. Anim. Sci. 38:194, 1958.

524. Nelson, W. A., and Slen, S. B.: Weight gains and wool growth in sheep infested with *Melophagus ovinus*. Exper. Parasitol. 22:223, 1968.

525. Nelson, W. A., and Weintraub, J.: *Hypoderma lineatum* (DeVill). (Diptera:Oestridae): Invasion of the bovine skin by newly hatched larvae. J. Parasitol. 58:614, 1972.

526. Nelson, W. A., and Kozub, G. C.: *Melophagus ovinus* (Diptera:Hippoboscidae): Evidence of local medication in acquired resistance of sheep to keds. J. Med. Entomol. 17:291, 1980.

527. Nemeseri, L., and Szeky, A.: Demodicosis in cattle. Acta Vet. Hung. Acad. Sci. 11:209, 1961.

528. Nemeseri, L., and Szeky, A.: Die Rinderdemodikose. Berl. Munch. Tierarztl. Wochenschr. 75:304, 1962.

529. Nemeseri, L., and Szeky, A.: Demodicosis of swine. Acta Vet. Hung. Acad. Sci. 16:251, 1966.

530. Nemeseri, L., and Szeky, A.: Demodicosis in sheep. Acta Vet. Hung. Acad. Sci. 16:53, 1966.
531. Nemeseri, L.: Untersuchungen uber die Haufigkeit von mikrofilarien pferdeaugen and ihre pathologische bedeutung. Acta Vet. Hung. Acad. Sci. 6:109, 1956.
532. Neville, E. M.: Preliminary report on the transmission of *Parafilaria bovicola* in South Africa. Onderstepoort J. Vet. Res. 42:41, 1975.
533. Nevill, E. M.: Experimental transmission of *Parafilaria bovicola* to cattle using *Musca* species as intermediate hosts. Onderstepoort J. Vet. Res. 46:51, 1979.
534. Nevill, E. M., and Viljoen, J. H.: The longevity of adult *Parafilaria bovicola* and the persistence of their associated carcass lesions in cattle in South Africa. Onderstepoort J. Vet. Res. 51:115, 1984.
535. Neville, E. M.: Seasonal abundance and distribution of *Parafilaria bovicola* ovipositional blood spots on cattle in South Africa. Onderstepoort J. Vet. Res. 51:107, 1984.
536. Nickel, E. A.: Experimentelle Untersuchungenuber Verlauf und Auswirkungen Grabmilbenraude der Schweine. Arch. Exp. Vet. Med. 37:617, 1983.
537. Niilo, L.: Bovine hemorrhagic filariasis in cattle imported into Canada. Can. Vet. J. 9:132, 1968.
538. Nilsson, N. G.: *Parafilaria bovicola*—rapport fran en arbetsgrupp. Svensk. Vet. 30:785, 1978.
539. Nishiyama, S.: Studies on habronemiasis in horses. Bull. Fac. Agric. Kagoshima Univ. 7, 1958.
540. Nolan, J., et al.: The potential of some synthetic pyrethroids for control of the cattle tick (*Boophilus microplus*). Aust. Vet. J. 55:463, 1979.
541. Nolan, J., et al.: Evaluation of the potential of systemic slow-release chemical treatments for control of the cattle tick (*Boophilus microplus*) using ivermectin. Aust. Vet. J. 57:493, 1981.
542. Nolan, J., et al.: The use of ivermectin to cleanse tick-infested cattle. Aust. Vet. J. 62:386, 1985.
543. Nolan, J., et al.: Resistance to synthetic pyrethroids in a DDT-resistant strain of *Boophilus microplus*. Pestic. Sci. 8:484, 1977.
544. Nooruddin, M., and Hoque, H. F.: Stephanofilariasis in cattle. Agri-Pract. 6:36, 1985.
545. Norris, K. R., and Murray, W. D.: The screw-worm problem. Aust. Vet. J. 40:148, 1964.
546. Norvall, J., and McPherson, E. A.: Dermatitis in the horse caused by *Acarus farinae*. Vet. Rec. 112:385, 1983.
547. Nusbaum, S. R., et al.: *Sarcoptes scabiei bovis*—a potential danger. JAVMA 166:252, 1975.
548. Nutting, W. B., et al.: Hair follicle mites (*Demodex* spp.) in New Zealand. N.Z. J. Zool. 2:219, 1975.
549. Nutting, W. B., et al.: Hair follicle mites (*Demodex* spp.) of medical and veterinary concern. Cornell Vet. 66:214, 1976.
550. Obasaju, M. F., and Otesile, E. B.: *Ctenocephalides canis* infestation of sheep and goats. Trop. Anim. Health Prod. 12:116, 1980.
551. O'Donnell, I. J., et al.: Immunoglobulin G antibodies to the antigens of *Lucilia cuprina* in the sera of fly struck sheep. Aust. J. Biol. Sci. 33:27, 1980.
552. O'Donnell, I. J., et al.: Immunization of sheep with larval antigens of *Lucilia cuprina*. Aust. J. Biol. Sci. 34:411, 1981.
553. Oberman, P. T., and Malan, F. S.: A new cause of cattle mange in South Africa: *Psorergates bos* Johnston. J. S. Afr. Vet. Assoc. 55:121, 1984.
554. Oduye, O. O.: Stephanofilarial dermatitis of cattle in Nigeria. J. Comp. Pathol. 81:581, 1971.
555. Oduye, O. O.: The pathology of bovine demodicosis in Nigeria. Bull. Anim. Health Prod. Afr. 23:45, 1975.
556. O'Kelly, J. C., and Spiers, W. G.: Resistance to *Boophilus microplus* (Canestrini) in genetically different types of calves in early life. J. Parasitol. 62:312, 1976.
557. Olander, H. J.: The migration of *Hypoderma lineatum* in the brain of a horse. Pathol. Vet. 4:477, 1967.
558. Oliveira, G. P.: *Raillietia auris* (Leidy, 1872) Trouessart, 1902 (Acari:Mesostigmata) em bovinos no estado de S. Paulo. Arq. Esc. Vet. 30:307, 1978.
559. Omar, M. S., et al.: The development of *Onchocerca ochengi* to the infective stage in *Simulium damnosum* with a note on the histochemical staining of the parasite. Tropenmed. Parasitol. 30:157, 1979.
560. Oormazdi, H., and Baker, K. P.: The effects of warble fly dressing using an organophosphate compound on bovine pediculosis. Vet. Parasitol. 3:85, 1977.
561. Oormazdi, H., and Baker, K. P.: Studies on the effects of lice on cattle. Br. Vet. J. 136:146, 1980.
562. Orkin, M., et al.: *Scabies and Pediculosis*. Philadelphia, J. B. Lippincott Co., 1977.
563. Ormerod, V. J., et al.: Propetamphos pour-on formulation for the control of lice on sheep: Effect of lice on weight gain and wool production. Res. Vet. Sci. 40:41, 1986.
564. Ostlind, D. A., et al.: Insecticidal activity of the antiparasitic avermectins. Vet. Rec. 105:168, 1979.
565. Ottley, M. L., and Moorehouse, D. E.: Laboratory transmission of *Onchocerca gibsoni* by *Forcipomyia* (*Lasiohela*) *townsvillensis*. Aust. Vet. J. 56:559, 1980.
566. Ottley, M. L., and Moorehouse, D. E.: Equine onchocerciasis. Aust. Vet. J. 54:545, 1978.
567. Ottley, M. L., and Moorehouse, D. E.: Bovine onchocerciasis: Aspects of carcase infection. Aust. Vet. J. 54:528, 1978.
568. Ottley, M. L., et al.: Equine onchocerciasis in Queensland and the Northern Territory of Australia. Aust. Vet. J. 60:200, 1983.
569. Ottley, M. L., and Moorehouse, D. E.: Morphological variations in *Onchocerca* sp. from atypical hosts and sites: The validity of *O. stilesi*. Ann. Parasitol. Hum. Comp. 57:389, 1982.
570. Pader, J.: Filariose du ligament suspenseur du boulet chez le cheval. Arch. Parasitol. 4:58, 1901.
571. Page, E. H.: Common skin diseases of the horse. Proc. Am. Assoc. Equine Pract. 18:385, 1972.
572. Pal, A. K., and Sinha, P. K.: *Stephanofilaria assamensis* as the cause of chronic ulcerated growth at the base of the dewclaw of cattle in West Bengal. Indian Vet. J. 48:190, 1971.
573. Pande, P. G.: On the identity of the nematode worm recovered from humpsore of cattle in India. Indian J. Vet. Sci. Anim. Husb. 6:346, 1936.
574. Pande, P. G.: The aetiology of humpsore in cattle: A preliminary report. Indian J. Vet. Sci. 5:332, 1936.
575. Panel Report: Skin conditions in horses. Mod. Vet. Pract. 56:363, 1975.
576. Panel Report: Dermatologic problems in horses. Mod. Vet. Pract. 62:75, 1981.
577. Panel Report: Dermatologic problems in cattle. Mod. Vet. Pract. 60:172, 1979.
578. Panel Report: Skin diseases in sheep. Mod. Vet. Pract. 64:340, 1983.
579. Panja, D.: Scabies in goats and rabbits communicable to man. Indian Med. Gazette 87:449, 1952.
580. Pannu, H. S.: Humpsore in Kutch. Indian Vet. J. 35:172, 1958.
581. Parent, J., and Belot, J.: Efficacité de l'ivermectine dans le traitement de la gale sarcoptique du porc au Senegal. Rev. Med. Vet. 136:469, 1985.
582. Pascoe, R. R.: Mites in "head shaker" horses. Vet. Rec. 107:234, 1980.
583. Pascoe, R. R.: The nature and treatment of skin conditions observed in horses in Queensland. Aust. Vet. J. 49:35, 1973.
584. Pascoe, R. R.: *Equine Dermatoses*. University of Sydney Post-Graduate Foundation in Veterinary Science, Veterinary Review No. 22, 1981.
585. Pasko, G. G., and Chotchaev, H. D.: Clinical and morphological features of sarcoptic mange in goats. Veterinariya (Moscow) 82:58, 1974.
586. Patid-Kukarni, V. G., et al.: Successful treatment of psoroptic mange in a horse with malathion emulsion. Indian Vet. J. 44:65, 1967.
587. Patnaik, B.: Studies on stephanofilariasis in Orissa. III. Life cycle of *S. assamensis* Pande, 1936. Z. Tropenmed. Parasitol. 24:457, 1973.
588. Patnaik, B., and Roy, S. P.: Studies on stephanofilariasis in Orissa. II. Dermatitis due to *S. assamensis* Pande, 1936, in the murrah buffalo and betal buck with remarks on the

morphology of the parasite. Indian J. Vet. Sci. Anim. Husb. 38:455, 1968.

589. Patnaik, B.: Studies on stephanofilariasis in Orissa. V. Treatment and control of "humpsore" in cattle due to *S. assamensis*. Indian J. Anim. Sci. 40:167, 1970.

590. Patnaik, B., and Roy, S. P.: On the life-cycle of the filarid *Stephanofilaria assamensis* Pande, 1936, in the arthropod vector Musca conducens Walker, 1859. Indian J. Anim. Health 5:91, 1966.

591. Patnayak, P. C., and Misra, S. C.: Studies on the epidemiology, biology, and control of bovine cutaneous myiasis. Orissa Vet. J. 11:52, 1977.

592. Pegram, R. G., and Lemche, J.: Observations on the efficacy of ivermectin in the control of cattle ticks in Zambia. Vet. Rec. 117:551, 1985.

593. Pecheur, M.: Protection du betail contre les mouches: Utilisation de boucles auriculaires impregnées de cypermethrine. Ann. Med. Vet. 129:215, 1985.

594. Perard, C., and Descazeaux, J.: Sur le parasite de la peribronchite nodulaire du cheval. Compt. Rend. Soc. Biol. 85:411, 1921.

595. Peterson, H. O., et al.: Anemia in cattle caused by heavy infestations of the blood-sucking louse, *Haematopinus eurysternus*. JAVMA 122:373, 1953.

596. Petrov, D., et al.: Epizootiology and economic importance of swine acariasis. Vet. Med. Nauki 14:61, 1977.

597. Pfister, K.: Epizootologische Betrachtungen zum Vorkommen von *Psoroptes-Raude* und andern Ektoparasiten beim Schaf im Kanton Bern. Schweiz. Arch. Tierheilkd. 120:561, 1978.

598. Pienaar, J. G., and van den Heever, L. W.: *Parafilaria bovicola* (Tubangui, 1934) in cattle in the Republic of South Africa. J. S. Afr. Vet. Med. Assoc. 35:181, 1964.

599. Pillars, A. W.: An exhibition of worms parasitic on equines, and remarks thereon. Vet. Rec. 27:234, 1914.

600. Pillars, A. W.: The parasitic origin of poll evil and fistulous withers. Vet. Rec. 44:1246, 1931.

601. Poliakov, D. K.: Demodicosis of horned cattle. Veterinariya (Moscow) 33:74, 1956.

602. Polley, L.: *Onchocerca* in horses from Western Canada and the Northwestern United States: An abattoir survey of the prevalence of infection. Can. Vet. J. 25:128, 1984.

602a. Pollitt, C. C., et al.: Treatment of equine onchocerciasis with ivermectin paste. Aust. Vet. J. 63:152, 1986.

603. Potemkin, V. I., and Vedernikov, N. T.: On the hypodermatosis of horses. Veterinariya (Moscow) 21:23, 1944.

604. Pouplard, L., and Detry, M.: Un progrès spectaculaire dans la lutte contre la gale bovine: Utilisation d'un nouvel agent antiparasitaire systemique: l'ivermectine. Ann. Med. Vet. 125:643, 1981.

605. Pruett, J. H., and Barrett, C. C.: Induction of intradermal skin reactions in the bovine by fractionated proteins of *Hypoderma lineatum*. Vet. Parasitol. 16:137, 1984.

606. Puccini, V., and Colella, G.: First report of *Demodex phylloides* infection of a pig in southeastern Italy. Acta Med. Vet. 21:65, 1975.

607. Purnell, R. E.: Tick-borne diseases. Br. Vet. J. 137:221, 1981.

608. Quintero, M. T.: Frecuencia de acaross *Demodex* en parpados de diferentes especies de animales domesticos. Vet. Max. 9:111, 1978.

609. Quintero, M. T. C., et al.: Hallazgo y description de *Raillietia caprae* sp. nov. (Acari:Mesostigmata:Raillietidae) en caprinos de Sinaloa, Mexico. Veterinaria (Mex. City) 11:17, 1980.

610. Quintero, T. C.: Frecuencia de *Demodex phylloides* en diversas regiones anatomicas de cerdos en el Estado de Mexico. Veterinaria (Mex. City) 7:42, 1977.

611. Rabalais, F. C., et al.: Survey for equine onchocerciasis in the midwestern United States. Am. J. Vet. Res. 35:125, 1974.

612. Rabalais, F. C., and Votava, C. L.: Cutaneous distribution of microfilariae of *Onchocerca cervicalis* in horses. Am. J. Vet. Res. 35:1369, 1974.

613. Radeleff, R. D., et al.: Benzene hexachloride poisoning of emaciated sheep. Vet. Med. 48:53, 1953.

614. Raebiger, H., and Ehrlich, K.: Zur Behandlung der Raude

bei Pferden und Rindern mittels Schwefeldioxyd. Dtsch. Tierarztl. Wochenschr. 28:1, 1920.

615. Rahman, A., and Khaleque, A.: Treatment of "humpsore" with Neguvon in local cattle of Bangladesh. Vet. Med. Rev. 4:379, 1974.

616. Railliet, M.: Contribution a l'étude de l'"esponja" ou plaies d'été des equides du Bresil. Rec. Med. Vet. 91:468, 1915.

617. Railliet, M., and Moussu, J.: La filaire des boutons hemorragiques observée chez l'ane; decouverte du male. Compt. Rend. Seanc. Soc. Biol. 44:545, 1892.

618. Ramachandran, C. L., and Tan, B. E.: Microfilaria of the genus *Onchocerca* from the skin snips of a domestic pig in Malaya. Malays. Vet. J. 4:159, 1967.

619. Ransom, B. H.: The occurrence of onchocerciasis in cattle in the United States. J. Parasitol. 7:98, 1920.

620. Rapeanu, M. D.: Afectarea impermeabilitatii cutunate prin modificari anatomo—histopathologice in psoropticoza ovina. Rev. Zootech. Med. Vet. 22:72, 1972.

621. Rawlins, S. C., and Mansingh, A.: Patterns of resistance to various acaricides in some Jamaican populations of *Boophilus microplus*. J. Econ. Entomol. 71:956, 1978.

622. Rebhun, W. C., et al.: Habronemic blepharoconjunctivitis in horses. JAVMA 179:469, 1981.

623. Reddy, A. B., et al.: Pathological changes due to *Habronema muscae* and *Draschia megastoma* infection in equine. Indian J. Anim. Sci. 46:207, 1976.

624. Reid, C. H.: Habronemiasis and *Corynebacterium* "chest" abscess in California horses. Vet. Med. Small Anim. Clin. 60:233, 1965.

625. Rhode, E. A., et al.: The occurrence of rhabiditis dermatitis in cattle. North Am. Vet. 34:634, 1953.

626. Rhodes, A. P.: Seminal degeneration associated with chorioptic mange of the scrotum of rams. Aust. Vet. J. 51:428, 1975.

627. Rhodes, A. P.: The effect of extensive chorioptic mange of the scrotum on reproductive function of the ram. Aust. Vet. J. 52:250, 1976.

628. Rich, G. B.: Post-treatment reactions in cattle during extensive field tests of systemic organophosphate insecticides. Can. J. Comp. Med. Vet. Sci. 29:30, 1965.

629. Rich, G. B., and Ireland, H. R.: An appraisal of Ruelene and Trolene against cattle grub infestations (Oestrida:Diptera). Can. J. Anim. Sci. 41:115, 1961.

630. Rich, G. B.: The economics of systemic insecticide treatment for reduction of slaughter trim loss caused by cattle grubs. Can. J. Anim. Sci. 50:301, 1970.

631. Richter, D.: Die Behundlung der Pferderaude mit Schwefligsaureanhydrid. Berl. Tierarztl. Wochenschr. 35:1, 1919.

632. Ridgway, J. R.: An unusual skin condition in Thoroughbred horses. Vet. Rec. 92:382, 1973.

633. Riek, R. F.: Allergic reaction in the horse to infestation with larvae of *Boophilus microplus*. Aust. Vet. J. 30:142, 1954.

634. Riek, R. F.: Studies on allergic dermatitis (Queensland itch) of the horse. The etiology of the disease. Aust. J. Agric. Res. 5:109, 1954.

635. Riek, R. F.: A note on the occurrence of *Onchocerca reticulata* (Diesing 1841) in the horse in Queensland. Aust. Vet. J. 30:178, 1954.

636. Riek, R. F.: Factors influencing the susceptibility of cattle to tick infestation. Aust. Vet. J. 32:204, 1956.

637. Riek, R. F.: Studies on the reactions of animals to infestation with ticks. VI. Resistance of cattle to infestation with the tick *Boophilus microplus* (Canestrini). Aust. J. Agric. Res. 13:532, 1962.

638. Roberts, F. H. S.: Onchocerciasis. Aust. Vet. J. 14:32, 1938.

639. Roberts, R. H. S.: *Insects Affecting Livestock*. Sydney, Angus and Robertson, 1952.

640. Roberts, I. H., et al.: Observations on the incidence of chorioptic acariasis of sheep in the United States. Am. J. Vet. Res. 25:478, 1964.

641. Roberts, I. H., and Meleney, W. P.: Psorergatic acariasis in cattle. JAVMA 146:17, 1965.

642. Roberts, I. H., et al.: Psorergatic acariasis on a New Mexico range ewe. JAVMA 146:24, 1965.

643. Roberts, I. H., et al.: Over summering locations of *Psoroptes ovis* on sheep. Ann. Entomol. Soc. Am. 64:105, 1971.

644. Roberts, I. H., and Meleney, W. P.: Variations among strains

of *Psoroptes ovis* (Acarina:Psoroptidae) on sheep and cattle. Ann. Entomol. Soc. Am. 64:109, 1971.

645. Roberts, I. H., et al.: Oral famphur for treatment of cattle lice, and against scabies mites and ear ticks of cattle and sheep. JAVMA 155:504, 1969.

646. Roberts, I. H., and Meleney, W. P.: Acaricidal treatments for protection of sheep against *Psoroptes ovis*. JAVMA 158:372, 1971.

647. Roberts, I. H., et al.: Evaluation of phosmet for the control of the common scabies mite on cattle. JAVMA 173:840, 1978.

648. Roberts, J. A.: Resistance of cattle to the tick *Boophilus microplus* (Canestrini). II. Stages of the life cycle of the parasite against which resistance is manifested. J. Parasitol. 54:667, 1968.

649. Roberts, J. A.: Acquisition of resistance by the host to the cattle tick, *Boophilus microplus* (Canestrini). J. Parasitol. 54:657, 1968.

650. Roberts, J. A.: Behaviour of larvae of the cattle tick, *Boophilus microplus* (Canestrini), on cattle of differing degrees of resistance. J. Parasitol. 57:651, 1971.

651. Roberts, J. A., and Kerr, J. D.: *Boophilus microplus*: Passive transfer of resistance in cattle. J. Parasitol. 62:485, 1976.

652. Roberts, M. C., and Seawright, A. A.: Amitraz-induced large intestinal impaction in the horse. Aust. Vet. J. 55:553, 1979.

652a. Roberts, M. C., and Argenzio, A.: Effects of amitraz, several opiate derivatives and anticholinergic agents on intestinal transit in ponies. Equine Vet. J. 18:256, 1986.

653. Roberts, S. R.: Etiology of equine periodic ophthalmia. Am. J. Ophthalmol. 55:1049, 1963.

654. Robson, J.: Filariasis of the withers in the horse. Vet. Rec. 31:348, 1918.

655. Rogoaff, W. M., and Kohler, P. H.: Effectiveness of Ruelene applied as localized pour-on and as spray for cattle grubs control. J. Econ. Entomol. 53:814, 1960.

656. Rohrer, H.: Demodikose bei Ziegen. Tierarztl. Rundsch. 41:291, 1935.

657. Ronald, N. C.: Muscoid flies of range cattle. *In*: Howard, J. L.: *Current Veterinary Therapy. Food Animal Practice.* Philadelphia, W. B. Saunders Co, 1981, p. 1153.

658. Rook, A., et al.: *Textbook of Dermatology III*. Oxford, Blackwell Scientific Publications, 1979.

659. Rosa, W. A. J., et al.: Informe sobre experiencias para investigar la presunta resistencia del *Psoroptes ovis* al hexachlorociclohexano. Gaceta Vet. 31:373, 1969.

660. Rosa, W. A. J., and Leukovich, R.: Experiencia con cepas de *Psoroptes* de tres arroyos. Banos con 87, 150 y 500 partes por million de isomero gamma y con 0.1% de diazinon. Rev. Med. Vet. 51:127, 1970.

661. Rosenberger, G.: Ein neuer Weg der Dasselbekumpfung erfolgreiche Behandlung der Rinder gegen die Wanderlarven. Dtsch. Tierarztl. Wochenschr. 64:441, 1957.

662. Roubaud, E., and Descazeaux, J.: Contribution a l'histoire de la mouche domestique comme agent vecteur des habronemoses des Equidés. Bull. Soc. Pathol. Exot. 14:471, 1921.

663. Roubaud, E., and Descazeaux, J.: Evolution de l'*Habronema muscae* Carter chez la mouche domestique et de l'*Habronema microstoma* Schneider chez le Stomoxe. Bull. Soc. Pathol. Exot. 15:572, 1921.

664. Roychaudhury, G. K., and Chakrabarty, A. K.: Otitis externa in bullocks due to stephanofilarial infection. Indian Vet. J. 46:79, 1969.

665. Runge, C.: Demodikose beim Schaf. Dtsch. Tierarztl. Wochenschr. 83:497, 1976.

666. Ruther, D.: Zur behandlung schwer heilbarer Raudeformen. Berl. Tierarztl. Wochenschr. 27:44, 1911.

667. Sabiiti, C. K., et al.: Sarcoptic mange in swine in Northwestern United States. JAVMA 175:818, 1979.

668. Sahai, B. N., et al.: Pathology of sarcoptic mange in goats. Indian J. Anim. Health 23:19, 1984.

669. Sahai, B. N., et al.: Chemotherapy of parafilariasis in bovines. Indian Vet. J. 42:881, 1965.

670. Salas-Auvert, R., et al.: Treatment of cutaneous equine habronemiasis with a beta-glycoside, aucubigenin. Equine Pract. 7:22, 1985.

671. Sandeman, R. M., et al.: Initial characterization of the sheep immune response to infections of *Lucilia cuprina*. Intl. J. Parasitol. 15:181, 1985.

672. Sayin, F., et al.: The use of Neguvon for control of grubs in Angora goats. Vet. Fak. Derg. Ank. Univ. 19:338, 1972.

673. Sayin, F., et al.: Ankara kecisi hypodermosisi uzeinide arastirmalar. I. *P. silenus* (Brauer) in biydojisi. Vet. Fak. Derg. Ank. Univ. 20:190, 1973.

674. Sayin, F., et al.: Ankara kecisi hypodermosis uzerinde arastirmalar. II. *P. silenus* (Brauer), *P. aegagri* (Brauer), ve *P. crossi* (Patton) arasindaki iliskiler. Vet. Fak. Derg. Ank. Univ. 20:262, 1973.

675. Sayin, F., et al.: Ankara kecisi hypodermosis uzerinde arastirmalar. III. *P. silenus* (Brauer) in yayilis durumu. Vet. Fak. Derg. Ank. Univ. 20:321, 1973.

676. Sayin, F., and Meric, I.: Dokme metodla uygulanan Hipolen-6 ve Tiguvon un sigir Hypodermosisine karsi etkisi uzerinde arastirmalar. Vet. Fak. Derg. Ank. Univ. 23:301, 1976.

677. Sayin, F., and Koseoglue, H.: Nitrozynil ve Ruelene 6-R, nin Ankara kecisinde hypodermosis uzerine etkileriyle ilgili arastirmalar. Vet. Fak. Derg. Ank. Univ. 24:171, 1977.

678. Sayin, F., et al.: Field trials with Tikas against cattle, sheep, goat, and dog ectoparasites of major importance in Turkey. Vet. Fak. Derg. Ank. Univ. 29:151, 1982.

679. Scharff, D. K., and Ludvig, P. D.: Cattle grub control with Ruelene as a dip and pour-on treatment. J. Econ. Entomol. 55:191, 1962.

680. Scharf, D. K.: An investigation of the cattle louse problem. J. Econ. Entomol. 55:684, 1962.

681. Scharff, D. K., et al.: Illness and death in calves induced by treatments with systemic insecticides for the control of cattle grubs. JAVMA 141:582, 1962.

682. Scharff, D. K.: Control of cattle grubs in horses. Vet. Med. Small Anim. Pract. 68:791, 1973.

683. Schillhorn Van Veen, T. W., and Mohammed, A. N.: Louse and flea infestation on small ruminants in the Zaire area. J. Nigerian Vet. Med. Assoc. 4:93, 1976.

684. Schimmelpfennig, K.: Neue Wege in der Praxis der Dasselbekampfung. Dtsch. Tierarztl. Wochenschr. 67:319, 1960.

685. Schleger, A. V., et al.: *Boophilus microplus*: Cellular responses to larval attachment and their relationship to host resistance. Aust. J. Biol. Sci. 29:499, 1976.

686. Schmidt, C. D., et al.: Evaluation of a synthetic pyrethroid for control of stable flies and horn flies on cattle. J. Econ. Entomol. 69:484, 1976.

687. Schmidt, G. M., et al.: Equine ocular onchocerciasis: Histopathologic study. Am. J. Vet. Res. 43:1371, 1982.

688. Schmidt, G. M., et al.: Equine onchocerciasis: Lesions in the nuchal ligament of midwestern U.S. horses. Vet. Pathol. 19:16, 1982.

689. Scholtens, R. G., et al.: Evidence of onchocerciasis in Georgia cattle: Prevalence at slaughter. Am. J. Vet. Res. 38:1093, 1977.

690. Schroder, J., et al.: Efficacy of invermectin against ectoparasites of cattle in South Africa. J. S. Afr. Vet. Assoc. 56:31, 1985.

691. Schultz, R. A., and Hoffmann, J.: Efficacy of a tylosin-ivermectin combination against *Streptococcus suis* infection with secondary mange. Agri-Pract. 7:44, 1986.

692. Schulze, W., and Reichel, K.: Demodikose in einer Karakal-Schafherde. Dtsch. Tierarztl. Wochenschr. 64:349, 1957.

693. Scott, D. W., and White, K. K.: Demodicosis associated with systemic glucocorticoid therapy in two horses. Equine Pract. 5:31, 1983.

693a. Scott, D. W.: Demodicosis. *In*: Robinson, N. E.: *Current Therapy in Equine Medicine II*. Philadelphia, W. B. Saunders Co., 1987, p. 626.

694. Scott, M. T.: Bionomics of *L. pedalis*. Aust. J. Agric. Res. 1:465, 1950.

695. SenGupta, C. M., et al.: Studies on myiasis and treatment. Indian Vet. J. 27:340, 1951.

696. Sekizawa, F., et al.: Therapeutic experience on porcine scabies. Jpn. J. Vet. Med. Assoc. 36:320, 1983.

697. Shanahan, G. J., and Hughes, P. B.: Larval implant studies with *Lucilia caprina*. Vet. Rec. 103:582, 1978.

698. Sharmadeorani, V. P.: Studies on the pathogenicity in ste-

phanofilarial humpsore among cattle in India. Indian J. Vet. Sci. 37:87, 1967.

699. Sharmadeorani, V. P., and Tewari, H. C.: Contribution to the parasitic part of the life-cycle of *Stephanofilaria assamensis* Pande, 1936. A skin parasite of the cattle in India. Arch. Vet. 5:11, 1968.

700. Shaw, J. G.: Ear mange in horses. N.Z. Vet. J. 14:127, 1966.

701. Sheahan, B. J.: Sarcoptic mange in Irish pigs: A survey. Irish Vet. J. 24:201, 1970.

702. Sheahan, B. J., et al.: Improved weight gains in pigs following treatment for sarcoptic mange. Vet. Rec. 95:169, 1974.

703. Sheahan, B. J.: Experimental *Sarcoptes scabiei* infection in pigs: Clinical signs and significance of infection. Vet. Rec. 94:202, 1974.

704. Sheahan, B. J.: Pathology of *Sarcoptes scabiei* infection in pigs. I. Naturally occurring and experimentally induced lesions. J. Comp. Pathol. 85:87, 1975.

705. Sheahan, B. J.: Pathology of *Sarcoptes scabiei* infection in pigs. II. Histological, histochemical, and ultrastructural changes at skin test sites. J. Comp. Pathol. 85:97, 1975.

706. Sheahan, B. J., and Hatch, C.: A method for isolating large numbers of *Sarcoptes scabiei* from lesions in the ears of pigs. J. Parasitol. 61:350, 1975.

707. Shergin, Y. K.: Warble-fly infestation of goats (migration of the larvae and pathomorphology). Veterinariya (Moscow) 45:70, 1968.

708. Shideler, R. K., and Hultine, J. D.: Eosinophilic granuloma removed from the equine prepuce. Vet. Med. Small Anim. Clin. 68:1330, 1973.

709. Simmons, S. W.: Some histopathological changes in the skin of cattle infested with larvae of *Hypoderma lineatum*. JAVMA 95:283, 1939.

710. Sinclair, A. N.: A field trial for the control of the itch mite (*Psorergates ovis*) of sheep. Aust. Vet. J. 34:405, 1958.

711. Sinclair, A. N.: Field trials with the jetting technique for applying insecticides to control itch mite (*Psorergates ovis*) of sheep. Aust. Vet. J. 37:211, 1961.

712. Sinclair, A. N., and Gibson, A. J. F.: Distribution of the itch mite (*Psorergates ovis*) on some Merino sheep. Aust. Vet. J. 46:311, 1970.

713. Sinclair, A. N.: The prevalence of fleece derangement in some Australian and New Zealand flocks infested with the sheep itch mite, *Psorergates ovis*. N.Z. Vet. J. 23:57, 1975.

714. Sinclair, A. N.: Fleece derangement of Merino sheep infested by the itch mite *Psorergates ovis*. N.Z. Vet. J. 24:149, 1976.

715. Sinclair, A. N., and Kirkwood, A. C.: Feeding behavior of *Psoroptes ovis*. Vet. Rec. 112:65, 1983.

716. Singh, B.: Sarcoptic mange in goats. Indian Vet. J. 27:128, 1950.

717 Singh, C. S. P., and Singh, D. K.: Studies on skin thickness of goats and its relation to body weight and resistance to mange. Indian Vet. J. 61:54, 1984.

718. Sinha, R. P., and Prasad, R. S.: Easy and simple technique of successful treatment and control of (sarcoptic) mange in goats (Savlon lotion and malathion). Indian Vet. J. 57:865, 1980.

719. Sinha, S. R. P., et al.: Sarcoptic mange in goats and its treatment. Indian J. Anim. Health 21:75, 1982.

720. Skerman, K. D., et al.: *Psorergates ovis*—the itch mite of sheep. A report to the Australian Veterinary Association by a Technical Committee. Aust. Vet. J. 36:317, 1960.

721. Slingenbergh, J., et al.: Studies on bovine demodicosis in Northern Nigeria. Specification and host-parasite relationships. Vet. Q. 2:90, 1980.

722. Smith, F.: "Bursattee." Vet. J. 9:300, 1879.

723. Smith, F.: The pathology of Bursattee. Vet. J. 19:16, 1884.

724. Smith, H. J.: A preliminary trial on efficacy of ciodrin against *Chorioptes bovis*. Can. Vet. J. 8:88, 1967.

725. Smith, H. J.: Demodicosis in a flock of goats. Can. Vet. J. 2:231, 1961.

726. Smith, H. J.: Bovine demodicosis. I. Incidence in Ontario. Can. J. Comp. Med. Vet. Sci. 25:165, 1961.

727. Smith, H. J.: Bovine demodicosis. II. Clinical manifestations in Ontario. Can. J. Comp. Med. Vet. Sci. 25:201, 1961.

728. Smith, H. J.: Bovine demodicosis. III. Its effect on hides and leather. Can. J. Comp. Med. Vet. Sci. 25:243, 1961.

729. Smith, J. P.: Fly infestations. *In*: Howard, J. L.: *Current Veterinary Therapy. Food Animal Practice*. Philadelphia, W. B. Saunders Co., 1981, p. 1148.

730. Smith, M. C.: Caprine dermatologic problems: A review. JAVMA 178:724, 1981.

731. Smith, M. C.: Dermatologic diseases of goats. Vet. Clin. North Am. Large Anim. Pract. 5:449, 1983.

732. Somorin, A. O.: Onchocerciasis. Intl. J. Dermatol. 22:182, 1983.

733. Soni, B. N.: Preliminary observations on the bionomics of the goat warble-fly (*H. crossi*, Patton). Indian J. Vet. Sci. 10:280, 1940.

734. Soulsby, E. J. L.: *Helminths, Arthropods, and Protozoa of Domesticated Animals*. London, Baillière Tindall, 1982.

735. Spence, T.: The latent phase of sheep scab: Its nature and relation to the eradication of the disease. J. Comp. Pathol. 59:305, 1949.

736. Sreenivasan, M. K., and Rizvi, S. W. H.: Demodectic mange of goats in India. Indian J. Vet. Sci. 15:287, 1946.

737. Srivastava, H. D., and Dutt, S. C.: Studies on the life history of *Stephanofilaria assamensis*, the causative parasite of "humpsore" of Indian cattle. Indian J. Vet. Sci. 33:173, 1963.

738. Srivastava, H. D., et al.: The pre-infective larval stage of *S. assamensis*, the causative parasite of humpsore of Indian cattle. Indian J. Helminthol. 19:81, 1967.

739. Srivastava, V. K., et al.: Chemotherapy of *Parafilaria bovicola* infection in cattle. Orissa Vet J. 7:151, 1972.

740. Stampa, S.: The control of the ectoparasites of Angora goats with Neguvon. Vet. Med. Rev. 1:5, 1964.

741. Stannard, A. A.: The skin. *In*: Catcott, E. J., and Smithcors, J. S.: *Equine Medicine and Surgery II*. Santa Barbara, CA, American Veterinary Publications, Inc., 1972, p. 381.

742. Stannard, A. A.: Equine dermatoses. Proc. Am. Assoc. Equine Pract. 22:273, 1976.

743. Stannard, A. A., and Cello, R. M.: *Onchocerca cervicalis* infection in horses from the western United States. Am. J. Vet. Res. 36:1029, 1975.

744. Stannard, A. A., and Scott, D. W.: Personal observations.

745. Steckel, R. R., et al.: Equine pulmonary habronemiasis with acute hemolytic anemia resulting from organophosphate treatment. Equine Pract. 5:35, 1983.

746. Steelman, C. D., et al.: Effects of mosquitoes on the average daily gain of feedlot steers in south Louisiana. J. Econ. Entomol. 65:462, 1972.

747. Steelman, C. D., et al.: Effects of mosquitoes on the average daily gain of Hereford and Brahman breed steers in south Louisiana. J. Econ. Entomol. 66:1081, 1973.

748. Steelman, C. D.: Effects of external and internal arthropod parasites on domestic livestock production. Ann. Rev. Entomol. 21:155, 1976.

749. Steward, J. S.: The occurrence of *Onchocerca gutturosa* Neumann in cattle in England, with an account of its life history and development in *Simulium ornatum*. Parasitol. 29:212, 1937.

750. Steward, J. S.: The diagnosis of onchocerciasis. Vet. Rec. 58:261, 1946.

751. Steward, J. S.: Fistulous withers and poll evil. Vet. Rec. 47:1563, 1935.

752. Stewart, T. B., et al.: Efficacy of ivermectin against five genera of swine nematodes and the hog louse, *Haematopinus suis*. Am. J. Vet. Res. 42:1425, 1981.

753. Stick, J. A.: Amputation of the equine urethral process affected with habronemiasis. Vet. Med. Small Anim. Clin. 74:1453, 1979.

754. Stick, J. A.: Surgical management of genital habronemiasis in a horse. Vet. Med. Small Anim. Clin. 76:410, 1981.

755. Stork, M. G.: The epidemiological and economic importance of fly infestation of meat and milk producing animals in Europe. Vet. Rec. 105:341, 1979.

756. Stresow, P.: Raudebehandlung mit Peruol. Berl. Tierarztl. Wochenschr. 36:607, 1920.

757. Strickland, R. K., and Gerrish, R. R.: Efficacy of coumaphos against *Psoroptes ovis*. JAVMA 148:553, 1966.

758. Strickland, R. K., et al.: Chloropyridyl phosphorothioate insecticide as dip and spray. Am. J. Vet. Res. 31:2135, 1970.

759. Strickland, R. K., and Gerrish, R. R.: Distribution of the tropical horse tick in the United States, and notes on associated cases of equine piroplasmosis. JAVMA 144:875, 1964.

759a. Strickland, R. K., and Gerrish, R. R.: Infestivity of *Psoroptes ovis* on invermectin-treated cattle. Am. J. Vet. Res. 48:342, 1987.

760. Stromberg, P. C., and Fisher, W. F.: Dermatopathology and immunity in experimental *Psoroptes ovis* (Acari:Psoroptidae) infestation of naive and previously exposed Hereford cattle. Am. J. Vet. Res. 47:1551, 1986.

760a. Stromberg, P. C., et al.: Systemic pathologic responses in experimental *Psoroptes ovis* infestation of Hereford calves. Am. J. Vet. Res. 47:1326, 1986.

761. Strother, G. R., et al.: Resistance of purebred Brahman, Hereford and Brahman cross Hereford crossbred cattle to the lone star tick, *Amblyoma americanum*. J. Med. Entomol. 11:559, 1974.

762. Subramanian, H., and Mohanan, K. R.: Incidence and etiology of cutaneous myiasis in domestic animals in Trichur. Kerala J. Vet. Sci. 11:80, 1980.

763. Supperer, R.: Uber das Vorkommen der Filarie *Onchocera gutturosa* Neumann in Rindern in Osterreich und ihre Entwicklung in der Krielbelmucke Odagmia Ornata. Wien. Tierarztl. Monatsschr. 39:173, 1952.

764. Supperer, R.: Filariosen der Pferde in Osterreich. Wien. Tierarztl. Monatsschr. 40:193, 1953.

765. Sutherst, R. W., et al.: Resistance in cattle to *Haemaphysalis longicornis*. Intl. J. Parasitol. 9:183, 1979.

766. Sutmoller, P.: Demodectin mange of goats and pigs in the Netherlands Antilles. Tijdschr. Diergeneeskd. 82:42, 1957.

767. Swan, G. E., et al.: Efficacy of ivermectin against *Parafilaria bovicola*. Vet. Rec. 113:260, 1983.

768. Swarup, D., et al.: A report on clinical trial with malathion against sarcoptic mange in Pashmina bearing goats. Indian Vet. J. 60:399, 1983.

769. Sweatman, G. K.: Seasonal variation in sites of infestation of *Chorioptes bovis*, a parasitic mite of cattle, with observations on the association with dermatitis. Can. J. Comp. Med. 20:321, 1956.

770. Sweatman, G. K.: Life history, nonspecificity, and revision of the genus *Chorioptes*, a parasitic mite of herbivores. Can. J. Zool. 35:641, 1957.

771. Sweatman, G. K.: On the life history and validity of the species in *Psoroptes*, a genus of mange mites. Can. J. Zool. 36:905, 1958.

772. Sweatman, G. K.: On the population reduction of chorioptic mange mites on cattle in summer. Can. J. Zool. 36:391, 1958.

773. Sweetman, H. L., et al.: Mange and fly control with lindane in a piggery. J. Econ. Entomol. 44:112, 1951.

774. Tarry, D. W.: Sheep scab: Its diagnosis and biology. Vet. Rec. 95:530, 1974.

775. Tarry, D. W., and Boreham, P. F. L.: Studies on the feeding patterns of the sheep headfly *Hydrotaea irritans* in Great Britain. Vet. Rec. 101:456, 1977.

776. Tarshis, I. B., and Ommert, W. D.: Control of the spinose ear tick, *Otobius megnini* (Duges), with an organic phosphate insecticide combined with a silica aerogel. JAVMA 138:665, 1961.

777. Tashiro, T., et al.: An outbreak of bovine demodectic mange in Kagoshima Prefecture J. Jpn. Vet. Med. Assoc. 32:30, 1979.

778. Tatchell, R. J., and Moorhouse, D. E.: The feeding processes of the cattle tick, *Boophilus microplus* (Canestrini). Part II. The sequence of host-tissue changes. Parasitology 58:441, 1968.

779. Taylor, D. J.: *Pig Diseases*. Cambridge, Burlington Press, 1979.

780. Taylor, S. M., et al.: Efficacy of pyrethroid-impregnated ear tags for prophylaxis of tick-borne diseases of cattle. Vet. Rec. 114:454, 1984.

781. Taylor, S. M., et al.: Cypermethrin concentrations in hair of cattle after application of impregnated ear tags. Vet. Rec. 116:620, 1985.

782. Testi, F., and Bravi, M. V.: Otocariasi psoroptica dei caprini. Atti. Soc. Ital. Sci. Vet. 23:885, 1969.

783. Theiler, G.: Zoological survey of the Union of South Africa: Tick survey. Onderstepoort. J. Vet. Sci. 24:34, 1950.

784. Thomas, A. D.: Microfilariasis in the horse. J. S. Afr. Vet. Med. Assoc. 24:17, 1963.

785. Thomsett, L. R.: Differential diagnosis of skin diseases of the horse. Equine Vet. J. 2:46, 1970.

786. Thomsett, L. R.: Skin diseases of the horse. In Pract. 1:15, 1979.

787. Thomson, J. R., and MacKenzie, C. P.: Demodectic mange in goats. Vet. Rec. 111:185, 1982.

788. Thornberry, H.: Control of *Hypoderma* larvae: Field trials with 2% Neguvon solution as a back wash and Ruelene 25E, 1961–1962. Irish Vet. J. 17:162, 1963.

789. Thornberry, H.: Warble fly eradication in Ireland. Irish Vet. J. 30:83, 1976.

790. Thorold, P. W.: Observations on the control of Angora goat lice, *Linognathus africanus* and *Damalinia caprae*. J. S. Afr. Vet. Med. Assoc. 34:59, 1963.

791. Tikaram, S. M., et al.,: Demodectosis in cattle and its treatment. Indian Vet. J. 61:986, 1984.

792. Tobin, W. C.: Cattle scabies can be costly. JAVMA 141:845, 1962.

793. Tontis, A.: Zur kutanen Myiasis des Schafes. Schweiz. Arch. Tierheilkd. 122:49, 1980.

794. Topacio, T.: Fatal suppurating abscess of the stomach caused by stomach worm (*Habronema megastoma*). Philippine J. Anim. Indust. 1:403, 1934.

795. Torres, C. A.: *Habronemose pulmonaire* (*Habronema muscae* Carter) experimentalement produit chez le cobaye. Compt. Rend. Soc. Biol. 88:242, 1924.

796. Tracey-Patte, P. D.: Effect of the bovine immune system on esterase deposited by *Boophilus microplus* larvae. Aust. Adv. Vet. Sci. 1979:78, 1979.

797. Tritschler, L. G.: Allergy in a horse due to *Amblyomma americanum*. Vet. Med. 60:219, 1965.

798. Trofimov, P. V., and Ermochenkov, P. N.: *Hypoderma* in sheep. Veterinariya (Moscow) 32:43, 1955.

799. Tubangui, M. A.: Nematodes in the collection of the Philippine Bureau of Science. II. Filaroidea. Philippine J. Sci. 55:115, 1934.

800. Turner, J. H.: Experimental strongyloidiasis in sheep and goats. II. Multiple infections: Development of acquired resistance. J. Parasitol. 45:76, 1959.

801. Turner, J. H., et al.: Experimental strongyloidiasis on sheep and goats. IV. Migration of *Strongyloides papillosus* in lambs and accompanying pathologic changes following percutaneous penetration. Am. J. Vet. Res. 20:536, 1960.

802. Ueno, H., and Chibana, T.: *Stephanofilaria okinawaensis* n. sp. from cutaneous lesions on the teats of cows in Japan. Natl. Inst. Anim. Health Q. 17:16, 1977.

803. Ueno, H., et al.: Occurrence of chronic dermatitis caused by *Stephanofilaria okinawaensis* on the teats of cows in Japan. Vet. Parasitol. 3:41, 1977.

804. Ueno, H., and Chigana, T.: Stephanofilariasis of cattle caused by *S. okinawaensis* in Japan. Trop. Agric. Res. Cent. Q. 12:152, 1978.

805. Ueno, H., and Chibana, T.: Clinical and parasitological evaluations of levamisole as a treatment for bovine stephanofilariasis. Vet. Parasitol. 7:59, 1980.

806. Uilenberg, G.: Notes sur les hematozoaires et tiques des animaux domestiques à Madagascar. Rev. Elev. Med. Vet. Pays Trop. 17:337, 1964.

807. Underwood, J. R.: Equine Dhobie itch a symptom of filariasis. A report of 56 cases. Vet. Bull. 28:227, 1934.

808. Utech, K. B. W., et al.: Biting cattle-louse infestations related to cattle nutrition. Aust. Vet. J. 45:414, 1969.

808a. Utech, K. B. W., et al.: Breeding Australian Illawarra Shorthorn cattle for resistance to *Boophilus microplus*. I. Factors affecting resistance. Aust. J. Agric. Res. 29:885, 1978.

809. Van den Heever, L. W., and Nevill, E. M.: Bovine parafilariasis. J. S. Afr. Vet. Med. Assoc. 44:333, 1973.

810. Vander Merwe, C. F.: Ear scab in sheep and goats. J. S. Afr. Vet. Med. Assoc. 20:93, 1949.

811. Van Emden, J. I.: The identity of the species of *Hypoderma* attacking goat. Bull. Entomol. Res. 41:223, 1950.

812. Van Heerden, A.: Sheep scab control and problems in South Africa. J. S. Afr. Vet. Assoc. 48:25, 1977.

813. Van Saceghem, R.: Cause étiologique et traitement de la dermite granuleuse. Bull. Soc. Pathol. Exot. 12:575, 1918.

814. Vasey, J. R.: Equine cutaneous habronemiasis. Compend. Cont. Educ. 3:S290, 1981.

815. Venkatesan, R. A., et al.: Occurrence and possible significance of demodectic mites, *Demodex caprae*, in the internal tissues of fetal and adult Indian goats. J. Am. Leather Chem. Assoc. 74:191, 1979.

816. Venugopal, G., and Nair, S. G.: Haematological studies in mange-infested goats. Kerala J. Vet. Sci. 6:89, 1975.

817. Verhulst, A.: *Tunga penetrans* (*Sarcopsylla penetrans*) as a cause of agalactia in sows in the Republic of Zaire. Vet. Rec. 98:384, 1976.

818. Verma, A. K.: Some photomicrographs depicting the pathology of filarial humpsore in cattle. Ceylon Vet. J. 4:11, 1956.

819. Villenberg, G., and Swart, D.: Skin nodules in East Coast fever. Res. Vet. Sci. 26:243, 1979.

820. Viljoen, J. H.: Studies on *parafilaria bovicola* (Tubangui 1934). I. Clinical observations and chemotherapy. J. S. Afr. Vet. Assoc. 47:161, 1976.

821. Viljoen, J. H., and Boomker, J. D. F.: Studies on *Parafilaria bovicola* (Tubangui 1934). II. Chemotherapy and pathology. Onderstepoort J. Vet. Res. 44:107, 1977.

822. Vural, A.: Treatment of mange in sheep with Asuntol. Vet. Med. Rev. 1:75, 1977.

823. Waddell, A. H.: A survey of *Habronema* spp. and the identification of third-stage larvae of *Habronema megastoma* and *Habronema muscae* in section. Aust. Vet. J. 45:20, 1969.

824. Wagland, B. M.: Host resistance to cattle tick (*Boophilus microplus*) in Brahman (*Bos indicus*) cattle. I. Responses of previously unexposed cattle to four infestations with 20,000 larvae. Aust. J. Agric. Res. 26:1073, 1975.

825. Wagland, B. M.: Host resistance to cattle tick (*Boophilus microplus*) in Brahman (*Bos indicus*) cattle. II. The dynamics of resistance in previously unexposed and exposed cattle. Aust. J. Agric. Res. 29:395, 1978.

826. Wagland, B. M.: Host resistance to cattle tic (*Boophilus microplus*) in Brahman (*Bos indicus*) cattle. IV. Ages of ticks rejected. Aust. J. Agric. Res. 30:211, 1979.

827. Walton, G. S.: The young pig. Ectoparasitic infestations. Vet. Rec. (80:Suppl.) 9:11, 1967.

828. Watts, J. E., et al.: The blowfly strike problem of sheep in New South Wales. Aust. Vet. J. 55:325, 1979.

829. Webster, W. A., and Wilkins, D. B.: The recovery of *Parafilaria bovicola* Tubangui, 1934, from an imported Charolais bull. Can. Vet. J. 1:13, 1970.

830. Webster, W. A., and Dukes, T. W.: Bovine and equine onchocerciasis in eastern North America with a discussion on cuticular morphology of *Onchocerca* spp. in cattle. Can. J. Comp. Med. 43:330, 1979.

831. Wellington, A. C.: The effect of nitroxynil on *Parafilaria bovicola* infestations in cattle. J. S. Afr. Vet. Assoc. 49:131, 1978.

832. Wellington, A. C.: *Parafilaria bovicola* in cattle and its control. J. S. Afr. Vet. Assoc. 51:243, 1980.

833. Wellington, A. C., and Van Schalkwyk, L.: The effect of a single injection of nitroxynil at 20 mg/kg live mass in the treatment of *Parafilaria bovicola* infestations in cattle. J. S. Afr. Vet. Assoc. 53:91, 1982.

834. Wetzel, R.: Zum Problem der Rinder-demodikose. Vortraygehaltem auf dem 43 Frankfurter Refereriabend. Dtsch. Tierärztl. Wochenschr. 65:156, 1958.

835. Wharton, R. H., and Roulston, W. J.: Resistance of ticks to chemicals. Ann. Rev. Entomol. 15:381, 1970.

836. Wheat, J. D.: Treatment of equine summer sores with systemic insecticide. Vet. Med. 56:477, 1961.

837. Whitten, L. K., and Elliot, D. C.: *Psorergates ovis* on New Zealand sheep. N.Z. Vet. J. 4:19, 1956.

838. Walladsen, P., et al.: Responses of cattle to allergens from *Boophilus microplus*. Intl. J. Parasitol. 8:89, 1978.

839. Weaver, D. B., et al.: Bovine parafilariasis at the Cato Ridge abattoir: Sex prevalence and districts of origin. J. S. Afr. Vet. Assoc. 54:254, 1983.

840. Wikel, S. K.: Immunomodulation of host responses to ecto-

841. Willadsen, P., et al.: The relation between histamine concentration, histamine sensitivity and the resistance of cattle to the tick, *Boophilus microplus*. Zeitschr. Parasitenk. 59:87, 1979.

841a. Willadsen, P., et al.: Responses of cattle to allergens from *Boophilus microplus*. Intl. J. Parasitol. 8:89, 1978.

842. Willadsen, P.: The relationship between immediate hypersensitivity reactions and resistance of cattle to the tick *Boophilus microplus*. Aust. Adv. Vet. Sc. 1979:77, 1979.

843. Willadsen, P.: Immunity to ticks. Adv. Parasitol. 18:293, 1980.

844. Williams, D. J., et al.: Insect stings in swine. Vet. Med. Small Anim. Clin. 74:1663, 1979.

845. Williams, H. E.: Haematidrosis in a horse. Vet. Rec. 65:386, 1953.

846. Williams, J. F., and Williams, C. S. F.: Demodicosis in dairy goats. JAVMA 180:168, 1982.

847. Williams, J. F., and Williams, C. S. F.: Psoroptic ear mites in dairy goats. JAVMA 173:1582, 1978.

848 Williamson, G., and Oxspring, G. E.: Demodectic scabies in the horse. Vet. J. 76:376, 1920.

849. Wilson, G. I., et al.: The infectivity of scabies (mange) mites. *Psoroptes ovis*, to sheep in naturally contaminated enclosures. Res. Vet. Sci. 22:292, 1977.

850. Wolfe, L. S.: Observations on the histopathologic changes caused by the larvae of *Hypoderma bovis* (*L.*) and *Hypoderma lineatum* (*DeVill.*) in tissues of cattle. Can. J. Anim. Sci. 39:145, 1959.

851. Wolffhugel, K.: Zur Schafraude (*Psoroptes*). Berl. Munch. Tierarztl. Wochenschr. 63:184, 1950.

852. Wood, J. C., et al.: The use of dieldrin, aldrin, and Delnav for the treatment of the sheep tick. Vet. Rec. 72:98, 1960.

853. Wood, J. C.: Parasitic skin diseases of large animals. Vet. Rec. 87:471, 1970.

854. Wooten, E. L., and Gaafar, S. M.: Detection of serum antibodies to sarcoptic mange mite antigens by the passive hemagglutination assay in pigs infested with *Sarcoptes scabiei var. suis*. Vet. Parasitol. 15:309, 1984.

855. Wooten, E. L., and Gaafar, S. M.: Hemagglutinating factor in an extract of *Sarcoptes scabiei var. suis* (de Geer). Vet. Parasitol. 15:317, 1984.

856. Wrich, M. J.: Horn fly and face fly control on beef cattle using backrubbers and dust bags containing coumaphos or fenthion. J. Econ. Entomol. 68:1123, 1970.

857. Wright, C. L., et al.: Insecticidal ear tags and sprays for the control of flies on cattle. Vet. Rec. 115:60, 1984.

858. Wright, F. C., and DeLoach, J. R.: Feeding of *Psoroptes ovis* (Acari-Psoroptidae) on cattle. J. Med. Entomol. 18:349, 1981.

859. Wright, F. C., et al.: Free amino acids in psoroptic mites. Southwest. Entomol. 5:187, 1980.

860. Wright, F. C., and DeLoach, J. R.: Feeding of *Psoroptes ovis* (Acari:Psoroptidae) on cattle. J. Med. Entomol. 18:149, 1981.

861. Wright, F. C., and Guillot, F. S.: Effect of invermectin in heifers on mortality and egg production of *Psoroptes ovis*. Am. J. Vet. Res. 45:2132, 1984.

862. Wright, F. C., and Guillot, F. S.: Infestation potential of *Psoroptes ovis* (Hering) from cattle injected with ivermectin. Am. J. Vet. Res. 45:228, 1984.

863. Yamahata, T., et al.: Porcine scabies and its treatment. Jpn. J. Vet. Med. Assoc. 35:510, 1982.

864. Yazwinski, T. A., et al.: Effectiveness of invermectin in the treatment of equine *Parascaris equorum* and *Oxyuris equi* infections. Am. J. Vet. Res. 43:1095, 1982.

865. Yeoman, G. H., and Bell, T. A.: Sheep blowfly breech strike control using aluminum alkoxide gellants. Vet. Rec. 103:337, 1978.

866. Yeruham, I., et al.: Psoroptic ear mange (*Psoroptes cuniculi*, Delafund, 1859) in domestic and wild ruminants in Israel. Vet. Parasitol. 17:349, 1985.

867. Zumpt, F.: Medical and veterinary importance of horse flies. S. Afr. Med. J. 23:359, 1949.

868 Zumpt, F.: *Myiasis in Man and Animals in the Old World*. London, Butterworth and Co., Ltd., 1965.

CHAPTER 10

IMMUNOLOGIC DISEASES

CUTANEOUS IMMUNOLOGY

In the past 20 years, there has been a phenomenal expansion of knowledge in basic and clinical immunology. It has become impossible to keep up with new information related to clinical immunodermatologic problems. A review of this information is decidedly beyond the scope of this chapter. For the practitioner, student, and academician interested in details, a plethora of basic and clinical immunology texts and review articles are available.* This section will be confined to a brief overview of basic and clinical immunodermatology.

The immune system and its inflammatory limb are complex models of biologic activity and interaction. There is a tendency to dissect the immune response into its individual components and discuss them as autonomous functional units. However, immune responses are delicately interwoven and interdependent, and manipulation of one component influences all others (Fig. 10–1).

Cutaneous Inflammation

Inflammation is defined as the changes occurring in living tissue when it is injured, provided that the injury is not severe enough to immediately kill all the cells. Inflammatory changes include both the processes of tissue damage induced by the initial stimulus and those induced by the autologous changes occurring after the initial stimulus. The intensity and duration of the inflammation are controlled to some extent by the nature of the stimulus and the severity of the damage.

Regardless of the injurious agent or the area involved, the inflammatory response is characterized by a certain number of tissue adjustments that involve mainly blood vessels and fluid and other cellular components of the

*References 3, 13, 15, 16, 22–24, 43, 52, 62, 63, 68, 75, 84, 122, 135, 156, 160, 161, 176, 189, 197, 199

blood as well as the surrounding connective tissue. Thus, very similar findings may accompany the skin's inflammatory response to bacteria, fungi, parasites, heat, cold, radiation, chemicals, mechanical trauma, or allergens.

To the clinician, cutaneous inflammation may be characterized by (1) redness (rubor) from vasodilatation, (2) swelling (tumor) due to increased capillary permeability resulting in edema, (3) heat (calor) from increased blood flow, and (4) pain (dolor), pruritus, or both, resulting from involvement of peripheral nerve fibers.

Overview of the Immune System

The immune response results from an integrated sequence of events involving antigens, lymphocytes, antibodies, lymphokines, mediator substances, and effector cells operating under genetic and physiologic controls to protect the host from harmful agents and to remove dead or injured tissue. Sometimes the immune response misfunctions by under-responding or over-responding. Under-response predisposes to infections and hinders the elimination of noxious substances. Over-response produces excessive inflammation and may lead to autoimmunity. Both under-response and over-response can lead to dermatologic disease.

CELLS INVOLVED IN THE IMMUNE RESPONSE

Lymphocytes are classically divided into two main types: B cells (bursa or bone marrow-derived) and T cells (thymus-dependent) (Fig. 10–1).[43, 135, 189]

B cells are characterized by surface immunoglobulins, Fc receptors, and C3b receptors. B cells differentiate into plasma cells, which produce the immunoglobulins (IgG, IgM, IgA, and IgE) and are responsible for humoral (antibody) immunity. The humoral immune system is instrumental in initiating immune and

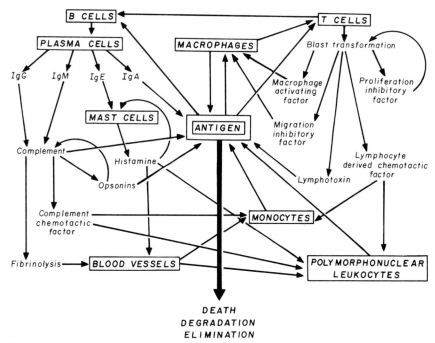

FIGURE 10-1. *The immune system—a complex system of interrelated components. Activity of one component often affects others. (Reproduced with permission from Dahl, M. V.: Clinical Immunodermatology. Copyright © 1981 by Year Book Medical Publishers, Inc., Chicago.)*

inflammatory responses. It is under genetic control and is also under the control of positive and negative feedback-control systems that modulate the amount of response. Humoral immunity provides the primary defense against invading bacteria and neutralization activity against circulating viruses.

T cells are responsible for cell-mediated immunity. Among the many functions attributable to T cells are (1) helping B cells make antibody (T-helper cells), (2) suppressing B-cell antibody production (T-suppressor cells), (3) directly damaging target cells, (4) mediating delayed-hypersensitivity reactions, (5) suppressing delayed-hypersensitivity reactions mediated by other T cells, (6) modulating the inflammatory response with lymphokines, (7) inducing graft rejection, and (8) producing graft-versus-host reactions. Cell-mediated immunity is specifically geared to defending against organisms that are intracellular or otherwise hidden from circulating or humoral factors (intracellular viruses, fungi, mycobacteria, and parasites). T cells seem to play a central role in orchestrating the immune response. They can force B cells to make greater or lesser quantities of antibodies or can reduce cell-mediated immune reactions. They can elaborate lymphokines that amplify or dampen phagocytic activity, collagen production, vas-

cular permeability, and coagulation phenomena. They themselves can kill, or they can recruit effector cells to perform this function.

Monocytes and *macrophages* (the mononuclear phagocyte system) have critical phagocytic, secretory, and antigen-processing functions (Table 10-1).[43, 135, 189] Mononuclear phagocytes are necessary for processing antigen to initiate immune responses and for secreting biologically active substances that mediate the immune and inflammatory responses.

Neutrophils have as their major role the containment of infection (Table 10-2).[43, 135, 189] However, because of their numerous chemoattractants (Table 10-3) and intracellular products (Table 10-4), they are omnipresent participants in virtually all immune and inflammatory reactions.

Eosinophils, effector cells in hypersensitivity reactions, also participate in the downgrading of inflammation (Tables 10-5 and 10-6).* In addition, they are phagocytic (immune complexes, mast cell granules, aggregated immunoglobulins, and certain bacteria and fungi) and play a unique role in the host's defense against extracellular parasitic infection.

Langerhans's cells are located in the epidermis. They are thought to be cells of the mon-

---

*References 15, 43, 66, 68, 122, 141, 142, 189

TABLE 10–1. Monocyte-Macrophage Functions

Antigen Processing
Phagocytosis
  Microorganisms
  Insoluble particles
  Kill antibody-coated cells
  Wound débridement
  Dead cells and remnant digestion
Secretion
  Enzymes
    Lysozyme
    Neutral proteases
      Plasminogen activator
      Collagenase
      Elastase
      Leukokinins
    Acid hydrolases
      Proteases
      Lipases
      Deoxyribonucleases
      Phosphatases
      Glucosidases
      Sulfatases
  Complement components
    C1, C2, C3, C4, C5
    All components of alternate pathway
  Enzyme inhibitors
    Plasmin inhibitors
    Alpha$_2$-macroglobulin
  Binding proteins
    Transferrin
    Fibronectin
  Endogenous pyrogens
  Reactive metabolites of oxygen
    Superoxide
    Hydrogen peroxide
    Hydroxyl radical
    Singlet oxygen
  Bioactive lipids
    Prostaglandins
    Thromboxanes
    Leukotrienes
    Platelet-activating factors
  Monokines
    Neutrophil chemotactic factor
    Lymphocyte-activating factors
    Lymphocyte-suppressor factors
    Colony-stimulating factor
    Interferon
    Fibroblast-stimulating factors
    Fibroblast-suppressor factors

TABLE 10–2. Neutrophil Functions

Phagocytosis (after opsonization)
Killing
  Nonoxidative (lysozyme, elastase, proteases)
  Oxidative (H_2O_2, singlet oxygen, hydroxyl radical, and superoxide)
Degranulation
Chemotaxis
Modulation of inflammation

zymes (Table 10–7). Ruminant mast cells are somewhat unique, as they contain dopamine.[24, 41, 52, 57] Mast cells probably have as their major role the recruitment of cells (eosinophils and neutrophils), immunoglobulins, and complement from the circulation. The actions of mast cell mediators can be divided into three broad categories: (1) to increase vascular permeability and contract smooth muscle, (2) to be chemotactic for, or activate, other inflammatory cells, and (3) to modulate the release of other mediators.

MEDIATOR SUBSTANCES

The changes observed in inflammation are mediated by substances derived from the plasma, from cells of the damaged tissue, and from infiltrating leukocytes. The interactions between cells and soluble mediators determine the inflammatory response. Some mediators augment inflammation, while others suppress it. Some mediators antagonize or destroy other mediators, while others amplify or generate other mediators. Normally, all mediators and cells act together in a harmonious fashion to maintain homeostasis and to protect the host

TABLE 10–3. Chemoattractants for Neutrophils

Bacterial products
C5a (derived from complement activation; tissue, virus, and bacterial enzymes cleave C5)
C3a
C567
Kallikrein
Denatured protein
Lymphokines
Monokines
Neutrophil chemotactic factor (NCF) from mast cells
Eosinophil chemotactic factor of anaphylaxis (ECF-A) from mast cells
Lipid chemotactic factors (e.g., HETE) from mast cells
Lysosomal proteases
Collagen breakdown products
Fibrin breakdown products
Plasminogen activator
Prostaglandins
Immune complexes

ocyte-macrophage series whose primary function is presentation of antigens to lymphocytes.[43, 122, 135, 189] The role of the Langerhans's cell in the mammalian epidermis probably is to process antigens absorbed through the skin.

Mast cells are believed to be of monocytogenous or mesenchymal origin.[43, 122, 135, 189] These cells serve as repositories for numerous inflammatory mediator substances, including histamine, leukotrienes, eosinophil chemotactic factor of anaphylaxis, and proteolytic en-

TABLE 10–4. Neutrophil Products

Antimicrobial enzymes
  Lysozyme
  Myeloperoxidase
Proteases
  Collagenase
  Collagenolytic proteinase
  Elastase
  Cathepsin G
  Leukokinins
Hydrolases
  Cathepsin B
  Cathepsin D
  N-acetyl-β-glucosaminidase
  β-glycerophosphatase
  β-glucuronidase
Others
  Lactoferrin
  Eosinophil chemotactic factor
  Leukotrienes
  Pyrogen
  Prostaglandins
  Thromboxanes

TABLE 10–6. Chemoattractants for Eosinophils

Factor	Source
Histamine	Mast cells
Eosinophil chemotactic factor of anaphylaxis (ECF-A)	Mast cells, neutrophils
Eosinophil stimulation promotor (ESP)	T lymphocytes
Immune complexes	—
C5a	Complement
C567	Complement
Hydroxy-eicosatetraenoic acid (HETE)	Platelets, mast cells, arachidonic acid

against infectious agents and other noxious substances.

Inflammatory mediator substances and their biologic actions are listed and cross-referenced in Table 10–8.* It is important to note that histamine appears to be a minor mediator of pruritus and cutaneous inflammation in domestic animals, as antihistamines are usually ineffective for controlling pruritic and inflammatory dermatoses in these species.[41, 51–53, 75, 81] Proteolytic enzymes appear to be the important pruritogenic mediators.

Interestingly, histamine has two types of effects on hypersensitivity reactions: proin-

---

*References 24, 41, 43, 50–52, 60, 62, 75, 78–81, 122, 143, 189, 199

flammatory and anti-inflammatory. Histamine's proinflammatory effects (Table 10–7) are mediated through histamine$_1$ (H$_1$) receptors and resultant decreases in intracellular cyclic AMP (Fig. 10–2). Histamine's anti-inflammatory effects (inhibition of the release of inflammatory mediator substances by mast cells, neutrophils, lymphocytes, and monocyte-macrophages) are mediated through H$_2$ receptors and resultant increases in cyclic AMP.

Complement is a series of several plasma proteins that induce and influence immunologic and inflammatory events (Table 10–9).[43, 122, 135, 189] The critical step in the generation of biologic activities from the complement proteins is in the cleavage of C3. There are two pathways for the cleavage of C3, the classic and the alternative (properidin), a pathway to amplify C3 cleavage, and an effector sequence. The biologic activities attributed to various complement components are listed in Table 10–10.

Lymphokines are proteins produced by activated T lymphocytes.[43, 122, 135, 189] More than 30 lymphokines have been described, but it is not clear if each plays a unique role or if a given lymphokine may play several different roles. In any case, lymphokines play a key role in inducing and modulating inflammatory reactions, especially in cell-mediated immune reactions and delayed-hypersensitivity reactions (Table 10–11).

Prostaglandins and *leukotrienes* play a central role, often acting synergistically with other mediators, both in the expression of the efferent limb of immune-based inflammatory responses and in acute inflammatory responses when specific immunity does not play a primary role.[24, 45, 60, 67, 75, 137] Prostaglandins and leukotrienes are produced by most, if not all, cells participating in the afferent and efferent limbs of the immune system as well as by keratinocytes, fibroblasts, and endothelial cells. Their formation depends on the deacy-

TABLE 10–5. Eosinophil Products and Their Function

Substance	Function
Acid phosphatase	Unknown
Arylsulfatase	Inactivates leukotrienes
Cationic protein	Inactivates heparin
Collagenase	Lyses collagen
Histaminase	Degrades histamine
Hydrogen peroxide	Cytotoxic
Kininase	Inactivates kinins
Major basic protein	Cytotoxic
Peroxidase	Stimulates mast cell secretion
Phospholipase	Inactivates platelet-activating factor (PAF)
Plasminogen	Lyses fibrin
Prostaglandins	Inhibit mast cell degranulation
Pyrogen	Produces fever
Superoxide	Cytotoxic
Zinc	Inhibits mast cell degranulation

TABLE 10-7. Mast Cell Products and Their Actions

Product	Action
Histamine	Smooth muscle contraction, increased vascular permeability, elevation of cyclic AMP, enhancement or inhibition of chemotaxis
Dopamine	Smooth muscle contraction, increased vascular permeability
Leukotrienes	Smooth muscle contraction, increased vascular permeability, neutrophil chemotaxis, epidermal hyperplasia
Platelet-activating factor (PAF)	Increased vascular permeability, platelet and neutrophil activation
Eosinophil chemotactic factor of anaphylaxis (ECF-A)	Chemoattraction of eosinopihils and neutrophils
Neutrophil chemotactic factor (NCF)	Chemoattraction of neutrophils
Lipid chemotactic factors (e.g., HETE)	Chemoattraction of eosinophils and neutrophils
Heparin	Anticoagulation, inhibition of complement activation, inhibition of proteolytic enzymes
Serotonin	Smooth muscle contraction, increased vascular permeability
Proteolytic enzymes	Proteolysis and hydrolysis

lation of arachidonic acid from cellular phospholipids, catalyzed by the activity of various phospholipases, and the subsequent utilization of arachidonic acid by cyclo-oxygenase and various lipoxygenase enzymes (Fig. 10-2). Cyclo-oxygenase converts free arachidonic acid to the endoperoxides that serve as precursors of the thromboxanes as well as the various prostaglandins and prostacyclin (PGI_2). The lipoxygenases form hydroperoxy-eicosatetraenoic acids (HPETEs), which are further metabolized to the hydroxy-eicosatetraenoic acids (HETEs) and leukotrienes. These arachidonic acid oxygenation products have numerous complex effects on the inflammatory response (Tables 10-7 and 10-8) and are currently the focus of much pathogenetic and therapeutic research.*

The Role of Cyclic Nucleotides in Inflammation

Szentivanyi proposed the β-adrenergic theory of atopic disease in 1968. He suggested that the heightened sensitivity of atopic human beings to various pharmacologic agents could be due to a blockage of β-adrenergic receptors in tissues. Since that time, there has been an explosion of investigative effort in the field of

*References 24, 41, 45, 51–53, 67, 75, 78–82, 101a, 137, 144

TABLE 10-8. Inflammatory Mediator Substances and Their Actions

Mediator	Action
Histamine	See Table 10-7
Serotonin	Smooth muscle contraction, increased vascular permeability
Leukotrienes	See Table 10-7
ECF-A	See Table 10-7
NCF	See Table 10-7
PAF	See Table 10-7
Heparin	See Table 10-7
Prostaglandins	Increase vascular permeability, potentiate itch and pain, modulate cAMP and the release of other mediators
Thromboxanes	Increase vascular permeability, potentiate itch and pain, modulate cAMP and the release of other mediators
Neutrophil proteases	Proteolysis and hydrolysis
Monocyte-macrophage proteases	Proteolysis and hydrolysis
Mast cell proteases	Proteolysis and hydrolysis
Eosinophil proteases	Proteolysis
Lymphokines	See Table 10-11
Monokines	See Table 10-11
Kallikrein and kinins	Smooth muscle contraction, increased vascular permeability, pain, neutrophil chemotaxis
Complement	See Table 10-9
Fibrin breakdown products (fibrinopeptides)	Increased vascular permeability, neutrophil chemotaxis
Dopamine	See Table 10-7

TABLE 10–9. Complement Function

Causes cell lysis
Kills certain bacteria and protozoa
Chemoattracts neutrophils, eosinophils, and monocyte-
  macrophages
Attaches antigens to phagocytes (immune adherence)
Opsonizes microorganisms and particles
Neutralizes certain viruses
Induces mast cell degranulation (anaphylatoxins)
Produces kinins
Activates clotting and fibrinolysis
Modulates inflammation by feedback mechanisms and
  interplay with inhibitors
Interacts with B lymphocytes
Mediates lysosome release

the cyclic nucleotides.[122, 189] In brief, the cyclic nucleotides, cyclic AMP (cAMP) and cyclic GMP (cGMP), appear to serve as the intracellular effectors of a variety of cellular events. Cyclic AMP and cyclic GMP are envisaged to impose opposing influences in a number of systems, the so-called yin-yang hypothesis of biologic control.

A number of pharmacologic agents are known to act via various cell receptors to influence intracellular levels of cAMP and cGMP (Fig. 10–3). In general, substances that elevate intracellular cAMP levels (β-adrenergic drugs, prostaglandin E, methylxanthines, histamine, and other mediator substances) or reduce intracellular cGMP levels (anticholinergic drugs) tend to stabilize the cells (lymphocytes, monocyte-macrophages, neutrophils, and mast cells) and inhibit the release of various inflammatory mediators. On the other hand, substances that reduce cAMP levels (α-adrenergic drugs) or elevate cGMP levels (cholinergic drugs, ascorbic acid, estrogen, and levamisole) tend to labilize the cells and promote the release of inflammatory mediators. Further studies in the area of cyclic nucleotides and biologic regulation may produce significant advances in the areas of pathologic mechanisms of disease and control of immunologic inflammation.

Types of Hypersensitivity Reactions

Immunology is the study of the mechanisms that preserve the biologic identity of animal organisms, or the "self" from the "not self." This function is carried out by a process characterized by two outstanding features: specificity and memory. If this process is effective, it is correctly called allergy.[13, 63, 122, 189] This specific, effective immunologic response, when protective, is called immunity. If this response is injurious, it is called hypersensitivity. In

TABLE 10–10. Biologic Actions of Complement Components

Factor	Action
C2-derived peptide (C kinin)	Increased vascular permeability
C3a	Anaphylatoxin (releases mediators from mast cells); chemotactic to neutrophils, eosinophils, and monocyte-macrophages
C3b	Immune adherence, enhanced phagocytosis, secretion of lysosomal enzymes
C5a	Anaphylatoxin; chemotactic to neutrophils and monocyte-macrophages; secretion of lysosomal enzymes
C$\overline{567}$	Chemotactic to neutrophils, eosinophils, and monocyte-macrophages
C5–C9	Lysis of membranes

TABLE 10–11. Lymphokines and Their Functions

Lymphokine	Function
Migration inhibition factor (MIF)	Inhibits macrophage movement
Leukocyte inhibition factor (LIF)	Inhibits neutrophil movement
Macrophage-activating factor	Increases macrophage adherence, phagocytosis, and protein synthesis
Macrophage-aggregating factor	Induces clumping of macrophages
Lymphocyte-derived chemotactic factor	Chemotactic to monocytes
Eosinophil stimulation (ES) promoter	Chemotactic to eosinophils
Skin reactive factor	Induces vascular permeability
Transfer factor	Educates unsensitized lymphocytes
Interferon	Defense against virus, modulates lymphocyte and macrophage functions
Lymphocyte blastogenic factor	Recruits unsensitized lymphocytes
Antibody production–enhancing factor	Increases antibody production
Antibody production–suppressing factor	Decreases antibody production
Proliferation inhibitory factor	Inhibits division of various cells
Lymphotoxin	Cytotoxic for various cells
Fibroblast stimulation factor	Increases collagen production
Lymph node permeability factor	Induces vascular permeability
Interleukin 2	Initiates and maintains T-lymphocyte proliferation

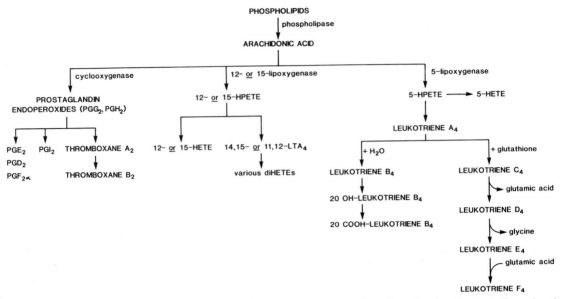

FIGURE 10–2. The pathways and products of arachidonic acid oxygenation. (From Davies, P., et al.: The role of arachidonic acid oxygenation products in pain and inflammation. Ann. Rev. Immunol. 2:335, 1984. Reproduced with permission from the Annual Review of Immunology, Vol. 2. © 1984 by Annual Reviews Inc.)

practice, the terms allergy and hypersensitivity are inappropriately used interchangeably.

Clinical hypersensitivity disorders have been divided by Gell and Coombs into four types on an immunopathologic basis:[63] (1) Type I, immediate (anaphylactic), (2) Type II, cytotoxic, (3) Type III, immune complex, and (4) Type IV, cell-mediated (delayed). Clearly, this scheme is oversimplified in light of the complex interrelationships that exist between the several events that constitute an inflammatory response. In most pathologic events, immunologically initiated events almost certainly involve multiple components of the inflammatory process. Realization of this simplistic approach to immunopathology has motivated other investigators to modify Gell and Coombs's original scheme, often to a seemingly hopeless degree of hair-splitting. In this section, we will briefly examine the classic Gell and Coombs classification of hypersensitivity disorders because (1) it is applicable to discussions on cutaneous hypersensitivity diseases, and (2) it is still the immunopathologic scheme used by most authors and by major immunologic and dermatologic texts.*

Type I (anaphylactic, immediate) hypersensitivity reactions are classically described as those involving genetic predilection, reaginic antibody (IgE), and mast cell degranulation. A genetically programmed individual inhales

*References 13, 22, 52, 53, 62, 63, 122, 135, 189, 197

(or possibly ingests or absorbs percutaneously) a complete antigen (e.g., ragweed pollen) and responds by producing a unique antibody (reagin, IgE). IgE is homocytotropic and avidly binds membrane receptors on tissue mast cells and blood basophils. When the eliciting antigen comes in contact with the specific reaginic antibody, a number of inflammatory mediator substances are released and cause tissue damage. It is important to note that older terms such as reaginic, homocytotropic, and skin-sensitizing antibodies are *not* strictly synonymous with IgE, as subclasses of IgG may also mediate Type I hypersensitivity reactions.[122, 169] Examples of Type I hypersensitivity reactions include urticaria, angioedema, anaphylaxis, milk allergy, insect hypersensitivity, atopy, and drug eruption.

Type II (cytotoxic) hypersensitivity reactions are characterized by the binding of antibody (IgG or IgM), with or without complement, to complete antigens on body tissues. This binding of antibody, with or without complement, results in cytotoxicity or cytolysis. Examples of Type II hypersensitivity reactions include pemphigus and drug eruption.

Type III (immune complex) hypersensitivity reactions are characterized by the deposition of circulating antigen-antibody complexes (in slight antigen excess) in blood vessel walls. These immune complexes (usually containing IgG or IgM) then fix complement, which attracts neutrophils. Proteolytic and hydrolytic enzymes released from the infiltrating neutrophils produce tissue damage. Studies have suggested that Type I hypersensitivity reactions and histamine release may be important in the initiation of immune complex deposition. Examples of Type III hypersensitivity reactions include lupus erythematosus, leukocytoclastic vasculitis, and drug eruption.

Type IV (cell-mediated, delayed) hypersensitivity reactions classically do not involve antibody-mediated injury. An incomplete antigen (hapten) interacts with a tissue protein (e.g., collagen) to form a complete antigen. This complete antigen is processed by monocyte-macrophages or Langerhans's cells (in contact hypersensitivity), after which it sensitizes T lymphocytes. These sensitized T lymphocytes respond to further antigenic challenge by releasing lymphokines that produce

tissue damage. It has been suggested that the term cell-mediated is an unfortunate misnomer for this type of immunologic reaction, since it is no more or less cell-mediated than antibody-dependent reactions that are ultimately due to the participation of a lymphocyte or plasma cell. Examples of Type IV hypersensitivity reactions include contact hypersensitivity and drug eruption.

Types I, II, and III hypersensitivity reactions together form the immediate-hypersensitivity reactions. All three are antibody-mediated, and thus, there is only a short delay (minutes to a few hours) before their tissue damaging effects become apparent. Type IV hypersensitivity is the delayed-hypersensitivity reaction. It is *not* antibody-mediated and classically requires 24 to 72 hours before becoming detectable.

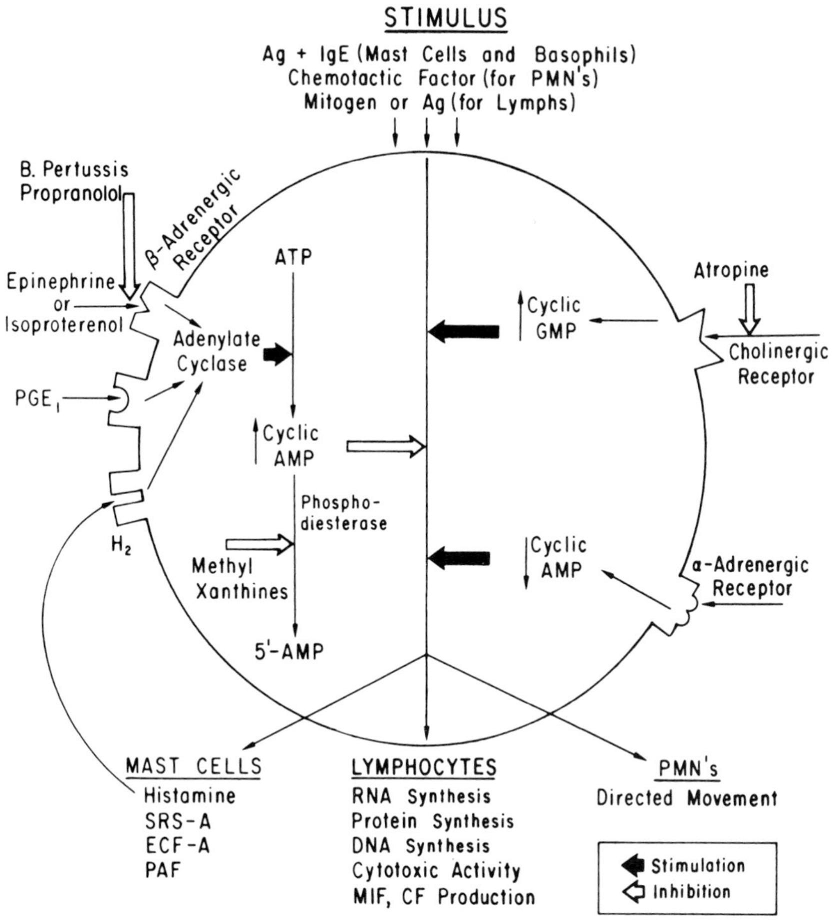

FIGURE 10-3. *Diagrammatic representation of pathways by which pharmacologic mediators might act on mast cell, lymphocyte, and PMN leukocyte membrane receptors to alter intracellular cyclic nucleotides, which in turn may either enhance or inhibit the function of those cells. Abbreviations include the following: Ag, antigen; PGE₁, prostaglandin E₁; SRS-A, slow-reacting substance of anaphylaxis; ECF-A, eosinophil chemotactic factor of anaphylaxis; PAF, platelet-activating factor; MIF, migration inhibitor factor; CF, chemotactic factor. (With permission from Hanifin, J. M., and Lobitz, W. C.: Newer concepts of atopic dermatitis. Arch. Dermatol. 113:663, 1977.)*

URTICARIA AND ANGIOEDEMA

Urticaria and angioedema are variably pruritic, edematous skin disorders. They are immunologic or nonimmunologic and are common in the horse but rare in ruminants and swine.

CAUSE AND PATHOGENESIS

Urticaria and angioedema can result from many stimuli, both immunologic and nonimmunologic (Table 10–12).[122] Immunologic mechanisms include Types I and III hypersensitivity reactions. Nonimmunologic factors that may precipitate or intensify urticaria and angioedema include physical forces (e.g., pressure, sunlight, heat, or exercise), psychologic stresses, genetic abnormalities, and various drugs and chemicals (e.g., aspirin, narcotics, foods, or food additives).

CLINICAL FEATURES

In general, no age, breed, or sex predilections have been reported for urticaria (hives, "humor spots," "heat bumps," "feed bumps") and angioedema in large animals. Clinical signs may be acute (most common) or chronic. In humans, acute urticaria and angioedema are empirically defined as those episodes lasting less than four to six weeks; those lasting several weeks or longer are termed chronic. Urticarial reactions are characterized by localized or generalized wheals, which may or may not be pruritic and which may or may not exhibit serum leakage or hemorrhage. The lesions are cold swellings that pit with digital pressure. Characteristically, the wheals are evanescent lesions, with each individual lesion persisting only a few hours. Urticarial lesions may occasionally assume bizarre patterns (serpiginous, linear, arciform, annular, or papular). Angioedematous reactions are characterized by localized or generalized large, edematous swellings, which may or may not be pruritic and exhibit serum leakage or hemorrhage.

A unique form of urticaria has been described in cattle, especially Jerseys and Guernseys, that become sensitized to the casein in their own milk.[38, 39] This autoallergy was shown to be a Type I hypersensitivity reaction by intradermal skin testing with autologous milk and by passive transfer studies.

In horses, urticaria is commonly seen, often just prior to races (perhaps psychogenic) or in association with insect or arthropod envenomation, various infections (strangles, dermatophytosis, dourine, babesiasis, surra, horsepox, or mal de caderas), intestinal parasitism, topical applications (especially parasiticidal sprays, dips, and pour-ons), systemic medicaments (especially penicillin, phenylbutazone, aspirin, guaiphenesin, phenothiazine, streptomycin, oxytetracycline, or iron-dextrans), feedstuffs (pasture plants, concentrates), physical trauma (dermatographism), contactants (saddle soaps, leather conditioners, or tack), various biologicals (strangles, encephalomyelitis, and salmonellosis vaccines; botulinum and tetanus toxoids), snake bites, hypodermiasis, inhalants (pollens, molds, chemicals), purpura hemorrhagica, and plants (stinging nettle).* Lesions occur anywhere on the body, especially on the face, neck, and trunk (Figs. 10–4 and 10–5).

In swine, urticaria has been reported in association with insect and arthropod stings and bites, infections (erysipelas), topical applications (especially parasiticides), feedstuffs, systemic medicaments, plants (stinging nettle), and biologicals.[30, 35, 100, 101, 125] Lesions are most commonly seen over the trunk and proximal limbs.

In *cattle*, urticaria has been reported in association with insect and arthropod stings and bites, infections, systemic medicaments (penicillin, streptomycin, oxytetracycline, chloramphenicol, neomycin, sulfonamides, diethylstilbestrol, carboxymethylcellulose, and hydroxypropyl methylcellulose), biologicals (various vaccines and toxoids, especially for leptospirosis, *Brucella abortus* strain 19, foot-and-mouth disease, shipping fever, salmonellosis, rinderpest, and contagious pleuropneumonia; horse serum), physical trauma (dermatographism), hypodermiasis, feedstuffs (pasture plants, moldy hay or straw, or potato and walnut leaves), and plants (stinging nettle).† Lesions are most commonly seen on the face, ears, and trunk. Milk allergy is a unique autoallergic disease of cattle, especially Jerseys and Guernseys.[28, 38, 39, 123] The disorder was estimated to have affected 0.5 percent of the dairy cattle in New York State in 1968.[39] It is believed to be familial and is triggered by circumstances that cause milk retention or unusual engorgement of the udder with milk.

---

*References 4, 5, 30, 33, 36, 53, 69, 72, 85, 98, 100, 109a, 114, 124, 138, 146, 179, 188, 197, 202

†References 20, 21, 23, 25, 29, 30, 32, 37, 52, 58, 59, 100, 120, 151, 179, 182, 197

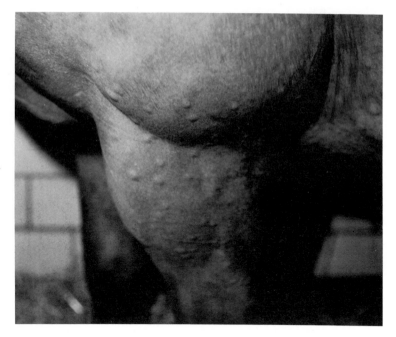

FIGURE 10–4. Equine urticaria. Multiple wheals on front leg.

Clinical signs include varying degrees of urticaria (Fig. 10–6) and respiratory distress.

DIAGNOSIS

The differential diagnosis includes cellulitis, vasculitis, lymphoreticular neoplasia, mast cell tumor, amyloidosis, erythema multiforme, and early dermatophytosis. Definitive diagnosis is based on history, physical examination, and pursuit of the etiologic factors just listed. A specific etiologic diagnosis can usually be made in acute cases, but chronic urticaria and angioedema are extremely frustrating diagnostic challenges, with 75 to 80 percent of such cases in human patients defying specific etiologic diagnosis.[122] Cattle with milk allergy may have a neutrophilia and eosinopenia.[39] Recurrent or chronic urticaria in horses may be a manifestation of atopy, wherein intradermal skin testing and hyposensitization may be beneficial (see Atopy below).[48a]

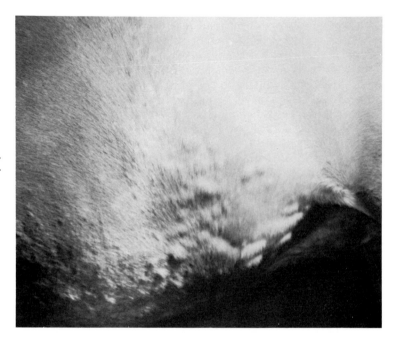

FIGURE 10–5. Equine urticaria. Multiple papules and wheals on abdomen.

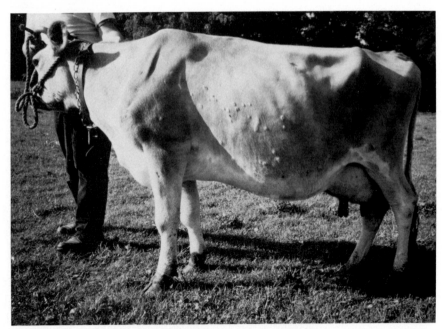

FIGURE 10–6. Bovine milk allergy. Multiple wheals on trunk. (Courtesy S. G. Campbell.)

Skin biopsy shows a variable, nondiagnostic pattern, from simple vascular dilatation and edema in the superficial and middle dermis to pure perivascular dermatitis with varying numbers of mononuclear cells, neutrophils, mast cells, and eosinophils (Fig. 10–7).* Cows with milk allergy develop positive intradermal skin test reactions within 30 minutes of the injection of 0.1 ml of autologous or homologous milk.[38, 39]

CLINICAL MANAGEMENT

The prognosis for urticarial reactions is good, since general health is not usually affected. The prognosis for angioedema varies with the severity and the location. Angioedematous reactions involving the nasal passages, pharynx, and larynx may be fatal.

Therapy includes (1) elimination and avoidance of known etiologic factors and (2) symptomatic treatment with systemic glucocorticoids (0.1 mg/kg dexamethasone, IV or IM, or 1 mg/kg prednisone or prednisolone, IV or IM) or nonsteroidal anti-inflammatory agents (aspirin, 5 mg/kg; phenylbutazone, 2.2 to 4.4 mg/kg; or diethylcarbamazine, 100 mg/kg; or flunixin meglumine, 1 to 2 mg/kg.† Antihistamines are rarely beneficial.[33, 41, 51–53, 72, 75]

Recently, hydroxyzine has been effective in the management of some horses with chronic urticaria when administered orally at a dosage of 200 to 400 mg b.i.d.[157] Epinephrine (3 to 5 ml of a 1:100 solution, SQ or IM) may be lifesaving in severe angioedematous reactions.

Milk allergy in cattle can be treated by milking out affected cows.[39] It can be prevented by managing milking times in a manner calculated to avoid over-filled udders and by drying cows off slowly.

ATOPY

Atopy is a genetically programmed pruritic dermatitis of horses and sheep, in which the affected animal becomes sensitized to inhaled environmental antigens.

CAUSE AND PATHOGENESIS

In humans and dogs, atopy is classified as a Type I hypersensitivity reaction.[122, 169] Genetically predisposed individuals inhale various allergens that provoke allergen-specific IgE or IgG production.[122, 169] The allergen-specific cytotropic antibodies fix to cutaneous mast cells. When mast cell–fixed cytotropic antibodies react with specific allergens, mast cell degranulation and release of many pharmacologically active compounds (see Table 10–7) ensue.

Atopy has not been conclusively docu-

*References 21, 33, 39, 52, 53, 165, 187, 193–195
†References 33, 36, 37, 41, 51–53, 72, 75, 81, 114, 124, 179

mented in large animals. However, it is well known that IgE, reaginic antibodies, and Type I hypersensitivity reactions occur in horses,* cattle,[22, 52, 74, 132, 189, 198] sheep,† swine,[10, 132, 189] and goats.[22, 132, 189] Thus, although atopy remains to be definitively documented in these species, they would all appear to be capable of manifesting atopic reactions.

CLINICAL FEATURES

Atopy-like dermatoses have been seen in horses[40, 47, 48a, 157, 175] and sheep.[169] Affected animals were examined for recurrent, seasonal or nonseasonal, pruritic skin disease. The face, ears, ventrum, and legs were most commonly affected (Figs. 10–8 and 10–9). The chief clinical sign was pruritus, and primary skin lesions were rarely seen. Some horses had chronic pruritic urticaria. Secondary lesions, developing over time, included excoriations, alopecia, lichenification, and hyperpigmentation. Affected animals were otherwise healthy. In

*References 49, 51, 73, 96, 132, 165, 184–187, 189, 199
†References 22, 50, 52, 54, 83, 162, 189

some animals, the signs were present in warm weather, whereas in others, the signs were present in winter. In one study of atopic horses manifesting recurrent urticaria,[48a] onset of clinical signs was usually at one and a half to four years of age, and Arabians and Thoroughbreds appeared predisposed.

DIAGNOSIS

The differential diagnosis includes numerous ectoparasitisms and food hypersensitivity. Definitive diagnosis is based on history, physical examination, ruling out other differentials, and intradermal skin testing. Peripheral and tissue eosinophilia are commonly found.[48a, 169, 175]

Intradermal Skin Testing. A tentative diagnosis of atopy can be made on the basis of history, clinical signs, and the ruling out of other diagnoses by tests. A definitive diagnosis of atopy and a revelation of the allergens involved can only be made with intradermal skin testing. Limited data on skin testing of horses[40, 48a, 56, 73, 114, 116, 157] and sheep[169] have been published. In general, techniques used in dogs[122] have also been used in large animals.

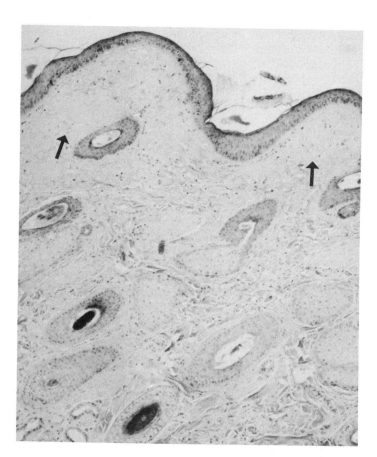

FIGURE 10–7. Equine urticaria. Marked superficial dermal edema (arrows) with minimal cellular infiltration.

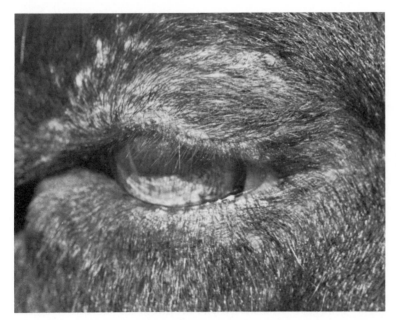

FIGURE 10–8. Periocular crusting in an atopic sheep.

The reader is referred to another text[122] for a detailed discussion of intradermal skin testing.

Allergen Selection. Allergen selection for skin testing is an important subject. There is such a regional variation in floral allergens that it is important to know the specific pollens in your particular locale. Consultations with local physician allergists, botany departments, pollen centers, and allergen firms, in addition to the use of national pollen charts, are essential.

It is important to select allergens from a reputable drug firm and to purchase from only one firm, if possible. Testing with allergen mixes is undesirable. Such mixes frequently result in false-negative reactions and also fail to include many important pollen and mold allergens. For these reasons, skin testing with commercial regional allergen kits is unsatisfactory. Molds, pollens, and dusts appear to be important allergens in horses.[40, 48a, 73, 116, 175] It

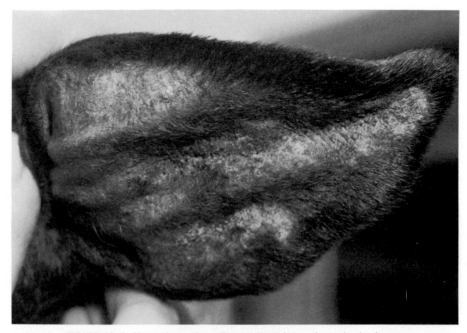

FIGURE 10–9. Alopecia and crusting on the pinna of an atopic sheep.

has been reported that grain mill dust, cottonseed, alfalfa, and black fly antigens may be primary irritants in horses, causing frequent false-positive reactions in normal horses.[56, 57]

It is essential to remember that a positive skin test reaction only means that the patient has skin-sensitizing antibody. It does not necessarily mean that the patient has clinical allergy to the allergen(s) injected. Thus, it is essential that positive skin test reactions be interpreted in light of the patient's history.

There are many factors that may lead to false-positive or false-negative skin test reactions (Tables 10–12 and 10–13). Clearly, intradermal skin testing is not a procedure to be taken lightly. It requires keen attention to details and possible pitfalls, together with experience and extensive practice. Clinicians who cannot do skin testing on a weekly basis will probably be unhappy with the results. When possible, difficult cases should be referred to clinicians who specialize in this field.

Procedure. The procedure of intradermal skin testing is as follows:

1. Make sure the patient is testable. One twentieth (0.05) ml of 1:100,000 histamine phosphate is injected intradermally. A wheal 15 to 20 mm in diameter should be present 15 to 30 minutes after injection. If the histamine wheal is small or absent, testing should be postponed, and the patient should be tested with histamine on a weekly or biweekly basis until the expected reaction is seen.

2. It is preferable to restrain the patient in a standing position. Fractious animals can be sedated with xylazine hydrochloride (Rompun). Phenothiazine tranquilizers should not be used, as they can inhibit skin test reactions.

TABLE 10–12. Reasons for False-Positive Intradermal Skin Test Reactions*

Irritant test allergens (especially those containing glycerin; also some house dust, feather, wool, mold, and food preparations)
Contaminated test allergens (bacteria, fungi)
Skin-sensitizing antibody only (prior clinical or present subclinical sensitivity)
Poor technique (traumatic placement of needle; dull or burred needle; too large a volume injected; air injected)
Substances that cause nonimmunologic histamine release (narcotics)
"Irritable" skin (large reactions seen to *all* injected substances, including saline control)
Dermatographism

*From Muller, G. H., et al.: *Small Animal Dermatology*, 3rd ed. Philadelphia, W. B. Saunders Co., 1983, p. 407.

TABLE 10–13. Reasons for False-Negative Intradermal Skin Test Reactions*

Subcutaneous injections
Too little allergen
  Testing with mixes
  Outdated allergens
  Allergens too dilute (1000 PNU/ml recommended)
  Too little volume of allergen injected
Drug interference
  Glucocorticoids
  Antihistamines
  Tranquilizers
  Progestational compounds
  Any drug that lowers blood pressure significantly
Anergy (testing during peak of hypersensitivity reaction)
Inherent host factors
  Estrus, pseudopregnancy
  Severe stress (systemic disease, fright, struggling)
Endo- or ectoparasitism? ("blocking" of mast cells with antiparasitic IgE?)
Off-season testing (testing more than one to two months after clinical signs have disappeared)
Histamine hyporeactivity

*From Muller, G. H., et al.: *Small Animal Dermatology*, 3rd ed. Philadelphia, W. B. Saunders Co., 1983, p. 407.

3. The skin over the lateral neck (horse) or lateral thorax (sheep) is the preferred test site. The hair or wool is gently clipped with a no. 40 blade, and no chemical preparation is used to clean the test site. A felt-tipped pen is used to mark each injection site. Injection sites are placed at least 2.5 cm apart, avoiding dermatitic areas.

4. Using a 25- to 26-gauge ⅜-in needle attached to a 1-ml disposable syringe, 0.05 ml of each test allergen (1000 protein nitrogen units [PNU]/ml or 1000 w/v strengths) is carefully injected intradermally. In addition, 0.05 ml of saline or diluent control (negative control) and 0.05 ml of 1:100,000 histamine phosphate (positive control) are injected intradermally. The test sites are read at 15 and 30 minutes and at four hours.

5. By convention, a "2-plus" or greater reaction is considered potentially significant and must be carefully correlated with the patient's history. With experience, positive reactions may be "guesstimated" by visual inspection (Fig. 10–10). However, it is strongly recommended that the novice *measure* in millimeters the diameter of each wheal. A positive skin test reaction may then be objectively defined as a wheal whose diameter is equal to or greater than the diameter that represents the halfway point between the saline and histamine controls.

The size of positive skin test reactions does not necessarily correlate with clinical impor-

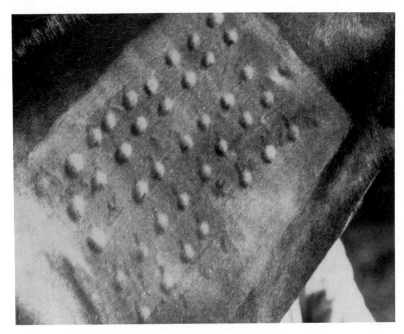

FIGURE 10–10. Positive skin test reactions on the neck of an atopic horse.

tance. Systemic reactions (urticaria, anaphylaxis) to intradermal skin testing are extremely rare.[114, 175]

HISTOPATHOLOGY

Skin biopsy reveals variable degrees of superficial or deep perivascular dermatitis with numerous eosinophils (Figs. 10–11 and 10–12).[48a, 169, 175, 187] Histopathologic findings consistent with secondary pyoderma (suppurative folliculitis, intraepidermal pustular dermatitis) may be seen.

CLINICAL MANAGEMENT

Therapy for atopy includes various combinations of avoidance, hyposensitization, and systemic glucocorticoids.

Avoidance. Avoidance of allergen(s) is fre-

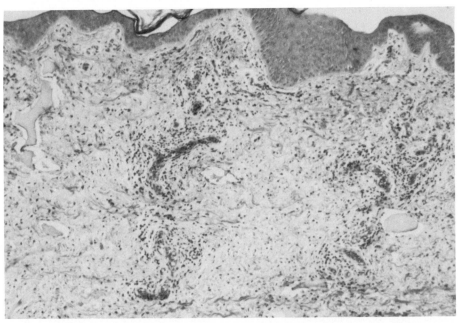

FIGURE 10–11. Ovine atopy. Hyperplastic superficial perivascular dermatitis.

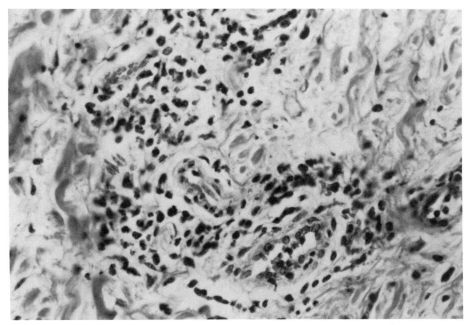

FIGURE 10–12. Ovine atopy. Perivascular eosinophils and lymphocytes.

quently impossible or impractical. However, such a tactic is impossible without having first identified the allergen(s) causing the atopy by intradermal skin testing.

Systemic Glucocorticoids. Systemic glucocorticoids are usually effective in the management of atopy. Prednisolone or prednisone are administered orally at 1 mg/kg s.i.d. for five to seven days, and then on an alternate-morning basis, as needed. The clinician must always strive for the lowest possible dose, at the least frequent interval, that will just control the pruritus.

Hyposensitization. Hyposensitization (immunotherapy) is indicated when avoidance is impossible and when the necessary regimens of glucocorticoids are unsatisfactory or contraindicated. The mechanism of action of hyposensitization is unclear. Various hypotheses include (1) humoral desensitization (reduced levels of IgE), (2) cellular desensitization (reduced reactivity of mast cells and basophils), (3) immunization (induction of blocking antibody), (4) generation of allergen-specific suppressor cells, or (5) some combination thereof.[122]

Experiences with hyposensitization in horses are limited[40, 48a, 56, 157, 175] and such experiences in sheep have not been reported. Some authors have utilized the hyposensitization schedules published for use in atopic dogs (Table 10–14).[56, 157] The author has employed the hyposensitization schedule outlined in Table 10–15.

By convention, no more than ten allergens are used at once for hyposensitization. If a beneficial response is not seen after six months of hyposensitization, the program is abandoned. For animals that derive benefit from hyposen-

TABLE 10–14. Hyposensitization Schedule for Aqueous Allergens*

Injection No.	Day No.	Vial 1† (100–200 PNU/ml)	Vial 2 (1000–2000 PNU/ml)	Vial 3 (10,000–20.000 PNU/ml)
1	1	0.1 ml		
2	2	0.2 ml		
3	4	0.4 ml		
4	6	0.8 ml		
5	8	1.0 ml		
6	10		0.1 ml	
7	12		0.2 ml	
8	14		0.4 ml	
9	16		0.8 ml	
10	18		1.0 ml	
11	20			0.1 ml
12	22			0.2 ml
13	24			0.4 ml
14	26			0.8 ml
15	28			1.0 ml
16	38			1.0 ml
17	48‡			1.0 ml

*Injections are given subcutaneously.

†Protein nitrogen unit (PNU) value of each vial represents the *total* of all allergens used.

‡Thereafter, repeat injections (1.0 ml) every 20 to 40 days, as needed.

(From Muller, G. H., et al.: *Small Animal Dermatology,* 3rd ed. Philadelphia, W. B. Saunders Co., 1983, p. 411.)

TABLE 10–15. Hyposensitization Schedule for Alum-Precipitated Allergens*

Injection No.	Week No.	Dose in PNU†
1	1	100
2	2	200
3	3	400
4	5	800
5	8	1,500
6	12	2,000
7	16	3,000
8	20	6,000
9‡	24	10,000

*Injections are given subcutaneously.
†Dose is per allergen.
‡Thereafter, repeat injections (10,000 PNU each allergen) every one to six months as needed.
(From Muller, G. H., et al.: *Small Animal Dermatology*, 3rd ed. Philadelphia, W. B. Saunders Co., 1983, p. 412.)

sitization, booster injections of allergen are administered as needed (when clinical signs first begin to reappear). Adverse reactions to hyposensitization (intensification of clinical signs; urticaria; and anaphylaxis) rarely occur and are treated symptomatically.

A number of drugs used to treat equine atopy have shown little or no success, including (1) antihistamines, (2) acetylsalicylic acid, (3) phenylbutazone, and (4) diethylcarbamazine. Recently, hydroxyzine has been reported to be effective in the management of some horses with chronic pruritus or urticaria, or both, when given orally at a dosage of 200 to 400 mg b.i.d.[157]

CONTACT HYPERSENSITIVITY

Contact hypersensitivity is a rare, variably pruritic dermatitis of large animals.

CAUSE AND PATHOGENESIS

Reports of naturally occurring contact hypersensitivity in large animals have not been documented by patch testing. Thus, the literature on naturally occurring contact hypersensitivity in these species is of dubious validity and value.

In most instances, contact hypersensitivity represents a Type IV hypersensitivity reaction.* The antigens (haptens) are substances of low molecular weight that penetrate the skin and form covalent bonds with cutaneous proteins. The resultant hypersensitivity reaction shows specificity for both the haptenic group and the protein carrier. Occasionally, contact hypersensitivity is due to a Type I hypersensitivity reaction.[110, 122]

Experimentally, Type IV hypersensitivity reactions have been induced and studied in the skin of cattle* and swine.[19, 107, 113]

CLINICAL FEATURES

Clinically, putative contact hypersensitivity is reported to occur with moderate frequency in the horse.† Rarely is the sensitizing contactant something new in the animal's environment. The most commonly incriminated contact sensitizers in horses include pasture plants, bedding, soaps, insect repellents, topical medicaments, and tack items (dyes and preservatives). Moisture is an important predisposing factor because it decreases the effectiveness of the normal skin barrier and increases the intimacy of contact between the agent and the skin surface. In this respect, the sweating horse is an ideal candidate for contact hypersensitivity.

Skin lesions are characterized by transient papules and vesicles, erythema, oozing, crusting, and variable pruritus, which may progress to alopecia, lichenification, and pigmentary changes. The area of the body affected often suggests the contactant: face, ears, neck (insect repellents and sprays); muzzle and extremities (pasture, bedding), face and trunk (tack). Again, because of the horse's ability to sweat profusely, contactants have access to the skin even in heavily haired areas.

DIAGNOSIS

The differential diagnosis includes primary irritant contact dermatitis (more probable), various ectoparasitisms, and other hypersensitivities. Definitive diagnosis is based on history, physical examination, provocative exposure, and patch testing.[33, 53, 87, 122, 124, 197] Provocative exposure involves avoiding contact with suspected allergenic substances for seven to ten days at a time. The animal is then re-exposed to these substances, on an individual basis, and observed for an exacerbation of

---

*References 3, 15, 22, 33, 53, 75, 110, 122, 136, 189, 197

*References 1, 31, 76, 91, 93, 118, 148, 177
†References 33, 36, 53, 87, 100, 109a, 124, 150, 178, 197

the dermatosis over a seven- to ten-day period. Provocative exposure is time-consuming, requires a patient, dedicated owner, and frequently is impossible to undertake. Additionally, provocative exposure does not distinguish between hypersensitivity and irritant skin reactions.

The patch test is the only test for documenting contact hypersensitivity.[110, 122] Classically, test substances are applied to pieces of cloth or soft paper that are then placed directly on intact skin, covered with an impermeable substance, and affixed to the skin with tape. After 48 hours, the patches are removed, and the condition of the underlying skin is assessed. Patch testing is rarely done because of (1) the logistic problems of applying and securing patch-testing substances to animals and (2) the absence of commercially available patch-testing kits that have been developed for, or shown to be effective in, large animals. Until patch testing becomes standardized for large animals, the diagnosis of contact hypersensitivity will remain elusive. The pitfalls of patch testing and its interpretation are many, and the interested reader is referred to other texts for details.[110, 122]

Skin biopsy findings in experimentally induced contact hypersensitivity in cattle[31, 76, 148, 177] and swine[110, 113] are characterized by spongiotic to hyperplastic superficial perivascular dermatitis with numerous lymphocytes and histiocytes and fewer eosinophils and neutrophils.

CLINICAL MANAGEMENT

Therapy for contact hypersensitivity may include avoidance of the allergen(s) or the use of glucocorticoids.[33, 53, 87, 122, 124, 197] Avoidance of the allergen(s) is preferable but may be impossible because of the nature of the allergen(s) or because the allergen(s) cannot be identified. In such instances, glucocorticoids may be very effective. Gentle cleansing and topical glucocorticoids may suffice. Other animals may require systemic glucocorticoids (prednisolone or prednisone, given orally at 1 mg/kg s.i.d. for five to seven days, then every other morning as needed).

FOOD HYPERSENSITIVITY

Food hypersensitivity is a rarely reported cause of pruritic skin disease in large animals.

CAUSE AND PATHOGENESIS

Diet has long been recognized as a cause of hypersensitivity-like skin reactions in dogs, cats, and humans.[122] Although the pathologic mechanism of food hypersensitivity is unclear, Type I hypersensitivity reactions are well documented, and Type III and Type IV reactions have been suspected.[122]

Food hypersensitivity has been rarely reported in horses,[36, 48a, 53, 72, 100, 124, 197] cattle,[23, 37, 100, 197] and swine.[65, 100, 102, 125] Incriminated substances have included (1) wheat, oats, concentrates, barley, bran, and tonics (horse),[72, 100, 124, 175, 197] (2) wheat, maize, soybeans, rice bran, and clover hay (cattle),[100, 197] and (3) pasture plants (swine).[65, 100, 125] The pathologic mechanism of these reactions is unclear.

CLINICAL FEATURES

Food hypersensitivity in horses and cattle has been characterized by generalized pruritus, with or without papules and plaques, or pruritic urticaria.[48a, 72, 100, 124, 175, 188, 197] In horses, food hypersensitivity may also be characterized by tail rubbing (pruritus ani).[124, 175] Swine with suspected food hypersensitivity manifested generalized erythema.[65, 125] Food hypersensitivity is usually a nonseasonal dermatosis and may be poorly responsive to systemic glucocorticoids.

DIAGNOSIS

The differential diagnosis includes atopy, drug eruptions, various ectoparasitisms, and the various causes of urticaria. In the tail-rubbing horse, the differential diagnosis includes insect hypersensitivity, chorioptic mange, pediculosis, oxyuriasis, and stable vice. Definitive diagnosis is based on history, physical examination, the ruling out of other diagnoses by laboratory tests, elimination diet, and test meal investigation.[122, 197] The animals are fed a hypoallergenic diet for three to four weeks. Hypoallergenic diets must be individualized for each patient, based on careful dietary history. A reasonable place to start is the elimination of all supplements and concentrates, feeding only oat hay for the first three to four weeks, then alfalfa hay for a second three- to four-week period.[48a] The major clinical sign being evaluated during the elimination diet is the pruritus. If the dermatosis resolves, the original diet is reinstituted so as to reproduce the clinical signs, thus confirming the diagnosis.

Skin biopsy is characterized by variable degrees of superficial perivascular dermatitis with eosinophils.[175]

CLINICAL MANAGEMENT

Therapy for food hypersensitivity consists of avoiding offending foods. Hypoallergenic diets are formulated by adding single foodstuffs to the diet, one at a time, and evaluating each item for seven days. When hypoallergenic diets are not feasible, systemic glucocorticoids may be used to suppress clinical signs. However, food hypersensitivity dermatitis may be poorly responsive to glucocorticoids.

DRUG ERUPTION

Drug eruption is a rare, variably pruritic, pleomorphic cutaneous or mucocutaneous reaction to a drug.

CAUSE AND PATHOGENESIS

Drugs responsible for skin eruptions may be administered orally, topically, or by injection or inhalation. The incidence of drug eruption in large animals is unknown. The pathologic mechanism of drug eruption is thought to involve Types I, II, III, and IV hypersensitivity reactions.*

Drugs reported to cause skin eruptions in large animals include penicillin, streptomycin, oxytetracycline, neomycin, chloramphenicol, sulfonamides, phenothiazines, phenylbutazone, guaifenesin, aspirin, iron-dextrans, diethylstilbestrol, glucocorticoids, and various topical parasiticides. Skin eruptions are also reported to be caused by various biologicals (antisera and vaccines for foot-and-mouth disease; bovine contagious pleuropneumonia; rabies; *Salmonella, Pasteurella,* and *Brucella abortus* strain 19 infections; leptospirosis; strangles; tetanus; botulism; encephalomyelitis; and rinderpest).†

CLINICAL FEATURES

Any drug may cause an eruption, and there is no specific type of reaction for any one drug.

Thus, drug eruption can mimic virtually any dermatosis (e.g., urticaria, papular dermatitis, generalized pruritus, or vesicular dermatitis). No breed, age, or sex predilections have been reported for large animal drug eruptions.

Because drug eruption can mimic so many different dermatoses, it is imperative to have all accurate information regarding the medications given to any patient with an obscure dermatosis. Drug eruption may occur after a drug has been given for days or years or a few days after drug therapy is stopped.

DIAGNOSIS

The differential diagnosis is complex, as the signs of drug eruption may resemble any dermatosis. In general, there are no specific or characteristic laboratory findings in drug eruption. Just as the clinical morphology of drug eruptions varies greatly, so do the histologic findings. Histopathologic patterns recognized with cutaneous drug eruptions include perivascular dermatitis, interface dermatitis, and intraepidermal or subepidermal vesicular dermatitis. The only reliable test for the diagnosis of drug eruption is to withdraw the drug and observe for the disappearance of the eruption in 10 to 14 days. Purposeful readministration of the offending drug to see whether the eruption is reproduced confirms the diagnosis but may be dangerous and produce anaphylaxis.

CLINICAL MANAGEMENT

Therapy for drug eruption includes (1) discontinuing the offending drug, (2) symptomatic topical and systemic medications, and (3) avoidance of chemically related drugs. Drug eruptions may be poorly responsive to glucocorticoids.

EQUINE INSECT HYPERSENSITIVITY

Equine insect hypersensitivity is a common, seasonal, pruritic dermatosis of horses, associated with a hypersensitivity to the bites of various *Culicoides* and *Simulium* species, *Stomoxys calcitrans,* and, possibly, *Haematobia (Lyperosia) irritans.*

CAUSE AND PATHOGENESIS

This disorder represents Type I and Type IV hypersensitivity reactions to salivary antigen(s) from numerous *Culicoides* (gnats) and

---

*References 22, 53, 75, 100, 122, 197, 199
†References 4, 5, 20–23, 29, 33, 36, 37, 52, 53, 58, 72, 98, 100, 114, 124, 138, 146, 151, 175, 197

Simulium (black flies) species, *Stomoxys calcitrans* (stable fly), and possibly Haematobia *(Lyperosia) irritans* (horn fly).* *Culicoides* gnats are the most important cause of this syndrome. Results of gnat-collection techniques, intradermal skin testing with gnat antigens, and passive cutaneous anaphylaxis trials have incriminated numerous *Culicoides* species: *C. brevitarsus (robertsi),* in Australia[138, 154]; *C. obsoletus,* in Canada[97]; *C. pulicaris,* in Great Britain†; *C. lupicaris, C. nubeculosus, C. punctatus, C. imicola,* and *C. circumscriptus,* in Israel[26]; and *C. variipenis, C. insignis, C. spinosus,* and *C. stellifer,* in the United States.[56, 70, 114, 115, 166] Clinical evidence strongly suggests that this disorder has familial and, therefore, genetic predilections.‡

In general, adult *Culicoides* gnats are most active when the ambient temperature is above 50°F, when humidity is high, and when there is no breeze. Because there are so many *Culicoides* species worldwide, biting times and sites are quite variable from region to region. Gnats are most numerous in swampy areas and wetlands.

CLINICAL FEATURES

Insect hypersensitivity is the most common hypersensitivity dermatosis and pruritic skin disease of the horse and is worldwide in distribution.§ It has been previously reported under a number of names, including "Dhobie itch," "Kasen," sweet itch, microfilarial pityriasis, summer sores, psoriasis, mange, Queensland itch, summer eczema, "lichen tropicus," summer itch, allergic urticaria, summer dermatitis, and allergic dermatitis. This disease is distinctly seasonal (warm weather) in colder climates but may be almost nonseasonal in warmer climates. The condition usually worsens with age. It may affect horses of any breed, age, or sex but is generally uncommon in horses younger than two years of age. Usually, only one or a few horses on any one premise are affected, and there may be a familial history of pruritic skin disease.

Affected horses may show one of three patterns of skin disease: (1) dorsal distribution,

(2) ventral distribution, and (3) some combination thereof. Dorsal insect hypersensitivity is characterized by an intensely pruritic, papulocrustous dermatitis of the head, ears, neck, withers, back, croup, and tailhead. Severely and chronically affected horses develop excoriations, alopecia, lichenification, pigmentary disturbances, and a rat-tail (Fig. 10–13) and "buzzed-off" mane (Fig. 10–14). Ventral insect hypersensitivity is characterized by an intensely pruritic, papulocrustous dermatitis that may affect the legs, groin, axillae, intermandibular space, ventral thorax, and ventral abdomen (Figs. 10–15 and 10–16). Combination insect hypersensitivity may have features of both of the first two distributions or may be truly generalized. Affected horses scratch and nibble at themselves and rub on environmental obstacles (e.g., doorways, posts, fences, walls, and tree stumps). These horses may be quite

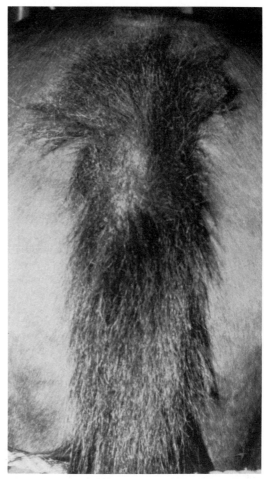

FIGURE 10–13. Equine insect hypersensitivity. Typical "rat-tailed" appearance with broken, disheveled tail hairs.

---

*References 7–9, 26, 33, 55, 56a, 88, 89, 97, 114, 115, 117, 125–128, 138, 147, 154, 157, 192

†References 8, 9, 111, 112, 117, 147, 190

‡References 8, 26, 55, 61, 88, 89, 97, 112, 125–128, 138, 152, 192

§References 8, 9, 26, 55, 56a, 61, 77, 85, 88, 89, 97, 103, 106, 109a, 111, 112, 114, 115, 117, 126–128, 138, 149, 152, 188, 191, 192

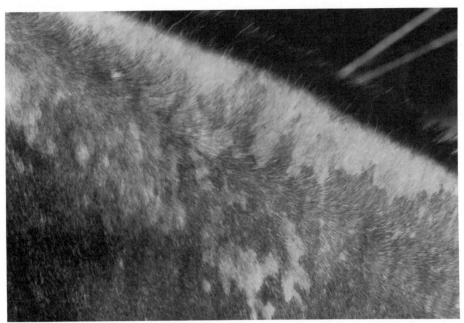

FIGURE 10–14. Equine insect hypersensitivity. Alopecia, crusting, and a "buzzed-off" mane.

anxious, nervous, and unfit for riding or working.

DIAGNOSIS

The differential diagnosis includes various ectoparasitisms and other hypersensitivity dermatoses. The definitive diagnosis is based on history, physical examination, the ruling out of other disease by laboratory tests, and the response to therapy.

Skin biopsy reveals variable degrees of superficial or superficial and deep perivascular dermatitis with eosinophilia (Fig. 10–17).[*] Focal areas of epidermal spongiosis, leukocytic exocytosis, and necrosis (epidermal nibbles) may be seen. In a few horses, small focal areas of collagen degeneration and eosinophilic granulomatous inflammation are seen. Eosinophilic folliculitis may be present.

Most horses with insect hypersensitivity are reported to have peripheral eosinophilia and elevated blood histamine levels.[†] However, neither of these findings has any particular diagnostic significance.

Intradermal skin testing has been reported to be very helpful in the diagnosis of insect hypersensitivity.[‡] The intradermal injection of aqueous whole insect antigens *(Culicoides* and *Simulium* species, Haematobia *[Lyperosia] irritans,* and *Stomoxys calcitrans)* has been reported to produce immediate and/or delayed reactions in affected horses. However, these antigens are not generally available commercially, and testing procedures require standardization and validation. Some investigators believe that grain mill dust, cottonseed, alfalfa, and black fly antigens may be primary irritants in horses, resulting in many false-positive reactions in normal horses.[56, 157] In one study,[56] the frequency of positive intradermal reactions to insect and mold antigens was found to increase with age in normal horses. The author has found the intradermal injection of 0.05 ml of commercial flea antigen (Flea Antigen 1:1000 w/v; Greer Laboratories) to be of no diagnostic value in horses with insect hypersensitivity.

CLINICAL MANAGEMENT

Treatment of insect hypersensitivity in horses involves (1) insect control and (2) systemic antipruritic drugs.[*] When it is feasible, protective housing is an effective preventive.[†] Insect-proof stables may be required during a

*References 8, 55, 56, 56a, 97, 115, 152, 175
†References 8, 55, 97, 114, 115, 128, 154, 155
‡References 8, 9, 26, 55, 56, 56a, 115, 128, 147, 154, 155, 157, 192

*References 8, 9, 55, 56a, 88, 97, 114, 115, 126–131, 138, 152–155, 175, 188
†References 8, 55, 56a, 88, 97, 114, 115, 117, 126–128, 138, 153, 154, 188

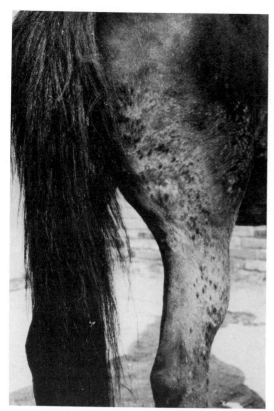

FIGURE 10–15. Patchy alopecia, crusts, and melanotrichia on the rear legs of a horse with insect hypersensitivity.

from crawling down these hairs to the skin.[8, 114, 188] However, such tactics are laborious, messy, and often ineffective.

Where protective housing and insecticidal treatments are inadequate or infeasible, systemic antipruritic agents are necessary. Systemic glucocorticoids are the agents of choice.* Prednisone or prednisolone is given orally at 1 mg/kg s.i.d. until the pruritus is controlled and then is tapered to the lowest alternate-morning dose that is effective. Antihistamines, tranquilizers, and diethylcarbamazine are usually ineffective.† Hydroxyzine was reported to be beneficial in some horses with insect hypersensitivity when administered orally at a dosage of 200 to 400 mg b.i.d.[157]

Hyposensitization has been attempted in horses with insect hypersensitivity.[56, 157]

---

*References 8, 55, 56a, 97, 109a, 114, 138, 175, 188
†References 41, 51, 53, 55, 75, 114, 126–130, 175

particular time of day or night or on a constant basis. *Culicoides* gnats are able to pass through mosquito netting and screens and require a smaller mesh screen (32 by 32). Housing and screens may be sprayed with residual insecticides as needed. In addition, time-operated spray-mist insecticide delivery mechanisms are useful.

Insect control often involves the use of insecticides on affected horses.* Weekly sprays with various pyrethroids or organophosphates are useful. In addition, cattle ear tags impregnated with various pyrethroid or organophosphate insecticides have been helpful when attached to halters or braided into the manes and tails of affected horses. Recently, a commercial bath oil (Skin-So-Soft) diluted with equal parts of water has achieved success as a wipe-on repellent.[56a] The maintenance of a continuous film of liquid paraffin or mineral oil on the skin and hairs of the mane and tail has been reported to prevent *Culicoides* gnats

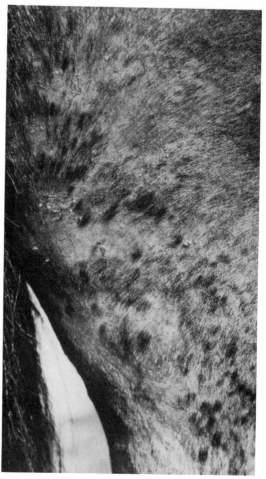

FIGURE 10–16. Patchy alopecia, crusting, and melanotrichia on the rear leg of a horse with insect hypersensitivity.

---

*References 8, 55, 56a, 88, 97, 114, 115, 117, 126–128, 131, 138, 153, 188

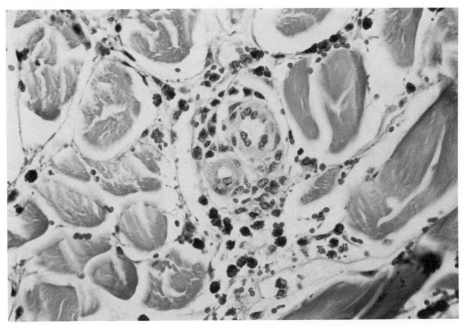

FIGURE 10–17. Equine insect hypersensitivity. Perivascular eosinophils.

Aqueous whole insect antigens were used, with a dosage and frequency schedule identical to that used in dogs (see discussion on atopy). Hyposensitization was consistently ineffective whenever *Culicoides* species were involved. A few horses with only mosquito or black fly hypersensitivity appeared to respond well.

The author[175] has successfully hyposensitized three of six horses with insect hypersensitivity (the precise insect(s) involved *not* determined by skin testing) with a commercial aqueous whole flea antigen (Flea Antigen 1:1000 w/v; Greer Laboratories). One ml was administered intradermally on a weekly basis until effective (three to eight weeks). Booster injections were given as needed (every one to two months). One of the three horses that was unsuccessfully treated developed generalized urticaria after the third injection, which recurred after the fourth injection, at which point hyposensitization was stopped.

MISCELLANEOUS PARASITE HYPERSENSITIVITIES

ONCHOCERCIASIS

Equine cutaneous onchocerciasis is believed to be a hypersensitivity reaction associated with the microfilariae of *Onchocerca cervicalis* (see Chapter 9, discussion on onchocerciasis).

INTESTINAL PARASITE HYPERSENSITIVITY

Various intestinal parasites have been suspected of being associated with pruritic and seborrheic allergic dermatoses in foals.[100, 197] The cause-and-effect relationship and pathologic mechanism of such reactions are unclear.

HABRONEMIASIS

Equine cutaneous habronemiasis is believed to be, in part, a hypersensitivity reaction to the larval stages of *Habronema muscae*, *H. majus*, and *Draschia megastoma* (see Chapter 9, discussion on habronemiasis).

PEMPHIGUS FOLIACEUS

Pemphigus foliaceus is a rare autoimmune dermatosis of horses and goats characterized by widespread vesicles, pustules, and crusts.

CAUSE AND PATHOGENESIS

Pemphigus is characterized histologically by intraepidermal acantholysis and immunologically by the presence of an autoantibody (pemphigus antibody) against the glycocalyx of keratinocytes.[122] The proposed pathologic mechanism of blister formation in pemphigus includes (1) the binding of pemphigus antibody

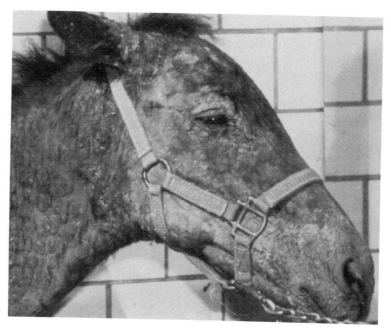

FIGURE 10–18. Equine pemphigus foliaceus. Severe crusting, scaling, and alopecia of the face and neck.

at the glycocalyx of keratinocytes, which results in an inhibition of cellular protein and RNA synthesis, and (2) resultant activation and release of a keratinocyte proteolytic enzyme (pemphigus acantholytic factor), which diffuses into the extracellular space and hydrolyzes the glycocalyx. The resultant loss of intercellular cohesion leads to acantholysis and blister formation within the epidermis. Pemphigus represents a Type II hypersensitivity reaction.

CLINICAL FEATURES

Pemphigus foliaceus has been reported in horses* and goats.[90, 171] There are no age or sex predilections, but Appaloosas may be predisposed.[174a] Lesions usually begin on the face or limbs (Figs. 10–18 and 10–19) and become widespread (see Plate 7). In some horses, only

*References 45a, 48, 64, 70a, 92, 109, 109a, 119, 124, 140, 145, 158, 159, 167, 172, 174a

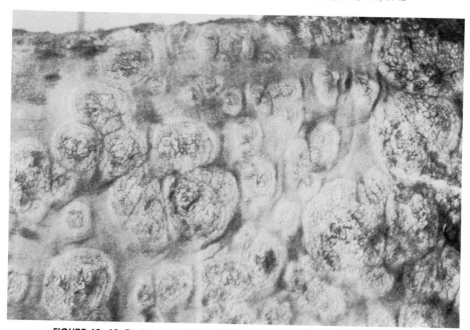

FIGURE 10–19. Equine pemphigus foliaceus. Annular, thick crusts over thorax.

the coronary bands are affected. The primary lesions are vesicles and pustules. However, these primary lesions are transient, and the clinician usually sees crusts, scales, oozing, and annular erosions bordered by epidermal collarettes. The Nikolsky sign may be present. Pruritus and pain are variable. Over 50 percent of the patients have concurrent signs of systemic illness (depression, weight loss, poor appetite, and pyrexia).

Diagnosis

The differential diagnosis includes dermatophytosis, dermatophilosis, bacterial folliculitis, zinc-responsive dermatosis (goat), sarcoidosis (horse), and equine exfoliative eosinophilic dermatitis and stomatitis. Definitive diagnosis is based on history, physical examination, direct smears, skin biopsy, and immunofluorescence testing.[109, 122, 172–174a] Results of routine laboratory examinations (hemogram, serum chemistry panel, and serum electrophoresis) are nondiagnostic, often revealing nonregenerative anemia (packed cell volume [PCV] 24 to 28), mild neutrophilia (7.5 to 10.3 thousand/ml), mild hypoalbuminemia (1.7 to 2.0 gm/dl), and mild to moderate elevations of $alpha_2$, beta, and gamma globulins.[174a]

Microscopic examination of direct smears from intact vesicles or pustules or from recent erosions often reveals numerous acanthocytes, numerous neutrophils (nondegenerate) or eosinophils, and no intracellular bacteria (Fig. 10–20). Occasional acanthocytes may be seen in any suppurative condition, but when present in clusters or large numbers in several microscopic fields, they are strongly indicative of pemphigus.

Skin biopsy may be diagnostic or strongly suggestive in pemphigus. Intact vesicles or pustules are essential. Because these lesions are so fragile and transient, it may be necessary to hospitalize the animal so that it can be carefully scrutinized every two to six hours for the presence of primary lesions. Multiple biopsies and serial sections will greatly increase the chances of demonstrating diagnostic histopathologic changes. Pemphigus foliaceus is characterized by intragranular to subcorneal acantholysis with resultant cleft and vesicle or pustule formation (Figs. 10–21 and 10–22).[167, 172–174a] Within the vesicle or pustule, cells from the stratum granulosum may be seen attached to the overlying stratum corneum (granular "cling-ons") (Fig. 10–23). Identical acantholytic lesions may be seen within hair follicles. Acantholytic granular cells may be seen at the surface of erosions (Fig. 10–24). Neutrophils or eosinophils may predominate within the vesicles and pustules.

Direct immunofluorescence testing[16, 167, 172–174a] reveals the diffuse intercellular deposition of immunoglobulin, and occasionally complement, within the epidermis (Fig. 10–25). It is important to sample intact vesicles and pus-

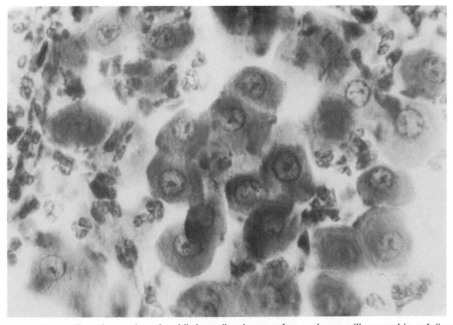

FIGURE 10–20. *Acanthocytes and neutrophils in a direct smear from a horse with pemphigus foliaceus.*

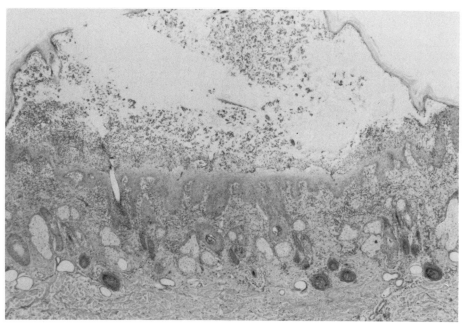

FIGURE 10–21. *Caprine pemphigus foliaceus. Intraepidermal (subcorneal) pustular dermatitis.*

tules and perilesional skin.[122, 172–174a] In addition, glucocorticoid therapy can produce false-negative results and should be stopped for three weeks prior to testing.[174a] Michel's fixative[16, 122, 158, 174a] has been shown to be a reliable fixative for skin specimens intended for direct immunofluorescence testing but must

be maintained at a pH of 7.0 to 7.2. Care must always be taken to correlate the findings of histopathologic and immunopathologic examinations, as direct immunofluorescence testing (intercellular pattern) has been reported to be positive in equine dermatophilosis as well.[170]

Indirect immunofluorescence testing[16, 122, 172–

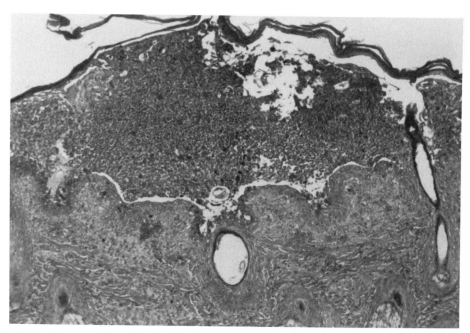

FIGURE 10–22. *Equine pemphigus foliaceus. Intraepidermal (subcorneal) pustular dermatitis with involvement of hair follicles.*

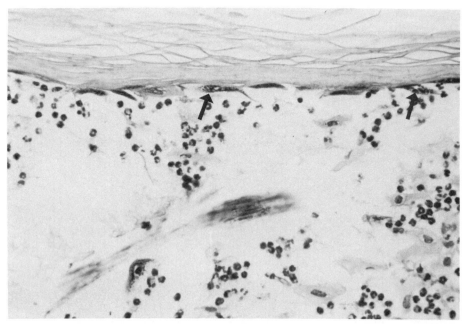

FIGURE 10–23. Caprine pemphigus foliaceus. Granular "cling-ons" (arrows) at the roof of a subcorneal pustule.

[174a] is frequently positive in equine pemphigus foliaceus (titers of 1:10 to 1:8000). However, here again, great caution is warranted when interpreting indirect immunofluorescence results in horses. Pemphigus-like antibodies have been demonstrated in the serum of normal horses and of horses with dermatophilosis and cutaneous lymphosarcoma.[170]

CLINICAL MANAGEMENT

Therapy for pemphigus foliaceus is often difficult, requiring high doses of systemic glucocorticoids, with or without other potent immunomodulating drugs. Additionally, therapy usually must be maintained for prolonged periods of time if not for life. Thus, the thera-

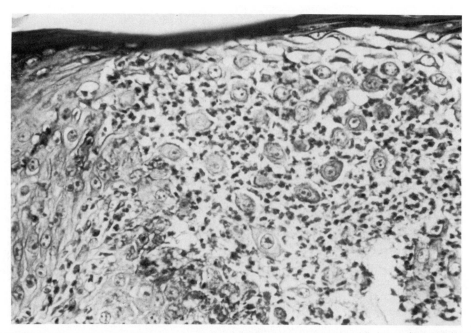

FIGURE 10–24. Equine pemphigus foliaceus. Numerous acanthocytes and neutrophils in a subcorneal pustule.

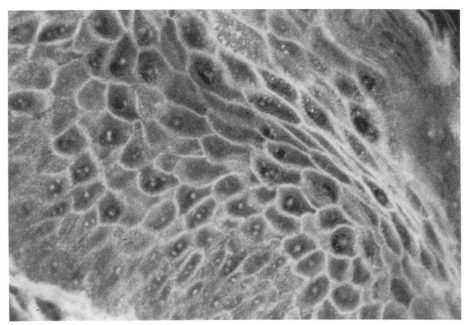

FIGURE 10–25. Caprine pemphigus foliaceus. Deposition of host immunoglobulin in the intercellular spaces of the epidermis on direct immunofluorescence testing.

peutic regimen must be individualized for each patient, and owner education is essential.

High doses of systemic glucocorticoids (1 mg/kg prednisone or prednisolone given orally b.i.d.; 0.2 mg/kg dexamethasone given orally s.i.d.) are the initial treatment of choice.[109, 109a, 119, 140, 173, 174a] Control of the dermatosis is usually achieved within seven to ten days, at which point alternate-morning therapy is begun and is slowly reduced to the lowest possible dosage.

When systemic glucocorticoids are unsatisfactory, the addition or substitution of other immunomodulating drugs may allow significant reduction or termination of glucocorticoid dosage and may result in superior management.[122, 172–174a] Chrysotherapy (gold compound) has been effective in the management of pemphigus foliaceus in horses[48, 70a, 109, 145, 174a] and goats.[171, 174a] Aurothioglucose (Solganal) is administered intramuscularly in two test doses a week apart: 5 and 10 mg for goats and 20 and 40 mg for horses. Patients are then given 1 mg/kg weekly until their disease begins to respond (6 to 12 weeks). Systemic glucocorticoids may be used concurrently with chrysotherapy during the "lag phase," if needed. Injections of gold are then given monthly. In humans, the side effects of chrysotherapy are legion (especially dermatitis and stomatitis) but rarely serious (blood dyscrasia, proteinuria).[122] Adverse reactions to chrysotherapy

have not been reported in horses and goats. It is recommended that a hemogram be checked every two weeks, and a urinalysis every week, during induction (weekly) therapy and then every two to three months during maintenance (monthly) therapy.

BULLOUS PEMPHIGOID

Bullous pemphigoid is a rare autoimmune vesicobullous, ulcerative disorder of skin or oral mucosa, or both, that has been reported in horses.

CAUSE AND PATHOGENESIS

Bullous pemphigoid is characterized histologically by subepidermal vesicle formation and immunologically by the presence of an autoantibody (pemphigoid antibody) against antigen(s) at the basement membrane zone of skin and mucosa.[108, 122] The proposed pathologic mechanism of blister formation in bullous pemphigoid includes (1) the binding of pemphigoid antibody at the basement membrane zone, (2) complement fixation, and (3) chemoattraction of neutrophils and eosinophils, whose release of proteolytic enzymes may disrupt dermoepidermal cohesion, resulting in dermoepidermal separation and vesicle formation.

CLINICAL FEATURES

Bullous pemphigoid has been rarely reported in horses.[64, 108, 124] It is a vesicobullous, ulcerative disorder that may affect the oral cavity, mucocutaneous junctions, skin, or any combination thereof (Figs. 10–26 and 10–27; see Plate 8). Cutaneous lesions occur most commonly in the axillae and groin. Vesicles and bullae are often fragile and transient. Thus, clinical lesions usually include crusts and ulcers bordered by epidermal collarettes. Pain and pruritus are variable. Severely affected horses may be anorectic, depressed, and febrile.

DIAGNOSIS

The differential diagnosis includes drug eruption, candidiasis, vesicular stomatitis, herpes coital exanthema, horsepox, and systemic lupus erythematosus. Definitive diagnosis is based on history, physical examination, skin (or mucosal) biopsy, and immunofluorescence testing.[64, 108, 122] Results of routine laboratory determinations (hemogram, serum chemistry panel, and serum protein electrophoresis) are nondiagnostic, often revealing mild to moderate neutrophilia, mild nonregenerative anemia, mild hypoalbuminemia, and mild to moderate elevations of alpha$_2$, beta, and gamma globulins.

Skin biopsy may be diagnostic or strongly suggestive in bullous pemphigoid. Intact vesicles or bullae are essential, and because of their transient nature, it may be necessary to hospitalize the horse so that it can be carefully scrutinized every two to six hours for the presence of primary lesions. Multiple biopsies and serial sections will greatly increase the chances of demonstrating diagnostic histologic changes. Bullous pemphigoid is characterized histologically by subepidermal vacuolar alteration (subepidermal "bubblies") and subepidermal cleft and vesicle formation (Fig. 10–28).[64, 108, 122] Inflammatory infiltrates are usually mild to moderate and perivascular.

Direct immunofluorescence testing[16, 64, 122] reveals the linear deposition of immunoglobulin and usually complement at the basement membrane zone of skin or mucosa (Fig. 10–29). It is important to sample intact vesicles and perilesional tissue and to withhold glucocorticoid therapy for three weeks prior to testing, if possible.

Indirect immunofluorescence testing[16, 64, 108, 122] may be positive in equine bullous pemphigoid.

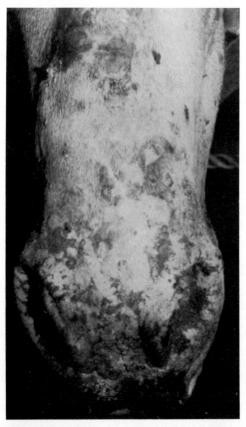

FIGURE 10–26. Multiple ulcers and crusts on the face of a horse with bullous pemphigoid.

CLINICAL MANAGEMENT

Therapy for bullous pemphigoid is often difficult, requiring high doses of systemic glucocorticoids, with or without other potent immunomodulating drugs. Additionally, therapy usually must be maintained for prolonged periods of time if not for life. Thus, the therapeutic regimen must be individualized for each patient, and owner education is essential.

High doses of systemic glucocorticoids (1 mg/kg prednisone or prednisolone given orally b.i.d.; 0.2 mg/kg dexamethasone given orally s.i.d.) are the initial treatment of choice.[108, 122] Maintenance therapy is achieved with the lowest alternate-morning dose possible. In humans and dogs,[108, 122] when systemic glucocorticoids are unsatisfactory, the addition or substitution of other immunomodulating drugs (azathioprine, chlorambucil) or of chrysotherapy may allow significant reduction in dosage or the termination of glucocorticoids and thus lead to

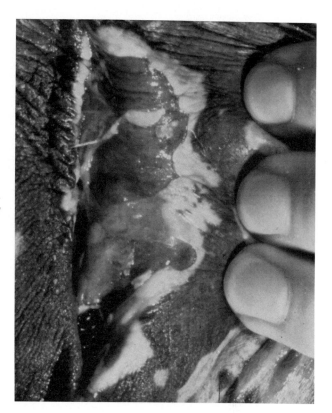

FIGURE 10–27. Ulceration and epidermal collarette at the mucocutaneous junction of the vulva in a horse with bullous pemphigoid.

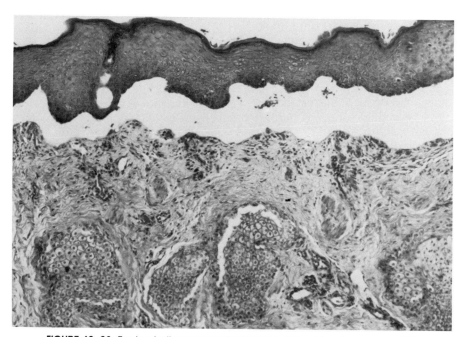

FIGURE 10–28. Equine bullous pemphigoid. Subepidermal vesicular dermatitis.

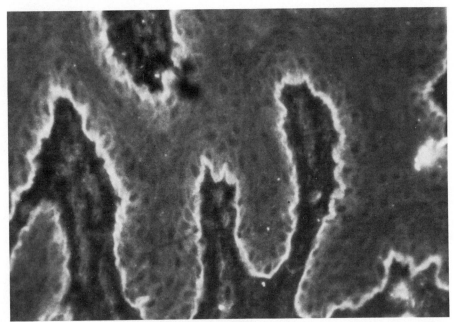

FIGURE 10–29. Equine bullous pemphigoid. Immunoglobulin deposited along the basement membrane zone on indirect immunofluorescence testing.

superior management. Such regimens have not been reported in horses.

SYSTEMIC LUPUS ERYTHEMATOSUS

Systemic lupus erythematosus is a rare multisystemic autoimmune disorder of horses.

CAUSE AND PATHOGENESIS

The etiology of systemic lupus erythematosus appears to be multifactorial, with genetic predilection, immunologic disorder (suppressor T-cell deficiency, B-cell hyperactivity), viral infection, hormones, and ultraviolet light modulation all playing a role.[122] B-cell hyperactivity results in a plethora of autoantibodies formed against numerous body constituents.

CLINICAL FEATURES

Systemic lupus erythematosus has been rarely recognized in horses.[175, 196] Cutaneous changes have included lymphedema of the extremities (Fig. 10–30), panniculitis (Fig. 10–31), and alopecia, leukoderma, and scaling of the face, neck, and trunk (Fig. 10–32). Extracutaneous abnormalities have included poly-arthritis, thrombocytopenia, proteinuria, fever, depression, and weight loss.

DIAGNOSIS

The differential diagnosis of systemic lupus erythematosus is lengthy because of the disorder's varied and changeable manifestations. Definitive diagnosis is based on history, physical examination, skin biopsy, positive antinuclear antibody test, and positive lupus erythematosus cell preparation.[122, 196] The most characteristic dermatohistopathologic finding is hydropic interface dermatitis (Fig. 10–33).

In humans and dogs,[122] direct immunofluorescence testing reveals the deposition of immunoglobulin or complement, or both, at the basement membrane zone. Such studies have not been reported in horses.

CLINICAL MANAGEMENT

The prognosis in systemic lupus erythematosus is, in general, unpredictable.[122] The initial therapeutic agents of choice are high doses of systemic glucocorticoids (1 mg/kg prednisone or prednisolone given orally b.i.d.; 0.2 mg/kg dexamethasone given orally s.i.d.).[175, 196] Maintenance therapy is achieved with the lowest possible alternate-morning dosage.

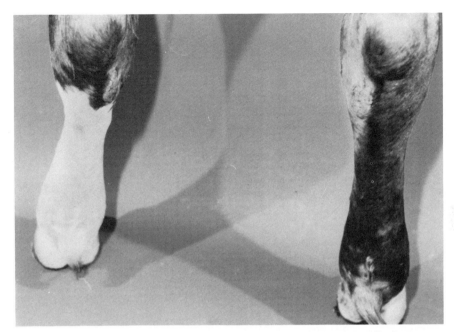

FIGURE 10–30. Equine systemic lupus erythematosus. Lymphedema of the legs.

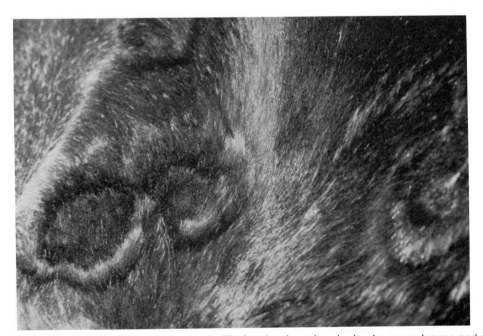

FIGURE 10–31. Equine lupus erythematosus panniculitis. Annular dermal and subcutaneous plaques and nodules over lateral thorax.

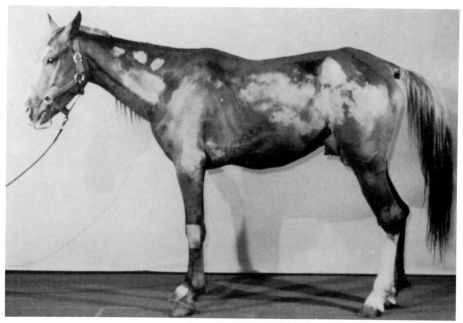

FIGURE 10–32. Equine systemic lupus erythematosus. Multifocal areas of alopecia, scaling, and leukoderma.

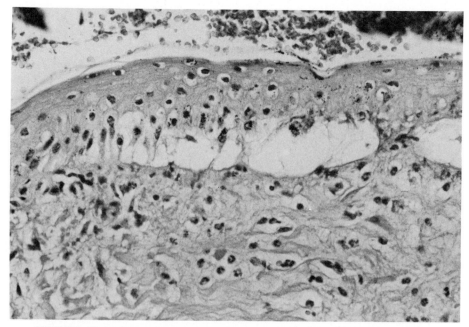

FIGURE 10–33. Equine systemic lupus erythematosus. Hydropic interface dermatitis.

DISCOID LUPUS ERYTHEMATOSUS

Discoid lupus erythematosus is a rare autoimmune dermatitis of horses that is usually confined to the head and neck.

CAUSE AND PATHOGENESIS

In discoid lupus erythematosus, thought to be a benign variant of systemic lupus erythematosus, systemic involvement is absent, and the disorder is confined to the skin.[122]

CLINICAL FEATURES

Discoid lupus erythematosus has been rarely recognized in horses.[175] Clinical signs include patchy erythema, scaling, alopecia, and crusting on the face, ears, and neck (Fig. 10–34). Leukoderma and leukotrichia may be seen within lesions. Affected horses are otherwise healthy.

DIAGNOSIS

The differential diagnosis includes dermatophytosis, onchocerciasis, vasculitis, occult sarcoid, and photodermatitis. Definite diagnosis is based on history, physical examination, skin biopsy, and immunofluorescence testing.[122] Skin biopsy reveals interface dermatitis (hydropic or lichenoid, or both) (Figs. 10–35 and 10–36). The antinuclear antibody and lupus erythematosus cell tests are negative.

Direct immunofluorescence testing reveals the deposition of immunoglobulin or complement, or both, at the basement membrane zone (Fig. 10–37).[122, 175] Indirect immunofluorescence testing is negative.

CLINICAL MANAGEMENT

Therapy for discoid lupus erythematosus must be geared to the individual. Mild cases may be controlled by, and all cases will benefit from, avoidance of exposure to intense sunlight (8:00 A.M. to 5:00 P.M.), the use of topical sunscreens, and the use of topical glucocorticoids (0.1 percent betamethasone-17-valerate; 1 percent hydrocortisone). For more severe or refractory cases, systemic glucocorticoids are usually effective (1 mg/kg prednisone or prednisolone given orally b.i.d.; 0.2 mg/kg dexamethasone given orally s.i.d.). Maintenance therapy is achieved with the lowest possible alternate-morning dosage.

GRAFT-VERSUS-HOST DISEASE

Graft-versus-host disease has been reported in horses given hepatic and thymus cells from fetuses or peripheral blood lymphocytes from unrelated horses.[6, 139] The pathogenesis of graft-versus-host disease is thought to involve cell-mediated as well as antibody-mediated damage to host tissues by donor immunocytes.[122]

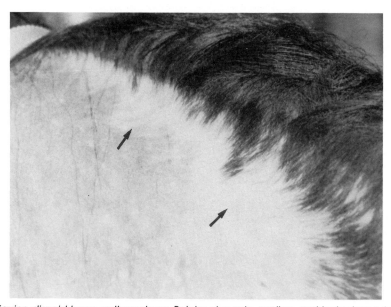

FIGURE 10–34. Equine discoid lupus erythematosus. Patchy alopecia, scaling, and leukoderma (arrows) on neck.

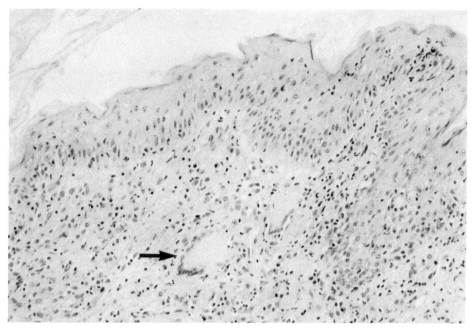

FIGURE 10–35. *Equine discoid lupus erythematosus. Lichenoid interface dermatitis with occasional multinucleated histiocytic giant cells (arrow).*

The principal target organs in graft-versus-host disease are the skin, liver, and alimentary tract.[6, 139] Affected horses develop an exfoliative to ulcerative dermatitis, ulcerative stomatitis, and diarrhea.

Diagnosis is based on history, physical examination, and skin biopsy. Skin biopsy reveals varying degrees of interface dermatitis (hydropic or lichenoid) with satellite-cell necrosis of keratinocytes.[6, 139]

Treatment of graft-versus-host disease emphasizes prevention (close histocompatibility matching) and immunosuppressive chemotherapy.

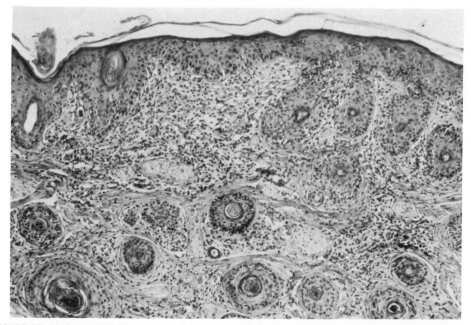

FIGURE 10–36. *Equine discoid lupus erythematosus. Hydropic and lichenoid interface dermatitis.*

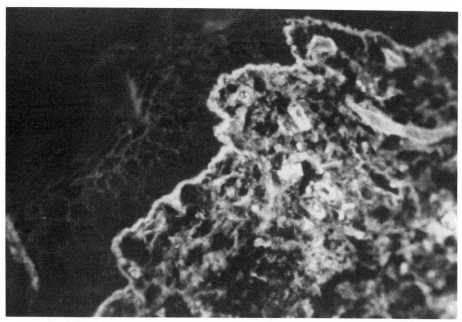

FIGURE 10–37. Equine discoid lupus erythematosus. Deposition of host IgG along the basement membrane zone on direct immunofluorescence testing.

ERYTHEMA MULTIFORME

Erythema multiforme is a rare, acute, self-limited urticarial, maculopapular, or vesicobullous dermatosis of horses and cattle.

CAUSE AND PATHOGENESIS

Despite the recognition of multiple etiologic and triggering causes, the pathogenesis of erythema multiforme is not fully understood.[122, 168, 174b] Recognized causes and precipitating factors of erythema multiforme in humans, dogs, and cats include infectious factors (viral, mycoplasmal, bacterial, and fungal), pregnancy, drugs, neoplasia, connective tissue disorders, and contact reactions. However, in about 50 percent of cases, no known provocative factor can be implicated. No cause has been established for erythema multiforme in horses[168, 174b] and cattle.[175]

Although the pathologic mechanism of erythema multiforme is unknown, it is believed to be a hypersensitivity reaction in a host with a specific immune response to diverse precipitating factors.[122, 168] In some cases of erythema multiforme in humans, direct immunofluorescence testing of lesional skin has revealed IgM and C3 in the walls of superficial blood vessels, and circulating immune complexes were demonstrated in sera.[122, 168]

CLINICAL FEATURES

Erythema multiforme has been recognized in horses[168, 174b] and cattle.[175] Cutaneous eruptions are usually asymptomatic. The clinical appearance of the cutaneous eruptions is variable but is usually monomorphous in any given patient. Eruptions are usually symmetric, often involve the trunk and limbs, and are characterized by maculopapular lesions, urticarial plaques, or vesicobullous lesions. These initial lesions exhibit fairly rapid peripheral expansion and central clearing, resulting in annular, arciform, and polycyclic shapes (Figs. 10–38 and 10–39). Unlike the individual wheals of urticaria, which disappear within hours, the individual wheals of erythema multiforme persist for days to weeks. Conspicuously absent in the maculopapular and urticarial forms of erythema multiforme are the scaling, crusting, and alopecia seen with other dermatoses that are commonly associated with superficial annular lesions (dermatophytosis, dermatophilosis, bacterial folliculitis, seborrhea, occult sarcoid, and pemphigus foliaceus).

DIAGNOSIS

The major differential diagnosis for erythema multiforme includes urticaria, amyloidosis, mastocytoma, lymphosarcoma, and ves-

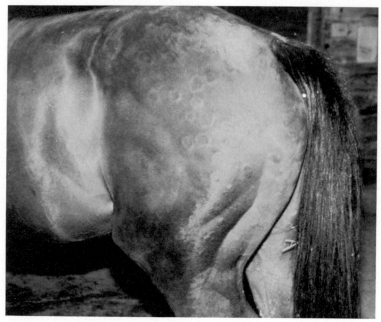

FIGURE 10–38. Erythema multiforme in a horse. Multiple annular, "donut-like" urticarial lesions on the hip.

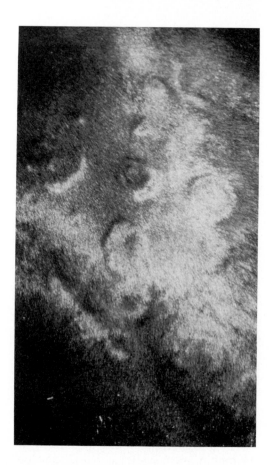

FIGURE 10–39. Equine erythema multiforme. Annular "donut-like" urticarial lesions on the lateral neck.

icular dermatoses. Definitive diagnosis is based on history, physical examination, and skin biopsy.[122, 168] Histologically, erythema multiforme is characterized by hydropic interface dermatitis and single cell necrosis of keratinocytes, with or without marked superficial dermal edema (Fig. 10–40). Vesicular lesions arise through either confluent full-thickness coagulation necrosis of the epidermis or massive subepidermal edema.

CLINICAL MANAGEMENT

The therapy for erythema multiforme is directed at the underlying cause, when found. Symptomatic therapy for the skin lesions is not usually required. Erythema multiforme usually runs a benign, self-limited course, with spontaneous remission occurring within three months.[168, 174b, 175]

VASCULITIS

Cutaneous vasculitis is an uncommon disorder in horses characterized by purpura, edema, necrosis, and ulceration of the extremities and oral mucosa.

CAUSE AND PATHOGENESIS

Vasculitides are often classified histologically into neutrophilic, lymphocytic, eosinophilic, and mixed forms, and the neutrophilic forms may be leukocytoclastic (neutrophil nuclei undergo karyorrhexis, resulting in nuclear dust) or nonleukocytoclastic.[104, 121, 122, 174b, 200] It has been postulated that differences in membrane receptors for immunoglobulin and complement on leukocytes may account for the different histologic appearances of vasculitides. The pathologic mechanism of most cutaneous vasculitides is assumed to involve Type I and Type III hypersensitivity reactions.

In horses, most cutaneous vasculitides have no known etiology. In some cases, especially purpura hemorrhagica, the inciting cause is presumed to be streptococcal infection (e.g., strangles) or various other viral (equine viral arteritis, equine influenza) or bacterial *(Corynebacterium pseudotuberculosis)* infections.[17, 25, 69, 134, 164] Purpura hemorrhagica has been compared with Henoch-Schönlein purpura in humans.[104, 164] In some instances, equine cutaneous vasculitides have been restricted to the white-skinned and haired areas of the pasterns and face, suggesting a photo-induced process.[174b, 180a]

CLINICAL FEATURES

In horses, idiopathic cutaneous vasculitis has no apparent age, breed, or sex predilections.[121, 174b, 200] Cutaneous lesions occur most commonly on the distal limbs, pinnae, lips, and periocular area. Lesions consist of purpura, edema, ery-

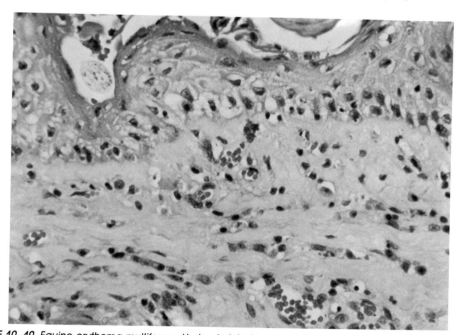

FIGURE 10–40. Equine erythema multiforme. Hydropic interface dermatitis with marked vascular congestion.

thema, necrosis, ulcers, and crusts (see Plate 8). Oral ulcers and occasional bullae may be seen. Affected horses may show signs of systemic illness, including pyrexia, depression, anorexia, and weight loss. Associated disorders have included *Corynebacterium equi* pneumonia, bronchopneumonia, and cholangiohepatitis.[174b]

Purpura hemorrhagica, an acute, noncontagious disease occurring chiefly in horses, is characterized by extensive edematous and hemorrhagic swellings in subcutaneous tissues, accompanied by hemorrhages in the mucosae and viscera.* Similar syndromes have been recorded in swine[25, 133, 163, 181] and cattle.[25] In horses, most cases follow respiratory infections due to *Streptococcus equi* (strangles) or equine influenza. The incidence of equine purpura hemorrhagica is generally low and sporadic. There are no apparent breed or sex predilections, and affected horses are usually over two years old. Clinical signs usually begin acutely within two to four weeks of a respiratory infection, and there may be substantial variation in severity and clinical course. Urticaria may be seen initially and is followed by pitting, edematous swellings of the distal limbs, ventrum, and head. Severe head edema may cause difficulty in breathing and eating. These swellings may progress to exudation and sloughing. Pruritus and pain are usually absent. Petechiae and ecchymoses may be present in visible mucous membranes. Affected horses are usually depressed, stiff, and reluctant to move, but their appetites and body temperatures usually remain normal. Some horses may develop colic or diarrhea, or both.

A syndrome of photoactivated vasculitis has recently been described in horses.[180a] Mature horses (there are no apparent breed or sex predilections) develop severe edema in the nonpigmented areas of the distal limbs during the summer.

DIAGNOSIS

The differential diagnosis includes bullous pemphigoid, systemic lupus erythematosus, equine viral arteritis, drug eruption, and toxicosis. The definitive diagnosis is based on history, physical examination, and biopsy. Skin biopsy reveals neutrophilic (leukocytoclastic), eosinophilic, lymphocytic, or mixed vasculitis (Fig. 10–41).[71, 95, 121, 164, 174b, 200] Fibrinoid degen-

eration and purpura are often present. The lesions most likely to show diagnostic changes are those from 8 to 24 hours old. Horses with purpura hemorrhagica often have mild to moderate anemia, neutrophilia with a mild to moderate left shift, hyperglobulinemia, and hyperfibrinogenemia.[18, 25, 34, 69, 164] Platelet counts and clotting function tests are usually normal.

Direct immunofluorescence testing may demonstrate immunoglobulin or complement, or both, in vessel walls (Fig. 10–42) and occasionally at the basement membrane zone.[121, 174b, 180a, 200] However, direct immunofluorescence is usually not needed, is not particularly useful for diagnosis, and, if it is performed, must be done within the first four hours after lesion formation. Once the diagnosis of cutaneous vasculitis has been established, it is imperative that underlying etiologic factors be sought and eliminated.

CLINICAL MANAGEMENT

It is difficult to predict the course of cutaneous vasculitis in any individual case. There may be only a single episode lasting a few weeks, or the disorder may be chronic or recurrent. The ultimate outcome is dependent upon the extent of internal organ involvement.[25, 69, 164, 174b]

Underlying diseases should be corrected when found and when possible. Some horses with idiopathic cutaneous vasculitis have responded well to systemic glucocorticoids (prednisone or prednisolone given orally at 1 mg/kg b.i.d. until effective, then at the lowest possible alternate-morning dosage).[121, 174b, 200]

In equine purpura hemorrhagica, the earlier that therapy is instituted, the better the prognosis.[25, 34, 69, 164] Death may occur because of secondary complications, such as pyoderma, pneumonia, myositis, or renal failure. Relapses may occur during convalescence. Therapy is directed at (1) correcting underlying bacterial infection (usually streptococcal), (2) correcting edema, and (3) inhibiting the hypersensitivity response. Penicillin is the antibiotic of choice (procaine penicillin G given intramuscularly at 20,000 IU/kg b.i.d.) and is continued for five to seven days after remission. Diuretics (furosemide at 1 mg/kg b.i.d. for two to four days) are useful for alleviating edema. Systemic glucocorticoids (prednisone or prednisolone given orally or intramuscularly at 1 mg/kg b.i.d.) are administered until remission. Hydrotherapy and gentle exercise are also beneficial therapeutic adjuncts.

---

*References 17, 18, 25, 34, 69, 71, 95, 109a, 164

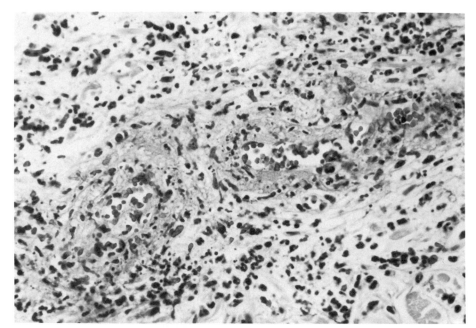

FIGURE 10–41. Equine cutaneous vasculitis. Leukocytoclasis and fibrinoid degeneration of vessel walls.

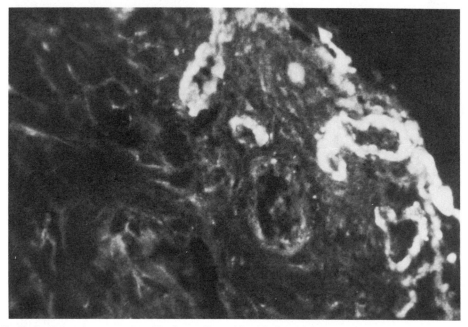

FIGURE 10–42. Equine cutaneous vasculitis. Deposition of host IgG in blood vessel walls on direct immunofluorescence testing.

Horses with photoactivated vasculitis benefit from sun avoidance and systemic glucocorticoids for 30 days.[180a] Most horses do not relapse.

EQUINE EXFOLIATIVE EOSINOPHILIC DERMATITIS AND STOMATITIS

This disorder is associated with exfoliative dermatitis, ulcerative stomatitis, severe wasting, and eosinophilic infiltration of epithelial tissues.

CAUSE AND PATHOGENESIS

The pathogenesis of this syndrome is unknown. However, the severe eosinophilic infiltration and granulomatous inflammation of affected tissues are suggestive of a hypersensitivity reaction.[105] Some authors have suspected a reaction to *Strongylus equinus* lar-

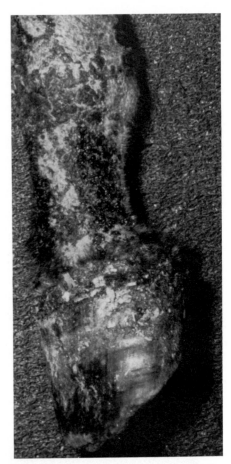

FIGURE 10–44. Equine exfoliative eosinophilic dermatitis and stomatitis. Extensive alopecia, scaling, crusting, and ulceration of leg. (Courtesy J. A. Yager.)

vae,[27] while others have suggested an epitheliotropic cell-associated virus.[201]

CLINICAL FEATURES

There are no apparent age, breed, or sex predilections. The dermatitis usually begins in winter with scaling, crusting, oozing, and fissures on the coronets or face (Figs. 10–43, 10–44, and 10–45). Oral ulceration is an early finding. The dermatosis then develops into a generalized exfoliative dermatitis, with easy epilation, alopecia, ulceration, and exudation. Pruritus is variable. Affected horses develop severe, progressive weight loss, despite a good to ravenous appetite and no diarrhea.

DIAGNOSIS

The differential diagnosis includes dermatophilosis, dermatophytosis, pemphigus foli-

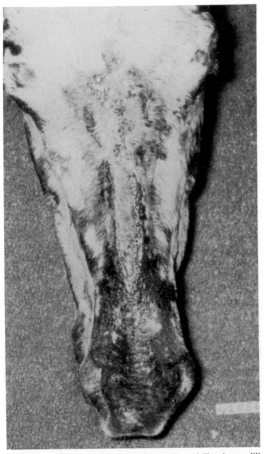

FIGURE 10–43. Equine exfoliative eosinophilic dermatitis and stomatitis. Extensive ulceration and crusting of face. (Courtesy J. A. Yager.)

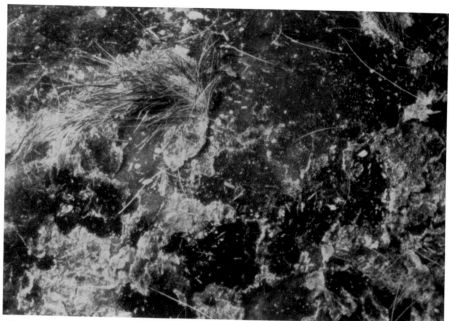

FIGURE 10–45. Equine exfoliative eosinophilic dermatitis and stomatitis. Severe alopecia, crusting, and ulceration over thorax. (Courtesy J. A. Yager.)

aceus, seborrhea, sarcoidosis, systemic lupus erythematosus, and toxicosis. Definitive diagnosis is based on history, physical examination, and skin biopsy. Peripheral eosinophilia is rare. Skin biopsy reveals a superficial and deep eosinophilic and lymphoplasmacytic dermatitis with marked irregular epidermal hyperplasia and orthokeratotic to parakeratotic hyperkeratosis (Fig. 10–46).[27, 105, 201] Exocytosis of eosinophils and lymphocytes, as well as satellite-cell necrosis of keratinocytes is seen.[175] Perivascular collagen degeneration, lymphoid nodules, and a lichenoid inflammatory infiltrate may be seen. In addition, eosinophilic infiltrations and

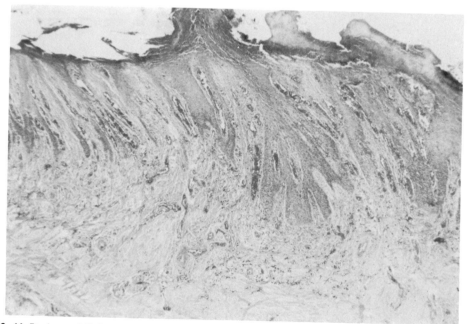

FIGURE 10–46. Equine exfoliative eosinophilic dermatitis and stomatitis. Severely hyperplastic superficial and deep perivascular eosinophilic dermatitis.

eosinophilic granulomas are present in other epithelial organs, including the pancreas, salivary glands, oral cavity, gastrointestinal tract, and bronchial and biliary epithelium. Direct immunofluorescence testing of affected skin has been negative.[27, 201]

CLINICAL MANAGEMENT

The prognosis is grave. Affected horses suffer a progressive dermatitis and wasting for two to four months and then are euthanized.[27, 105, 201] High doses of systemic glucocorticoids (2 mg/kg/day prednisone or prednisolone) have been ineffective.

EQUINE SARCOIDOSIS

This disorder is associated with exfoliative dermatitis, severe wasting, and sarcoidal granulomatous inflammation of multiple organ systems.

CAUSE AND PATHOGENESIS

The pathogenesis of this syndrome is unknown. Pathologically, it closely resembles sarcoidosis in humans. The cause of human sarcoidosis is also unknown, although the disease is thought to represent a pattern of reaction to an infectious agent or allergen.[94]

CLINICAL FEATURES

There are no apparent age, breed, or sex predilections.[124, 175, 180] The dermatitis usually begins as scaling, crusting, and alopecia on the face or limbs and progresses to a generalized exfoliative dermatitis (Fig. 10–47). Peripheral lymph nodes may be palpably enlarged. Affected horses eventually develop a wasting syndrome, characterized by weight loss, poor appetite, exercise intolerance, and persistent low-grade fever.

DIAGNOSIS

The differential diagnosis includes dermatophilosis, dermatophytosis, pemphigus foliaceus, seborrhea, systemic lupus erythematosus, toxicosis, and exfoliative eosinophilic dermatitis and stomatitis. Definitive diagnosis is based on history, physical examination, and skin biopsy. Skin biopsy reveals perifollicular and mid-dermal sarcoidal granulomatous dermatitis with frequent multinucleated histiocytic giant cells (Figs. 10–48 and 10–49). In addition, sarcoidal granulomas are present in other organs, including mesenteric and thoracic lymph nodes, the lungs, gastrointestinal tract, liver, and spleen. Direct immunofluorescence testing of affected skin has been negative. Attempts to isolate bacteria, fungi, and viruses have been unsuccessful, as have electron mi-

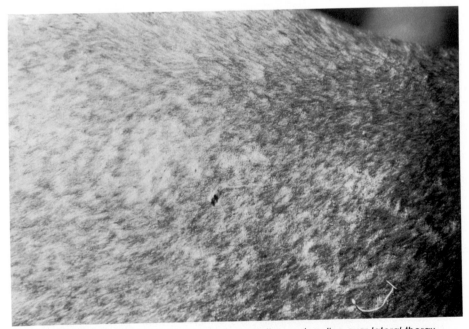

FIGURE 10–47. Equine sarcoidosis. Extensive crusting and scaling over lateral thorax.

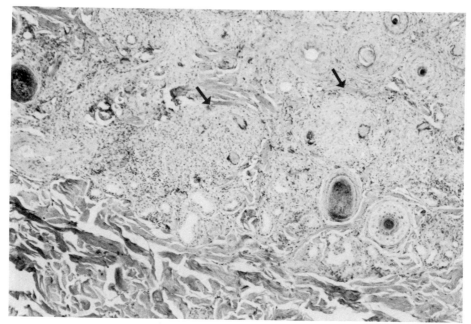

FIGURE 10–48. Equine sarcoidosis. Perifollicular epithelioid granulomas (arrows).

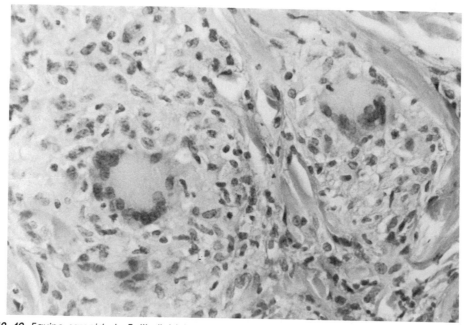

FIGURE 10–49. Equine sarcoidosis. Epithelioid (sarcoidal) granulomas containing multinucleated histiocytic giant cells.

croscopic examinations and animal inoculation studies.[175, 180]

CLINICAL MANAGEMENT

The prognosis is grave. Affected horses suffer a progressive dermatitis and wasting over the course of weeks to months and are eventually euthanized.[124, 175, 180] High doses of systemic glucocorticoids (2 mg/kg/day of prednisone or prednisolone) have occasionally been effective if administered early in the course of the disease and continued on an alternate-morning basis for several weeks. A few horses have experienced spontaneous remissions.

EQUINE CUTANEOUS AMYLOIDOSIS

Amyloidosis is a rare papulonodular disorder of the skin and upper respiratory mucosa of horses.

CAUSE AND PATHOGENESIS

Amyloid is a precise group of proteins with certain physiochemical properties.[42, 104] Although the pathogenesis of amyloidosis is unclear, morphologically, it is related to cells of the mononuclear phagocytic system and plasma cells. Functional studies suggest that such cells play at least a partial role in the genesis of amyloidosis. While immune function in humans is abnormal,[42] these abnormalities do not fully explain why amyloid forms.

In horses, cutaneous amyloidosis rarely, if ever, occurs in conjunction with underlying disease or with visceral involvement.[114, 124, 175, 179] Equine cutaneous amyloidosis closely resembles nodular cutaneous amyloidosis in humans.[42, 104]

CLINICAL FEATURES

There are no apparent age, breed, or sex predilections. Cutaneous lesions include papules, nodules, and plaques, which are most common on the head, neck, shoulders, and pectoral region (Fig. 10–50).[114, 124, 175, 179, 183] The lesions are multiple, firm, well circumscribed, 0.5 to 10 cm in diameter, nonpainful, and nonpruritic. The overlying skin is normal. In some horses, the lesions have an initial rapid onset and urticarial appearance. Such lesions may regress spontaneously or in conjunction with systemic glucocorticoid treatment, only

to recur and assume a chronic, progressive course.

Some horses develop concurrent diffuse or nodular deposits of amyloid in the upper respiratory mucosa, especially the nasal mucosa.[114, 124, 179] Although affected horses are usually healthy otherwise, severe upper respiratory involvement can produce severe dyspnea.

DIAGNOSIS

The differential diagnosis of equine cutaneous amyloidosis includes other asymptomatic nodular skin diseases, such as equine eosinophilic granuloma, mastocytoma, and certain infectious granulomas. The definitive diagnosis is based on history, physical examination, and skin biopsy.[114, 124, 179, 183] Biopsy reveals granulomatous dermatitis with numerous multinucleated histiocytic giant cells (Fig. 10–51). Amyloid is present as a homogeneous, amorphous, hyaline, eosinophilic substance in extra- and intracellular locations (Fig. 10–52). Larger extracellular deposits of amyloid often

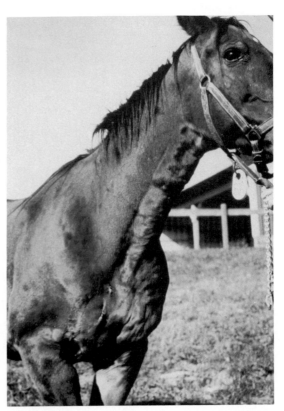

FIGURE 10–50. Equine cutaneous amyloidosis. Multiple nodules on neck and chest.

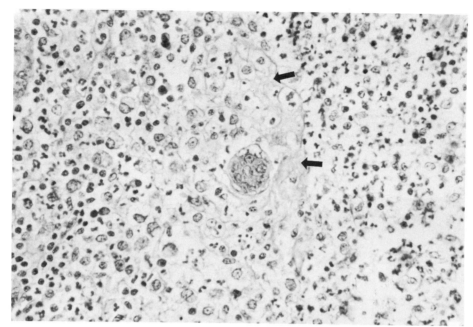

FIGURE 10–51. Equine cutaneous amyloidosis. Pyogranulomatous dermatitis and small amount of extracellular amyloid (arrows).

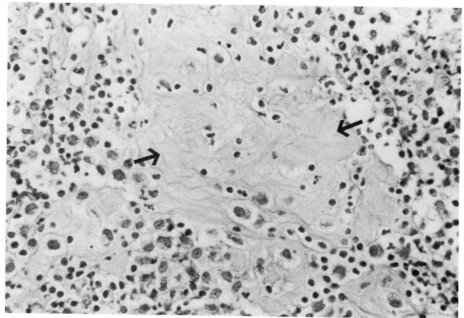

FIGURE 10–52. Equine cutaneous amyloidosis. Pyogranulomatous dermatitis and large extracellular amyloid deposit (arrows).

contain clefts or fractures. Special stains such as Congo red, crystal violet, and thioflavin T are useful in demonstrating that the deposits are amyloid. When Congo red–stained sections are viewed in the polarizing microscope, a unique green birefringence is present.[42, 104] This is the single most useful light microscopic procedure for establishing the presence of amyloid. Electron microscopy reveals typical amyloid filaments, 6 to 10 nm thick, which are straight and nonbranching.[104]

CLINICAL MANAGEMENT

Equine cutaneous amyloidosis usually follows a prolonged and progressive course.[114, 124, 179] There is no effective treatment. Because some forms of cutaneous amyloidosis in humans are inherited,[42, 104] it may not be advisable to use affected horses for breeding.[179]

BOVINE EXFOLIATIVE ERYTHRODERMA

A cow with severe exfoliative erythroderma was studied.[11] Her calves and an unrelated calf that were fed her colostrum developed exfoliative erythroderma. From their birth to four days of age, the calves developed erythema and vesicles on the muzzle. Between 4 and 50 days of age, the calves developed generalized erythema, scaling, easy epilation, and alopecia. By four months of age the calves had recovered. Skin biopsies revealed intraepidermal pustular dermatitis with neutrophils. An immune-mediated disorder associated with colostrum was postulated.

REFERENCES

1. Aitken, M. E., et al.: Investigation of a cutaneous delayed hypersensitivity response as a means of detecting *Salmonella dublin* infection in cattle. Res. Vet. Sci. 24:370, 1978.
2. Alexander, F., et al.: Effects of anaphylaxis and chemical histamine liberators in sheep. J. Comp. Pathol. 83:19, 1970.
3. Alexander, J. W., and Good, R. A.: *Fundamentals of Clinical Immunology.* Philadelphia, W. B. Saunders Co., 1977.
4. Anderson, I. L.: An unusual reaction in a horse during anaesthesia. N. Z. Vet. J. 31:85, 1983.
5. Anderson, W. I., et al.: Adverse reaction to penicillin in horses. Mod. Vet. Pract. 64:928, 1983.
6. Ardans, A. A., et al.: Immunotherapy in two foals with combined immunodeficiency, resulting in graft-versus-host reaction. JAVMA 1970:167, 1977.
7. Baker, K. P.: Sweet itch in horses. Vet. Rec. 93:617, 1973.
8. Baker, K. P., and Quinn, P. J.: A report on clinical aspects and histopathology of sweet itch. Equine Vet. J. 10:243, 1973.
9. Baker, K. P.: The pathogenesis of insect hypersensitivity. Vet. Dermatol. News. 8:11, 1983.
10. Barratt, M. E. J.: Immediate hypersensitivity to *Metastrongylus* spp. infection in the pig. 1. The passive transfer of skin sensitivity to uninfected recipients. Immunology 22:601, 1972.
11. Bassett, H.: Bovine exfoliative dermatitis: A new bovine skin disease transferred by colostrum. Irish Vet. J. 39:106, 1985.
12. Becker, W.: Uber Vorkommer, Ursacheu und Behandlung des sogenannten "Sommerekzems" bei Ponys. Berl. Munch. Tierarztl. Wochenschr. 77:120, 1964.
13. Bellanti, J. A.: *Immunology II.* Philadelphia, W. B. Saunders Co., 1978.
14. Bellocq, P., and Guilhem, P.: Guérison spectaculaire d'un cas de dermite estivale des équidés. Rec. Med. Vet. 136:663, 1960.
15. Benacerraf, B.: *Textbook of Immunology.* Baltimore, Williams & Wilkins Co., 1979.
16. Beutner, E. H., et al.: *Immunopathology of the Skin II.* New York, John Wiley & Sons, 1979.
17. Biggers, J. D., and Ingram, P. L.: Studies on equine purpura haemorrhagica. Review of the literature. Vet. J. 104:214, 1948.
18. Biggers, J. D., et al.: Studies on equine purpura haemorrhagica. Article No. 4—haematology. Br. Vet. J. 105:191, 1949.
19. Bilski, A. J., and Thomson, D. S.: Allergic contact dermatitis in the domestic pig. A new model for evaluating the typical anti-inflammatory activity of drugs and their formulations. Br. J. Dermatol. 111:143, 1984.
20. Black, L., and Pay, T. W. F.: The evaluation of hypersensitivity in cattle after foot-and-mouth disease vaccination. J. Hygiene 74:169, 1975.
21. Black, L.: Allergic skin disease. *In:* Howard, J. L.: *Current Veterinary Therapy. Food Animal Practice.* Philadelphia, W. B. Saunders Co., 1981, p. 1126.
22. Black, L.: Hypersensitivity in cattle. Part I. Mechanisms of causation. Vet. Bull. 49:1, 1979.
23. Black, L.: Hypersensitivity in cattle. Part II. Clinical reactions. Vet. Bull. 49:77, 1979.
24. Black, L., and Burlea, J. F.: Hypersensitivity in cattle. Part III. The mediators of anaphylaxis. Vet. Bull. 49:303, 1979.
25. Blood, D. C., et al.: *Veterinary Medicine VI.* London, Baillière Tindall, 1983.
26. Braverman, Y., et al.: Epidemiological and immunological studies of sweet itch in horses in Israel. Vet. Rec. 112:521, 1983.
27. Breider, M. A., et al.: Chronic eosinophilic pancreatitis and ulcerative colitis in a horse. JAVMA 186:809, 1985.
28. Brewer, R. L.: An allergic condition in Jersey cows. JAVMA 130:181, 1957.
29. Brisbane, W. P.: Antibiotic reactions in cattle. Can. Vet. J. 4:234, 1963.
30. Brownlee, A. J.: Allergy in the domestic animals. J. Comp. Pathol. Ther. 53:55, 1940.
31. Brummerstedt, E., and Basse, A.: Cutaneous hypersensitivity to 2,4-dinitrochlorobenzene in calves. Nord. Vet. Med. 25:392, 1973.
32. Burghardt, H. F., et al.: Dermatitis in cattle due to *Simulium* (black flies). Cornell Vet. 41:311, 1951.
33. Byars, D. T.: Allergic skin diseases in the horse. Vet. Clin. North Am. Large Anim. Pract. 6:87, 1984.
34. Byars, T. D., and Divers, T. J.: Equine purpura haemorrhagica. Georgia Vet. 32:14, 1980.
35. Cameron, R. D. A.: *Skin Diseases of the Pig.* University of Sydney Post-Graduate Foundation in Veterinary Science, Review No. 23, 1984.
36. Campbell, S. G.: Sporadic allergies in the horse. *In:* Catcott, E. J., and Smithcors, J. F.: *Equine Medicine and Surgery II.* Santa Barbara, CA, American Veterinary Publications, Inc., 1972, p. 227.
37. Campbell, S. G.: Allergic reactions. *In:* Gibbons, W. J., et al.: *Bovine Medicine and Surgery.* Santa Barbara, CA, American Veterinary Publications, Inc., 170, p. 317.
38. Campbell, S. G.: The milk proteins responsible for milk allergy, an autoallergic disease of cattle. J. Allergy Clin. Immunol. 48:230, 1971.
39. Campbell, S. G.: Milk allergy, an autoallergic disease of cattle. Cornell Vet. 60:684, 1970.

40. Carr, S. H.: A practitioner report: Equine allergic dermatitis. Florida Vet. J. 10:1, 1981.
41. Chand, N., and Eyre, P.: Nonsteroidal anti-inflammatory drugs: a review. New applications in hypersensitivity reactions of cattle and horses. Can. J. Comp. Med. 41:233, 1977.
42. Cohen, A. S.: An update of clinical, pathologic, and biochemical aspects of amyloidosis. Intl. J. Dermatol. 20:515, 1981.
43. Dahl, M. V.: Immunodermatology. Chicago, Year Book Medical Publishers, 1981.
44. Datta, S.: Microfilarial pityriasis in equines. Vet. J. 95:213, 1939.
45. Davies, P., et al.: The role of arachidonic acid oxygenation products in pain and inflammation. Annu. Rev. Immunol. 2:335, 1984.
45a. Day, M. J., and Penhale, W. J.: Immunodiagnosis of autoimmune skin disease in the dog, cat, and horse. Aust. Vet. J. 63:65, 1986.
46. Dikmans, G.: Skin lesions of domestic animals in the United States due to nematode infestation. Cornell Vet. 38:3, 1948.
47. Elliott, F. A.: Allergens—apparent cause of "summer itch" (equine). Calif. Vet. 13:29, 1970.
48. Edmond, R. J., and Frevert, C.: Pemphigus foliaceus in a horse. Mod. Vet. Pract. 67:527, 1986.
48a. Evans, A. G.: Recurrent urticaria due to inhaled allergens. In: Robinson, N. E.: Current Therapy in Equine Medicine II. Philadelphia, W. B. Saunders Co., 1987, p. 619.
49. Eyre, P.: Anaphylactic (skin-sensitizing) antibodies in the horse. Vet. Rec. 88:36, 1972.
50. Eyre, P.: Cutaneous vascular permeability factors (histamine; 5-hydroxytryptamine; bradykinin) and passive cutaneous anaphylaxis in sheep. J. Pharmacol. Pharm. 22:104, 1970.
51. Eyre, P.: Preliminary studies of pharmacological antagonism of anaphylaxis in the horse. Can. J. Comp. Med. 40:149, 1976.
52. Eyre, P., and Burka, J. F.: Hypersensitivity in cattle and sheep: A pharmacological review. J. Vet. Pharmacol. Ther. 1:97, 1978.
53. Eyre, P., and Hanna, C. J.: Equine allergies. Equine Pract. 2:40, 1980.
54. Eyre, P., and Deline, T. R.: Anaphylactic hypersensitivity in sheep lung in vitro: Vascular Schultz-Dale response and biogenic amine liberation. Arch. Intl. Pharmacodyn. Ther. 222:141, 1976.
55. Fadok, V. A., and Mullowney, P. C.: Dermatologic diseases of horses, part 1. Parasitic dermatoses of the horse. Compend. Cont. Educ. 5:S615, 1983.
56. Fadok, V. A.: Equine pruritus: Results of intradermal skin testing. Proc. Annu. Meet. Am. Acad. Vet. Dermatol. & Am. Coll. Vet. Dermatol. New Orleans, 1986.
56a. Fadok, V. A.: Culicoides hypersensitivity. In: Robinson, N. E.: Current Therapy in Equine Medicine II. Philadelphia, W. B. Saunders Co., 1987, p. 624.
57. Falck, B., et al.: Dopamine and mast cells in ruminants. Acta Pharmacol. Toxicol. 21:51, 1964.
58. Ficarelli, R., et al.: Eczema ad insorgenza ritardata dopo vaccina zione antiaftosa del bovino e loro terapia. Clin. Vet. Milano 94:173, 1971.
59. Fincher, M. G.: Anaphylaxis and related reactions in cattle. Allied Vet. 31:135, 1960.
60. Ford-Hutchinson, A. W., and Chan, C. C.: Pharmacological actions of leukotrienes in the skin. Br. J. Dermatol. 113:95, 1985.
61. Frost, R. D. I.: Sweet itch. Vet. Rec. 94:28, 1974.
62. Fudenberg, H. H., et al.: Basic and Clinical Immunology III. Lange Medical Publications, Los Altos, CA, 1980.
63. Gell, P. G. H., et al.: Clinical Aspects of Immunology III. Oxford, Blackwell Scientific Publications, 1975.
64. George, L. W., and White, S. L.: Autoimmune skin disease of large animals. Vet. Clin. North Am. Large Anim. Pract. 6:79, 1984.
65. Gibbon, W. J.: Skin diseases. Mod. Vet. Pract. 43:76, 1962.
66. Gleich, G. J., and Loegering, D. A.: Immunobiology of eosinophils. Annu. Rev. Immunol. 2:429, 1984.
67. Goldyne, M. E.: Leukotrienes: Clinical significance. J. Am. Acad. Dermatol. 10:659, 1984.
68. Golub, E. S.: The Cellular Basis of the Immune Response: An Approach to Immunobiology. Sunderland, MA, Sinauer Associates, 1978.
69. Greatorex, J. C.: Urticaria, blue nose and purpura haemorrhagica in horses. Equine Vet. J. 1:157, 1969.
70. Greiner, E. C., and Fadok, V. A.: Determination of the Culicoides spp. associated with hypersensitivity in horses. Proc. Annu. Meet. Am. Acad. Vet. Dermatol. & Am. Coll. Vet. Dermatol. Orlando, 1985.
70a. Griffith, G.: Pemphigus foliaceus in a Welsh pony. Compend. Cont. Educ. 9:347, 1987.
71. Gunson, D. E., and Rooney, J. R.: Anaphylactoid purpura in a horse. Vet. Pathol. 14:325, 1977.
72. Halliwell, R. E.: Urticaria and angioedema. In: Robinson, N. E.: Current Therapy in Equine Medicine. Philadelphia, W. B. Saunders Co., 1983, p. 535.
73. Halliwell, R. E. W., et al.: The role of allergy in chronic pulmonary disease of horses. JAVMA 174:277, 1979.
74. Hammer, D. K., et al.: Detection of homocytotropic antibody associated with a unique immunoglobulin class in the bovine species. Eur. J. Immunol. 1:249, 1971.
75. Hanna, C. J., et al.: Equine immunology 2: Immunopharmacology—biochemical basis of hypersensitivity. Equine Vet. J. 14:16, 1982.
76. Hanrahan, L. A., et al.: Experimentally induced Cooperia oncophora infection in calves: Lymphocyte blastogenic and delayed hypersensitivity responses. Am. J. Vet. Res. 45:855, 1984.
77. Henry, A., and Bory, L.: Dermatose estivale recidivante du cheval. Rec. Med. Vet. 113:65, 1937.
78. Higgins, A. J., and Lees, P.: Arachidonic acid metabolites in carrageenin-induced equine inflammatory exudate. J. Vet. Pharmacol. Ther. 7:65, 1984.
79. Higgins, A. J., and Lees, P.: Detection of leukotriene B4 in equine inflammatory exudate. Vet. Rec. 115:275, 1984.
80. Higgins, A. J., et al.: The detection of protaglandin-like activity in equine inflammatory exudate—a preliminary report. Equine Vet. J. 16:71, 1984.
81. Higgins, A. J., et al.: Influence of phenylbutazone on eicosanoid levels in equine acute inflammatory exudate. Cornell Vet. 74:198, 1984.
82. Higgs, G. A., and Moncada, S.: Leukotrienes in disease. Implications for drug development. Drugs 30:1, 1985.
83. Hogarth-Scott, R. S.: Homocytotropic antibody in sheep. Immunology 16:543, 1969.
84. Hood, L. E., et al.: Immunology. Menlo Park, CA, Benjamin-Cummings Publishing Company, 1978.
85. Hopes, R.: Skin diseases of the horse. Vet. Dermatol. News. 1:4, 1976.
86. Hupka, E.: Uber gehaufte exanthematische Hauterkrankungen nach Verfutterung von Reismehl bei Kuhen. Dtsch. Tierarztl. Wochenschr. 37:183, 1929.
87. Ihrke, P. J.: Contact dermatitis. In: Robinson, N. E.: Current Therapy in Equine Medicine. Philadelphia, W. B. Saunders Co., 1983, p. 547.
88. Isharo, T., and Ueno, H.: Studies on summer mange ("Kassen" disease) of the horse. IV. Etiology considered from prevention and treatment. Bull. Natl. Inst. Anim. Health (Tokyo) 34:105, 1958.
89. Ishihara, A., and Ueno, H.: Genetical study on predisposition for summer mange. Bull. Natl. Inst. Anim. Health (Tokyo) 32:179, 1957.
90. Jackson, P. G. G., et al.: Pemphigus foliaceus in a goat. Vet. Rec. 114:479, 1984.
91. Jacobs, R., et al.: Cutaneous response to PHA-M and hematological changes in corticosteroid-treated cows. Can. J. Comp. Med. 45:385, 1981.
92. Johnson, M. E., et al.: Pemphigus foliaceus in the horse. Equine Pract. 3:40, 1981.
93. Kelley, K. W., et al.: Delayed-type hypersensitivity, contact sensitivity, and phytohemagglutinin skin-test responses of heat- and cold-stressed calves. Am. J. Vet. Res. 43:775, 1982.
94. Kerdel, F. A., and Moschella, S. L.: Sarcoidosis. An updated review. J. Am. Acad. Dermatol. 11:1, 1984.

95. King, A. S.: Studies on equine purpura haemorrhagica. Article No. 3–morbid anatomy and histology. Br. Vet. J. 105:35, 1949.

96. Kings, M. A., and deWeck, A. L.: Pharmacological and immunological aspects of histamine release from horse leucocytes. Intl. Arch. Allergy Appl. Immunol. 62:397, 1980.

97. Kleider, N., and Lees, M. J.: *Culicoides* hypersensitivity in the horse: 15 cases in southwestern British Columbia. Can. Vet. J. 25:26, 1984.

98. Klein, L.: Urticaria in the horse after anesthesia. N.Z. Vet. J. 31:206, 1983.

99. Konig, H.: Untersuchungen uber Solaninwirkung bei Rind und Schaf im Zusammenhang mit Kartoffelkrant-Futterung. Schweiz. Arch. Tierheilkd. 95:97, 1953.

100. Kral, F., and Schwartzman, R. M.: *Veterinary and Comparative Dermatology*. Philadelphia, J. B. Lippincott Co., 1964.

101. Kust, D.: Ein Fallvon Urticaria beim Schwein nach verfuttern von verdorbenen Kohlrabikanserven. Dtsch. Tierarztl. Wochenschr. 30:191, 1922.

101a. Lees, P., et al.: Eicosanoids and equine leucocyte locomotion in vitro. Equine Vet. J. 18:493, 1986.

102. Leman, A. D., et al.: *Diseases of Swine V.* Ames, Iowa State University Press, 1981.

103. LeSeach, G.: La dermatite estivale des équidés en Algérie. Rec. Med. Vet. 122:442, 1946.

104. Leven, W. F., and Schaumburg-Lever, G.: *Histopathology of the Skin VI.* Philadelphia, J. B. Lippincott Co., 1983.

105. Lindberg, R., et al.: Clinical and pathophysiological features of granulomatous enteritis and eosinophilic granulomatosis in the horse. Zbl. Vet. Med. A 32:526, 1985.

106. Lowe, J. E.: Heat bumps, sweet feed bumps, sweet itch. *In:* Robinson, N. E.: *Current Therapy in Equine Medicine.* Philadelphia, W. B. Saunders Co., 1983, p. 110.

107. Mann, D., and Hargis, J. W.: Intradermal testing of swine to monitor changes in delayed hypersensitivity response. Am. J. Vet. Res. 46:2363, 1985.

108. Manning, T. O., et al.: Pemphigus-pemphigoid in a horse. Equine Pract. 3:38, 1981.

109. Manning, T. O.: Pemphigus foliaceus. *In:* Robinson, N. E.: *Current Therapy in Equine Medicine.* Philadelphia, W. B. Saunders Co., 1983, p. 541.

109a. Manning, T., and Sweeney, C.: Immune-mediated equine skin diseases. Compend. Cont. Educ. 8:879, 1986.

110. Marzulli, F. N., and Maibach, H. I.: *Dermatotoxicology and Pharmacology.* New York, John Wiley & Sons, 1977.

111. McCraig, J.: Recent thought on sweet itch. Vet. Annu. 15:204, 1975.

112. McCraig, J.: A survey to establish the incidence of sweet itch in ponies in the United Kingdom. Vet. Rec. 93:444, 1973.

113. McFarlin, D. E., and Balfour, B.: Contact sensitivity in the pig. Immunol 25:995, 1973.

114. McMullen, W. C.: The skin. *In:* Mansmann, R. A., et al.: *Equine Medicine and Surgery III.* Santa Barbara, CA, American Veterinary Publications, Inc., 1982, p. 793.

115. McMullen, W. C.: Allergic dermatitis in the equine. Southwest. Vet. 24:121, 1971.

116. McPherson, F. A., et al.: Chronic obstructive pulmonary disease (COPD) in horses: Aetiological studies: Responses to intradermal and inhalation antigenic challenge. Equine Vet. J. 11:159, 1979.

117. Mellor, P. S., and McCraig, J.: The probable cause of "sweet itch" in England. Vet. Rec. 95:411, 1974.

118. Merritt, F. F., et al.: Relationship of cutaneous delayed hypersensitivity to protection from challenge exposure with *Salmonella typhimurium* in calves. Am. J. Vet. Res. 45:1081, 1984.

119. Messer, N. T., and Knight, A. P.: Pemphigus foliaceus in a horse. JAVMA 180:938, 1982.

120. Moorhouse, D. E.: Cutaneous lesions on cattle caused by stable fly. Aust. Vet. J. 48:643, 1972.

121. Morris, D. D., et al.: Chronic necrotizing vasculitis in a horse. JAVMA 183:579, 1983.

122. Muller, G. H., et al.: *Small Animal Dermatology III.* Philadelphia, W. B. Saunders Co., 1983.

123. Mullins, J.: Milk allergy. N.Z. Vet. J. 8:68, 1960.

124. Mullowney, P. C.: Dermatologic diseases of horses part V. Allergic, immune-mediated, and miscellaneous skin diseases. Compend. Cont. Educ. 7:S217, 1985.

125. Mullowney, P. C., and Hall, R. F.: Skin diseases of swine. Vet. Clin. North Am. Large Anim. Pract. 6:107, 1984.

126. Nakamura, R., et al.: Studies on "Kasen" of horses of Hokkaido. I. Results obtained in 1953. Jpn. J. Vet. Res. 2:109, 1954.

127. Nakamura, R., and Maisuhashi, A.: Studies on "Kasen" of horses in Hokkaido. II. Studies in 1954. Jpn. J. Vet. Res. 3:73, 1955.

128. Nakamura, R., et al.: Studies on "Kasen" of horses in Hokkaido. III. Research on the actual state of the disease. Jpn. J. Vet. Res. 4:81, 1956.

129. Nakamura, R., et al.: Studies on "Kasen" of horses in Hokkaido. V. Preliminary experiments concerning the effects of antiallergic drugs applied to horses with the disease. Jpn. J. Vet. Res. 5:97, 1957.

130. Nakamura, R., et al.: Studies on "Kasen" of horses in Hokkaido. VI. Therapeutic significance of antihistaminic preparations for horses affected with the disease. Jpn. J. Vet. Res. 6:123, 1958.

131. Nakamura, R., et al.: Studies on "Kasen" of horses in Hokkaido. VII. Applications of repellents against "Kasen" in 1958 and 1959. Jpn. J. Vet. Res. 8:53, 1960.

132. Nielsen, K. H.: Bovine reaginic antibody III. Cross-reaction of antihuman IgE and antibovine reaginic immunoglobulin antisera with sera from several species of mammals. Can. J. Comp. Med. 41:345, 1977.

133. Nordstoga, K.: Thrombocytopenic purpura in baby pigs caused by maternal isoimmunization. Pathol. Vet. 2:601, 1965.

134. O'Dea, J. C.: Comments on vaccination against strangles. JAVMA 155:427, 1969.

135. Olsen, R. G., and Krakowka, S.: *Immunology and Immunopathology of Domestic Animals.* Springfield, Charles C Thomas Publisher, 1979.

136. Olson, G. B., and Drube, C. G.: Passive transfer of delayed-type hypersensitivity with fractions of sera of sensitized animals. Clin. Immunol. Immunopathol. 19:19, 1981.

137. Ophir, J., et al.: Leukotrienes. Intl. J. Dermatol. 24:199, 1985.

138. Pascoe, R. R.: *Equine Dermatoses.* University of Sydney Post-Graduate Foundation in Veterinary Science, Review No. 22, 1981.

139. Perryman, L. E., and Liu, I. K. M.: Graft-versus-host reactions in foals with combined immunodeficiency. Am. J. Vet. Res. 41:187, 1980.

140. Peter, J. E., et al.: Pemphigus in a Thoroughbred. Vet. Med. Small Anim. Clin. 76:1203, 1981.

141. Pincus, S. H.: Hydrogen peroxide release from eosinophils: Quantitative, comparative studies of human and guinea pig eosinophils. J. Invest. Dermatol. 80:278, 1983.

142. Pincus, S. H., et al.: Superoxide production by eosinophils: Activation by histamine. J. Invest. Dermatol. 79:53, 1982.

143. Pirotzky, E., et al.: A role for Paf-acether (platelet-activating factor) in acute skin inflammation? Br. J. Dermatol. 113:91, 1985.

144. Potter, K. A., et al.: Stimulation of equine eosinophil migration by hydroxyacid metabolites of arachidonic acid. Am. J. Pathol. 121:361, 1985.

145. Power, H. T., et al.: Use of a gold compound for the treatment of pemphigus foliaceus in a foal. JAVMA 180:400, 1982.

146. Prickett, M. E.: The untoward reaction of the horse to injection of antigenic substances. JAVMA 155:258, 1969.

147. Quinn, P. J., et al.: Sweet itch: Responses of clinically normal and affected horses to intradermal challenge with extracts of biting insects. Equine Vet. J. 15:266, 1983.

148. Radosevich, J. K., et al.: Delayed-type hypersensitivity responses induced by bovine colostral components. Am. J. Vet. Res. 46:875, 1985.

149. Ralbag, E. D.: Allergic urticaria in horses. Refuah Vet. 11:166, 1954.

150. Reddin, L., and Steven, D. W.: Allergic contact dermatitis. North Am. Vet. 27:561, 1946.

151. Reinhardt, G., et al.: Reacciones de hipersensibilidad en

vacunacion antiaftosa. I. Manifestaciones clinicas. Arch. Med. Vet. 9:18, 1977.

152. Riek, R. F.: Studies on allergic dermatitis ("Queensland itch") of the horse. I. Description, distribution, symptoms and pathology. Aust. Vet. J. 29:177, 1953.

153. Riek, R. F.: Studies on allergic dermatitis of the horse. II. Treatment and control. Aust. Vet. J. 29:185, 1953.

154. Riek, R. F.: Studies on allergic dermatitis (Queensland itch) of the horse: The aetiology of the disease. Aust. J. Agric. Res. 5:109, 1954.

155. Riek, R. F.: Studies on allergic dermatitis ("Queensland itch") of the horse: The origin and significance of histamine in the blood and its distribution in the tissues. Aust. J. Agric. Res. 6:161, 1955.

156. Roitt, I. M.: *Essential Immunology IV*. Philadelphia, J. B. Lippincott Co., 1981.

157. Rosenkrantz, W., and Griffin, C.: Treatment of equine urticaria and pruritus with hyposensitization and antihistamines. Proc. Annu. Meet. Am. Acad. Vet. Dermatol. & Am. Coll. Vet. Dermatol. New Orleans, 1986.

158. Rosser, E. J., et al.: The duration and quality of positive direct immunofluorescence in skin biopsies using Michel's fixative on a case of equine pemphigus foliaceus. J. Equine Vet. Sci. 3:14, 1983.

159. Rothwell, T. L. W., et al.: Possible pemphigus foliaceus in a horse. Aust. Vet. J. 62:429, 1985.

160. Rumbaugh, G. E., and Ardans, A. A.: Immunologic diseases. *In*: Robinson, N. E.: *Therapy in Equine Medicine*. Philadelphia, W. B. Saunders Co., 1983, p. 321.

161. Safai, B., and Good, R. A.: *Immunodermatology. Comprehensive Immunology. Vol. 7*. New York, Plenum Publishing Corp., 1980.

162. Sanderman, R. M., et al.: Initial characterization of the sheep immune response to infections of *Lucilia cuprina*. Intl. J. Parasitol. 15:181, 1985.

163. Saunders, C. N., et al.: Thrombocytopenic purpura in pigs. Vet. Rec. 79:549, 1966.

164. Schalm, O. W., and Carlson, G. P.: The blood and blood-forming organs. *In*: Mansmann, R. A., et al.: *Equine Medicine and Surgery III*. Santa Barbara, CA, American Veterinary Publications, Inc., 1982, p. 377.

165. Schatzmann, U., et al.: Active and passive cutaneous anaphylaxis in the horse following immunization with benzyl-penicilloyl-bovine gamma globulin. Res. Vet. Sci. 15:347, 1973.

166. Schmidtmann, E. T., et al.: Comparative host-seeking activity of *Culicoides* species (Diptera: Ceratopogonidae) attracted to pastured livestock in Central New York State, U. S. A. J. Med. Entomol. 17:221, 1980.

167. Scott, D. W., et al.: The comparative pathology of nonviral bullous skin diseases in domestic animals. Vet. Pathol. 17:257, 1980.

168. Scott, D. W., et al.: Erythema multiforme in a horse. Equine Pract. 6:26, 1984.

169. Scott, D. W., and Campbell, S. G.: A seasonal pruritic dermatitis in sheep resembling atopy. Agri-Pract. (In press).

170. Scott, D. W., et al.: Pitfalls in immunofluorescence testing in dermatology. III. Pemphigus-like antibodies in the horse and direct immunofluorescence testing in equine dermatophilosis. Cornell Vet. 74:305, 1984.

171. Scott, D. W., et al.: Pemphigus foliaceus in a goat. Agri-Pract. 5:38, 1984.

172. Scott, D. W.: Pemphigus in domestic animals. Clin. Dermatol. 1:141, 1983.

173. Scott, D. W., et al.: Pemphigus and pemphigoid in dogs, cats, and horses. Ann. N.Y. Acad. Sci. 420:353, 1983.

174a. Scott, D. W., et al.: Immune-mediated dermatoses in domestic animals: Ten years after—part I. Compend. Cont. Educ. 9:426, 1987.

174b. Scott, D. W., et al.: Immune-mediated dermatoses in domestic animals: Ten years after—part II. Compend. Cont. Educ. (in press).

175. Scott, D. W.: Unpublished data. New York State College of Veterinary Medicine, 1986.

176. Sell, S.: *Immunology, Immunopathology and Immunity III*. New York, Harper & Row, 1980.

177. Snider, T. G., et al.: Dermal responses to Ostertagia ostertagi in *Ostertagia ostertagi*- and *Cooperia punctata*-inoculated calves. Am. J. Vet. Res. 46:887, 1985.

178. Stannard, A. A.: The skin. *Equine Medicine and Surgery II*. Santa Barbara, CA, American Veterinary Publications, Inc., 1972, p. 381.

179. Stannard, A. A.: Equine dermatology. Proc. Am. Assoc. Equine Practit. 22:273, 1976.

180. Stannard, A. A.: Generalized granulomatous disease. *In*: Robinson, N. E.: *Current Therapy in Equine Medicine II*. Philadelphia, W. B. Saunders Co., 1987, p. 645.

180a. Stannard, A. A.: Photoactivated vasculitis. *In*: Robinson, N. E.: *Current Therapy in Equine Medicine II*. Philadelphia, W. B. Saunders Co., 1987, p. 647.

181. Stormorken, H., et al.: Thrombocytopenic bleedings in young pigs due to maternal isoimmunization. Nature 198:1116, 1963.

182. Stroble, C. P., and Glenn, M. W.: A fatal case of bovine anaphylaxis. JAVMA 126:227, 1955.

183. Stunzi, H., et al.: Systemische Hautund Unterhautamyloidose beim Pferd. Vet. Pathol. 12:405, 1975.

184. Suter, M., and Fey, H.: Isolation and characterisation of equine IgE. Zbl. Vet. Med. B28:414, 1981.

185. Suter, M., and Fey, H.: Allergen-specific ELISA for horse IgE. Vet. Immunol. Immunopathol. 4:555, 1983.

186. Suter, M., and Fey, H.: Further purification and characterisation of horse IgE. Vet. Immunol. Immunopathol. 4:545, 1983.

187. Suter, M., et al.: Histologische und morphologische Charakterisierung von Pferde-Reagin (IgE) mittels Prausnitz-Kustner-Technik. Schweiz. Arch. Tierheilkd. 123:647, 1981.

188. Thomsett, L. R.: Skin diseases of the horse. In Pract. 1:15, 1979.

189. Tizard, I. R.: *An Introduction to Veterinary Immunology II*. Philadelphia, W. B. Saunders Co., 1982.

190. Townley, P., et al.: Preferential landing and engorging sites of *Culicoides* species landing on a horse in Ireland. Equine Vet. J. 16:117, 1984.

191. Underwood, J. R.: Equine Dhobie itch, a symptom of filariasis. Vet. Bull. U.S. Army 28:227, 1934.

192. Ueno, H., and Ishihara, I.: Studies on summer mange ("Kassen" disease) of the horse in Japan. III. Skin sensitivity tests with insect allergens. Bull. Natl. Inst. Anim. Health (Tokyo) 32:217, 1957.

193. Vegad, J. L., and Lancaster, M. C.: Eosinophil leukocyte-attracting effect of histamine in sheep skin. Indian J. Exp. Biol. 10:147, 1972.

194. Vegad, J. L., and Lancaster, M. C.: Cutaneous antigen-antibody reactions in the sheep. N.Z. Vet. J. 20:103, 1972.

195. Vegad, J. L.: Leukocyte emigration following intradermal injection of histamine, 5-hydroxytryptamine and bradykinin in the sheep. Indian J. Exp. Biol. 9:113, 1971.

196. Vrins, A., and Feldman, B. F.: Lupus erythematosus–like syndrome in a horse. Equine Pract. 5:18, 1983.

197. Walton, G. S.: Allergic responses involving the skin of domestic animals. Adv. Vet. Sci. Comp. Med. 15:201, 1970.

198. Weil, A. J., and Reddin, L.: Dermal hypersensitivity, heat-labile, and heat-stable antibody against ragweed in cattle. J. Immunol. 47:345, 1943.

199. Wells, P. W., et al.: Equine immunology: An introductory review. Equine Vet. J. 13:218, 1981.

200. Werner, L. L., et al.: Acute necrotizing vasculitis and thrombocytopenia in a horse. JAVMA 185:87, 1984.

201. Wilkie, J. S. N., et al.: Chronic eosinophilic dermatitis: A manifestation of a multisystemic, eosinophilic, epitheliotropic disease in five horses. Vet. Pathol. 22:297, 1985.

202. Wirth, D., and Kuscher, A.: Streifenartige urtikarielle Hauterkrankung (Strefenurtikaria) bei Pferden. Wien. Tierarztl. Monatsschr. 37:449, 1950.

CHAPTER 11

CONGENITAL AND HEREDITARY DISEASES

HYPOTRICHOSIS

Hypotrichosis implies a less than normal amount of hair. The condition may be regional or multifocal but is usually generalized. It has been reported most commonly in cattle,* frequently in swine,† and rarely in sheep,[49, 56, 168, 185] goats,[46, 124] and horses.[178]

Cattle

Many types of hypotrichosis have been described in cattle.

Lethal Hypotrichosis. This condition has been described in Holstein-Friesians and is inherited as a simple autosomal recessive trait.[105, 106, 159, 205] Affected calves die within a few hours after birth. They have hair only on the muzzle, eyelids, ears, tail, and pasterns. Skin biopsy reveals normal numbers of hypoplastic hair follicles that do not form hairs. Sebaceous glands and arrector pili muscles appear normal, but apocrine sweat gland ducts lack lumina and undergo cystic degeneration.

Semihairlessness. This condition has been described in Herefords and Polled Herefords and is inherited as a simple autosomal recessive trait.[43, 105, 106, 123, 205, 252] Affected calves are fully viable but at birth show a thin coat of short, fine, curly hair. At later stages, there is a sparse coat of coarse, wiry hair that is thicker and longer on the legs than elsewhere. The coat appears patchy, and the skin is wrinkled and scaly. Some animals do not grow well, and many have a wild temperament. Skin biopsy reveals dysplastic follicles that do not produce hairs.

Hypotrichosis and Anodontia. This condition has been described in male Maine-Anjou-Normandy mixed cattle and is thought to be inherited as a sex-linked recessive trait.[60, 105, 106, 205] Affected calves were completely hairless and toothless at birth but developed a coat of fine, downy hair and partial dentition after several weeks. A long, thick, protruding tongue (macroglossia), defective horns, and hypoplastic testicles were additional findings. Even with special care and soft feed, these calves did not survive beyond six months of age. Skin biopsy revealed deformed dermal papillae that lacked a normal vascular network and cystic degeneration of apocrine sweat glands associated with a lack of ducts.

Viable Hypotrichosis. This condition has been reported in Guernseys, Jerseys, Holsteins (Fig. 11–1), and one Hereford and is inherited as a simple autosomal recessive trait.* Affected calves are nearly hairless at birth, except for the legs, tail, eyelids, and ears. At later ages, the animals have, at times, varying amounts of hair on the chest and belly. Skin biopsy reveals dysplastic hair follicles that produce no hair or hairs that are thinner than normal. Apocrine sweat glands are hypoplastic and may undergo cystic degeneration. Dermal arteriovenous anastomoses are larger and more complex than normal, causing one group of investigators to postulate that the arteriovenous anomaly produces vascular insufficiency to, and resultant hypoplasia of, the follicles and apocrine glands.[200]

Hypotrichosis and Missing Incisors. This condition has been reported in Holstein-Friesians, but the mode of inheritance is unknown.[38, 105, 106, 173a, 205] Affected calves had patchy hypotrichosis on the face and neck and lacked four to six incisors. The condition was apparently viable.

Streaked Hypotrichosis. This condition has been described in female Holstein-Friesians

---

*References 21, 99, 100, 105, 106, 111, 112, 184, 200, 205
†References 45, 46, 54, 62, 157, 190, 196, 203

*References 15, 103, 105, 106, 152, 200, 223

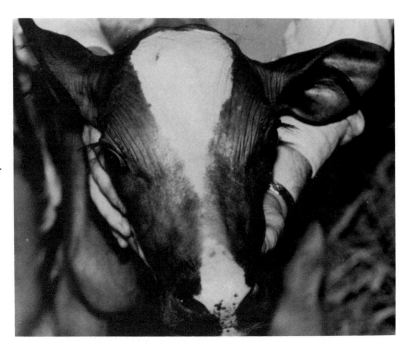

FIGURE 11–1. Viable hypotrichosis in a Holstein calf.

and appears to be inherited as a sex-linked dominant trait, which is lethal to males.[65, 105, 106, 205] Affected animals lacked hair in vertical streaks over the hips and sometimes on the sides and legs.

Tardive Hypotrichosis. This condition has been reported in female Friesians and is believed to be inherited as a sex-linked recessive trait.[98, 205] Affected cattle were normal until six weeks to six months of age, when a progressive, symmetric loss of hair began on the face and neck and spread caudally and down the legs. The cattle were otherwise healthy. Skin biopsy revealed follicular keratosis and absence of hair shafts.

Baldy Calf Syndrome. This condition has been recognized in female Holsteins and is inherited as an autosomal recessive trait.[1, 21] The homozygous state is apparently lethal to males. Affected calves are normal at birth but rarely survive beyond six to eight months of age. At one to two months of age, they begin to lose condition and develop generalized hair loss and patchy areas of scaly, thickened, wrinkled skin, especially over the neck, shoulders, axillae, stifles, hocks, elbows, and periocular region. The tips of the ears may curl medially (Fig. 11–2). Affected cattle also develop persistent salivation, become severely emaciated, and eventually die.

Hypotrichosis with hypophyseal hypoplasia has been reported in Jerseys and Guernseys.[21, 99] Hypotrichosis was recently reported in several United States Polled and Horned Herefords.[22, 112] The condition is believed to be inherited as a simple autosomal dominant gene, and affected animals had variable degrees of generalized hypotrichosis from birth. The skin was thin, and the hairs were thin, soft, curly, and easily broken and epilated (Fig. 11–3). Hoof development was impaired in a few of the animals. Skin biopsies revealed

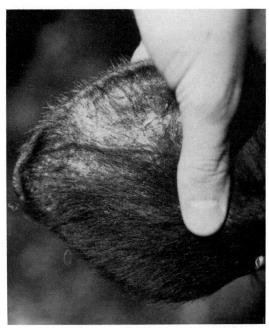

FIGURE 11–2. Medial curling of ear tip and pinnal alopecia in a Holstein with baldy calf syndrome.

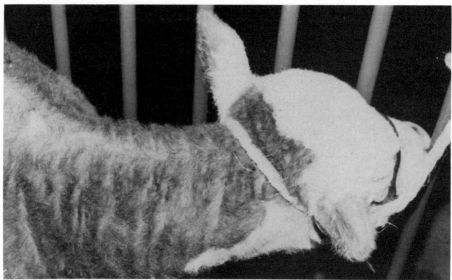

FIGURE 11–3. *Viable hypotrichosis in a polled Hereford calf.*

hypoplastic follicles and arrector pili muscles, absent or degenerate hair shafts, vacuolization, necrosis, and abnormally large trichohyalin granules in Huxley's and Henle's layers of the inner root sheath (Fig. 11–4). Electron microscopic examination showed that the megalotrichohyalin granules did not possess the microfilaments associated with normal trichohyalin granules. The absence of arginine-converting enzyme was suggested as a cause of this syndrome[193] but was later rejected.[22] Hairs from these hypotrichotic Herefords are more soluble than hairs from healthy cattle.[194]

The skin of hypotrichotic cattle is reported to be susceptible to sunburn, dermatophytosis, and superficial pyodermas.[112, 121, 123, 200, 205] In addition, tolerance to cold is diminished.

Other Species

A viable hypotrichosis, believed to be a simple autosomal recessive trait, was described in Polled Dorset sheep.[56] Affected animals were hypotrichotic at birth, especially over the face and legs. Skin biopsy revealed hypoplastic follicles that were often devoid of hairs but filled with keratosebaceous material (Fig. 11–5). Other congenitally hypotrichotic sheep have been described.[50, 51]

Hypotrichosis has been reported in swine and was thought to be inherited as a simple autosomal recessive trait.[190] Skin biopsy revealed hypoplastic hair follicles, sebaceous glands, and apocrine sweat glands. Hypotrichosis, as seen in the Mexican hairless swine

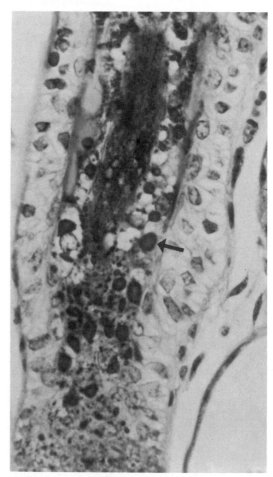

FIGURE 11–4. *Viable hypotrichosis in Herefords. Megalotrichohyalin granules (arrow) and degeneration of the inner root sheath.*

and German swine, is thought to be autosomal dominant in inheritance.[45, 157] Histologic findings in the skin of Mexican hairless swine included follicular hypoplasia and rudimentary sebaceous and apocrine sweat glands.[45]

Reports of hypotrichosis in goats and horses are anecdotal and sketchy.[45, 124, 178]

HYPERTRICHOSIS

Hypertrichosis (hirsutism) implies a more than normal amount of hair. Hypertrichosis in European Friesian cattle is inherited as an autosomal dominant trait.[92] The condition is associated with a considerable reduction in productivity and with polypnea during hot weather.

Hair whorls may be seen on the neck, rump, loin, and topline of newborn piglets.[42, 171, 236] The condition is believed to be autosomal recessive in inheritance.

Maternal hyperthermia has been shown to be a cause of hypertrichosis, low birth weight, and increased mortality in lambs.[147, 207] However, no histologic abnormalities of the skin could be detected.[32]

Border disease is a congenital togavirus infection of sheep and is characterized by a long, coarse birthcoat and neurologic disorders (hairy shaker disease).[12, 31, 52, 100, 174, 175] The main lesion is an enlargement (hyperplasia) of the primary wool follicles (Fig. 11–6), and the abnormal birthcoat results from the presence of enlarged primary wool fibers, a relatively high proportion of which are medullated. There is no obvious inflammatory reaction in the skin, and the pathogenesis of the lesion is unknown.

CURLY COAT

Abnormal curliness of the hair coat has been reported as an autosomal dominant trait in Ayrshire cattle[64] and an autosomal recessive in Swedish cattle.[117] Curly hair coat has been reported as a phenotypic marker for cardiomyopathy in Polled Hereford calves in Australia.[162] The condition is thought to be inherited as an autosomal recessive trait. Curly coat has been recognized in Percheron horses as an autosomal recessive trait[153] and in other horse breeds, such as the Missouri Fox Trotting and the Bashkin.[153] Curly coat (woolly hair) has also been reported in swine.[203]

MANE AND TAIL DYSTROPHY

Mane and tail dystrophy has been recognized in horses.[204a] Affected hairs are short, stubbled, brittle, and dull. The pathologic mechanism of the defect is unknown. No effective therapy exists.

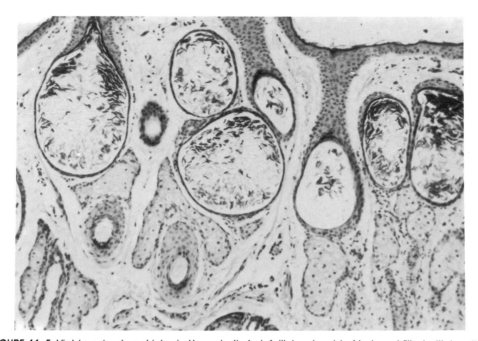

FIGURE 11–5. *Viable ovine hypotrichosis. Hypoplastic hair follicles devoid of hair and filled with keratin.*

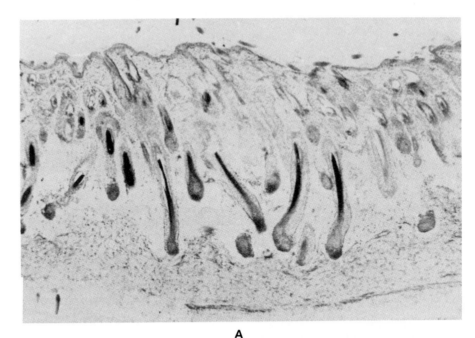

A

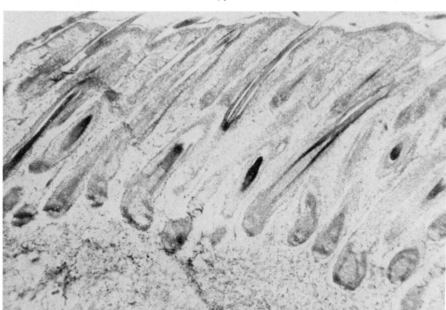

B

FIGURE 11–6. A, *Vertical section of skin from a control fetus at 115 days' gestation (× 50, Mercury Orange). B, Vertical section of skin from a fetus affected by Border disease at 115 days' gestation (× 50, Mercury Orange).*
In both cases, primary fibers have grown above the skin surface. In Border disease, primary follicle hypertrophy is evident, and the primary fibers are heavily medullated. Note the positive reaction in the keratogenous zone of each fiber. In Border disease, the zone appears to be situated nearer the skin surface, although its length relative to the follicle length is similar to that of the control. (With permission from Orr, M. B., et al.: Histological and histochemical studies of fetal skin follicles in Border disease of sheep. Res. Vet. Sci. 22:56, 1977.)

BLACK AND WHITE HAIR FOLLICLE DYSTROPHIES

Black and white hair follicle dystrophies have been recognized in horses.[204a] Affected horses have dystrophic hairs in either black- or white-haired areas. Affected hairs are stubbled, brittle, and dull, and the affected areas may be hypotrichotic. The pathologic mechanism is unknown. No effective therapy is known.

ICHTHYOSIS

Ichthyosiform dermatoses (fish scale disease) consists of a heterogeneous group of hereditary disorders characterized by the accumulation of large amounts of scales on the cutaneous surface.[69, 121]

Cause and Pathogenesis

In humans, these dermatoses differ in their mode of inheritance, clinical expression, and dermatohistopathologic findings.[69, 192] Suggested pathogenetic mechanisms include (1) increased hyperplasia of the stratum basale and epidermal turnover time, (2) increased adhesiveness of the stratum corneum cells, or failure of normal separation, and (3) alteration of lipid metabolism.

Clinical Features

Ichthyosis has been reported in cattle* and swine.[172] In cattle, two clinical forms of ichthyosis have been recognized. Ichthyosis fetalis is a severe clinical form reported in Norwegian Red Poll, English Friesian, and United States Brown Swiss cattle.[11, 61, 233, 241] Affected calves either are dead at birth or die within a few hours or days. The entire skin is alopecic and covered with thick, scaly, horny epithelium that is divided into plates by deep fissures (Fig. 11–7). The skin around the lips (eclabium), eyelids (ectropion), and other body orifices tends to be everted. Ichthyosis fetalis is analogous to human lamellar ichthyosis, with the production of so-called collodion babies and harlequin fetuses.[69, 192] Both the bovine and the human forms are inherited as simple autosomal recessive traits.

Ichthyosis congenita is a milder clinical form

---

*References 61, 100, 121, 122, 137, 145, 167, 213, 233, 241

reported in German Pinzgauer, Canadian Holstein, and United States Chianina calves.[122, 137, 145] Affected calves are born with, or develop over the course of several weeks, variable degrees of generalized hyperkeratosis and alopecia. This condition may be associated with microtia and cataracts and is inherited as a sublethal simple autosomal recessive trait.

Diagnosis

Diagnosis is based on history, physical examination, and skin biopsy. Dermatohistopathologic findings in ichthyosis include variable, though often spectacular, degrees of orthokeratotic hyperkeratosis as well as follicular keratosis (Fig. 11–8).[120–122, 167, 233] The keratinization abnormality may also involve the ducts of sebaceous and apocrine sweat glands. Hairs are usually absent or hypoplastic. Variable degrees of epidermal hyperplasia and superficial perivascular dermatitis may be present.

Clinical Management

Although various ichthyosiform dermatoses in humans have been successfully managed with topical agents such as propylene glycol and lactic acid or with systemic retinoids, such therapy would appear to be impractical for cattle and swine.[69, 192]

LINEAR KERATOSIS

Linear keratosis is a characteristic focal keratinization defect of the skin of the horse.[108, 153] It is distinguished by one or more linear, usually vertically oriented bands of keratinous crusting and alopecia. The striking predilection of this disease for quarter horses and its occurrence in closely related animals have suggested an inherited basis, but this has not been proved. See Chapter 16, discussion on linear keratosis, for further details.

CUTANEOUS ASTHENIA

Cutaneous asthenia (dermatosparaxis, cutis hyperelastica, Ehlers-Danlos syndrome) is a group of inherited, congenital connective tissue dysplasias characterized by loose, hyperextensible, abnormally fragile skin that is easily torn by minor trauma.[69, 158, 164, 192]

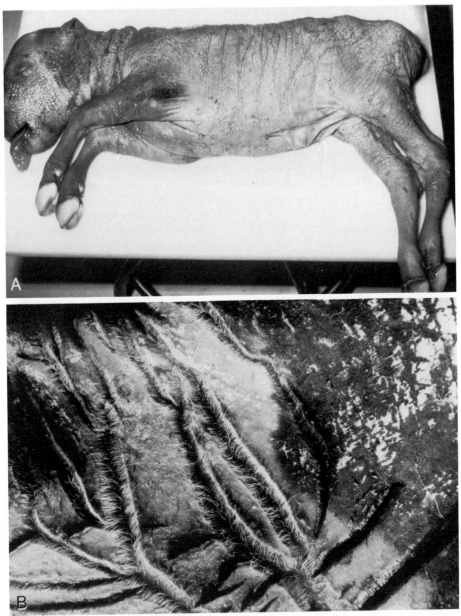

FIGURE 11–7. A, Bovine congenital ichthyosis. Generalized hyperkeratosis and fissures (Courtesy J. M. King). B, Bovine congenital ichthyosis. Severe hyperkeratosis, ridges, and fissures. (Courtesy J. M. King.)

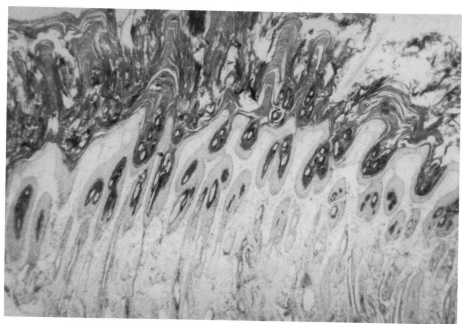

FIGURE 11–8. Bovine congenital ichthyosis. Marked orthokeratotic hyperkeratosis.

Cause and Pathogenesis

This disease complex resembles the Ehlers-Danlos syndrome of humans, which consists of at least seven different disorders that are distinguishable clinically and genetically.[69, 192] In most cattle and sheep, cutaneous asthenia is inherited as a lethal autosomal recessive trait, and is associated with a deficiency in aminopropeptidase (procollagen peptidase, procollagen N-protease) activity.* The deficiency in the enzymatic activity of aminopropeptidase results in the inadequate removal of the aminopropeptide extensions of the collagen precursor, procollagen. In addition, dermatosparactic fibroblasts fail to retract a collagen gel.[48] Abnormal structure and function of collagenous tissues is the end result.

In Australian Border Leicester–Southdown crossbred lambs with cutaneous asthenia, skin contained about one third of the normal amount of collagen but no increased amount of procollagen. Thus, this form is not associated with aminopropeptidase deficiency.[13] An abnormality in the packing of collagen fibrils was found.[13] The mode of inheritance and the biochemical defect in equine and porcine cutaneous asthenia are not known.

Light microscopic studies of one horse[85] revealed decreased collagen as well as fragmentation and disorientation of collagen fibers. Electron microscopic examination revealed that many collagen fibers had discrete foci of degradation, in which collagen fibrils were fragmented, loosely packed, and widely separated by granular material. Collagen fibril fragments were present in secondary lysosomes of dermal fibroblasts. Findings suggested that a noninflammatory degradation and phagocytosis of collagen had occurred.

Clinical Features

Bovine cutaneous asthenia has been reported in Belgian, Charolais, Hereford, Holstein-Friesian, Simmental, and crossbred cattle.* From birth, affected cattle show variable degrees of cutaneous friability and hyperextensibility as well as joint laxity. The skin is thin and easily torn, resulting in gaping (fishmouth) wounds that heal with thin, papyraceous (cigarette paper–thin) scars. Wound healing may be delayed. In about one third of cases, cutaneous edema develops soon after birth, especially involving the eyelids, dewlap, and distal limbs.

Ovine cutaneous asthenia has been reported in Norwegian Dala, Border Leicester–Southdown crossbred, Finnish crossbred Merino, and Romney sheep† (Figs. 11–9 and 11–10).

*References 10, 16, 17, 33–36, 70, 74, 75, 111, 114, 128–130, 141–143, 158, 173, 187, 208, 210, 215, 224, 231, 242, 245, 251

*References 89, 111, 114, 137, 173, 219, 220, 248
†References 9, 14, 37, 70, 93, 154, 187, 198

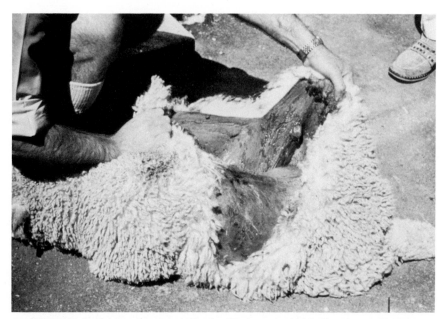

FIGURE 11–9. Ovine cutaneous asthenia. Skin tears on back. (Courtesy J. M. King.)

Clinical findings were essentially as previously described for cattle. In addition, many lambs had fragile internal organs, especially gastrointestinal tracts and arteries.

Porcine cutaneous asthenia was reported in a litter of Large White–Essex crossbred swine.[177] About one half of the litter were affected. Skin lesions consisted of a few to several circular to oval, shallow depressions (dimples), 3 to 7 cm in diameter, especially over the back, flanks, and thighs. Affected skin was very hyperextensible but not fragile. No joint abnormalities were reported.

Equine cutaneous asthenia has been re-

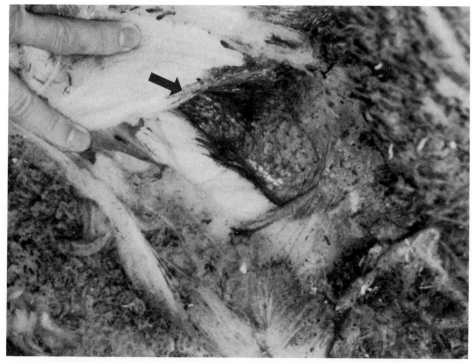

FIGURE 11–10. Ovine cutaneous asthenia. Large skin tear over neck (arrow).

ported in quarter horses[144, 153, 214] and an Arabian crossbred.[85] Lesions are usually noticed at 6 to 12 months of age and are characterized by multiple well-circumscribed areas, 2 to 8 cm in diameter, where the skin is hyperextensible, velvety to the touch, and depressed 1 to 2 mm below the normal skin surface. Lesions are most common over the thorax and back. These areas tend to tear with minor trauma, heal slowly, hold sutures poorly, and develop scars.

Diagnosis

The differential diagnosis includes aplasia cutis, epidermolysis bullosa (sheep), and familial acantholysis (cattle). Definitive diagnosis is based on history, physical examination, and histopathologic studies. Skin biopsies from cattle and sheep usually reveal small, fragmented, disorganized, loosely packed collagen fibers in an edematous and myxedematous dermis (Fig. 11–11).* Collagen fibers may or may not exhibit a normal staining affinity for Masson's trichrome stain. Collagenous tissues throughout the body may show similar changes. Dermal elastin fibers appear normal.

Electron microscopic examination reveals disorganized and structurally abnormal collagen fibrils.* Parallel packing of collagen fibrils within collagen fibers is disturbed, and cross-sectional views of collagen fibrils reveal misshapen, hieroglyphic-like structures instead of the normal round appearance (Fig. 11–12).

The cutaneous asthenia described in Romney lambs[37] had light microscopic findings similar to those just described, but the morphology of collagen fibrils appeared normal on electron microscopic examination. In addition, elastin fibers in the aorta of these lambs appeared fragmented. In the cutaneous asthenia described in swine,[177] the skin was reported to appear normal on light microscopic examination, except for an increase in the amount of dermal elastin. As no photomicrographs were offered, it cannot be ascertained whether the increased elastin was real or relative.

In the cutaneous asthenia described in quarter horses, a thin dermis was the only reported abnormality,[144] while a similarly affected Arabian crossbred showed disorganization and fragmentation of collagen fibers as well as foci of degradation and phagocytosis of collagen fibrils (see preceding).

*References 6, 7, 13, 70, 114, 137, 154, 187, 219, 245

*References 14, 70, 114, 137, 173, 187, 211

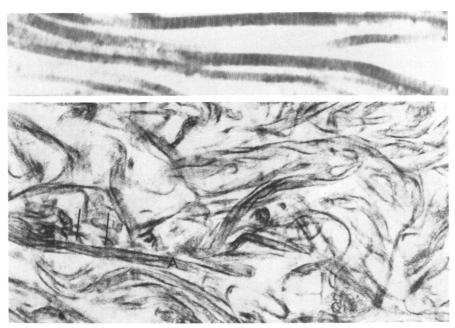

FIGURE 11–11. Bottom, *Dermal collagen fibrils are randomly distributed. One fiber is composed of three fibrils, which are wound in a loose helix. Faint cross striations (arrows) having spacings similar to those of normal fibers are visible. Top, Normal calf dermal collagen (× 49,400, uranyl acetate and lead citrate). (With permission from O'Hara, P. J., et al.: A collagenous tissue dysplasia of calves. Lab. Invest. 23:307, 1970, and © 1970, The International Academy of Pathology.)*

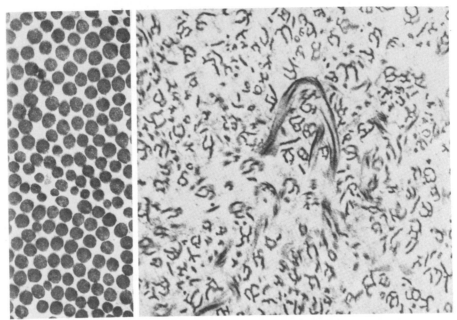

FIGURE 11–12. Right, Dermal collagen in cross section. The bizarre patterns are apparently the result of inadequate packing of fibrils. The amorphous and finely granular background material is the connective tissue matrix. Left, Normal calf dermal collagen (× 49,400, uranyl acetate and lead citrate). (With permission from O'Hara, P. J., et al.: A collagenous tissue dysplasia of calves. Lab. Invest. 23:307, 1970, and © 1970, The International Academy of Pathology.)

Clinical Management

The cutaneous asthenias of cattle and sheep are usually severe and fatal. However, those of horses and swine are usually a mild to moderate inconvenience, and affected animals are quite viable. There is no effective therapy, and affected animals and their relatives should not be used for breeding.

APLASIA CUTIS

Aplasia cutis (epitheliogenesis imperfecta) is an inherited congenital discontinuity of squamous epithelium.[21, 111, 121, 213, 250] It is thought to be a simple autosomal recessive trait in cattle, horses, swine, and sheep.[86, 87, 104, 121, 205, 250] Although its pathogenesis is not completely understood, a primary failure of embryonic ectodermal differentiation is probable.

Aplasia cutis is characterized by areas of abrupt absence of epithelium, with resultant ulcers. It has been reported in several breeds of cattle, including Holstein-Friesian, Ayrshire, Jersey, Shorthorn, Angus, Dutch Black Pied, Swedish Red Pied, and German Yellow Pied.* The lesions in cattle tend to be exten-

sive, affecting the distal limbs, pinnae, muzzle, nostrils, tongue, hard palate, and cheeks. One or more hooves may be deformed or absent. Bovine aplasia cutis may also be associated with brachygnathia, atresia ani, and dental, genitourinary, and ocular abnormalities.[86, 87, 188, 205, 247]

Aplasia cutis is also seen in several breeds of swine.* Lesions vary in number, size (most are 3 to 8 cm in diameter), and shape (most are round or elliptic) and are most commonly present over the back, loins, and thighs (Fig. 11–13). Hydroureter and hydronephrosis and skull and ear defects have also been observed in association with porcine aplasia cutis.[169, 229]

Aplasia cutis has been reported in several breeds of horses.† Lesions are most common on the limbs (Fig. 11–14), followed by the head and tongue. The hooves may slough in severe cases.

Aplasia cutis is comparatively rare in sheep.[111, 121, 166, 198] Affected sheep have had lesions of the distal limbs, tongue, and hard palate and separation of the hooves.

The major differential diagnoses include cutaneous asthenia, epidermolysis bullosa

---

*References 86, 87, 104, 114, 121, 137, 138, 148, 222, 247

*References 18, 20, 30, 62, 66, 67, 82, 102, 111, 121, 140, 160, 165, 169, 197, 203, 229, 230
†References 19, 28, 44, 60a, 84, 101, 111, 121, 153, 221

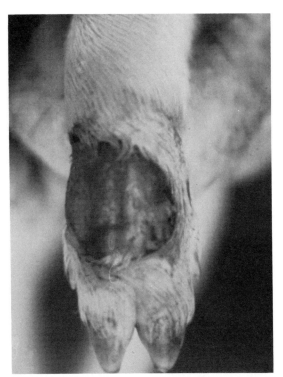

FIGURE 11–13. Porcine aplasia cutis. Well-demarcated ulcer on leg. (Courtesy R. D. Cameron.)

(sheep), and familial acantholysis (cattle). Skin biopsy in aplasia cutis reveals complete absence of epidermis, hair follicles, and glands from the ulcerated areas.

The prognosis varies with the severity of the condition. Moderately to severely affected animals usually die within the first few days of life, as a result of septicemia, other associated developmental anomalies, or both. Mildly affected animals may develop normally, their ulcers healing by scar formation.

FOCAL CUTANEOUS HYPOPLASIA

Focal cutaneous hypoplasia (erroneously described as congenital ectodermal defect) was reported in Essex, Large White, and Essex–Large White crossbred swine.[177] The animals had congenital, shallow cutaneous depressions, especially over the thorax and flank. The depressions were multiple (2 to 12 per pig), irregular in shape, 2 to 5 cm in diameter, and devoid of hair and pigment. Skin biopsy revealed epidermal hypoplasia, a thin dermis containing loosely packed collagen fibers, and absence of hair follicles and seba-

ceous glands. The mode of inheritance is not known.

SUBCUTANEOUS HYPOPLASIA

Subcutaneous hypoplasia was recognized in a Large White male piglet at birth.[177] Irregular, shallow depressions, 4 to 6 cm in diameter, were present on the skin over the flanks and thighs. Affected skin was neither fragile nor hyperextensible. Skin biopsy revealed focal areas of subcutaneous fat hypoplasia. Further details were not available.

EPIDERMOLYSIS BULLOSA

Epidermolysis bullosa (red foot disease) is a group of hereditary mechanobullous diseases characterized by cutaneous blisters in response to trauma.[69, 164, 192]

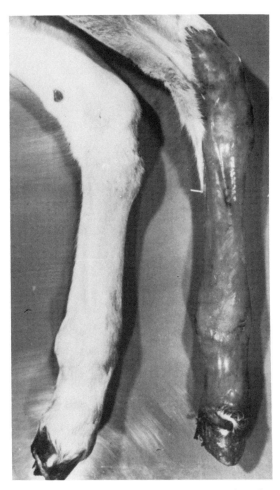

FIGURE 11–14. Equine aplasia cutis. Extensive ulceration of hind leg. (Courtesy J. M. King.)

Cause and Pathogenesis

Epidermolysis bullosa is a heterogeneous group of chronic hereditary blistering disorders with different patterns of inheritance and clinical manifestations.[69, 164, 192] Its pathogenesis is incompletely understood. In humans, studies have demonstrated increased collagenase activity in organ cultures of blistered skin and increased tissue levels of immunoreactive collagenase in both blistered and nonblistered skin. In addition, recent studies indicate that increased synthesis of a structurally altered collagenase is expressed in cultured skin fibroblasts as a genetically specific trait. The demonstration that the intracutaneous injection of bacterial collagenase results in rapid dermoepidermal separation lends support to the concept that collagenase may play an important role in the production of blisters in epidermolysis bullosa.

Clinical Features

Epidermolysis bullosa has been reported in Suffolk and South Dorset Down sheep in New Zealand,[2] Scottish Blackface sheep and their crosses in Great Britain,[156] Simmental calves in Great Britain,[13] and Brangus calves in the United States.[227] The disorder is probably hereditary, but the mode of inheritance is unknown. Lesions were present at birth or developed after a few days or weeks of life. Vesicles and bullae evolved into ulcers on the gums, palate, tongue, lips, nasolabium, distal limbs, and pinnae (Fig. 11–15). Often, hooves and horns were shed. Death resulting from septicemia was the inevitable outcome.

Diagnosis

The differential diagnosis includes cutaneous asthenia and aplasia cutis. Definitive diagnosis is based on history, physical examination, the ruling out of other diseases by laboratory testing, skin biopsy, and creation of new lesions with friction. Dermatohistopathologic findings include subepidermal vesicle formation as a result of dermoepidermal separation below the basement membrane zone (Fig. 11–16). Inflammation is minimal except when ulceration and secondary infection are present. In humans and dogs, clinical lesions may be reproduced on normal skin by briskly rubbing the skin for one minute with a pencil eraser or paper clip.[164]

Clinical Management

Although vitamin E, phenytoin, and glucocorticoids have been used systemically with variable degrees of success in managing humans and dogs with epidermolysis bullosa,[164] such therapy appears to be impractical in sheep and cattle.

FAMILIAL ACANTHOLYSIS

Familial acantholysis was reported in New Zealand Angus calves.[119] It is thought to be inherited as an autosomal recessive trait. Affected calves developed erosions and ulcers with epithelial collarettes in areas subjected to trauma, especially the lips, nasolabium, tongue, gingivae, hard and soft palates, carpus, metacarpophalangeal joints, phalanges, and coronets (Fig. 11–17). Some calves developed partial separation of the hooves. The disorder was present at birth or developed within the first two weeks of life and ended in death. Skin biopsy revealed acantholysis at varying levels within the stratum spinosum (Fig. 11–18). Electron microscopy suggested anomalous development of desmosomes and tonofilaments.

HEREDITARY ZINC DEFICIENCY

Hereditary zinc deficiency (hereditary parakeratosis, lethal trait A46, Adema disease, hereditary thymic hypoplasia) in cattle is characterized by a symmetric scaling or crusting dermatitis and a wasting syndrome resulting from intestinal malabsorption of zinc.[8, 25, 126, 160, 235, 238]

Cause and Pathogenesis

Hereditary zinc deficiency is inherited as a simple autosomal recessive trait and is associated with intestinal malabsorption of zinc.[4, 5, 25, 72] It is analogous to acrodermatitis enteropathica in humans.[69, 192, 238] Zinc has myriad physiologic effects, including maintenance of normal keratogenesis and immunity (see Chapter 12, discussion on zinc). Zinc-deficient cattle develop parakeratosis as well as hypoplasia of the thymus, spleen, and lymph nodes, which results in marked cellular and humoral immunodeficiency.[25] Chromosome analysis reveals a number of structural abnormalities, the most common being gaps, breakages, and rearrangements.[94]

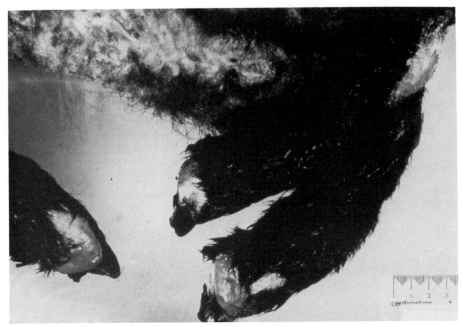

FIGURE 11-15. Ovine epidermolysis bullosa. Ulceration and sloughing of feet. (Courtesy M. R. Alley.)

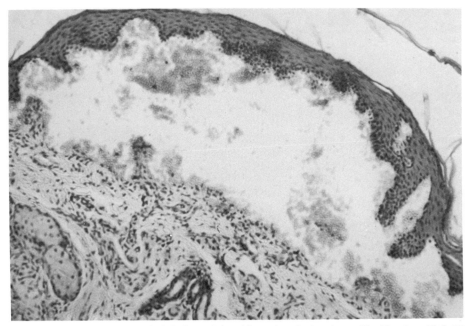

FIGURE 11-16. Ovine epidermolysis bullosa. Subepidermal vesicular dermatitis. (Courtesy M. R. Alley.)

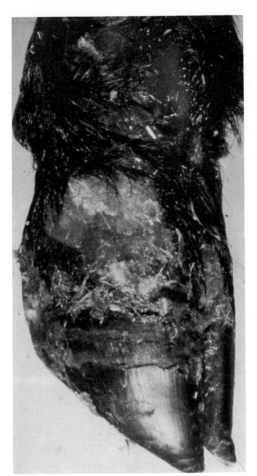

FIGURE 11–17. Bovine familial acantholysis. Ulceration of distal leg. (Courtesy M. R. Alley.)

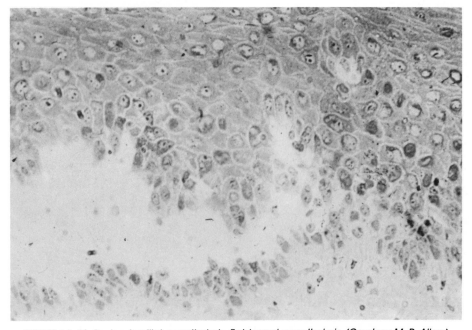

FIGURE 11–18. Bovine familial acantholysis. Epidermal acantholysis. (Courtesy M. R. Alley.)

Clinical Features

Hereditary zinc deficiency has been recognized in European Friesian and Black Pied cattle since the 1950's.* The animals appear normal at birth, but characteristic skin lesions begin at four to eight weeks of age. Erythema, scaling, oozing, crusting, and alopecia are prominent on the face and distal limbs and around mucocutaneous junctions. Many animals suffer from conjunctivitis, rhinitis, bronchopneumonia, and diarrhea. If untreated, the disease runs a fatal course in four to eight weeks.

Diagnosis

The differential diagnosis includes ichthyosis, dermatophytosis, streptothricosis, and demodicosis. Definitive diagnosis is based on history, physical examination, the ruling out of other diseases by laboratory tests, skin biopsy, serum zinc levels, and necropsy findings. Skin biopsy reveals hyperplastic superficial perivascular dermatitis with marked diffuse parakeratotic hyperkeratosis.[25, 232, 238] Serum alkaline phosphatase and zinc levels (less than 50 μg/dl) are decreased (see Chapter 12, discussion on zinc).[71, 72, 126, 139, 217, 238]

Affected cattle have poor intestinal uptake of zinc.[71, 72, 228] In addition, decreased humoral responses to tetanus toxoid and decreased delayed hypersensitivity responses to *Mycobacterium tuberculosis* and dinitrochlorobenzene (DNCB) have been reported.[25, 27, 238] Although blood lymphocyte counts are normal, necropsy findings include hypoplasia and lymphocytic depletion of the thymus, spleen, lymph nodes, and gut-associated lymphoid tissue (GALT).[25, 27]

Clinical Management

Hereditary zinc deficiency responds rapidly and completely to zinc replacement therapy.[25, 26, 71, 238] Calves given 0.5 gm of zinc oxide (ZnO) orally per day showed improvement within seven to ten days and complete recovery within one to two months.[26, 126] Other investigators reported success with 2 gm of zinc sulfate (ZnSO₄) orally per week.[132] However, when zinc therapy is discontinued, relapse occurs within a few weeks.

Flagstad[71] reported that oral oxyquinolines improved intestinal zinc absorption, restored serum zinc levels to normal, and resulted in clinical recovery of calves with hereditary zinc deficiency. Similar responses have been documented in children with acrodermatitis enteropathica.[69, 192] Oxyquinolines appear to facilitate intestinal zinc uptake.

DERMATOSIS VEGETANS

Dermatosis vegetans is a hereditary and often congenital disorder of swine characterized by a symmetric erythematous maculopapular dermatitis, coronary band and hoof lesions, giant cell pneumonia, and a usually fatal course.*

Cause and Pathogenesis

Dermatosis vegetans is inherited as a simple autosomal recessive trait.[73, 118, 131, 180] However, the pathogenesis of the skin and lung lesions is not understood. No significant microorganisms have been recovered from affected pigs.[179, 180]

Clinical Features

Dermatosis vegetans has been reported in Landrace pigs in Sweden, Norway, England, Austria, Switzerland, and Canada.† There is no sex predilection. Skin and hoof lesions are often present at birth but occasionally develop after two to three weeks of age. An erythematous maculopapular dermatitis develops on the ventral abdomen and medial thighs. The lesions tend to expand peripherally and develop a dry, brownish-black papillomatous crust (Fig. 11–19). The coronary band becomes erythematous and edematous and then is covered with a yellowish-brown greasy substance. The hooves become irregularly ridged and deformed (Fig. 11–20).

The general condition of the piglets is initially good, but then a gradual deterioration and stunted growth is observed. Most piglets die by five to six weeks of age. Some piglets are febrile. Respiratory signs (acute or chronic interstitial pneumonia or bronchopneumonia) precede death. Some piglets recover spontaneously but remain stunted.

Diagnosis

The differential diagnosis includes juvenile pustular psoriasiform dermatitis, swinepox,

---

*References 4, 5, 8, 79, 83, 126, 155, 216, 217, 234, 235, 243

*References 59, 73, 96, 97, 116, 118, 179, 180
†References 59, 73, 81, 88, 96, 97, 180

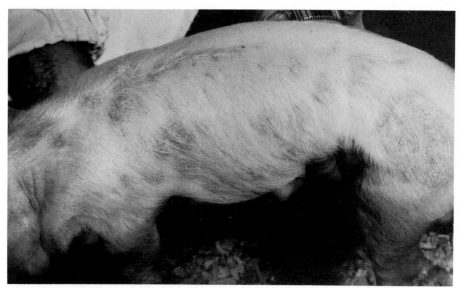

FIGURE 11–19. *Porcine dermatosis vegetans. Multiple annular areas of hyperkeratosis and crusting. (Courtesy D. H. Percy.)*

biotin deficiency, and folliculitis. Definitive diagnosis is based on history, physical examination, the ruling out of other diseases by laboratory tests, and skin biopsy. Skin biopsy in early cases reveals intraepidermal pustular dermatitis (Fig. 11–21). Epidermal microabscesses contain many eosinophils and neutrophils. Parakeratotic hyperkeratosis is usually prominent. Older skin lesions show predominantly hyperplastic superficial perivascular dermatitis with increasing numbers of multinucle-

ated giant cells in the dermis.[116, 180, 182] Bone marrow examination may reveal twice the normal number of eosinophils.[182] The characteristic necropsy finding is giant cell pneumonia.[97, 116, 181]

Clinical Management

No effective therapy is known. Sows and boars known to have produced affected progeny should not be used for breeding.

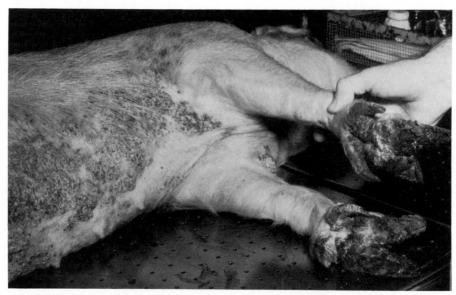

FIGURE 11–20. *Porcine dermatosis vegetans. Hyperkeratotic papules and plaques on trunk, and dystrophic hooves. (Courtesy D. H. Percy.)*

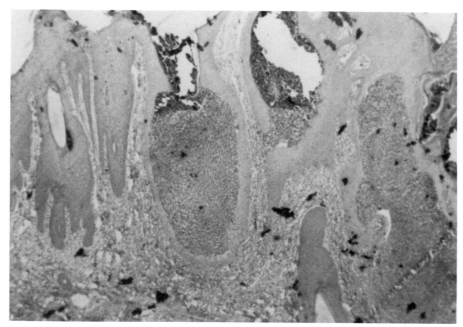

FIGURE 11–21. *Porcine dermatosis vegetans. Intraepidermal pustular dermatitis and irregular epidermal hyperplasia.*

PORCINE JUVENILE PUSTULAR PSORIASIFORM DERMATITIS

Pustular psoriasiform dermatitis is a self-limited, symmetric, usually asymptomatic maculopapular dermatitis of young pigs.*

Cause and Pathogenesis

Although the mode of inheritance is not simple, it is clear that swine that have had juvenile pustular psoriasiform dermatitis are more likely to produce affected progeny.† In one study of 231 litters of swine,[240] juvenile pustular psoriasiform dermatitis was observed only in animals related to others that had had the disorder. In another study,[40] 72 of 120 litters sired by a specific Landrace boar were affected with juvenile pustular psoriasiform dermatitis. Attempts to transmit the disease by contact or inoculation or to demonstrate any significant microorganisms have been unsuccessful, and juvenile pustular psoriasiform dermatitis occurs in piglets delivered by cesarean section and reared in isolation.‡ Although this condition had been previously called pityriasis rosea, clinically and pathologically it is nothing like human pityriasis rosea, and this unfortunate terminology should be abandoned.[63]

Clinical Features

Pustular psoriasiform dermatitis (pityriasis rosea, pseudoringworm) is a cosmopolitan disease affecting 3- to 14-week-old piglets of either sex.* The disorder is most common in the white breeds, especially the Landrace. One or most of the piglets in a given litter may be affected.

A symmetric, usually asymptomatic, erythematous maculopapular dermatitis begins on the ventral abdomen and medial thighs. The lesions tend to spread peripherally, developing first a central crater and then a central area of branlike scaling, and eventually heal completely. As a result, the ventrum and, occasionally, the lateral and dorsal aspects of the body are covered with numerous annular, arciform, serpiginous, and polycyclic erythematous skin lesions (see Plate 8). Occasionally, the skin lesions are preceded by decreased appetite, vomiting, and diarrhea, which subside when the dermatitis appears. The dermatitis is self-limited, usually resolving spontaneously after a course of three to ten weeks.

Diagnosis

The differential diagnosis includes dermatophytosis, folliculitis, dermatosis vegetans, and swinepox. Definitive diagnosis is based on

---

*References 21, 29, 47, 62, 77, 127, 140
†References 29, 47, 58, 62, 95, 140, 239, 240
‡References 21, 58, 62, 95, 125, 151, 239, 240

---

*References 21, 29, 30, 62, 77, 80, 127, 140, 149, 228

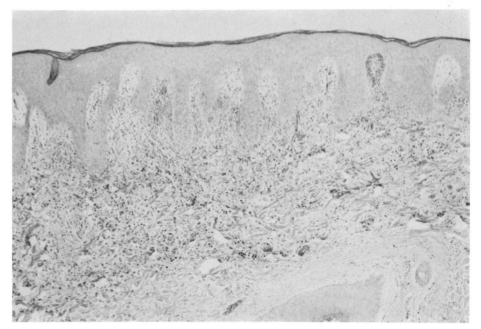

FIGURE 11–22. Porcine juvenile pustular and psoriasiform dermatitis. Psoriasiform epidermal hyperplasia and superficial perivascular dermatitis.

history, physical examination, the ruling out of other diseases by laboratory tests, and skin biopsy. Skin biopsy reveals superficial perivascular dermatitis with psoriasiform epidermal hyperplasia (Fig. 11–22). The superficial dermis usually shows mild to moderate mucinous degeneration, and eosinophils and neutrophils are the predominant inflammatory cell types. Intraepidermal pustules containing eosinophils and neutrophils are prominent in early lesions. Parakeratotic hyperkeratosis is usually prominent.

Clinical Management

Because juvenile pustular psoriasiform dermatitis is usually asymptomatic and always self-limited, no therapy is needed. If the condition is associated with a particular boar or sow, it would be best not to use the animal for future breeding.

LYMPHEDEMA

Lymphedema (primary or secondary) is swelling of some part of the body due to a lymphatic system disorder.[164, 192] Primary lymphedema is caused by developmental defects in lymphatics and lymph nodes. Secondary lymphedema occurs as a result of the obstruc-

tion of lymphatic flow by inflammation or neoplastic disease. Detailed histopathologic and lymphangiographic studies usually reveal primary lymphedema to be characterized by (1) lymphatic hypoplasia, with or without hypoplasia or absence of the regional lymph nodes, or (2) lymphatic hyperplasia and dilatation.

Primary lymphedema has been recognized as a simple autosomal recessive inherited disorder in Ayrshire cattle.[57, 161] Calves are affected at birth to varying degrees of severity. Milder cases show pitting edema of the face, ears, tail, or distal limbs. Severely affected animals have anasarca and die. Detailed histopathologic and lymphangiographic studies that elucidate the lymphatic disorder involved have not been reported.

ALBINISM

Complete and partial albinism has been reported in several breeds of cattle and in horses.* Both autosomal dominant and recessive forms have been described. See Chapter 14, discussion on albinism, for further details.

---

*References 78, 111, 115, 133–136, 183, 195, 201, 237, 246

CHÉDIAK-HIGASHI SYNDROME

The Chédiak-Higashi syndrome has been described in cattle and is associated with partial albinism, increased susceptibility to infection, and abnormally large membrane-bound organelles in various cell types.[176] It is inherited as an autosomal recessive trait. See Chapter 14, discussion on Chédiak-Higashi syndrome, for further details.

VITILIGO

Vitiligo (Arabian fading syndrome, pinky syndrome) is an idiopathic, noninflammatory, symmetric depigmentation of the skin on the face and occasionally elsewhere.[153, 178] Because the disorder occurs frequently in Arabian horses and related animals, there may be an inherited basis. See Chapter 14, discussion on vitiligo, for further details.

LETHAL WHITE FOALS

Lethal white foals represent hereditary abnormalities in pigmentation and intestinal tract development. Dominant and recessive forms are recognized. See Chapter 14, discussion on lethal white foals, for further details.

PORPHYRIA

Bovine erythropoietic porphyria has been described in several breeds of cattle.[21, 204] The disorder is inherited as a simple autosomal recessive trait and is associated with a deficiency of uroporphyrinogen III cosynthetase activity. It is characterized by retarded growth, discolored teeth and urine, and photodermatitis. See Chapter 4, discussion on bovine erythropoietic porphyria, for further details.

Bovine protoporphyria is believed to be inherited as a simple autosomal recessive trait.[24] It is associated with a deficiency of heme synthetase (ferrochelatase) activity and is characterized by photodermatitis. See Chapter 4, discussion on bovine protoporphyria, for further details.

HEREDITARY PHOTOSENSITIVITY AND HYPERBILIRUBINEMIA

Congenital and hereditary photosensitivity and hyperbilirubinemia have been reported in Southdown sheep.[21, 41] The condition is inherited as an autosomal recessive, sublethal trait. See Chapter 4, discussion on porphyria, for further details.

HEREDITARY GOITER AND HYPOTHYROIDISM

Inherited, congenital goiter with hypothyroidism has been described in Merino sheep,[186] Afrikander cattle,[109] and Saanen-Dwarf crossbreds.[53, 189] The conditions are presumed to be autosomal recessive in inheritance and are associated with defective thyroglobulin synthesis. See Chapter 13, discussion on hypothyroidism, for further details.

PORCINE WATTLES

Wattles (tassels) are reported to occur with some frequency in swine.[39, 62, 68, 146, 191] There is no apparent breed or sex predilection, and the condition appears to be inherited as an autosomal dominant trait. Wattles appear as asymptomatic, cylindric, teatlike appendages, 5 to 7 cm long, hanging from the ventral mandibular region. Histologically, wattles are characterized by a central core of fibrocartilaginous tissue covered with dense connective tissue and skin.[191]

CYSTS AND NEOPLASMS

Congenital and hereditary cysts and neoplasms of the skin have been reported in large animals. Reported cysts include epidermoid (atheroma) and dermoid (conchal sinus, temporal teratoma, dentigerous cyst) in horses[153, 163, 178] and dermoid and branchial cleft (wattle cyst) cysts in goats.[76, 244] Reported neoplasms include (1) papilloma, hemangioma, melanoma, and mast cell tumor in horses,[153, 163, 178, 199] (2) melanoma, hemangioma, histiocytosis, apocrine sweat gland adenoma, fibroid polyp, and nephroblastoma in swine,[163, 170, 177, 225] and (3) melanoma, hemangioma, and neurofibromatosis in cattle.[21, 163, 212, 249] See Chapter 17 for further details.

REFERENCES

1. Ackerman, L.: Inheritance of baldy calf syndrome. Mod. Vet. Pract. 64:807, 1983.
2. Alley, M. R., et al.: An epidermolysis bullosa of sheep. N.Z. Vet. J. 22:55, 1974.

3. Amstutz, H. E.: *Bovine Medicine and Surgery II*. Santa Barbara, CA, American Veterinary Publications, Inc., 1980.

4. Andresen, E., et al.: Lethal trait A46 in cattle: Additional genetic investigations. Nord. Vet. Med. 26:275, 1974.

5. Andresen, E., et al.: Evidence of a lethal trait, A46, in Black Pied Danish cattle of Friesian descent. Nord. Vet. Med. 22:473, 1970.

6. Ansay, M., et al.: La dermatosparaxie héréditaire des bovidés: Biochimie descriptive de la peau. Ann. Med. Vet. 112:449, 1968.

7. Ansay, M., et al.: La dermatosparaxie des bovidés: Observations complémentaires sur le collagene et les mucopolysaccharides. Ann. Med. Vet. 112:465, 1968.

8. Ansay, M.: Le syndrome héréditaire A46 (déficience héréditaire en zinc) dans le bétail pie-noir d'origine hollandaise: Une déficience de l'immunité de type cellulaire? Ann. Med. Vet. 119:479, 1975.

9. Atroshi, F., et al.: A heritable disorder of collagen tissue in Finnish cross-bred sheep. Zbl. Vet. Med. A 30:233, 1983.

10. Bailey, A. J., and Lapiere, C. M.: Effect of an additional peptide extension of the N-terminus of collagen from dermatosparactic calves on the cross-linking of the collagen fibers. Eur. J. Biochem. 34:91, 1973.

11. Baker, J. R., and Ward, W. R.: Ichthyosis in domestic animals: A review of the literature and a case report. Br. Vet. J. 14:1, 1985.

12. Barlow, R. M.: Border disease of sheep: The diagnostic significance of medullated wool fibre scores and counts of glial cells in the spinal cord. Res. Vet. Sci. 13:236, 1972.

13. Bassett, H.: Skin fragility of calves. Vet. Rec. 106:43, 1980.

14. Bavington, J. H., et al.: A morphologic study of a mild form of ovine dermatosparaxis. J. Invest. Dermatol. 84:391, 1985.

15. Becker, R. B., et al.: Hairless Guernsey cattle. Hypotrichosis—a nonlethal character. J. Hered. 54:1, 1963.

16. Becker, U., et al.: NH2-terminal extensions on skin collagen from sheep with a genetic defect in conversion of procollagen into collagen. Biochem. 15:2853, 1976.

17. Becker, U., Helle, O., and Timpl, R.: Characterization of the amino-terminal segment in procollagen p-alpha-2 chain from dermatosparactic sheep. FEBS Lett 73:197, 1977.

18. Bentinck-Smith, J.: A congenital epithelial defect in a herd of Berkshire swine. Cornell Vet. 41:47, 1951.

19. Berthelsen, H., and Eriksson, K.: Epitheliogenesis imperfecta neonatorum in a foal possibly of a hereditary nature. J. Comp. Pathol. 48:285, 1935.

20. Bille, N., and Nielsen, N. C.: Congenital malformations in pigs in a postmortem material. Nord. Vet. Med. 29:128, 1977.

21. Blood, D. C., et al.: *Veterinary Medicine V*. Baltimore, Williams & Wilkins Co., 1979.

22. Bracho, G. A., et al.: Further studies of congenital hypotrichosis in Hereford calves. Zbl. Vet. Med. A 31:72, 1984.

23. Bradley, R.: Pityriasis rosea in pigs. Vet. Rec. 76:1479, 1964.

24. Brenner, D. A., and Bloomer, J. R.: Comparison of human and bovine protoporphyria. Yale J. Biol. Med. 52:449, 1979.

25. Brummerstedt, E., et al.: Lethal trait A46 in cattle (hereditary parakeratosis, hereditary thymic hypoplasia, hereditary zinc deficiency). Am. J. Pathol. 87:725, 1977.

26. Brummerstedt, E., et al.: The effect of zinc on calves with hereditary thymus hypoplasia (lethal trait A46). Acta Pathol. Microbiol. Scand. 79:686, 1971.

27. Brummerstedt, E., et al.: Lethal trait A46 in cattle: Immunological investigations. Nord. Vet. Med. 26:279, 1974.

28. Butz, H.: Epitheliogenesis imperfecta neonatorum equinum. Dtsch. Tierarztl. Wochenschr. 47:305, 1939.

29. Cameron, R. D. A.: Skin diseases of the pig. Proc. Univ. Sydney Post-Grad. Comm. Vet. Sci. 56:445, 1981.

30. Cameron, R. D. A.: *Skin Diseases of the Pig*. Sydney, University of Sydney Post-Graduate Foundation in Veterinary Science, Veterinary Review No. 23, 1984.

31. Carter, H. B., et al.: Experimental border disease of sheep: Effect of infection on primary follicle differentiation in the skin of Dorset Horn lambs. Br. Vet. J. 128:421, 1972.

32. Cartwright, G. A.: The influence of high ambient temperature during gestation on the development of wool follicles in the fetal lamb. J. Reprod. Fertil. 28:151, 1972.

33. Cassidy, K., et al.: X-ray diffraction of collagen fibril structure in dermatosparactic lamb tissues. Lab. Invest. 43:542, 1980.

34. Cassidy, K., et al.: Low angle x-ray diffraction of dermatosparactic lamb skin. Biophys. J. 25:238a, 1979.

35. Church, R. L., et al.: Identification of two distinct species of procollagen synthesized by a clonal line of calf dermatosparactic cells. Nature 244:188, 1973.

36. Church, R. L., et al.: Isolation and partial characterization of procollagen fractions produced by a clonal line of calf dermatosparactic cells. J. Mol. Biol. 86:785, 1974.

37. Clark, R. G., et al.: A fragile skin condition in Romney lambs. N.Z. Vet. J. 25:213, 1977.

38. Cole, L. J.: A defect of hair and teeth in cattle, probably hereditary. J. Hered. 10:303, 1919.

39. Cook, R., and Baty, C.: Wattled pigs in Panama. J. Hered. 30:216, 1939.

40. Corcoran, C. J.: Pityriasis rosea in pigs. Vet. Rec. 76:1407, 1964.

41. Cornelius, C. E., and Gronwall, R. R.: Congenital photosensitivity and hyperbilirubinemia in Southdown sheep in the United States. Am. J. Vet. Res. 29:291, 1968.

42. Craft, W. A.: Inheritance of hair whorls. Proc. Okla. Acad. Sci. 12:7, 1931.

43. Craft, W. A., and Blizzard, W. L.: The inheritance of semihairlessness in cattle. J. Hered. 25:385, 1934.

44. Crowell, W. A., et al.: Epitheliogenesis imperfecta in a foal. JAVMA 168:56, 1976.

45. David, L. T.: Histology of the skin of the Mexican hairless swine *(Sus srofa)*. Am. J. Anat. 50:283, 1932.

46. David, L. T.: The external expression and comparative dermal histology of hereditary hairlessness in mammals. Zeitschr. Zellforsch. Mikro. Anat. 14:616, 1932.

47. Davis, G. B., and Kyle, M. G.: Pityriasis rosea in pigs. N.Z. Vet. J. 17:71, 1969.

48. Delvoye, P., et al.: The capacity of retracting a collagen matrix is lost by dermatosparactic skin fibroblasts. J. Invest. Dermatol. 81:267, 1983.

49. Dennis, S. M., and Leipold, H. W.: Diagnosing congenital defects in sheep. Zuchthygiene (Berl.) 11:105, 1976.

50. Dennis, S. M.: A survey of congenital defects of sheep. Vet. Rec. 95:488, 1974.

51. Dennis, S. M.: Perinatal lamb mortality in Western Australia. VII. Congenital defects. Aust. Vet. J. 51:80, 1975.

52. Derbyshire, M. B., and Barlow, R. M.: Experiments in border disease. IX. The pathogenesis of the skin lesion. J. Comp. Pathol. 86:557, 1976.

53. deViglder, J. J. M., et al.: Hereditary congenital goiter with thyroglobulin deficiency in a breed of goats. Endocrinology 102:1214, 1978.

54. Deyoe, G. P., and Krider, J. L.: *Raising Swine*. New York, McGraw-Hill Book Co., 1952.

55. Dodd, D. C.: Pityriasis rosea in pigs. N.Z. Vet. J. 18:95, 1970.

56. Dolling, C. H. S., and Brooker, M. G.: A viable hypotrichosis in poll Dorset sheep. J. Hered. 57:87, 1966.

57. Donald, H. P., et al.: Genetical analysis of the incidence of dropsical calves in herds of Ayrshire cattle. Br. Vet. J. 108:227, 1952.

58. Done, J. T.: Pityriasis rosea in pigs. Vet. Rec. 76:1507, 1964.

59. Done, J. T., et al.: Dermatosis vegetans in pigs. Vet. Rec. 80:292, 1967.

60. Drieux, H., et al.: Hypotrichose congénitale avec anodontie, acerie, et macroglossie chez le veau. Rec. Med. Vet. 126:385, 1950.

60a. Dubielzig, R. R., et al.: Dental dysplasia and epitheliogenesis imperfecta in a foal. Vet. Pathol. 23:325, 1986.

61. Dunlap, G. L.: Congenital hypertrophic keratinizing dermatosis in a calf. JAVMA 94:45, 1939.

62. Dunne, H. W.: *Diseases of Swine IV*. Ames, Iowa State University Press, 1975.

63. Dunstan, R. W., et al.: Does pityriasis rosea occur in pigs? Proc. Ann. Meet. Am. Acad. Vet. Dermatol. & Am. Coll. Vet. Dermatol., Orlando, FL, 1985.

64. Eldridge, F. E., et al.: Inheritance of a Karakul-type curliness in the hair of Ayrshire cattle. J. Hered. 40:205, 1949.
65. Eldridge, F. E., and Atkeson, F. W.: Streaked hairlessness in Holstein-Friesian cattle. J. Hered. 44:265, 1953.
66. Fischer, H.: Epitheliogenesis imperfekta neonatorum suis. Tierarztl. Umsch. 9:372, 1954.
67. Fischer, H.: Die Letalfaktoren des Pferdes und Schweines. Tierarztl. Umsch. 9:50, 1954.
68. Fischer, H.: Ein Beitrag zur Genetik von Gesaugeanomallen und "Glokchen" bein Schwein. Zuchthyg. Fortp. Besamung. Haut. 1:172, 1957.
69. Fitzpatrick, T. B., et al.: *Dermatology in General Medicine II.* New York, McGraw-Hill Book Co., 1979.
70. Fjolstad, M., and Helle, O.: A hereditary dysplasia of collagen tissues in sheep. J. Pathol. 112:183, 1974.
71. Flagstad, T.: Intestinal absorption of ^{65}zinc in A46 (Adema disease) after treatment with oxychinolines. Nord. Vet. Med. 29:96, 1977.
72. Flagstad, T.: Lethal trait A46 in cattle: Intestinal zinc absorption. Nord. Vet. Med. 28:160, 1976.
73. Flatla, J. L., et al.: Dermatosis vegetans in pigs. Symptomatology and genetics. Zbl. Vet. Med. A 8:25, 1961.
74. Fujii, K., et al.: Collagen fibrogenesis and the form of complex crosslinks. J. Mol. Biol. 106:223, 1976.
75. Furthmayer, H., et al.: Chemical properties of the peptide extension in the p-alpha-1 chain of dermatosparactic skin procollagen. FEBS Lett 28:247, 1974.
76. Gamlem, T., and Crawford, T. B.: Dermoid cysts in identical locations in a doe goat and her kid. Vet. Med. Small Anim. Clin. 72:616, 1974.
77. Gatti, R., et al.: Pityriasis rosea in swine. Clin. Vet. 99:599, 1976.
78. Gelatt, K. N., et al.: Ocular anomalies of incomplete albinism in cattle: Ophthalmoscopic examination. Am. J. Vet. Res. 30:1313, 1969.
79. Gentile, S.: Suliper-paracheratosi dei bovini. Nuova Vet. 45:113, 1969.
80. Glasser, K., et al.: *Die Krankheiten des Schweines V.* Hanover, M. and H. Schaper, 1950.
81. Glawischnig, E., et al.: Zum Vorkommen der Dermatosis vegetans des Schweines in Osterreich. Dtsch. Tierarztl. Wochensch. 81:5, 1974.
82. Gotze, R.: *Lehrbuch der Tiergebartschilfe.* Berlin, Richard Schoetz, 1950.
83. Gronborg-Pedersen, H.: Morbus ademae. En ny sygdom hos SDM-Kalve-med 74. genetisk baggrund. Medlemsbl. Danske Dyrlaeg. 53:143, 1970.
84. Grunth, P.: Klinische Mitteilungen. Monatsschr. Tierheilkd. 24:259, 1913.
85. Gunson, D. E., et al.: Dermal collagen degradation and phagocytosis. Occurrence in a horse with hyperextensible fragile skin. Arch. Dermatol. 120:599, 1984.
86. Hadley, F. B., and Warwick, B. L.: Inherited defects of livestock. JAVMA 70:492, 1926.
87. Hadley, F. B.: Congenital epithelial defects of calves. Epitheliogenesis imperfecta neonatorum bovis—a recessive brought to light by inbreeding. J. Hered. 18:487, 1927.
88. Hani, H.: Zum Vorkommen der Dermatosis vegetans des Schweines in der Schweiz. Schweiz. Arch. Tierheilkd. 122:117, 1980.
89. Hanset, R., and Ansay, M.: Dermatosparaxie (peau dechirée) chez le veau: Un defaut general du tissue conjonctif de nature hereditaire. Ann. Med. Vet. 11:451, 1967.
90. Hanset, R., and Lapiere, C. M.: Inheritance of dermatosparaxis in the calf. A genetic defect of connective tissues. J. Hered. 65:356, 1974.
91. Hanset, R.: Dermatosparaxis of the calf, a genetic defect of connective tissue. 1. Genetic aspects. Hoppe Seylers Z. Physiol. Chem. 352:13, 1971.
92. Helbig, K.: Untersuchungen uber die Wirtschaftliche Bedeutung und die Erblichkeit der Langhaarigkeit beim Schwarzbuten Niederungsrind. Dtsch. Tierarztl. Wochenschr. 65:431, 1958.
93. Helle, O., and Nes, N. N.: A hereditary skin defect in sheep. Acta Vet. Scand. 13:443, 1972.
94. Herzog, A., and Hohn, H.: Chromosome defects in hereditary parakeratosis of Black Pied calves. Preliminary report. Giess. Beit. Erbpath. Zuchthyg. 3:1, 1971.
95. Heuner, F.: Weitere Beobachtungen uber das Auftreten der Bauchflechte (Pityriasis rosea) der Ferkel. Tierarztl. Umsch. 12:354, 1957.
96. Hjarre, A.: Vegetierende Dermatosen mit Riesenzellenpneumonia beim Schwein. Dtsch. Tierarztl. Wochenschr. 60:105, 1953.
97. Hjarre, A., et al.: Riesenzellenpneumonia bei Tieren. Schweiz. Z. Allg. Pathol. Bakteriol. 15:566, 1952.
98. Holmes, J. R., and Young, G. B.: Symmetrical alopecia in cattle. Vet. Rec. 66:704, 1954.
99. Hosokawa, K.: Studies on congenital semihairless calves together with other malformations occurring in Hokkaido. Res. Bull. Obihiro Univ. 10:617, 1977.
100. Howard, J. L. (ed): *Current Veterinary Therapy. Food Animal Practice.* Philadelphia, W. B. Saunders Co., 1981.
101. Huston, R., et al.: Congenital defects in foals. Equine J. Med. Surg. 1:146, 1977.
102. Huston, R., et al.: Congenital defects in pigs. Vet. Bull. 48:645, 1978.
103. Hutt, F. B., and Saunders, L. Z.: Viable genetic hypotrichosis in Guernsey cattle. J. Hered. 44:97, 1953.
104. Hutt, F. B., and Frost, J. N.: Hereditary epithelial defects in Ayrshire cattle. J. Hered. 39:131, 1948.
105. Hutt, F. B.: A note on six kinds of genetic hypotrichosis in cattle. J. Hered. 54:186, 1963.
106. Hutt, F. B.: *Animal Genetics.* New York, Ronald Press Co., 1964.
107. Hutyra, F.: *Special Pathology and Therapeutics of the Diseases of Domestic Animals V.* Chicago, Eger, 1946.
108. Ihrke, P. J.: Diseases of abnormal keratinization (seborrhea). In: Robinson, N. E. (ed.): *Current Therapy in Equine Medicine.* Philadelphia, W. B. Saunders Co., 1983, p. 546.
109. Jaarsveld, P., et al.: Afrikander cattle congenital goiter: Purification and partial identification of the complex iodoprotein pattern. Endocrinology 91:470, 1972.
110. Jackson, T. A., et al.: Experimental production of hairy fleece and chorea in California lambs. Vet. Rec. 89:223, 1972.
111. Jayasekara, M. U., and Leipold, H. W.: Congenital defects of the skin. Vet. Med. Small Anim. Clin. 77:1461, 1982.
112. Jayasekera, M. Y., et al.: Pathological changes in congenital hypotrichosis in Hereford cattle. Zbl. Vet. Med. A 26:744, 1979.
113. Jayasekera, M. U., and Leipold, H. W.: Epitheliogenesis imperfecta in Shorthorn and Angus cattle. Zbl. Vet. Med. A 26:497, 1979.
114. Jayasekara, M. U., et al.: Ehlers-Danlos' syndrome in cattle. Zchr. Tierzuchtung Zuchtungsbiol. 96:100, 1979.
115. Jayasekara, M. U., and Leipold, H. W.: Albinism in Charolais cattle. Ann. Genet. Sel. Anim. 13:213, 1982.
116. Jericho, K. W. F.: Dermatosis vegetans—giant cell pneumonitis in pigs: Further observations and interpretations. Res. Vet. Sci. 16:176, 1974.
117. Johansson, I.: Reduced phalanges and curly goat, two mutant characters in native Swedish cattle. Hereditas 28:278, 1942.
118. Johansson, I.: Hereditary defects in farm animals. World Rev. Anim. Prod. 3:19, 1965.
119. Jolly, R. D., et al.: Familial acantholysis of Angus calves. Vet. Pathol. 10:473, 1973.
120. Jones, T. C., and Hunt, R. D.: *Veterinary Pathology V.* Philadelphia, Lea & Febiger, 1983.
121. Jubb, K. V. F., and Kennedy, P. C.: *Pathology of Domestic Animals II.* New York, Academic Press, 1970.
122. Julian, R. J.: Ichthyosis congenita in cattle. Vet. Med. 55:35, 1960.
123. Kidwell, J. F., and Guilbert, H. R.: A recurrence of the semihairless gene in cattle. J. Hered. 41:190, 1950.
124. Kislovsky, D.: Inherited hairlessness in the goat. J. Hered. 28:265, 1937.
125. Kral, F., and Schwartzman, R. M.: *Veterinary and Comparative Dermatology.* Philadelphia, J. B. Lippincott Co., 1964.
126. Kroneman, J., et al.: Hereditary zinc deficiency in Dutch Friesian cattle. Zbl. Vet. Med. A 22:201, 1975.
127. Kwon, N. S.: Pityriasis rosea in the pig: A case report. Korean J. Vet. Res. 19:159, 1979.
128. Lapiere, C. M., and Hanset, R.: Les enzymes intervenant

dans le metabolisme des proteines fibreuses des tissus conjonctifs. Bull. Acad. R. Med. Belg. 11:747, 1971.

129. Lapiere, C. M., et al.: Procollagen peptidase: An enzyme excising the coordination peptides of collagen. Proc. Natl. Acad. Sci. USA 68:3054, 1971.

130. Lapiere, C. M., and Nusegens, B.: Polymerization of procollagen in vitro. Biochim. Biophys. Acta 400:121, 1975.

131. Larsson, E. L.: "Klumpfotgrisar." Svenska Svinavels. Tidskr. 1:1 1953.

132. Legg, S. P., and Sears, L.: Zinc sulphate treatment of parakeratosis in cattle. Nature 186:1061, 1960.

133. Leipold, H. W., and Huston, K.: A herd of glass-eyed albino cattle. J. Hered. 57:179, 1966.

134. Leipold, H. W., et al.: Complete albinism in a Guernsey calf. J. Hered. 59:223, 1968.

135. Leipold, H. W., and Huston, K.: Dominant incomplete albinism in cattle. J. Hered. 59:223, 1968.

136. Leipold, H. W., and Huston, K.: Incomplete albinism and heterochromia irides in Herefords. J. Hered. 59:2, 1968.

137. Leipold, H. W.: Diagnosis of congenital disease of the bovine skin. Am. Assoc. Vet. Lab. Diag. 22:69, 1979.

138. Leipold, H. W., et al.: Epitheliogenesis imperfecta in Holstein-Friesian calves. Can. Vet. J. 14:114, 1973.

139. Lekeux, P., et al.: Parakeratose de la peau chez un veau. Ann. Med. Vet. 124:185, 1980.

140. Leman, A. D., et al.: Diseases of Swine V. Ames, Iowa State University Press, 1981.

141. Lenaers, A., et al.: Collagen made of extended alpha-chains, procollagen, in genetically defective dermatosparaxic calves. Eur. J. Biochem. 23:533, 1971.

142. Lenaers, A., and Lapiere, C. M.: Type III procollagen and collagen in skin. Biochim. Biophys. Acta 400:121, 1975.

143. Lenaers, A., et al.: Dermatosparaxis of the calf, a genetic defect of connective tissue. 3. The abnormal collagen. Hoppe Seylers Z. Physiol. Chem. 352:14, 1971.

144. Lerner, D. J., and McCracken, M. D.: Hyperelastosis cutis in two horses. J. Equine Med. Surg. 2:350, 1978.

145. Lueps, P.: Die fischschuppen krankheit Ichthyosis Universalis Congenita, eine in Bayern Beobachtete Erbkrankheit des Rindes. Berl. Munch. Tierarztl. Wochenschr. 76:204, 1963.

146. Lush, J. L.: Inheritance of horns, wattles, and color. J. Hered. 17:72, 1926.

147. Lyne, A. G., et al.: Effects of experimentally produced local subdermal temperature changes on skin temperature and wool growth in the sheep. J. Agric. Sci. Camb. 74:83, 1974.

148. Manning, T. O.: Noninfectious skin diseases of cattle. Vet. Clin. North Am. Large Anim. Pract. 6:175, 1984.

149. Matschullat, G.: Pityriasis rosea beim Schwein. Dtsch. Tierarztl. Wochenschr. 89:42, 1982.

150. Mayo, G. M. E., and Mulhearn, C. J.: Inheritance of congenital goitre due to a thyroid defect in Merino sheep. Aust. J. Agric. Res. 20:533, 1969.

151. McDermid, K. A.: Ontario certified herd policy for swine. Can. Vet. J. 5:95, 1964.

152. McGavin, M. D., and Alexander, G. I.: Viable hypotrichosis in a Jersey calf. Queensland J. Agric. Sci. 18:105, 1961.

153. McMullan, W. C.: The skin. In: Mansmann, R. A., et al. (eds.): Equine Medicine and Surgery III. Santa Barbara, CA, American Veterinary Publications, Inc., 1982, p. 789.

154. McOrist, S., et al.: Ovine skin collagen dysplasia. Aust. Vet. J. 59:189, 1982.

155. McPherson, E. A., et al.: An inherited defect in Friesian calves. Nord. Vet. Med. 16:533, 1964.

156. McTaggart, H. S., et al.: Red foot disease of lambs. Vet. Rec. 94:153, 1974.

157. Meyer, V. H., and Drommer, W.: Erbliche Hypotrichie beim Schwein. Dtsch. Tierarztl. Wochenschr. 75:13, 1968.

158. Minor, R. R.: Collagen metabolism. Am. J. Pathol. 98:227, 1980.

159. Mohr, O. L., and Wreidt, C.: Hairless, a new recessive lethal in cattle. J. Genet. 19:315, 1928.

160. Monlux, W. S., and Peckham, J. C.: Common skin lesions in baby pigs. Iowa State Vet. 23:137, 1961.

161. Morris, B., et al.: Congenital lymphatic edema in Ayrshire calves. Aust. J. Exp. Biol. Med. Sci. 32:265, 1954.

162. Morrow, C. J., and McOrist, S.: Cardiomyopathy associated with a curly haircoat in Poll Hereford calves in Australia. Vet. Rec. 117:312, 1985.

163. Moulton, J. E.: Tumors in Domestic Animals II. Berkeley, University of California Press, 1978.

164. Muller, G. H., et al.: Small Animal Dermatology III. Philadelphia, W. B. Saunders Co., 1983.

165. Mulley, R. C., and Edwards, M. J.: Prevalence of congenital abnormalities in pigs. Aust. Vet. J. 61:116, 1984.

166. Munday, B. L.: Epitheliogenesis imperfecta in lambs and kittens. Br. Vet. J. 126:xlvii, 1970.

167. Nieberle, K., and Cohrs, P.: Textbook of the Special Pathological Anatomy of Domestic Animals. Oxford, Pergamon Press, 1967.

168. Niel, J. A.: Hypotrichosis congenita in Karakul sheep. S. Afr. J. Agric. Sci. 7:875, 1964.

169. Nordby, J. E.: Congenital skin, ear, and skull defects in a pig. Anat. Rec. 42:267, 1929.

170. Nordby, J. E.: Congenital melanotic skin tumors in swine. J. Hered. 24:361, 1933.

171. Norby, J. E.: Inheritance of whorls in the hair of swine. J. Hered. 23:397, 1932.

172. Nusshag, W.: Ichthyosis beim Schwein. Tierarztl. Rdsch. 42:233, 1936.

173. O'Hara, P. J., et al.: A collagenous tissue dysplasia of calves. Lab. Invest. 23:307, 1971.

173a. Ojo, S. A., et al.: The characteristics of bovine congenital hypodontia. Vet. Med. 82:192, 1987.

174. Orr, M. B., et al.: Histological and histochemical studies of fetal skin follicles in Border disease of sheep. Res. Vet. Sci. 22:56, 1977.

175. Osburn, B. I., et al.: Unthriftiness, hairy fleece, and tremors in new-born lambs. JAVMA 160:442, 1972.

176. Padgett, G. A., et al.: The Chédiak-Higashi syndrome: A comparative review. Curr. Top. Pathol. 51:175, 1970.

177. Parish, W. E., and Done, J. T.: Seven apparently congenital, noninfectious conditions of the skin of the pig, resembling congenital defects in man. J. Comp. Pathol. 72:286, 1962.

178. Pascoe, R. R.: Equine Dermatoses. Sydney, University of Sydney Post-Graduate Foundation in Veterinary Science, Veterinary Review No. 22, 1981.

179. Percy, D. H.: Studies on dermatosis vegetans in pigs. MS Thesis, University of Guelph, 1966.

180. Percy, D. H., and Hulland, T. J.: Dermatosis vegetans (vegetative dermatosis) in Canadian swine. Can. Vet. J. 8:3, 1967.

181. Percy, D. H., and Hulland, T. J.: Evolution of multinucleate giant cells in dermatosis vegetans in swine. Pathol. Vet. 5:419, 1968.

182. Percy, D. H., and Hulland, T. J.: The histopathological changes in the skin of pigs with dermatosis vegetans. Can. J. Comp. Med. 33:48, 1969.

183. Peterson, W. E., et al.: Albinism in cattle. J. Hered. 35:135, 1944.

184. Pirchner, F., and Gruneberg, W.: Alopecia in Pinzgauer cattle. Ann. Genet. Sel. Anim. 2:129, 1970.

185. Popova-Wassina, E. T. A.: A naked lamb. J. Hered. 22:90, 1931.

186. Rac, R., et al.: Congenital goitre in Merino sheep due to inherited defect in the biosynthesis of thyroid hormone. Res. Vet. Sci. 9:209, 1968.

187. Ramshaw, J. A. M., et al.: Ovine dermatosparaxis. Aust. Vet. J. 60:149, 1983.

188. Regan, W. M., et al.: An inherited skin-defect in cattle. J. Hered. 26:357, 1935.

189. Rijnberk, A., et al.: Congenital defect in iodothyronine synthesis. Clinical aspects of iodine metabolism in goats with congenital goitre and hypothyroidism. Br. Vet. J. 133:495, 1977.

190. Roberts, E., and Carroll, W. E.: The inheritance of hairlessness in swine. J. Hered. 22:125, 1931.

191. Roberts, E., and Morrill, C. C.: Inheritance and histology of wattles in swine. J. Hered. 35:14, 1944.

192. Rook, A., et al.: *Textbook of Dermatology III.* Oxford, Blackwell Scientific Publications, Inc., 1979.
193. Rose, R., et al.: Role of arginine-converting enzyme in hypotrichosis of Hereford cattle. Zbl. Vet. Med. A 30:369, 1983.
194. Rose, R., et al.: Increased solubility of hair from hypotrichotic Herefords. Zbl. Vet. Med. A 30:363, 1983.
195. Roy, J. S.: Observation on the albinism in a breeding bull in Uttarapradesh. Indian Vet. J. 51:654, 1974.
196. Ryley, J. W., et al.: Neonatal maldevelopment in a litter of Large White pigs. Queensland J. Agric. Sci. 12:61, 1955.
197. Sailer, J.: Epitheliogenesis imperfekta neonatorum beim Schwein. Tierarztl. Umsch. 10:215, 1955.
198. Saperstein, G., et al.: Congenital defects of sheep. JAVMA 167:314, 1975.
199. Sartin, E. A., and Hodge, T. G.: Congenital hemangioendothelioma in two foals. Vet. Pathol. 19:569, 1982.
200. Schleger, A. V., et al.: Histopathology of hypotrichosis in calves. Aust. J. Biol. Sci. 20:661, 1967.
201. Schleger, W.: Auftreten eines Albinokalbes beder Murbodnerrasse. Wien. Tierarztl. Monatsschr. 46:196, 1959.
202. Schlerka, G., and Baumgartner, W.: Parakeratosis in a Simmental calf. Wien. Tierarztl. Monatsschr. 63:19, 1976.
203. Schumann, H.: Erbliche Hautkrankheiten und Anomalien des Haarkleides beim Schwein. Dtsch. Tierarztl. Wochenschr. 63:459, 1956.
204. Scott, D. W., et al.: Dermatohistopathologic changes in bovine congenital porphyria. Cornell Vet. 69:145, 1979.
204a. Scott, D. W.: Unpublished observations.
205. Selmanowitz, V. J.: Ectodermal dysplasias in cattle. Analogues in man. Br. J. Dermatol. 84:258, 1970.
206. Shand, A., and Young, G. B.: A note on congenital alopecia in a Friesian herd. Vet. Rec. 76:907, 1964.
207. Shelton, M.: Relation of environmental temperature during gestation to birth weight and mortality of lambs. J. Anim. Sci. 23:360, 1964.
208. Shinkai, H., and Lapiere, C. M.: Characterization of oligosaccharide units of P-N-collagen type III from dermatosparactic bovine skin. Biochim. Biophys. Acta 758:30, 1983.
209. Shortridge, E. H., and Cordes, D. O.: Pityriasis rosea in pigs. N.Z. Vet. J. 18:95, 1970.
210. Shoshan, S., et al.: Normal characteristics of dermatosparactic calf skin collagen fibers following their subcutaneous implantation within a diffusion chamber into a normal calf. FEBS Lett 41:269, 1974.
211. Simar, L. J., and Betz, E. H.: Dermatosparaxis of the calf, a genetic defect of the connective tissue. 2. Ultrastructural study of the skin. Hoppe Seylers Z. Physiol. Chem. 352:13, 1971.
212. Slanina, L., et al.: Hromadny vyskyt kongenitalnej koznej neurofibromatozy u teliat. Veterinarstvi 26:245, 1976.
213. Smith, H. A., and Jones, J. T.: *Veterinary Pathology V.* Philadelphia, Lea & Febiger, 1975.
214. Solomons, B.: Equine cutis hyperelastica. Equine Vet. J. 16:541, 1984.
215. Stark, M. A., et al.: Elektronoptical studies of procollagen from the skin of dermatosparaxic calves. FEBS Lett 18:225, 1971.
216. Stober, M., et al.: Hereditary parakeratosis of Black Pied Lowland calves. Zbl. Vet. Med. A 20:165, 1974.
217. Stober, M.: Parakeratose beim Schwartzbunten Niederungskalb. I. Klinisches Bild und Atiologie. Dtsch. Tierarztl. Wochenschr. 78:257, 1971.
218. Stober, M.: Osservazioni cliniche sulla dermatoressia dei vitelli pezzati neri. Atti Scoc. Ital. Buiatria 13:243, 1981.
219. Stober, M., et al.: Ubermaffige Dehnbarkeit und Verletzlichkeit der Haut beim Schwarzbunten Niederungsrind (Bindegewebsschwache, Dermatosparaxie). Prakt. Tierarztl. 53:139, 1982.
220. Stober, M., and Scholz, D.: Ubermassige Dehnbarkeit und Zerreisslichkeit der Haut beim Schwarzbunten Niederungskalb. Dtsch. Tierarztl. Wochenschr. 91:230, 1984.
221. Stoss, A.: Eine seliene Pferdemissbildung. Monatsschr. Tierheilkd. 7:456, 1896.
222. Straub, O. C.: Epitheliogenesis Imperfekta bein einem Kalb. Vet. Med. Nach. 3:189, 1969.
223. Surrarrer, T. C.: Bulldog and hairless calves. J. Hered. 34:175, 1943.
224. Tanzer, M. L., et al.: Procollagen. Intermediate form containing several types of peptide chains and noncollagen peptide extensions at NH_2 and COOH ends. Proc. Natl. Acad. Sci. USA 71:3009, 1974.
225. Teredesai, A.: Kongenitale Histioztyose der Haut beim Ferkel. Berl. Munch. Tierarztl. Wochenschr. 87:253, 1974.
226. Terlicki, S.: Border disease: A viral teratogen of farm animals. Vet. Annu. 17:74, 1977.
227. Thompson, K. G., et al.: A mechanobullous disease with sub-basilar separation in Brangus calves. Vet. Pathol. 22:283, 1985.
228. Thomson, R.: Pityriasis rosea in a herd of swine. Can. Vet. J. 1:449, 1960.
229. Thoonen, J., and Hoorens, J.: Epitheliogenesis imperfecta neonatorum in the pig. Vlaams Diergeneeskd. Tijdschr. 25:239, 1956.
230. Thoonen, J., et al.: Epitheeldefekten op tougen kroonrand bij biggen. Vlaams Diergeneeskd. Tijdschr. 33:197, 1964.
231. Timpe, R., et al.: Immunochemical properties of procollagen from dermatosparaxic calves. Eur. J. Biochem. 32:584, 1973.
232. Trautwein, G.: Parakeratose beim schwarzbunten Niederungskalb. 2. Pathologisch-anatomische Befunde. Dtsch. Tierarztl. Wochenschr. 78:265, 1971.
233. Tuff, P., and Gledish, L. A.: Ichthyosis congenita hos kalveren arvelig letal defect. Nord. Vet. Med. 1:619, 1949.
234. van Adrichem, P. W. M., et al.: Parakeratosis of the skin in calves. Neth. J. Vet. Sci. 1:57, 1971.
235. van Adrichem, P. W. M., et al.: Parakeratose van de huidbij kalveren. Tijdschr. Diergeneeskd. 95:1170, 1970.
236. Warwich, E. J., et al.: Some anomalies in pigs. J. Hered. 34:349, 1943.
237. Weber, W., et al.: Albinisms hereditaire en race tachettee rouge de Suisse. Schweiz. Arch. Tierheilkd. 115:142, 1973.
238. Weisman, K., and Flagstad, T.: Hereditary zinc deficiency (Adema disease) in cattle, an animal parallel to acrodermatitis enteropathica. Acta Derm. Venereol. (Stockh.) 56:151, 1976.
239. Wellman, G.: Beobachtungen uber die Bauchflechte (Pityriasis rosea) der Ferkel und die Erblichkeit der Disposition dazu. Tierarztl. Umsch. 8:292, 1954.
240. Wellman, G.: Weitere Beobachtungen uber die Erblichkeit der Disposition zur Bauchflechte (Pityriasis rosea) der Ferkel. Berl. Munch. Tierarztl. Wochenschr. 76:107, 1963.
241. Wettimuny, S. G., and Jainudeen, M. R.: Ichthyosis foetalis in a calf. Ceylon Vet. J. 10:102, 1962.
242. Wick, G., et al.: Immunohistologic analysis of fetal and dermatosparactic calf and sheep skin with antisera to procollagen and collagen type I. Lab. Invest. 39:151, 1978.
243. Wiesner, E., and Willer, S.: *Veterinarmedizinische Pathogenetik.* Jena, VEB Gustav Fischer Verlag, 1974.
244. Williams, C. S. F.: Differential diagnosis of caseous lymphadenitis in the goat. Vet. Med. Small Anim. Clin. 75:1165, 1980.
245. Winand, R. J., and Nusgens, B.: Dermatosparaxis of the calf, a genetic defect of the connective tissue. 4. The modified glycosaminoglycans and proteoglycans. Hoppe Seylers Z. Physiol. Chem. 352:14, 1971.
246. Winzenreid, H. U., and Lauvergne, J. J.: Spontanes Auftreten von Albinos in der Schweizer ischen Braunviehrasse. Schweiz. Arch. Tierheilkd. 12:581, 1970.
247. Wipprecht, C., and Horlacher, W. R.: A lethal gene in Jersey cattle. J. Hered. 26:363, 1935.
248. Witzig, P., et al.: Dermatosparaxie bei einem Fohlen und einem Rind—eine seltene Krankheit? Schweiz. Arch. Tierheilkd. 126:589, 1984.
249. Wiseman, A., et al.: Melanotic neuroectodermal tumor of infancy (melanotic progonoma) in two calves. Vet. Rec. 101:264, 1977.
250. Wright, B. G.: Epitheliogenesis imperfecta: Understanding this rare skin anomaly. Vet. Med. 81:246, 1986.
251. Yaeger, J. A., et al.: Structure of cultured fibroblasts from dermatosparaxic calves. Vet. Pathol. 12:16, 1975.
252. Young, J. B.: A note on the occurrence of an epithelial defect in a grade Hereford herd. Aust. Vet. J. 9:298, 1953.

CHAPTER 12

NUTRITIONAL DISEASES

INTRODUCTION

The nutritional factors that influence the health of the skin are exceedingly complex.* However, it is obvious that for proper skin health and functioning, the diet must be complete in all essential nutrients. Deficiencies that are produced experimentally often result in cutaneous disorders, but these are seldom characteristic enough to allow specific diagnosis. Furthermore, the interaction of nutrients is such that a deficiency of one item may upset delicate balances, and the resulting skin disorder may be the product of the imbalance rather than the initial deficiency.

General malnutrition (protein and calorie deficiency), whether strictly dietary in origin or secondary to debilitating diseases, causes the skin to become dry, scaly, thin, and inelastic.† The skin may become more susceptible to infection and may show hemorrhagic tendencies and pigmentary disturbances. The hair coat becomes dull, dry, brittle, and thin. In sheep, it has been shown that underfeeding pregnant ewes results in reduced secondary hair follicle initiation and maturation in their fetuses.[40, 68, 159, 186] Malnutrition can develop via interference with intake, absorption, or utilization of nutrients; via increased requirements or excretion of nutrients; or via inhibition.

Specific nutritional factors are most difficult to evaluate. A great many nutrients have been determined to have an influence on skin health, including protein, essential fatty acids, vitamins, and minerals.

PROTEIN DEFICIENCY

Protein deficiency may be produced by starvation, inanition, or diets very low in protein.[13, 17, 39, 91, 139, 191] Hair is 95 per cent protein, with a high percentage of sulfur-containing amino acids. The normal growth of hair and the keratinization of skin require 25 to 30 percent of the animal's daily protein requirement. Animals with protein deficiency may have hyperkeratosis, cutaneous atrophy, and pigmentary disturbances of skin and hair coat. The hair coat may be dry, dull, brittle, thin, and easily epilated. Hair growth is retarded, and shedding may be prolonged. Paradoxically, swine fed a ration low in protein and calories often develop a longer, thicker, and heavier hair coat.[17, 91] Dermatohistopathologic findings include orthokeratotic hyperkeratosis, diffuse dermal edema, atrophy and disorganization of dermal collagen, and curled hairs.

It has been shown that maternal underfeeding of sheep during pregnancy results in inhibition of secondary hair follicle development in fetuses and shorter and finer fleeces in newborn lambs.[40, 68, 160, 186] This could result in poorer insulation by the birthcoat,[2, 3, 159] which would add to the hazards that lambs must overcome if they are to survive.

The growth rate and the strength of wool fibers are particularly sensitive to the amounts and proportions of amino acids available to the wool follicle.[45, 146] The omission of either methionine or lysine from a mixture of amino acids infused into the abomasum of sheep inhibits wool growth and weakens wool fibers.[147, 148]

The inhibitory effects of amino acids and their analogues on wool growth may have an application in research aimed at discovering new methods for harvesting wool from sheep.[51, 149, 152, 152a] Many agents that weaken wool are known to inhibit the synthesis of high-tyrosine proteins in wool.[42, 43] Ethionine, an analogue of methionine, is an inhibitor of wool growth and may cause shedding of the fleece.[150] Mimosine has also been shown to be an effective depilatory agent in sheep.[151]

---

*References 5, 13, 18, 33, 39, 72, 91, 101, 139, 178, 179, 191

†References 13, 17, 33, 72, 91, 101, 139, 191

ESSENTIAL FATTY ACID DEFICIENCY

Fatty acid deficiency may occur when animals are given feed low in fat or feed whose fats have been destroyed during storage, especially as a result of rancidity in the absence of adequate antioxidants. Fatty acid deficiency in a number of species produces abnormal keratinization, resulting in orthokeratotic hyperkeratosis, hypergranulosis, and epidermal hyperplasia.[94, 142] This abnormal keratinization is thought to be due to arachidonic acid deficiency, with resultant prostaglandin E deficiency, which causes aberrations in the ratios of epidermal cyclic AMP ($cAMP$) to cyclic GMP ($cGMP$) and in DNA synthesis.

Fatty acid deficiency has been produced in swine through the use of experimental diets containing 0.06 percent fat.[18, 19, 33, 39, 87, 190] Cutaneous changes included diffuse scaling and alopecia. Brownish exudate tended to accumulate on the ears, axillae, and flanks, and the skin seemed more prone to infection and necrosis. Poor growth was also observed. It was concluded that swine had a linoleic acid requirement approximating 1 percent of their caloric intake and that practical rations would not be low enough in essential fatty acids to produce deficiency symptoms. Others recommend that fats constitute 1.0 per cent of the total ration for swine.[39, 79] It has been suggested that swine parakeratosis may also be, in part, a manifestation of fatty acid deficiency.[58]

VITAMIN DEFICIENCIES

Vitamin A. Vitamin A maintains the structural and functional integrity of epithelial tissues. Vitamin A deficiency is most likely to occur when swine and cattle are fed grain diets and have no access to green feed or are not given vitamin A supplements. It is most prevalent in desert and arid regions of the world. This deficiency results in hyperkeratosis and a tendency toward squamous metaplasia of secretory epithelia.[13]

Vitamin A deficiency has been produced experimentally and has occurred under field conditions in swine, cattle, sheep, and goats.* It was also seen in association with chlorinated naphthalene poisoning in cattle (see Chapter 4, discussion on chlorinated naphthalene toxicosis). Early clinical signs include night blindness and excessive lacrimation. These are followed by neurologic disorders (e.g., head tilt, ataxia, paralysis, and convulsions), corneal changes (e.g., ulcers and xerophthalmia), skeletal abnormalities, and reproductive disorders (e.g., infertility, abortion, and congenital anomalies). Cutaneous changes include a rough, dry, shaggy, often faded hair coat and seborrheic skin disease.

Clinical vitamin A deficiency is usually associated with plasma vitamin A levels lower than 10 µg/dl and liver vitamin A levels lower than 5 µg/gm dry matter liver.[5, 13] Recommended daily doses for swine and cattle, depending on physiologic status, are about 40 IU/kg and 60 IU/kg, respectively.[39] Therapeutic recommendations for cattle include 440 IU aqueous vitamin A/kg orally or intramuscularly[13, 13a] and 50,000 IU to 500,000 IU intramuscularly or intrarumenally.[5] If dietary supplementation with good-quality hay is impractical, intramuscular injection of vitamin A at 3000 to 6000 IU/kg every 50 to 60 days is recommended.[13a] Adult steers were found to be fairly resistant to vitamin A intoxication, consuming, in feed, levels as high as 2,500,000 IU/day for 170 days with no obvious harmful effects.[5]

Biotin. Biotin is a component of several enzyme systems. Deficiency syndromes have occurred naturally and have been produced with experimental diets in swine.* Clinical signs included hind leg spasticity; generalized alopecia; pustules, scaling, and crusting; ulcers on the thighs and abdomen; transverse cracking, erosion, and bleeding of the toes, side walls, and heels; and stomatitis (furry tongue). Biotin supplementation was reported to reduce the incidence and severity of heel cracks, heel-horn junction cracks, and side-wall horn cracks in sows, as well as to increase the number of hairs/cm² skin.[15a] Dermatohistopathologic findings included epidermal hyperplasia and orthokeratotic and parakeratotic hyperkeratosis, along with focal epidermal necrosis, intraepidermal pustular dermatitis, and folliculitis.[45–47] Plasma biotin levels of less than 40 ng/dl have been associated with clinical signs.[47] Biotin requirements for swine are in the range of 55 to 220 µg/kg/day.[103]

Niacin (Nicotinic Acid). Niacin is a component of several enzyme systems. Deficiency syndromes have occurred naturally and have been produced with special diets in swine.†

---

*References 5, 13, 13a, 20, 33, 34, 36, 46a, 57, 60, 91, 100, 130

*References 13, 15, 18–20, 26, 28, 33, 34, 45–48, 90, 91
†References 13, 18, 19, 23, 29–34, 65, 91, 97

Clinical signs included anorexia, diarrhea, emaciation, neurologic disorders, anemia, and a generalized scaling, crusting dermatitis. Characteristic necropsy findings included thickening and friability of the wall of the colon and cecum. Niacin requirements for growth and maintenance of swine are 0.6 to 1.0 mg/kg/day and 0.1 to 0.4 mg/kg/day, respectively.[13, 33, 34, 39, 65, 91] Recommended therapy is 100 to 200 mg/day orally (10 to 20 gm/T feed).

Pantothenic Acid. Pantothenic acid is a coenzyme in many biochemical reactions and is involved in the metabolism and synthesis of fats, carbohydrates, and many other compounds. Deficiency syndromes have occurred in the field and have been produced in swine on experimental diets.* Clinical signs included anorexia, poor growth, diarrhea, coughing, locomotive incoordination (goose-stepping), reproductive disorders, and patchy alopecia with the accumulation of dark brown exudate around the eyes. Characteristic necropsy findings included edema, hyperemia, inflammation of the colon, and degeneration of peripheral nerves and funiculi of the spinal cord.[166] Pantothenic acid administered at 500 µg/kg/day (10 to 12 gm/T feed) is effective for therapy and prevention.[13, 28, 33, 34, 38, 67]

Riboflavin (Vitamin B₂). Riboflavin is required by all living cells. It is a constituent of several enzymes and functions in oxidative processes. Deficiency syndromes have been produced with experimental diets in swine and cattle.† Cattle exhibited anorexia, poor growth, hypersalivation, excessive lacrimation, diarrhea, and generalized alopecia. In swine, the symptoms included poor growth, vomiting, stiffness of gait, cataracts, anemia, neurologic disorders, reproductive disorders, and a generalized scaling and ulcerative dermatitis.

The suggested daily riboflavin requirement for swine is 60 to 80 µg/kg (2 to 3 gm/T feed), and this requirement may increase with a colder environment.‡

Vitamin C (Ascorbic Acid). Vitamin C is involved in collagen metabolism and the antagonism of histamine.[1, 8, 21] Farm animals are presumed to have no dietary requirement for this vitamin,[13] and studies with the microsomal fraction of cow liver incubated with ascorbic

acid precursors showed the ability to synthesize 50 ± 6 mg ascorbic acid/mg of protein/hour.[21]

A vitamin C–responsive dermatosis has been described in dairy calves.[13, 24, 100, 157, 163] The syndrome was seen in 16- to 75-day-old barn-fed calves in the northeastern United States during fall and winter. No common dietary or environmental abnormalities were detected. Occasional calves had a history of a febrile and/or diarrheal illness a few weeks previously. Clinical signs included moderate to severe scaling, alopecia, easy epilation of hairs, and crusting beginning over the head and/or limbs (Fig. 12–1). The extremities were usually erythematous and purpuric (Figs. 12–2 and 12–3). Pain and pruritus were not observed. Some calves showed depression and poor growth, and rare calves developed bronchopneumonia and died.

Dermatohistopathologic findings included orthokeratotic hyperkeratosis, follicular keratosis, curlicue hairs, vascular dilatation and congestion, and perifollicular purpura (Figs. 12–4 and 12–5).[163] Necropsy findings included macroscopic and microscopic hemorrhages in the lungs, endocardium, myocardium, and intima of the pulmonary vessels and aorta.[163] Plasma ascorbic acid levels in affected calves ranged from 0.07 to 0.09 mg/dl, as compared with 0.24 to 0.38 mg/dl in normal and recovered calves.[24]

Spontaneous recovery was reported to occur after a period of two months.[24] Recovered calves often failed to grow at a normal rate and appeared unthrifty. Treatment with one to two subcutaneous injections of 3 gm of ascorbic acid resulted in immediate improvement and rapid recovery.[24, 163]

The pathogenesis of this syndrome in calves is not known. It has been theorized that it may represent a temporary vitamin C deficiency in growing calves, analogous to the situation in swine parakeratosis.[163]

Vitamin E. A dermatosis responsive to vitamin E and selenium has been recognized in goats.[164, 168] In goat herds on a selenium-deficient diet and with an undetermined vitamin E intake, both young and adult goats developed periorbital alopecia and generalized seborrheic skin disease. The skin was very scaly, with occasional crusts, and the hair coat was dry, dull, and brittle (Fig. 12–6). Usually, the goats were otherwise healthy, although some were moderately depressed and not feeding well.

Skin biopsies revealed marked orthokeratotic hyperkeratosis and a mild superficial perivascular accumulation of mononuclear cells

---

*References 13, 18, 19, 28, 33, 34, 38, 49, 67, 91, 166, 177, 185, 187, 189

†References 5, 13, 18, 19, 33, 34, 66, 89, 91, 108, 109, 126, 187

‡References 33, 34, 39, 66, 91, 108, 109, 126

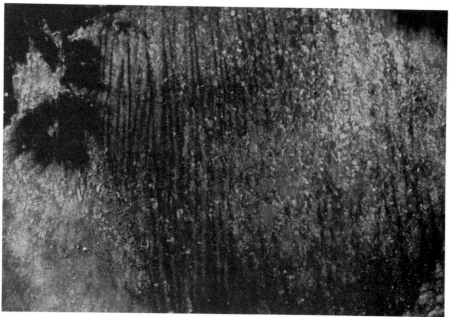

FIGURE 12–1. Vitamin C–responsive dermatosis in a calf. Alopecia and scaling of lateral thorax.

(Fig. 12–7). Affected goats responded well to an injection of vitamin E and selenium (BoSe), 3 ml/50 kg. A good response was seen in two to four weeks. Injections of vitamin E and selenium every six months was an effective preventive.

A deficiency of vitamin E in swine is associated with liver necrosis, muscular dystrophy, mulberry heart disease, and yellow fat disease.[91] In addition, scurfy skin has been observed in affected newborn piglets. Vitamin E–selenium deficiency was suspected in an outbreak of porcine ear necrosis.[52] Dietary supplementation with sodium selenate was curative.

MINERAL DEFICIENCIES

Cobalt. Cobalt (Co) is an essential trace element in ruminant nutrition that is stored in the body in limited amounts and must be continually present in the feed.[13, 178, 179] When the concentration of cobalt in rumen fluid falls below a critical level, the rate of vitamin B_{12} synthesis by rumen organisms is reduced below the animal's needs. Deficiency syndromes have occurred on pastures containing less than 0.04 to 0.07 ppm Cobalt/dry matter.[13, 100, 179] Clinical signs usually occur after six months on pasture and include severe reduction in growth, lactation, and wool production and a rough, faded hair coat. The wool in sheep may be tender

and broken. Tests for cobalt (less than 0.10 ppm/dry matter liver) or vitamin B_{12} (less than 0.10 μg/gm wet weight liver) are diagnostically the most valuable.[13, 179]

Therapy includes the use of cobalt sulfate ($CoSO_4$) orally (1 mg cobalt/day), and response is rapid.[13] Dietary levels of 0.06 mg/cobalt/kg dry matter feed or topdressing-defi-

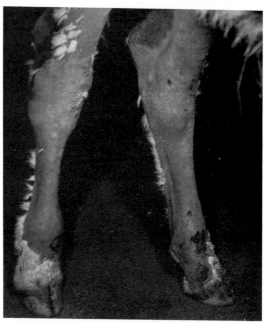

FIGURE 12–2. Vitamin C–responsive dermatosis in a calf. Alopecia, erythema, and purpura of rear legs.

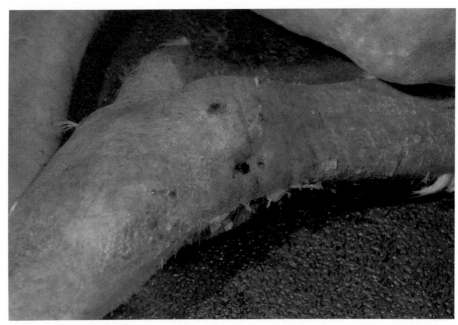

FIGURE 12–3. Vitamin C–responsive dermatosis in a calf. Alopecia, erythema, purpura, and scaling of leg.

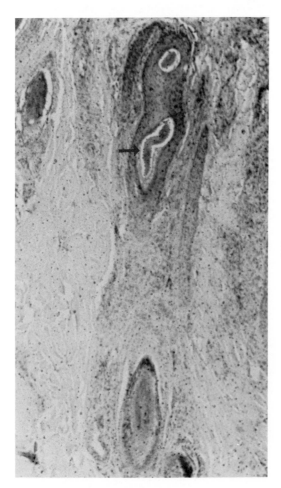

FIGURE 12–4. Vitamin C–responsive dermatosis in a calf. "Curlycue" hair (arrow).

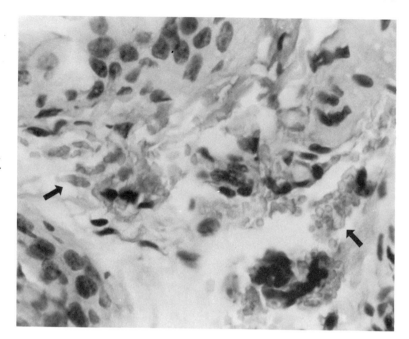

FIGURE 12–5. Vitamin C–responsive dermatosis. Perifollicular purpura (arrows).

cient pastures with 150 gm of cobalt sulfate per acre applied annually are recommended for prevention.[13, 39, 179] Although treatment and prevention with vitamin B_{12} are also effective, they are less convenient and more expensive.

Copper. Copper (Cu) is an essential component of many oxidative enzymes, such as tyrosinase, uricase, ascorbic acid oxidase, lysyl oxidase, and cytochrome oxidase.[13b, 158, 179]

Copper deficiency (hypocuprosis) may occur in cattle and sheep owing to a dietary deficiency or secondary to molybdenum poisoning (molybdenosis) (see Chapter 4, discussion on molybdenosis).* Zinc or cadmium interfere with the absorption of copper. Clinical signs

*References 4, 5, 13, 13b, 22, 92, 100, 125, 158, 174, 178, 179

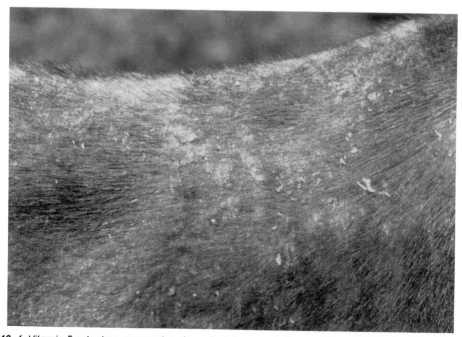

FIGURE 12–6. Vitamin E-selenium–responsive dermatosis in a goat. Generalized scaling and thinning of the coat.

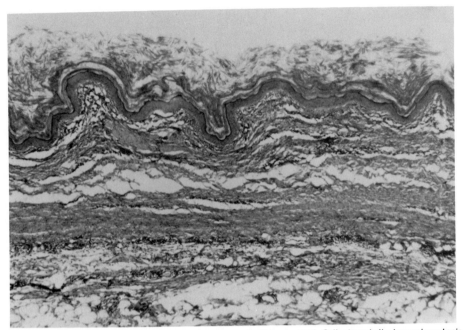

FIGURE 12–7. Vitamin E-selenium–responsive dermatosis in a goat. Orthokeratotic hyperkeratosis.

include stunted growth, diarrhea, infertility, anemia, bone disorders, heart failure, a rough, brittle, faded hair coat, and varying degrees of itching and hair-licking. Black hairs often turn red or gray, especially around the eyes, producing a "spectacled" appearance. (Fig. 12–8.) A breakdown in the conversion of tyrosine to melanin is the probable explanation of this failure of pigmentation, since this conversion is catalyzed by copper-containing polyphenyl oxidases.[179]

In sheep, wool loses its crimp, becoming straight and steely in appearance. The tensile strength of the wool is reduced, and the elastic properties are abnormal. The characteristic physical properties of wool, including crimp, are dependent on the presence of disulfide groups that provide the cross-linkages of keratin and on the alignment of long-chain keratin fibrillae in the fiber. Both of these are adversely affected in copper deficiency.[179]

Dairy cattle herds that are copper-deficient often have a history of lameness associated with exfoliative pododermatitis and heel cracks.[158] The correlation between copper concentrations in blood, liver, and hair and clinical signs is relatively poor.[22, 174, 179]

In general, clinical hypocuprosis is associated with blood copper levels lower than 0.7 μg/ml and liver levels lower than 20 ppm/dry matter liver.[13, 92, 158, 179] A number of acute and chronic disorders elevate blood copper levels.[179]

The copper requirement for cattle and sheep has been reported to be approximately 8 to 9 mg/kg dry matter feed.[39, 178, 179] Treatment with 1.5 gm (sheep) or 4 gm (cattle) copper sulfate ($CuSO_4$) orally per week or 40 mg (sheep) or 120 mg (cattle) copper glycinate intramuscularly is reported to be effective.[5, 13, 92, 158, 179] Salt licks containing 0.5 to 1.0 percent copper sulfate are reported to be effective for prevention.[5, 13, 179] Twenty-five to 50 ppm copper in cattle rations has been reported to be preventive.[158] Copper toxicity, characterized by jaundice, hemoglobinuria, and methemoglobinemia, was produced in calves fed rations containing 500 ppm copper sulfate for several months or given 12 gm orally.[5, 13, 13b, 179]

Iodine. Iodine is required for the proper development and function of the thyroid gland and is an indispensable component of the thyroid hormones, which control metabolism. Dietary iodine deficiency resulting in goitrous neonates has been reported in cattle, sheep, swine, goats, and horses.* Certain soils and pastures are known to be iodine-deficient, such as those in the Great Lakes, Northern Plains, and Pacific Northwest regions of the United

*References 5, 6, 9, 10, 13, 18, 19, 33, 34, 41, 70, 75, 81, 91–93, 101, 127, 136, 144, 167, 179, 180, 182, 183

States. In addition, goitrogens such as thiocyanates, perchlorates, rubidium salts, and arsenic are known to interfere with thyroidal iodine uptake.[179] Clinical signs include newborn animals with generalized alopecia and thickened, puffy (myxedematous) skin. Animals may be alive at birth but usually die within a few hours. Goiter may or may not be visible externally.

Dermatohistopathologic findings include epidermal atrophy, sebaceous gland hypoplasia, diffuse mucinous degeneration (myxedema), and scarce hair follicles that are hypoplastic.[71, 127] Blood levels of thyroid hormones are reported to be low.[9, 13, 127, 136, 180] Thyroid glands are enlarged and may be hemorrhagic.[13, 134]

Iodine supplied in fertilizer or in salt or mineral mixtures is effective for prevention.[13, 179] An organic iodide, ethylenediamine dihydroiodine (EDDI), has been recommended as a food additive for cattle (50 mg/head/day in feed), sheep (12 mg/head/day in feed), and swine (250 to 500 mg/head/day for one week).[16] Salt licks containing potassium iodate at a level of 0.01 percent iodine are also effective.[39, 92, 179] The daily iodine requirements for swine, cattle, and horses have been estimated to be 8 μg/kg, 400 to 800 μg/head, and 1 to 2.6 mg/head, respectively.[39, 101] Iodine toxicity (iodism) is characterized by coughing, seromucoid nasal discharge, excessive lacrimation, and generalized scaling of the skin (see Chapter 4, discussion on iodism).[13, 16] The minimum toxic iodine (as calcium iodate) intake for cattle is about 50 to 100 ppm, whereas in swine, it is about 400 to 800 ppm.[179]

Zinc. Zinc (Zn) has many functions in body metabolism.[82, 106, 107, 121, 124, 179] It is needed for muscle and bone growth, feed utilization, normal reproductive function, taste and smell acuity, normal leukocyte function, and normal keratogenesis and wound healing and is a component of over 70 metalloenzymes. Deficiency syndromes have occurred in the field and have been extensively studied using experimental diets in cattle, sheep, and goats.* The nature of the diet is important because calcium, phytates, and other chelating agents and feedstuffs affect zinc absorption and requirements.

Clinical signs of zinc deficiency are remarkably similar in cattle, sheep, and goats. The sequence of clinical signs is not consistent and includes decreased feed consumption and growth rate, depraved appetite (wool eating), wool break, listlessness, shivering, testicular atrophy, stiff or swollen joints, bowing of the hind legs, and decreased resistance to infec-

---

*References 5, 12, 13, 80, 82, 99, 106, 111, 112, 114, 115, 117, 120, 122, 129, 131, 133, 137, 138, 161, 164, 172, 178, 179

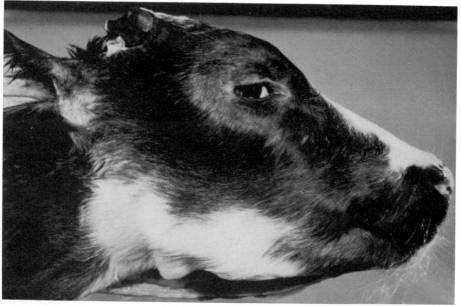

FIGURE 12–8. Bovine copper deficiency. Periocular lightening of hair creating a spectacled appearance. (Courtesy J. M. King.)

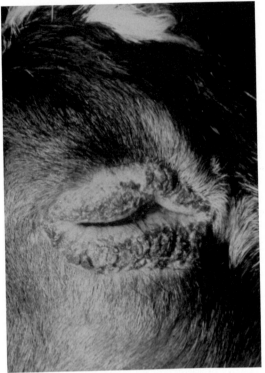

FIGURE 12–9. *Zinc-responsive dermatosis in a goat. Periocular crusts.*

tions. The nasal and oral mucosae become inflamed, and submucosal hemorrhages and horny overgrowths are seen on the lips and dental pads. Cutaneous changes include a dull, rough hair coat, with scaling, crusting, and alopecia developing over the face, ears, neck, distal limbs, and mucocutaneous junctions and with variable pruritus (Fig. 12–9). The coronary bands become inflamed, crusted, and fissured (Fig. 12–10). Hooves may become deformed and twisted. Wound healing is prolonged.[12, 104, 115, 118–120, 179] It has been suggested that low zinc levels predispose to infectious pododermatitis in cattle.[82]

A syndrome called itching tail root eczema has been described in cattle.[53–56] The syndrome was particularly common in young, nonlactating cattle and in dairy cows during the dry period, especially when rations were high in calcium. Affected cattle would lick and bite themselves, especially over the tailhead (which became excoriated and crusted), twitch their tails, and have decreased appetites, fertility, and milk production. Affected cattle had much higher urinary calcium levels and lower urinary magnesium levels than do normal cattle, and they had very low levels of serum alkaline phosphatase. These abnormalities returned to normal during zinc therapy. Treatment with 800 mg of zinc chloride ($ZnCl_2$)/cow/day or 240 mg of zinc oxide (ZnO)/cow/day resulted in clinical remission within 3 to 14 days. Cessation of zinc therapy was followed by relapse within 14 days. Diets containing 45 ppm of zinc were found to be protective. This syndrome was produced in 12.5 percent of all normal test cattle with diets containing 0.5 percent calcium, less than 45 ppm of zinc, and 2 to 11 ppm of copper.[54, 55] The syndrome could also be produced with diets containing 80 to 100 ppm zinc, but with a calcium content greater than 0.5 percent and a copper content less than 4 ppm.

Zinc-deficient cattle, sheep, and goats generally have low levels of serum alkaline phosphatase (may be low in "normal" cows) and dermatohistopathologic findings that include marked parakeratotic hyperkeratosis, epidermal hyperplasia, and a superficial perivascular accumulation of mononuclear cells and eosinophils (Fig. 12–11).* Some animals may show

---

*References 5, 12, 13, 80, 82, 113, 114, 120, 122, 131, 133, 137

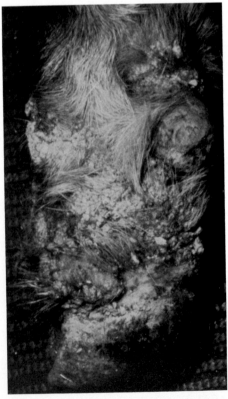

FIGURE 12–10. *Zinc-responsive dermatosis in a goat. Marked crusting of distal leg.*

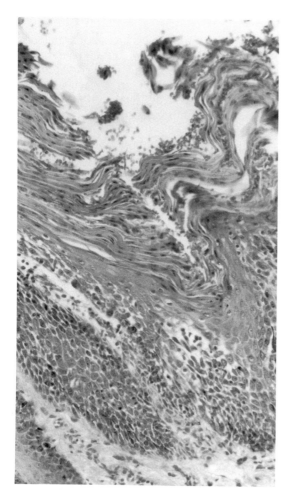

FIGURE 12–11. Zinc-responsive dermatosis in a goat. Hyperplastic superficial perivascular dermatitis with parakeratotic hyperkeratosis.

only orthokeratotic hyperkeratosis, or alternating parakeratotic and orthokeratotic hyperkeratosis.[106] Although serum or plasma zinc levels are usually low (lower than 50 μg/dl; normal range 100 to 200 μg/dl), these are not sufficiently accurate to be of general diagnostic worth.* Plasma zinc levels were decreased with several diseases in sheep and cattle.[25, 30, 82, 86, 179, 181] Zinc levels in hair and wool also were not found to be a suitable indicator of zinc status in dairy cows and lambs, respectively.[137, 162, 179] Scanning electron microscopic examination of wool fibers from zinc-deficient lambs revealed a variety of defects, including irregular or absent cortical scale pattern, separation of cortical cells, and breaking, fraying, and distortion of fibers.[106]

Because of the inherent difficulties associated with assessing zinc levels in cattle, sheep, and goats, it has been suggested that the best diagnostic indicator is the response to zinc therapy.[5, 12, 13, 122] Therapeutic recommendations include 2 to 5 gm of zinc sulfate ($ZnSO_4$)/day for cattle[5, 13]; 800 mg of zinc chloride or 240 mg of zinc oxide/day for cattle[53]; 0.5 gm zinc salts/500 kg for cattle[5]; 40 mg of zinc sulfate/day for sheep[129] and 100 mg zinc/kg diet for sheep.[131] Oral treatment is not always effective when there are problems with absorption, and a single intramuscular injection of either zinc oxide or metallic zinc powder has been shown to be both effective and quick-acting.[82–85] The dose rates commonly used are 300 mg of zinc metal (in 5 ml of an oily suspension) for adult sheep and goats and 600 mg (in 10 ml) for adult cattle. The author and others[129] have treated zinc-responsive skin disease in goats and sheep with 0.25 to 0.5 gm of zinc sulfate/day. This condition has *not* been associated with dietary deficiency, has affected individual animals, and has required constant therapy. In general, a dietary level of about 10 ppm zinc is sufficient for ruminant growth and maintenance.[39, 179] Cattle and sheep appear to have a relatively high tolerance for zinc, with no toxic effects being produced by diets containing 500 ppm of zinc.[5, 12, 13, 120, 179] Diets containing 700 to 1500 ppm zinc produced reduced weight gain, reduced feed efficiency, and perinatal deaths in sheep.[179] Diets containing 900 ppm of zinc resulted in reduced weight gain and feed efficiency in cattle.[179] Poor appetite, weight loss, decreased milk production, and abortions were reported in cattle and sheep given zinc sulfate.[169, 170] Recent studies[51a, 51b] have indicated that preruminants (veal calves) are more susceptible to zinc toxicosis (clinical signs included pneumonia, ocular disease, anorexia, bloat, cardiac arrhythmias) and that zinc concentrations should not exceed 100 μg/kg of diet in these animals.

Selenium (Se). Selenium is an essential mineral.[178, 179] Selenium deficiency was reported in a 60-cow dairy herd suffering from retained placentas, pyometra, poor conception rates, foot and leg problems, respiratory disease, and dermatitis around the base of the tail.[74] Serum calcium and zinc levels were normal, but serum selenium levels were low (0.036 to 0.061 ppm; in normal cattle, 0.077 to 0.160 ppm). Dietary selenium supplementation resulted in a resolution of the disorders within two months.

*References 5, 12, 13, 25, 82, 99, 122, 129, 162, 179, 181

SWINE PARAKERATOSIS

Parakeratosis is a self-limited, nutrition-related metabolic disorder of growing pigs characterized by a generalized nonpruritic crusting dermatosis.[13, 18, 19, 34, 78, 91]

CAUSE AND PATHOGENESIS

The exact cause of swine parakeratosis is unknown. The condition was originally observed in the late 1940's, coinciding with the increasing introduction of dry-meal feeding.[13, 34, 58, 78, 91, 135] Parakeratosis occurs rarely, if ever, in pigs whose diets include pasture grasses. An identical syndrome can be induced by dietary zinc deficiency, and zinc therapy is known to be curative in the naturally occurring disease.* In addition, high levels of dietary calcium, phytates, and other minerals and chelators will exacerbate the disorder.†

Hanson and colleagues[58] reported that a deficiency of essential fatty acids in swine produced a syndrome very similar to parakeratosis. These authors found fatty acids to be equally as effective as zinc in the treatment and prevention of swine parakeratosis. They postulated that parakeratosis was associated with periods of extremely rapid growth and the inability of essential fatty acid biosynthesis to keep up with metabolic demands. Hvidsten and associates[69] reported that the serum levels of unsaturated fatty acids in parakeratotic and normal pigs were identical.

Pigs with intestinal infections (transmissible gastroenteritis virus, *Clostridium perfringens*) develop more severe forms of zinc deficiency and parakeratosis.[102, 184] In addition, a parakeratosis-like syndrome was induced in swine fed methylthiouracil (a thyroid antagonist) for several days.[44, 59] The gross and histologic appearance of the skin was typical for swine parakeratosis, but the swine also had typical iodine-deficient goitrous thyroid glands on gross and histologic examination. The zinc content of the hair and bone was reduced.

It is probably best to think of swine parakeratosis as a temporary, nutrition-related metabolic disorder of rapidly growing pigs, in which dietary zinc, essential fatty acids, calcium, other chelating agents, and other disease conditions play a role.

CLINICAL FEATURES

Swine parakeratosis is a cosmopolitan disease that usually affects housed feeder pigs between the ages of 7 and 20 weeks, regardless of breed or sex.[13, 18, 34, 78, 91] It is usually seen in 20 to 80 percent of the pigs in affected herds and is more common in winter and early spring in the northeastern United States.

Early clinical signs consist of erythematous macules and papules on the ventral abdomen and medial thighs. The dermatitis spreads and evolves into hard, dry crusts, especially on the distal limbs, face, ears, tail, and ventrum (Fig. 12–12). Pruritus is absent, and greasiness is minimal to absent. Secondary skin infections, especially hock abscesses, are fairly common.

Parakeratotic swine frequently exhibit reduced appetite, growth rate, and feed utilization efficiency.[13, 18, 34, 78, 91, 110] Death is rare, and any economic losses are associated with the growth retardation, which is directly related to the severity of the disease. Mild to moderately severe diarrhea and occasional vomiting may also be seen.[18, 19, 24, 34, 91, 105] Pigs with experimental zinc deficiency had retarded thymic and testicular development.[110, 123, 124, 179, 184]

DIAGNOSIS

Diagnosis is based on history, physical examination, and laboratory evaluation. Skin biopsy reveals hyperplastic superficial perivascular dermatitis with marked diffuse parakeratotic hyperkeratosis.* The superficial dermis is edematous, and a perivascular accumulation of mononuclear cells and eosinophils is seen. Electron microscopy reveals injury to keratinocyte tonofibrils and desmosomes.[76] Although the total mucopolysaccharide content of parakeratotic skin is unchanged, the hyaluronic acid component is increased.[175]

Serum alkaline phosphatase levels and serum zinc levels (mean of 17 μg/dl; in normal pigs, mean of 60 μg/dl) are decreased.† However, for reasons previously discussed (see discussion on zinc), fluctuations in serum zinc levels are modulated by many factors and are unlikely to be of significant benefit in the field.

CLINICAL MANAGEMENT

Swine parakeratosis is a self-limited disorder. Mildly to moderately affected animals and

---

*References 13, 18, 34, 76–78, 91, 110, 123, 124, 139, 153, 165, 171, 173, 175, 176, 179
†References 13, 18, 34, 61, 63, 91, 95, 110, 123, 124, 153, 154, 178, 179

---

*References 13, 76, 78, 91, 139, 175, 176, 191
†References 11, 13, 34, 61, 63, 64, 91, 96, 110, 124, 140, 154, 155, 179

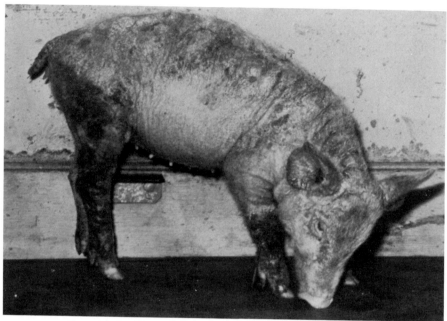

FIGURE 12–12. Swine parakeratosis. Generalized hyperkeratosis and crusting. (Courtesy J. Runnels.)

severely affected animals usually recover in 10 to 14 days or 30 to 45 days, respectively, even without therapy.[13, 18, 34, 91] Therapy and prevention revolve around dietary correction.* Calcium intake should be kept at 0.65 to 0.75 percent of the total ration. Zinc salts should be supplemented at 0.02 percent, or 100 ppm, or the caloric ration (e.g., 0.4 pound of zinc sulfate or zinc carbonate/T feed). Fats should comprise 1.0 percent of the total ration.[39, 79, 190]

Zinc toxicity has been produced in piglets,[14, 179] but the margin of safety is wide. When zinc was supplemented at an amount greater than 1000 ppm of the ration, piglets developed growth retardation, arthritis, gastritis, and enteritis.

DERMATOSIS ASSOCIATED WITH HIGH-FAT MILK REPLACERS IN CALVES

A dermatosis characterized by alopecia and scaling has been reported in calves receiving high-fat (15 to 20 percent) milk replacers.[7, 31, 50, 98, 141] Clinical signs were observed within two to three weeks after calves were placed on various proprietary milk substitutes. The cutaneous changes were particularly severe on the muzzle, periocular region, base of the pinnae, and the limbs. In addition, many calves developed signs of muscular dystrophy (muscle weakness and stiffness, tachycardia).

Affected calves had adequate selenium levels, as assessed by erythrocyte glutathione peroxidase activity, but had low levels of plasma vitamin E (0.2 to 1.3 μg/ml, with levels higher than 1.5 μg/ml being normal).[141]

Some calves were treated with a single dose of a vitamin E–selenium preparation, which resulted in a rapid recovery.[141] Thereafter, all calves were given vitamin E and selenium at about one week of age, and no further cases of the syndrome were seen. In other cases, the calves were switched to a lower-fat milk powder (10 percent), which also resulted in rapid recovery.[141]

The pathogenesis of this syndrome is not understood, but the similarities, in some respects, to muscular dystrophy resulting from a deficiency of vitamin E and selenium are intriguing.

REFERENCES

1. Alfano, M. C., et al.: Effect of ascorbic acid deficiency on the permeability and collagen biosynthesis of oral mucosal epithelium. Ann. N.Y. Acad. Sci. 258:253, 1975.
2. Alexander, G.: Temperature regulation in the newborn lamb. Aust. J. Agric. Res. 13:82, 1962.
3. Alexander, G.: Heat production of newborn lambs in relation to type of birth coat. Proc. Aust. Soc. Anim. Prod. 2:10, 1958.
4. Allcroft, R., and Lewis, G.: Relationships of copper, molybdenum and inorganic sulfate content of feeding stuffs to

*References 13, 18, 34, 58, 91, 124, 165, 171, 178, 179

the occurrence of copper deficiency in sheep and cattle. Landbouwkd Tijdschr. 68:711, 1956.

5. Amstutz, H. E.: *Bovine Medicine and Surgery II*. Santa Barbara, CA, American Veterinary Publications, Inc., 1980.

6. Andrews, F. N., et al.: Iodine deficiency in newborn sheep and swine. J. Anim. Sci. 7:298, 1948.

7. Anonymous: Alopecia in calves. Mod. Vet. Pract. 65:6, 1984.

8. Barnes, M. J.: Function of ascorbic acid in collagen metabolism. Ann. N.Y. Acad. Sci. 258:264, 1975.

9. Bath, G. F., et al.: Cretinism in Angora goats. J. S. Afr. Vet. Assoc. 50:237, 1979.

10. Baumann, R.: Goitre and myxoedema in newborn goats. Wien. Tierarztl. Monatsschr. 35:585, 1948.

11. Beardsley, D. W., and Forbes, R. M.: Growth and chemical studies of zinc deficiency in the baby pig. J. Anim. Sci. 16:1038, 1957.

12. Blackmon, D. M., et al.: Zinc deficiency in ruminants: Occurrence, effects, diagnosis, treatments. Vet. Med. Small Anim. Clin. 62:265, 1967.

13. Blood, D. C., Henderson, J. A., and Radostits, O. M.: *Veterinary Medicine V*. Philadelphia, Lea & Febiger, 1979.

13a. Booth, A., et al.: Hypovitaminosis A in feedlot cattle. JAVMA 191:1305, 1987.

13b. Brewer, N. R.: Comparative metabolism of copper. JAVMA 190:654, 1987.

14. Brink, M. F., et al.: Zinc toxicity in the weanling pig. J. Anim. Sci. 18:83, 1959.

15. Brooks, P. H., et al.: Biotin supplementation of diets. The incidence of foot lesions, and the reproductive performance of sows. Vet. Rec. 101:46, 1977.

15a. Bryant, K. L., et al.: Supplemental biotin for swine. III. Influence of supplementation to corn- and wheat-based diets on the incidence and severity of toe lesions, hair and skin characteristics, and structural soundness of sows housed in confinement during parities. J. Anim. Sci. 60:154, 1985.

16. Buck, W. B.: Iodine. *In*: Howard, J. L. (ed.): *Current Veterinary Therapy. Food Animal Practice*. Philadelphia, W. B. Saunders Co., 1981, p. 398.

17. Cabak, V., et al.: Severe undernutrition in growing and adult animals. X. The skin and hair of the pigs. Br. J. Nutr. 16:635, 1962.

18. Cameron, R. D. A.: *Skin diseases of the pig*. Proc. Univ. Sydney Post-Grad. Comm. Vet. Sci. 56:445, 1981.

19. Cameron, R. D. A. *Skin Diseases of the Pig*. Sydney, University of Sydney Post-Graduate Foundation in Veterinary Science, Veterinary Review No. 23, 1984.

20. Cargill, C. F.: Noninfectious preweaning health problems. Proc. Univ. Sydney Post-Grad. Comm. Vet. Sci. 56:75, 1981.

21. Chatterjee, I. B., et al.: Synthesis and some major functions of vitamin C in animals. Ann. N.Y. Acad. Sci. 258:24, 1975.

22. Chauvaux, G., et al.: Cuivre et manganese chez les bovins, méthodes de dosage et signification biologique du cuivre et du manganese dans les poils. Ann. Med. Vet. 109:174, 1965.

23. Chick, H., et al.: Curative action of nicotinic acid on pigs suffering from the effects of a diet consisting largely of maize. Biochem. J. 32:10, 1938.

24. Cole, C. L., et al.: Dermatosis of the ears, cheeks, neck, and shoulders in young calves. Vet. Med. 39:204, 1944.

25. Corrigall, W., et al.: Modulation of plasma copper and zinc concentrations by disease states in ruminants. Vet. Rec. 99:396, 1976.

26. Cunha, J. J., et al.: Biotin deficiency syndrome in pigs fed desiccated egg white. J. Anim. Sci. 5:219, 1946.

27. Cunha, J. J., et al.: Further observations on the dietary insufficiency of a corn-soybean ration for reproduction of swine. J. Anim. Sci. 3:415, 1944.

28. Cuthbertson, W. F. J.: Vitamins in animal feeding-stuffs. Vet. Rec. 69:192, 1957.

29. Davis, G. K., and Freeman, V. A.: Studies upon the relation of nutrition to the development of necrotic enteritis in young pigs fed massive doses of *S. choleraesuis*. Proc. Am. Assoc. Anim. Prod. 1940.

30. Depelchin, B. O., et al.: Clinical and experimental modifi-

31. Dirksen, G., and Hoffman, W.: Actual health problems in the rearing and fattening of calves—a review. Vet. Med. Rev. 1:3, 1974.

32. Dunne, H. W., et al.: The pathology of niacin deficiency in swine. Am. J. Vet. Res. 10:351, 1949.

33. Dunne, H. W.: *Diseases of Swine III*. Ames, Iowa State University Press, 1970.

34. Dunne, H. W., and Leman, A. D.: *Diseases of Swine IV*. Ames, Iowa State University Press, 1975.

35. Dutt, B., and Kehar, N. D.: Incidence of goitre in goats and sheep in India. Br. Vet. J. 115:176, 1959.

36. Dutt, B., and Majumdar, B. N.: Epithelial metaplasia in experimental vitamin A deficient goats. Indian Vet. J. 46:789, 1969.

37. Dynna, O., and Havre, G. N.: Interrelationship of zinc and copper in the nutrition of cattle. A complex zinc-copper deficiency. Acta Vet. Scand. 4:197, 1963.

38. Ellis, N. R.: The vitamin requirements of swine. Nutr. Abst. Rev. 16:1, 1946.

39. Ensminger, M. E., and Olentine, C. G.: *Feeds and Nutrition—Complete*. Clovis, CA, Ensminger Publishing Co., 1978.

40. Everitt, G. C.: Residual effects of prenatal nutrition on the postnatal performance of Merino sheep. Proc. N.Z. Soc. Anim. Prod. 27:52, 1967.

41. Evvard, J. M.: Iodine deficiency symptoms and their significance in animal nutrition and pathology. Endocrinology 12:539, 1928.

42. Frenkel, M. J., et al.: Factors influencing the biosynthesis of the tyrosine-rich proteins of wool. Aust. J. Biol. Sci. 27:31, 1974.

43. Frenkel, M. J., et al.: Studies on the inhibition of synthesis of the tyrosine-rich proteins of wool. Aust. J. Biol. Sci. 28:331, 1975.

44. Gabrasanski, P., and Nedkova, L.: Neki novi pogledi etiopatogeneze parakeratoze prasadi. Vet. Glasnik. 29:485, 1975.

45. Geyer, H., et al.: Morphologische und histochemische Untersuchungen von Haut, Schleimhauten und Klauen bei Schweinen mit experimentellem Biotinmangel. Zbl. Vet. Med. A 28:574, 1981.

46. Geyer, H., et al.: Der Einfluss des experimentellen Biotinmangels auf Morphologie und Histochemie von Haut und Klauen des Schweines. Zbl. Vet. Med. A 31:519, 1984.

46a. Ghanem, Y. S., and Farid, M. F. A.: Vitamin A deficiency and supplementation in desert sheep. Deficiency symptoms, plasma concentrations, and body growth. World Rev. Anim. Prod. 18:69, 1982.

47. Glattli, H. R., et al.: Klinischne und morphologische Befunde beim experimentellen Biotinmangel. Zbl. Vet. Med. A 22:102, 1975.

48. Glattli, H. R.: Zur Klinik des experimentell erzeugten Biotinmangels beim Schwein und Mitteilung erster Ergebnisse aus Feldversuchen. Schweiz. Arch. Tierheilkd. 117:135, 1975.

49. Goodwin, R. F. W.: Some clinical and experimental observations on naturally occurring pantothenic acid deficiency in pigs. J. Comp. Pathol. 72:214, 1962.

50. Grunder, H. D.: Alopezie beim Kalb-Ursachen und Behandlung. Prakt. Tierarztl. 58:84, 1977.

51. Gordon, A. J., and Donnel, J. B.: The potential for harvesting weakened wool. Aust. J. Agric. Res. 30:949, 1979.

51a. Graham, T. W., et al.: Economic losses from an episode of zinc toxicosis on a California veal calf operation using a zinc sulfate–supplemented milk replacer. JAVMA 190:668, 1987.

51b. Graham, T. W., et al.: An epidemiologic study of mortality in veal calves subsequent to an episode of zinc toxicosis on a California veal calf operation using zinc sulfate–supplemented milk replacer. JAVMA 190:1296, 1987.

52. Gutwein, G. M. L.: Ear necrosis in swine. Mod. Vet. Pract. 64:143, 1983.

53. Haaranen, S.: The effect of zinc on itching tail root eczema in cattle. Nord. Vet. Med. 14:265, 1962.

54. Haaranen, S.: Some observations on the zinc requirement of cattle for the prevention of itch and hair licking with

cations of plasma iron and zinc concentrations in cattle. Vet. Rec. 116:519, 1985.

different calcium levels in the feed. Nord. Vet. Med. 15:536, 1963.

55. Haaranen, S.: Some observations on the occurrence of itch and hair licking in cattle at different zinc and copper levels in the feed. Nord. Vet. Med. 17:36, 1965.

56. Haaranen, S.: Zinc requirements of dairy cattle for removal of deficiency symptoms. Feedstuffs 35:17, 1963.

57. Hale, F.: The relation of vitamin A to anophthalmos in pigs. Am. J. Ophthalmol. 18:1087, 1935.

58. Hanson, L. J., et al.: Essential fatty acid deficiency—its role in parakeratosis. Am. J. Vet. Res. 19:921, 1958.

59. Hennig, A., et al.: Die Parakeratose des Schweines. 4. Mitteilung: Methylthiouracil als Parakeratosenoxe. Arch. Exp. Vet. Med. 23:911, 1969.

60. Hentges, J. F., et al.: Experimental avitaminosis A in young pigs. JAVMA 120:213, 1952.

61. Hoefer, J. A., et al.: Interrelationships between calcium, zinc, iron, and copper in swine feeding. J. Anim. Sci. 19:249, 1960.

62. Hoekstra, W. G.: Parakeratosis in swine. Vet. Sci. News Univ. Wics. 9:1, 1955.

63. Hoekstra, W. G., et al.: The relationship of parakeratosis, supplemental calcium and zinc to the zinc content of certain body components of swine. J. Anim. Sci. 15:752, 1956.

64. Hoekstra, W. G., et al.: Zinc deficiency in reproducing gilts fed a diet high in calcium and its effect on tissue zinc and blood serum alkaline phosphatase. J. Anim. Sci. 26:1348, 1967.

65. Hughes, E. H.: The minimum requirement of nicotinic acid for the growing pig. J. Anim. Sci. 2:23, 1943.

66. Hughes, E. H.: The minimum requirement of riboflavin for the growing pig. J. Nutr. 20:233, 1940.

67. Hughes, E. H., and Ittner, N. R.: The minimum requirement of pantothenic acid for the growing pig. J. Anim. Sci. 1:116, 1942.

68. Hutchinson, G., and Mellor, D. J.: Effects of maternal nutrition on the initiation of secondary wool follicles in foetal sheep. J. Comp. Pathol. 93:577, 1983.

69. Hvidsten, H., et al.: Unsaturated fatty acids of blood stream from pigs with and without parakeratosis. Proc. Soc. Exp. Biol. Med. 89:454, 1955.

70. Irvine, C. H. G., and Evans, M. J.: Hypothyroidism in foals. N.Z. Vet. J. 25:354, 1977.

71. Itakura, C., et al.: Histopathologic features of the skin of hairless newborn pigs with goiter. Am. J. Vet. Res. 40:111, 1979.

72. Jensen, R., and Swift, B. L.: Diseases of Sheep II. Philadelphia, Lea & Febiger, 1982.

73. Johnson, W. S.: Vitamins A and C as factors affecting skin condition in experimental piglets. Vet. Rec. 79:363, 1966.

74. Jones, G.: Selenium deficiency in a dairy herd. Mod. Vet. Pract. 65:868, 1984.

75. Jovanovic, M., et al.: Goitre in domestic animals in Serbia. Acta Vet. (Belgr.) 3:31, 1953.

76. Kapp, P., and Simon, F.: Ultrastructural cutaneous changes in zinc-depleted pigs. Acta Vet. Acad. Sci. Hung. 28:463, 1980.

77. Keith, T. B., et al.: Nutritional deficiencies of a concentrate mixture composed of corn, tankage, soybean oil meal, and alfalfa meal for growing pigs. J. Anim. Sci. 1:120, 1942.

78. Kernkamp, H. C. H., and Ferrin, E. F.: Parakeratosis in swine. JAVMA 123:217, 1953.

79. King, J. O. L.: Veterinary Dietetics. Baltimore, Williams & Wilkins Company, 1961.

80. Kirchgessner, M., and Schwarz, W. A.: Beziehungen zwischen klinischen Zinkmangelsymptomen und Zinkstatus bei laktierenden Kuhen. Zbl. Vet. Med. A22:572, 1975.

81. Lall, H. K.: A case of congenital goitre in kids. Indian Vet. J. 29:133, 1952.

82. Lamand, M.: Zinc deficiency in ruminants. Irish Vet. J. 38:40, 1984.

83. Lamand, M.: Copper and zinc deficiencies treatment by intramuscular injections in sheep. Ann. Rech. Vet. 9:495, 1978.

84. Lamand, M., et al.: A zinc-deficient diet for ruminants: Diagnosis and treatment of deficiency. Ann. Rech. Vet. 14:211, 1983.

85. Lamand, M., et al.: Comparison of the efficiency of zinc injected as metal or oxide for zinc deficiency treatment in sheep. Ann. Rech. Vet. 11:147, 1980.

86. Lamand, M., and Levieux, D.: Effects of infection on plasma levels of copper and zinc in ewes. Ann. Rech. Vet. 12:113, 1981.

87. Leat, W. M. F.: Studies on pig diets containing different amounts of linoleic acid. Br. J. Nutr. 16:559, 1962.

88. Legg, S. P., and Sears, L.: Zinc sulphate treatment of parakeratosis in cattle. Nature 186:1061, 1960.

89. Lehrer, W. P., and Wiese, A. C.: Riboflavin deficiency in baby pigs. J. Anim. Sci. 11:244, 1952.

90. Lehrer, W. P., et al.: Biotin deficiency in suckling pigs. J. Anim. Sci. 11:245, 1952.

91. Leman, A. D., et al.: Diseases of Swine V. Ames, Iowa State University Press, 1981.

92. Lofstedt, J.: Dermatologic diseases of sheep. Vet. Clin. North Am. Large Anim. Pract. 5:427, 1983.

93. Love, W. G.: Parenchymatous goiter in newborn goats and sheep. JAVMA 101:484, 1942.

94. Lowe, N. J., and DeQuoy, P. R.: Linoleic acid effects on epidermal DNA synthesis and cutaneous prostaglandin levels in essential fatty acid deficiency. J. Invest. Dermatol. 70:200, 1978.

95. Luecke, R. W., et al.: Mineral interrelationships in parakeratosis in swine. J. Anim. Sci. 15:347, 1956.

96. Luecke, R. W., et al.: Calcium and zinc in parakeratosis of swine. J. Anim. Sci. 16:3, 1957.

97. Madison, L. C., et al.: Nicotinic acid in swine nutrition. Science 89:490, 1939.

98. Maidment, D. C. J.: The feeding of stored bovine colostrum to calves. Br. Vet. J. 137:268, 1981.

99. Mahmoud, O. M., et al.: Zinc deficiency in Sudanese desert sheep. J. Comp. Pathol. 93:591, 1983.

100. Manning, T. O.: Noninfectious skin diseases of cattle. Vet. Clin. North Am. Large Anim. Pract. 6:175, 1984.

101. Mansmann, R. A., McAllister, E. S., and Pratt, P. W.: Equine Medicine and Surgery III. Santa Barbara, CA, American Veterinary Publications, Inc., 1982.

102. Mansson, I.: The intestinal flora in pigs with parakeratosis. I. The intestinal flora with special reference to an atypical Clostridium perfringens and clinical observations. Acta Vet. Scand. 5:279, 1964.

103. Marks, J.: A Guide to the Vitamins, Their Role in Health and Disease. Lancaster, Medical and Technical Publishing, 1975.

104. Martin, Y. G., et al.: Wound healing, hair growth, and biochemical measures as affected by subnormal protein and energy intake in young cattle. Am. J. Vet. Res. 30:355, 1969.

105. Martinsson, K., and Ekman, L.: Behandlingsforsok med zink aveseende s.k. pellar bland avvanda grisar. Svensk. Vet. 26:824, 1974.

106. Masters, D. G., et al.: Effects of zinc deficiency on the wool growth, skin, and wool follicles of pre-ruminant lambs. Aust. J. Biol. Sci. 38:355, 1985.

107. Michaelsson, G., et al.: Effects of oral zinc and vitamin A in acne. Arch. Dermatol. 113:31, 1977.

108. Miller, C. O., et al.: The riboflavin requirement of swine for reproduction. J. Nutr. 51:163, 1953.

109. Miller, E. R., et al.: The riboflavin requirement of the baby pig. J. Nutr. 52:405, 1954.

110. Miller, E. R., et al.: Biochemical, skeletal and allometric changes due to zinc deficiency in the baby pig. J. Nutr. 95:278, 1968.

111. Miller, J. K., and Miller, W. J.: Development of zinc deficiency in Holstein calves fed a purified diet. J. Dairy Sci. 43:1854, 1960.

112. Miller, J. K., and Miller, W. J.: Experimental zinc deficiency and recovery of calves. J. Nutr. 76:467, 1961.

113. Miller, W. J., and Miller, J. K.: Photomicrographs of skin from zinc-deficient calves. J. Dairy Sci. 46:1285, 1963.

114. Miller, W. J., et al.: Experimentally produced zinc deficiency in the goat. J. Dairy Sci. 47:556, 1964.

115. Miller, W. J., et al.: Effect of zinc deficiency and restricted feeding on wound healing in the bovine. Proc. Soc. Exp. Biol. Med. 118:427, 1965.

116. Miller, W. J., et al.: Influence of zinc deficiency on zinc and dry matter content of ruminant tissues and excretion of zinc. J. Dairy Sci. 49:1446, 1966.

117. Miller, W. J.: Calfhood zinc deficiency and limited feed intake on subsequent reproduction in bulls. Feedstuffs 39:18, 1967.

118. Miller, W. J., et al.: Effects of adding two forms of supplemental zinc to a practical diet on skin regeneration in Holstein heifers and evaluation of a procedure for determining rate of wound healing. J. Dairy Sci. 50:715, 1967.

119. Miller, W. J., et al.: Effect of high protein diets with normal and low energy intake on wound healing, hair growth, hair and serum zinc, and serum alkaline phosphatase in dairy heifers. J. Nutr. 98:411, 1969.

120. Miller, W. J.: Zinc nutrition of cattle: A review. J. Dairy Sci. 53:1123, 1970.

121. Mills, C. F., et al.: Metabolic role of zinc. Am. J. Clin. Nutr. 22:1240, 1969.

122. Mills, C. F., et al.: Zinc deficiency and the zinc requirements of calves and lambs. Br. J. Nutrit. 21:751, 1967.

123. Mills, C. F.: Metabolic interrelationships in the utilization of trace elements. Proc. Nutr. Soc. 23:38, 1964.

124. Mills, C. F.: *Trace Element Metabolism in Animals*. Edinburgh, E. and S. Livingston, 1970.

125. Mills, C. F., et al.: Biochemical and pathological changes in tissues of Friesian cattle during experimental induction of copper deficiency. Br. J. Nutr. 35:309, 1976.

126. Mitchell, H. H., et al.: The riboflavin requirement of the growing pig at two environmental temperatures. J. Nutr. 41:317, 1950.

127. Nagae, K., et al.: An outbreak of alopecia in newborn piglets. J. Jpn. Vet. Med. Assoc. 33:333, 1980.

128. Neathery, M. W., et al.: Performance and milk zinc from low-zinc intake in Holstein cows. J. Dairy Sci. 56:212, 1973.

129. Nelson, D. R., et al.: Zinc deficiency in sheep and goats: Three field cases. JAVMA 184:1480, 1984.

130. Nelson, E. C., et al.: Effect of vitamin A intake on some biochemical and physiological changes in swine. J. Nutr. 76:325, 1962.

131. Ott, E. A., et al.: Zinc deficiency syndrome in the young lamb. J. Nutr. 82:41, 1964.

132. Ott, E. A., et al.: Zinc requirement of the growing lamb fed a purified diet. J. Nutr. 87:459, 1965.

133. Ott, E. A., et al.: Zinc deficiency syndrome in the young calf. J. Anim. Sci. 24:735, 1965.

134. Pantic, V., and Jovanovic, M.: Histology of the thyroid in endemic goitre in domestic animals. Acta Vet. (Belgr.) 5:13, 1955.

135. Pepere, L., and Placidi, L.: "Parakeratose" syndrome de déséquilibre alimentaire chez le porc. Rec. Med. Vet. 132:913, 1956.

136. Piel, H. P.: Goitre chez le veau: Mise en évidence et traitement d'une carence en iode sur un troupeau de bovins en combrailles (France). Rec. Med. Vet. 155:605, 1979.

137. Pierson, R. E.: Zinc deficiency in young lambs. JAVMA 149:1279, 1966.

138. Pitts, W. J., et al.: Effect of zinc deficiency and restricted feeding from two to five months of age on reproduction in Holstein bulls. J. Dairy Sci. 49:995, 1966.

139. Platt, B. S.: Nutritional influences on the skin: Experimental evidence. *In*: Rook, A. J., and Walton, G. S. (eds.): *Comparative Physiology and Pathology of the Skin*. Oxford, Blackwell Scientific Publications, 1965, p. 245.

140. Pond, W. G., et al.: Influence of dietary zinc, corn oil, and cadmium on certain blood components, weight gain, and parakeratosis in weanling pigs. J. Anim. Sci. 23:16, 1964.

141. Pritchard, G. C., et al.: Alopecia in calves associated with milk substitute feeding. Vet. Rec. 112:435, 1983.

142. Prottey, C., et al.: Correction of the cutaneous manifestations of essential fatty acid deficiency in man by application of sunflower seed oil to the skin. J. Invest. Dermatol. 64:228, 1975.

143. Pryor, W. J.: Plasma zinc status of dairy cattle in the periparturient period. N.Z. Vet. J. 24:57, 1976.

144. Rajkumar, S. S.: A case of congenital goiter in kids. Indian Vet. J. 47:133, 1970.

145. Reis, P. J.: Effects of amino acids on the growth and properties of wool. *In* Black, J. L., and Reis, P. J. (eds.): *Physiological and Environmental Limitations to Wool Growth*. Armidale, University of New England Publishing Unit, 1979, p. 223.

146. Reis, P. J., et al.: Investigations of some amino acid analogues and metabolites as inhibitors of wool and hair growth. Aust. J. Biol. Sci. 36:157, 1983.

147. Reis, P. J., and Tunks, D. A.: The influence of abomasal supplements of zinc and some amino acids on wool growth rate and plasma amino acids. J. Agric. Sci. 86:475, 1976.

148. Reis, P. J., and Tunks, D. A.: Effects on wool growth of the infusion of mixtures of amino acids into the abomasum of sheep. J. Agric. Sci. 90:173, 1978.

149. Reis, P. J., and Panaretto, B. A.: Chemical defleecing as a method of harvesting wool from sheep. World Anim. Rev. 30:36, 1979.

150. Reis, P. J., and Tunks, D. A.: Inhibiting effects of ethionine, an analogue of methionine, on wool growth. Aust. J. Biol. Sci. 35:49, 1982.

151. Reis, P. J., et al.: Effects of mimosine, a potential chemical defleecing agent on wool growth and the skin of sheep. Aust. J. Biol. Sci. 28:69, 1975.

152. Reis, P. J., and Gillespie, J. M.: Effects of phenylalanine and analogues of methionine and phenylalanine on the composition of wool and mouse hair. Aust. J. Biol. Sci. 38:151, 1985.

152a. Reis, P. J., et al.: Effects of methoxinine, an analogue of methionine, on the growth and morphology of wool fibres. Aust. J. Biol. Sci. 39:209, 1986.

153. Ritchie, H. D., et al.: Copper and zinc interrelationship in swine feeding. J. Anim. Sci. 20:950, 1961.

154. Ritchie, H. D., et al.: Copper and zinc interrelationships in the pig. J. Nutr. 79:117, 1963.

155. Roberts, H. F., et al.: Significance of zinc in high calcium diets for reproducing gilts. J. Anim. Sci. 21:1011, 1962.

156. Robinson, W. L.: Solvent extracted cottonseed meal as a protein concentrate for pigs in dry lot. J. Anim. Sci. 7:531, 1948.

157. Rydell, R. O.: Dermatosis in calves. JAVMA 112:59, 1948.

158. Sanders, D. E.: Copper deficiency in food animals. Compend. Cont. Educ. 5:S404, 1983.

159. Samson, D. E., and Slee, J.: Factors affecting resistance to induced body cooling in newborn lambs of 10 breeds. Anim. Prod. 33:65, 1981.

160. Schinckel, P. G., and Short, B. F.: The influence of nutritional level during prenatal and postnatal life on adult fleece and body characters. Aust. J. Agric. Res. 12:176, 1961.

161. Schulze, A., and Ustdal, K. M.: Mogliche Ursachen der Alopezie turkischer Angora-Ziegen. Berl. Munch. tierarztl. Wochenschr. 88:66, 1975.

162. Schwarz, W. A., and Kirchgessner, M.: Zur Zinkkonzentration in Rinderhaar bei Zinkmangel. Dtsch. Tierarztl. Wochenschr. 82:141, 1975.

163. Scott, D. W.: Vitamin C–responsive dermatosis in calves. Bovine Pract. 2:22, 1981.

164. Scott, D. W., et al.: Caprine dermatology. II. Viral, nutritional, environmental, and congenitohereditary disorders. Compend. Cont. Educ. 6:S473, 1984.

165. Shanklin, S. H., et al.: Zinc requirements of baby pigs on casein diets. J. Nutr. 96:101, 1968.

166. Sharma, G. L., et al.: A study of the pathology of the intestine and other organs of weanling pigs when fed a ration of natural feedstuffs low in pantothenic acid. Am. J. Vet. Res. 13:298, 1952.

167. Slatter, E. E.: Mild iodine deficiency and losses of newborn pigs. JAVMA 127:149, 1955.

168. Smith, M. C.: Caprine dermatologic problems: A review. JAVMA 178:724, 1981.

169. Smith, B. L., et al.: The protective effect of zinc sulphate in experimental sporidesmin poisoning of sheep. N.Z. Vet. J. 25:124, 1977.

170. Smith, B. L.: Toxicity of zinc in ruminants. N.Z. Vet. J. 25:310, 1977.

171. Smith, W. H., et al.: Zinc requirements of the growing pig fed isolated soybean protein semi-purified rations. J. Anim. Sci. 20:128, 1961.

172. Spias, A. G., and Papasteriadis, A. A.: Zinc deficiency in

cattle under Greek conditions. *In*: Hoekstra, W.: *Trace Element Metabolism in Animals II*. Baltimore, University Park Press, 1974, p. 628.

173. Stevenson, J. W., and Earle, I. P.: Studies on parakeratosis in swine. J. Anim. Sci. 15:1036, 1956.

174. Suttle, N. F., and Angus, K. W.: Experimental copper deficiency in the calf. J. Comp. Pathol. 86:595, 1976.

175. Thompson, R. W., and Gilbreath, R. L.: Alteration of porcine skin acid mucopolysaccharides in zinc deficiency. J. Nutr. 105:154, 1975.

176. Tucker, H. F., and Salmon, W. D.: Parakeratosis or zinc deficiency disease in the pig. Proc. Soc. Exp. Biol. Med. 88:613, 1955.

177. Ullrey, D. E., et al.: Dietary levels of pantothenic acid and reproductive performance of female swine. J. Nutr. 57:401, 1955.

178. Underwood, E. J.: *Trace Elements in Human and Animal Nutrition III*. New York, Academic, 1971.

179. Underwood, E. J.: *Trace Elements in Human and Animal Nutrition IV*. New York, Academic Press, 1977.

180. Walton, E. A., and Humphrey, J. D.: Endemic goitre of sheep in the highlands of Papua, New Guinea. Aust. Vet. J. 55:43, 1979.

181. Wegner, T. N., et al.: Effect of stress on serum, zinc, and plasma corticoids in dairy cattle. J. Dairy Sci. 56:748, 1973.

182. Welch, H.: Hairlessness and goiter in newborn domestic animals. Bull. 119, Agric. Exp. Stat., Univ. Montana, 1917.

183. Welch, H.: Goiter in farm animals. Bull. 214, Agric. Exp. Stat., Univ. Montana, 1928.

184. Whitenack, D. L., et al.: Influence of enteric infection on zinc utilization and clinical signs and lesions of zinc deficiency in young swine. Am. J. Vet. Res. 39:1447, 1978.

185. Wiese, A. C., et al.: Pantothenic acid deficiency in baby pigs. J. Anim. Sci. 10:80, 1951.

186. Williams, P. M., and Hendersen, A. E.: Effect of nutrition of the dam on wool follicle development of Corriedale lambs. Proc. N.Z. Soc. Anim. Prod. 31:114, 1971

187. Wintrobe, M. M., et al.: Sensory neuron degeneration in pigs. J. Nutr. 24:345, 1942.

188. Wintrobe, M. M., et al.: Riboflavin deficiency in swine. Johns Hopkins Hosp. Bull. 75:102, 1944.

189. Wintrobe, M. M., et al.: Pantothenic acid deficiency in swine with particular reference to the effects on growth and on the alimentary tract. Johns Hopkins Hosp. Bull. 73:313, 1943.

190. Witz, W. M., and Beeson, W. M.: The physiological effects of a fat-deficient diet on the pig. J. Anim. Sci. 10:112, 1951.

191. Worden, A. N.: Nutritional influences on the skin of domestic animals. *In*: Rook, A. J., and Walton, G. S. (eds): *Comparative Physiology and Pathology of the Skin*. Oxford, Blackwell Scientific Publications, 1965, p. 261.

CHAPTER 13

ENDOCRINE DISEASES

CUTANEOUS ENDOCRINOLOGY

Hormones regulate physiologic processes by modifications of existing activities rather than by initiation of new reactions. Thus, in the skin, as elsewhere, excesses or deficiencies of hormones generally result in quantitative rather than qualitative changes in cutaneous function and morphology. However, the expression of altered hormonal balance is determined, to some extent, by intrinsic properties of the skin in various areas. The capacity of cutaneous structures to respond, local hemodynamics, and extrinsic factors such as light and trauma influence the distribution as well as the quantity of hormonally induced changes in the skin.

Many hormones affect the skin and adnexa. Although this chapter is limited to endocrine influences on the skin, it must be remembered that hormones also have effects on the rest of the body. The specific actions of many hormonal imbalances, either proved or alleged, on the skin are often poorly understood. Additionally, confusion is intensified by (1) species differences, (2) lack of adequate standardized or readily available diagnostic tests, (3) conflicting data in the literature, and (4) the complex physiologic and pathophysiologic interrelationships between the endocrine glands and their hormonal products.

Clinically, bilaterally symmetric alopecia is often associated with hormonal disorders. The hair coat is often dull, dry, and easily epilated and fails to regrow after clipping. Bilaterally symmetric pigmentary disturbances may accompany the alopecia. Endocrine dermatoses are classically nonpruritic. Secondary seborrheic skin disease or pyoderma, or both, are frequent complications.

Functional Anatomy of the Endocrine Hypothalamus and Hypophysis

Anatomically and functionally, the hypothalamus and hypophysis (pituitary gland) are best thought of together as "the master gland."[29, 39, 144, 175] The important portion of the hypophysis, in regard to dermatology, is the adenohypophysis (anterior pituitary, pars distalis).

The hypothalamus contains a number of specialized cells that combine neural and secretory activity: the endocrine neurons. The endocrine hypothalamus produces hormones (adenohypophysiotropic-releasing and inhibiting factors), which are transported as unstainable neurosecretions to the pituitary portal system and then to the adenohypophysis. On the basis of biologic assays of hypothalamic extracts, there is good evidence for biologic activities corresponding to ten hypophysiotropic (releasing) factors: (1) ACTH-releasing factor (corticotropin-releasing factor, CRF), (2) TSH-releasing factor (thyrotropin-releasing factor, TRF, TRH), (3) GH-releasing factor (growth hormone–releasing factor, GHRF; somatotropin-releasing factor, SRF), (4) LH-releasing factor (luteinizing hormone–releasing factor, LHRF), (5) FSH-releasing factor (follicle-stimulating hormone–releasing factor, FSHRF), (6) Prolactin-releasing factor (PRF), (7) Prolactin-inhibiting factor (PIF), (8) GH-inhibiting factor (GHIF; somatotropin-inhibiting factor, SIF; somatostatin), (9) MSH-releasing factor (melanocyte-stimulating hormone–releasing factor, MSHRF), (10) MSH-inhibiting factor (melanocyte-stimulating hormone–inhibiting factor, MSHIF).

These hypophysiotropic factors are thought to be regulated by higher brain centers, adenohypophyseal hormones ("short-loop" feedback system), and target endocrine gland hormones ("long-loop" feedback system).

The adenohypophysis consists of six functional cell types: five chromophils and one chromophobe.[39] Of the five chromophil cell types, two are acidophils (making GH and prolactin) and three are basophils (making TSH, ACTH, and a combined FSH and LH). When these chromophil cells become hypersecretory, they usually discharge their store of granulation and become chromophobes. The adenohypophyseal tropic hormones are released into the systemic blood vasculature and regulate the functions of their distant target endocrine glands. The release of adenohypophyseal hormones is thought to be regulated by hypophysiotropic factors from the hypothalamus and by negative feedback by target endocrine gland hormones.

Assay of Hormones

The assay procedures used to determine the level of a specific hormone vary in specificity and sensitivity.[140, 145, 175] Older, less desirable hormonal assay techniques include bioassay, column chromatography, fluorometry, and competitive protein-binding methods. In recent years, the use of radioimmunoassay has initiated a new era in the diagnosis and management of endocrine disorders. Radioimmunoassay procedures are the most sensitive, specific, and precise in measuring the minute quantities of circulating hormones in domestic animals. However, even radioimmunoassay techniques must be specifically validated for the species being tested, and thus the use, for veterinary purposes, of laboratories that assay human sera with techniques developed for human hormones is unsatisfactory.

Glucocorticoids

Glucocorticoids, produced by the zona fasciculata of the adrenal cortex, are probably the most commonly used therapeutic agents in veterinary medicine. Hyperglucocorticoidism may be produced by hypersecretion of ACTH or ACTH-like substances (idiopathic, functional pituitary tumor, ectopic); hypersecretion of endogenous glucocorticoids (functional adrenal tumor); and exogenous glucocorticoid administration (iatrogenic).

Glucocorticoids and the Skin

The skin is a rather sensitive and specific indicator of hyperglucocorticoidism, reflecting both internal disease and inappropriate therapy. The protein catabolic, antienzymatic, and antimitotic effects of glucocorticoids are manifested in numerous ways in animal skin: (1) the epidermis becomes thin and hyperkeratotic (suppressed DNA synthesis, decreased mitoses, keratinization abnormalities), (2) the basement membrane zone becomes thin and disrupted, (3) pilosebaceous atrophy becomes pronounced, (4) the dermis becomes thin, and dermal vasculature becomes fragile (inhibition of fibroblast proliferation and collagen and ground substance production), and (5) wound healing is delayed.[9, 18, 26, 31, 44, 92] Additionally, as a result of the broad-spectrum anti-inflammatory and immunosuppressive effects of excessive glucocorticoids, patients have increased susceptibility to cutaneous infections.[9, 26]

Clinically, hyperglucocorticoidism is characterized by (1) thin, hypotonic skin, (2) easy bruising (petechiae and ecchymoses), (3) poor wound healing, (4) seborrhea sicca, and (5) increased susceptibility to pyoderma.[9, 18, 26, 44] In horses, as in humans, hypertrichosis is a feature of hyperglucocorticoidism.[9, 26, 45, 126, 149] In sheep, experimental hyperglucocorticoidism resulted in decreased wool production, increased shedding, and wool fibers that were shorter and of reduced diameter compared with normal fibers.*

Histologically, hyperglucocorticoidism is characterized by orthokeratotic hyperkeratosis, follicular keratosis, epidermal and follicular atrophy, telogenization of hair follicles, sebaceous gland atrophy, decreased size of arrector pili muscles, thin dermis, and telangiectasia.†

Adrenal Function Tests

Adrenal function tests are basically of two types: those that are single measurements of basal glucocorticoid levels in blood or urine and those that are provocative, dynamic response tests. Single measurements of basal glucocorticoid levels, while cheaper and easier to perform, are unreliable.[9, 26, 126, 175]

BLOOD CORTISOL

Radioimmunoassay (RIA) is the method of choice for determining blood cortisol levels.[145, 175] Basal blood cortisol levels by competitive protein-binding or RIA in normal large animals approximate 1 to 10 µg/dl.‡

Important considerations to keep in mind when interpreting blood cortisol levels include the following: (1) different laboratories may differ in their normal and abnormal values, (2) stress can markedly elevate blood cortisol lev-

---

*References 18, 43, 44, 93, 128, 163, 164
†References 18, 31, 43, 44, 91, 93, 163, 164
‡References 7, 9, 26, 46–48, 65, 76, 89, 94, 100, 103, 108, 125, 126, 155, 171, 184

els, (3) episodic daily secretion of cortisol occurs, and (4) single measurements of blood cortisol are of limited value in the diagnosis of hyperglucocorticoidism.* The clinical significance of diurnal cortisol rhythms in large animals is unclear. In the horse and the pig, blood cortisol levels are highest in the morning and lowest at night.† In cattle and sheep, most studies have demonstrated no diurnal variation,[7, 65, 103, 160, 184] whereas others have reported peak cortisol levels at night[48] or in the morning.[108]

CORTISOL RESPONSE TESTS

To overcome the unreliability of basal blood cortisol levels, various provocative tests have been developed. The ACTH response test usually confirms a diagnosis of naturally occurring or iatrogenic hyperadrenocorticism in the horse.[9, 26, 101, 112, 122, 126] Two commonly used ACTH response test procedures for the horse are as follows: (1) plasma or serum cortisol determinations are made before and eight hours after the intramuscular injection of 1 IU/kg of ACTH gel (Adrenomone, Acthar Gel) or (2) plasma or serum cortisol determinations are made before and two hours after the intravenous injection of 100 IU synthetic aqueous ACTH (Cortrosyn). By either procedure, normal horses will show double to triple their basal cortisol levels, whereas horses with pituitary-dependent hyperadrenocorticism will have exaggerated responses.‡

The dexamethasone suppression test is a less sensitive indicator of adrenocortical function in horses than it is in dogs and humans.§ In horses, dexamethasone does *not* have the suppressive effect seen in dogs and humans, presumably because the hypersecretion of ACTH is from the pars intermedia (rather than the pars distalis) and is relatively insensitive to glucocorticoid negative feedback. In normal horses, the dexamethasone suppression test is often performed by measuring plasma or serum cortisol before and six hours after the intramuscular administration of 20 mg dexamethasone. Normal horses respond with an 80 percent decrease in basal cortisol levels at six hours.[9, 35]

---

*References 6, 8, 9, 26, 28, 33, 46–49, 52, 61, 62, 66, 76, 89, 94, 100, 108, 125–127, 133, 137, 140a, 151, 155, 171
†References 6, 8, 16, 33, 61, 72, 87, 89, 191
‡References 9, 10a, 34, 53, 61, 62, 72, 112, 122, 126
§References 9, 10a, 26, 112, 116, 119, 122, 123, 188

BLOOD ACTH

Plasma ACTH levels have been measured by radioimmunoassay in normal horses and horses with pituitary-dependent hyperadrenocorticism.[9, 112, 122, 123, 188] The mean value for normal horses was 32 ± 5 pg/ml, whereas horses with Cushing's syndrome had markedly elevated levels, 470 to 4350 pg/ml.

Blood for ACTH determinations must be handled quickly because the disappearance rate of ACTH from fresh whole blood is rapid. Contact with glass should be avoided during blood collection and separation. At present, plasma ACTH assays are neither generally available nor economically feasible.

Thyroid Hormones

Naturally occurring hypothyroidism is rare in large animals. The most commonly recognized causes of hypothyroidism in large animals include iodine deficiency (see Chapter 12) and inherited abnormalities of thyroglobulin synthesis (see Chapter 11).

Thyroid Hormones and the Skin

Thyroid hormones play a dominant role in controlling metabolism and are essential for normal growth and development.[82, 83, 175] The primary mechanisms of action of thyroid hormones are stimulation of cytoplasmic protein synthesis and increasing tissue oxygen consumption. These effects are thought to be initiated by the binding of thyroid hormones to nuclear chromatin and the augmentation of the transcription of genetic information.[121, 170, 175] Available data suggest that thyroid hormones play a pivotal role in differentiation and maturation of mammalian skin as well as in the maintenance of normal cutaneous function.[45, 149]

Hypothyroidism results in epidermal atrophy and abnormal keratinization as a result of decreased protein synthesis, mitotic activity, and oxygen consumption.[45, 64, 73] Epidermal melanosis may be seen, but the pathologic mechanism is unclear.[45, 149] Sebaceous gland atrophy occurs, and sebum excretion rates are reduced.[32, 45, 51, 135] Thyroid hormones are necessary for the initiation of the anagen phase of the hair follicle cycle.* In hypothyroid individuals, anagen is not initiated, resulting in the

---

*References 1, 45, 74, 88, 102, 150, 152, 154

hair follicles being retained in telogen and leading to failure of hair growth and alopecia.

Hypothyroidism results in the accumulation of hyaluronic acid in the dermis, leading to an increase in the interstitial ground substance and a thick, myxedematous dermis.[1, 45, 165, 166] The exact cause of this tissue myxedema is unknown, although evidence suggests that (1) elevated levels of TSH in primary hypothyroidism result in an increased synthesis of ground substance and (2) the transcapillary albumin escape rate is increased while lymphatic drainage is inadequate in myxedema.[1, 45, 88, 129]

Thyroid hormone has been reported to heal the ulcers and reduce the scarring associated with chronic radiodermatitis in humans[50] and to improve the healing of deep dermal burns in rats.[109] These effects were thought to be due to thyroid hormone actions on the proliferation and metabolism of fibroblasts and collagen synthesis. Not surprisingly, the skin of hypothyroid dogs and humans exhibits poor wound healing and easy bruising.[45, 88, 116]

Clinically, hypothyroidism is characterized by (1) a dull, dry, thin hair coat, (2) skin that is often thickened and puffy or spongy (myxedema), and (3) frequent seborrheic skin disease.*

Histologically, hypothyroidism is characterized by orthokeratotic hyperkeratosis and follicular keratosis, follicular atrophy, telogenization of follicles, sebaceous gland atrophy, and diffuse mucinous degeneration (myxedema).[19, 42-44, 77, 165, 166]

Thyroid Function Tests

No single area of veterinary diagnostics is more misunderstood, confused, and abused than thyroid function testing. For the most part, this situation is referable to the failure to recognize the significance of (1) the euthyroid sick syndrome, (2) the unreliability of basal serum thyroid hormone levels, and (3) the unsatisfactory results obtained by sending samples to laboratories geared to testing human sera.

Thyroid function tests (e.g., basal metabolic rate; radioactive iodine uptake; protein-bound iodine; butanol-extractable iodine; thyroxine (T_4) by competitive protein-binding or column chromatography; triiodothyronine (T_3) resin uptake; and free thyroxine index, T_7 test) are either inaccurate, impractical, or inferior to

---

*References 82, 98, 99, 106, 147, 162, 165, 166, 190

modern techniques and will not be discussed here.*

SERUM T_4 AND T_3

Radioimmunoassay is the method of choice for determining serum levels of T_4 and T_3.[82, 117, 140, 145] However, radioimmunoassay techniques that were developed to measure thyroid hormone levels in human sera are unsatisfactory for large animals. Reported basal levels of serum T_4 and T_3 in large animals are summarized in Table 13–1. However, even laboratories utilizing radioimmunoassay procedures adapted to large animals may vary in their normal ranges of serum T_4 and T_3, so one must exercise caution when attempting to compare published data.

Other factors to consider when assessing basal serum T_4 and T_3 levels include the following: (1) T_4 and T_3 levels are lower in euthyroid patients with the euthyroid sick syndrome (discussed later), (2) T_4 and T_3 levels are lower in euthyroid patients associated with recent drug therapy (e.g., glucocorticoids, anabolic steroids, phenylbutazone),[9, 27, 55, 113, 124] (3) normal T_4 and T_3 levels may be lower during warm weather,[38, 66, 117] (4) normal T_4 and T_3 levels tend to be lower in horses in training,[70, 80, 98] and (5) normal T_4 and T_3 levels are higher in neonates.†

In humans, rodents, and dogs, it is well known that a number of conditions (chronic illness, acute illnesses, surgical trauma, fasting, starvation, and fever) produce moderate to marked reductions in serum T_3 and T_4 levels.‡ Under these circumstances, the patients are euthyroid and in no need of thyroid medication. This situation is referred to as the euthyroid sick syndrome and is a common source of misdiagnosis regarding basal serum T_4 and T_3 levels. It is thought that this metabolic switch

---

*References 57-60, 69, 70, 80-83, 96, 115, 134, 136, 138, 141, 142, 173-175, 179, 189
†References 20, 24, 67, 78, 80, 81, 83, 98, 118, 130, 161
‡References 90, 110, 116, 153, 172, 176, 187

TABLE 13–1. Approximate Normal Ranges for Basal Serum T_4 and T_3 Levels in Large Animals

Species	T4 (µ/dl)	T3 (ng/dl)
Horse	1–3	30–170
Cattle	2–7	30–170
Sheep	2–6	60–160
Goat	3–10	80–200
Swine	1.5–5	40–150

in the sick patient is protective by counteracting the excessive calorigenic effects of T_3 in catabolic states. Although not studied as extensively, the euthyroid sick syndrome also occurs in large animals. Spuriously low basal serum T_4 and T_3 levels have been reported in starving cattle, sheep, and swine[3, 3a, 14, 15, 180] and in horses with Cushing's syndrome.[9]

In summary, basal serum levels of T_4 and T_3 are significantly influenced by numerous conditions that have nothing to do with thyroidal disease and hypothyroidism. In the absence of classic historical, clinical, and clinicopathologic evidence of thyroid hormone deficiency, low basal serum T_4 and T_3 levels are unreliable for a diagnosis of hypothyroidism.

TSH RESPONSE TEST

Because of the unreliability of basal serum T_4 and T_3 determinations, the TSH response has been widely used in dogs, cats, and humans.[116] Methodology of the TSH response test in horses varies considerably from one report to another, and there are no data suggesting that one method is superior to another.* Morris and Garcia[113] reported that equine serum T_4 and T_3 responses to 5, 10, or 20 IU of TSH were similar. The recommended procedure for the TSH response test in horses is as follows: (1) plasma or serum T_4 levels measured before and 6 to 12 hours after the intramuscular injection of 5 IU TSH (Dermathycin) or (2) plasma or serum T_4 levels measured before and four hours after the intravenous administration of 5 IU of TSH.[113, 120] In normal horses, basal T_4 levels should at least double. In humans and small animals, the TSH response test achieves normal poststimulation serum T_4 levels in individuals with drug-related low basal T_4 levels.[116] The same is probably true for horses. It has been reported that the TSH response is normal in horses with low basal serum T_4 and T_3 levels associated with phenylbutazone administration.[113, 114]

TRH RESPONSE TEST

The thyrotropin-releasing hormone response test is reported to be a valuable indicator of equine thyroid function.[97] TRH given intravenously at a dose of 0.5 to 1 mg was reported to cause maximal increases in serum T_4 and T_3 levels within four and two hours, respectively,

after injection. Plasma T_4 and T_3 levels in cattle were reported to peak 12 hours after the intravenous injection of 0.2 mg TRH.[84a]

CLINICAL ASPECTS OF ENDOCRINE SKIN DISEASES

Equine Hyperadrenocorticism

Hyperadrenocorticism (Cushing's disease, Cushing's syndrome, equine hirsutism), an uncommon disorder of the horse, is associated with excessive endogenous glucocorticoids and characterized by polydipsia, polyuria, polyphagia, muscle wasting, weight loss, and hirsutism.

Cause and Pathogenesis

Equine hyperadrenocorticism is usually associated with functional chromophobe adenomas of the pars intermedia of the hypophysis.* Hypersecretion of ACTH results in bilateral adrenocortical hyperplasia that may be diffuse or nodular, or both.†

Several immunoreactive ACTH-related proopiolipomelanocortin (proOLMC) peptides have been distinguished in plasma and pituitary tissues from normal horses and horses with Cushing's syndrome.[36, 122, 123, 188] In horses, adenomas of the pars intermedia secrete ACTH and other proOLMC peptides, such as α-MSH, β-MSH, corticotropin-like intermediate lobe peptide, and β-endorphin. Secretion of these peptides is very resistant to glucocorticoid suppression but can be inhibited by the administration of dopaminergic agonists.

The pathogenesis of the hirsutism is unknown. It has been postulated that increased production of androgens by the hyperplastic adrenal cortices may be the cause.[45, 63, 149]

Clinical Features

Hyperadrenocorticism is most common in aged horses, with females being affected twice as frequently as males.[9, 26, 53, 112] Often, attention is first drawn to the disease when the horse exhibits a rapid regrowth of long hair after a normal shed or fails to shed a longer than normal winter coat.[9, 26, 131] This hirsutism is characterized by a usually symmetric shaggy

---

*References 9, 80, 82, 99, 113, 145, 185

*References 4, 9, 13, 17, 26, 36, 53, 63, 112, 131, 132, 181
†References 9, 26, 53, 77, 112, 122, 123

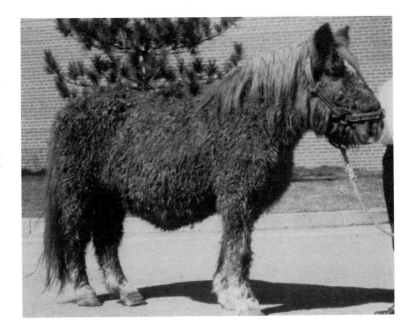

FIGURE 13–1. Equine hyperadrenocorticism. Hirsutism, swayback, and potbelly.

or wavy coat up to 10 to 12 cm in length (Fig. 13–1). The mane and tail are unaffected. The skin may be dry and scaly or greasy. Superficial skin infections (e.g., dermatophilosis) are common.[9, 26] Some horses have episodic hyperhidrosis.[9, 26, 63, 112] Wound healing is delayed. Rarely, papular and nodular xanthomas are seen over the thorax[158] (Figs. 13–2 and 13–3).

The most common clinical signs seen with equine hyperadrenocorticism are polydipsia and polyuria.[9, 26, 53, 112, 131] Some horses will drink in excess of 80 L of water a day. Other common clinical signs include muscle wasting, weight loss, and lethargy.[9, 26, 53, 131] Skeletal muscle wasting often leads to a swayback appearance, pendulous abdomen, and flaccid musculature.

Occasionally, horses will develop neurologic disorders, blindness, and thermoregulatory disorders, presumably associated with pressure

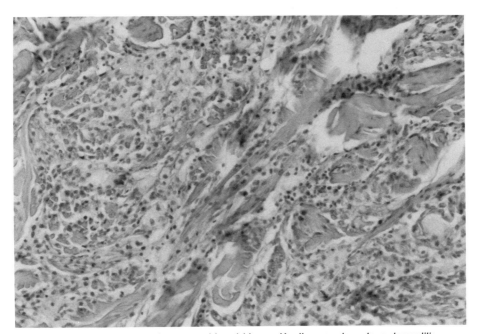

FIGURE 13–2. Xanthoma from a cushingoid horse. Xanthogranulomatous dermatitis.

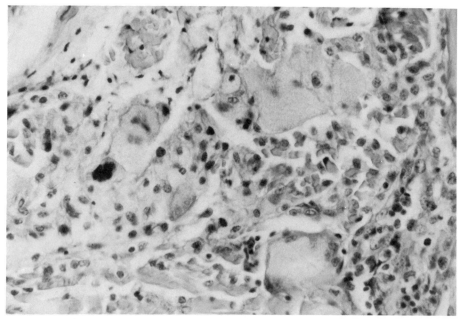

FIGURE 13–3. Xanthoma from a cushingoid horse. Typical xanthoma cells.

on the hypothalamus and optic chiasm by an enlarging pituitary neoplasm.[9, 26, 53, 63] Chronic infections, such as abscesses, sinusitis, pneumonia, and fistulae, are common.[9, 26]

Diagnosis

The major differential diagnoses include parasitism, inadequate nutrition, poor dentition, chronic infections, chronic renal or liver disease, chronic arsenic poisoning, and pheochromocytoma.[9, 26, 37, 107, 131] Retention of the long winter coat can be seen in horses with chronic illnesses and dietary deficiencies.[9, 26, 107] Definitive diagnosis is based on history, physical examination, hemogram, urinalysis, serum chemistries, and adrenal function tests.

Hemograms may reveal various combinations of neutrophilia, lymphopenia, and eosinopenia.[9, 26, 53, 131] The total white blood cell count is usually normal, unless secondary infections are present. A mild nonregenerative anemia is common.

Urinalysis usually reveals a low specific gravity (1.005 to 1.017).[9, 26, 53, 131] Horses with hyperglycemia may also have glucosuria. Water deprivation tests may result in a marked increase in urine specific gravity, but the administration of exogenous antidiuretic hormone (ADH) does not.[9, 26, 112]

Serum chemistry panel abnormalities may include mild to marked insulin-resistant hyperglycemia, hypercholesterolemia, and lipemia.[*] Plasma insulin levels are elevated.[10] Basal thyroid hormone levels (T_4 and T_3) are usually low.[9] These spuriously low thyroid hormone levels are caused by glucocorticoids (see preceding discussion on thyroid hormones) and do *not* usually indicate concurrent hypothyroidism. TSH response tests are usually normal.

Adrenal Function Tests

Adrenal function tests are basically of two types: those that are single measurements of basal glucocorticoids in blood and those that are provocative, dynamic response tests. Single measurements of basal glucocorticoid levels, while cheaper and easier to perform, are unreliable (see preceding discussion on glucocorticoids).

The ACTH response test usually confirms a diagnosis of equine hyperadrenocorticism.[9, 10a, 26, 112, 126] Two commonly used ACTH response test protocols are as follows: (1) plasma or serum cortisol determinations are collected before and eight hours after the intramuscular injection of 1 IU/kg of ACTH gel or (2) plasma or serum cortisol determinations are made before and two hours after the intravenous

---

[*]References 5, 9, 10, 26, 53, 63, 85, 95, 111, 112, 131, 177

on serum thyroxine levels of pregnant or growing swine. J. Nutr. 108:1546, 1978.

3a. Aceves, C., et al.: Thyroid hormone profile in dairy cattle acclimated to cold or hot environmental temperatures. Acta Endocrinol. 114:201, 1987.

3b. Amann, J. F., et al.: Distribution and implications of β-endorphin and ACTH-immunoreactive cells in the intermediate lobe of the hypophysis in healthy equids. Am. J. Vet. Res. 48:323, 1987.

4. Backstrom, G.: Hirsutism associated with pituitary tumors in horses. Nord. Vet. Med. 15:778, 1963.

5. Baker, J. R., and Richie, H. E.: Diabetes mellitus in the horse: A case report and review of the literature. Equine Vet. J. 6:7, 1974.

6. Barnett, J. L., et al.: Effects of photoperiod and feeding on plasma corticosteroid concentrations and maximum corticosteroid-binding capacity in pigs. Aust. J. Biol. Sci. 34:577, 1981.

7. Bassett, J. M.: Diurnal patterns of plasma insulin, growth hormone, corticosteroid, and metabolite concentrations in fed and fasted sheep. Aust. J. Biol. Sci. 27:167, 1976.

8. Becker, B. A., et al.: Effects of transportation on cortisol concentrations and on the circadian rhythm of cortisol in gilts. Am. J. Vet. Res. 46:1457, 1985.

9. Beech, J.: Tumors of the pituitary gland (pars intermedia). *In* Robinson, N. E. (ed.): *Current Therapy in Equine Medicine.* Philadelphia, W. B. Saunders Co., 1983, p. 164.

10. Beech, J., and Garcia, M.: Hormonal response to thyrotropin-releasing hormone in healthy horses and in horses with pituitary adenoma. Am. J. Vet. Res. 46:1941, 1985.

10a. Beech, J.: Tumors of the pituitary gland (pars intermedia). *In*: Robinson, N. E. (ed.): Current Therapy in Equine Medicine II. Philadelphia, W. B. Saunders Co., 1987, p. 182.

11. Belonje, P. C.: A report of some long-term effects of thyroparathyroidectomy in a Merino wether. J. S. Afr. Vet. Med. Assoc. 38:225, 1967.

12. Blackmore, D. J., et al.: Observations on thyroid hormones in the blood of thoroughbreds. Res. Vet. Sci. 25:294, 1978.

13. Blood, D. C., et al.: *Veterinary Medicine V.* Baltimore, Williams & Wilkins, 1979.

14. Blum, J. W., et al.: Thyroid hormone levels relative to energy and nitrogen balance during weight loss and regain in adult sheep. Acta Endocrinol. 93:440, 1980.

15. Blum, J. W., and Kunz, P.: Effects of fasting on thyroid hormone levels and kinetics of reverse triiodothyronine in cattle. Acta Endocrinol. 98:234, 1981.

16. Bottoms, G. D., et al.: Circadian variation in plasma cortisol and corticosterone in pigs and mares. Am. J. Vet. Res. 33:785, 1972.

17. Brandt, A. J.: Uber Hyphophysenadenome bei Hund und Pferd. Skand. Vet. Tidskrift. 30:875, 1940.

18. Chapman, R. E., and Bassett, J. M.: The effects of prolonged administration of cortisol on the skin of sheep on different planes of nutrition. J. Endocrinol. 48:649, 1970.

19. Chapman, R. E., et al.: The effects of fetal thyroidectomy and thyroxine administration on the development of the skin and wool follicles of sheep fetuses. J. Anat. 117:419, 1974.

20. Chen, C. L., and Riley, A. M.: Serum thyroxine and triiodothyronine concentrations in neonatal foals and mature horses. Am. J. Vet. Res. 42:1415, 1981.

20a. Chen, D. C. L., and Li, O. W. I: Hypothyroidism. *In*: Robinson, N. E. (ed.): Current Therapy in Equine Medicine II. Philadelphia, W. B. Saunders Co., 1987, p. 185.

21. Convey, E. M., et al.: Serum thyrotropin and thyroxine after thyrotropin-releasing hormone in dairy cows fed varying amounts of iodine. J. Dairy Sci. 60:975, 1977.

22. Convey, E. M., et al.: Serum thyrotropin, thyroxine, and triiodothyronine in dairy cows fed varying amounts of iodine. J. Dairy Sci. 61:771, 1978.

23. Cornelius, C. E., and Kaneko, J. J.: *Clinical Biochemistry of Domestic Animals II.* New York, Academic Press, 1970.

24. Curtis, R. J., and Abrams, J. T.: Circadian rhythms in the concentration of thyroid hormone in the plasma of normal calves. Br. Vet. J. 133:134, 1977.

25. Davis, R. B.: Inherited goitre in sheep. N.Z. Vet. J. 25:213, 1977.

26. Deem, D. A., and Whitlock, R. H.: The pituitary gland. *In*: Mansmann, R. A., et al. (eds.): *Equine Medicine and Surgery II.* Santa Barbara, CA, American Veterinary Publications, Inc., 1982, p. 885.

27. DeGroot, L. J., and Hoye, K.: Dexamethasone suppression of serum T$_3$ and T$_4$. J. Clin. Endocrinol. Metab. 42:976, 1976.

28. DeSilva, A. W. M. V., et al.: Comparison of serum prolactin and cortisol in sheep bled by two methods. J. Anim. Sci. 53:306, 1981.

29. Dickson, W. M.: Endocrine glands. *In*: Swenson, M. J. (ed.): *Duke's Physiology of Domestic Animals,* 9th ed. Ithaca, Comstock Publishing Co., 1977, pp. 731–771.

30. de Vijlder, J. J. M., et al.: Hereditary congenital goiter with thyroglobulin deficiency in a breed of goats. Endocrinology 102:1214, 1978.

31. Downes, A. M., and Wallace, A. L. C.: Local effects on wool growth of intradermal injections of hormones. *In* Lyne, A. G., and Short, B. F. (eds.): *Biology of the Skin and Hair Growth.* New York, American Elsevier Publishing Co., Inc., 1965, p. 679.

32. Ebling, F. J.: Hormonal control and methods of measuring sebaceous gland activity. J. Invest. Dermatol. 62:161, 1974.

33. Edqvist, L. E., et al.: Diurnal variations in peripheral plasma levels of testosterone, androsterone and cortisol in boars. Acta Vet. Scand. 21:451, 1980.

34. Eiler, H., et al.: Adrenal gland function in the horse: Effects of cosyntropin (synthetic) and corticotropin (natural) stimulation. Am. J. Vet. Res. 40:724, 1979.

35. Eiler, H., et al.: Adrenal gland function in the horse: Effect of dexamethasone on hydrocortisone secretion and blood cellularity and plasma electrolyte concentrations. Am. J. Vet. Res. 40:727, 1979.

36. Ericksson, K., et al.: A case of hirsutism in connection with hypophyseal tumor in a horse. Nord. Vet. Med. 8:807, 1956.

37. Evans, L. H., et al.: Clinicopathologic conference. JAVMA 159:209, 1971.

38. Evans, S. E., and Ingram, D. L.: The effect of ambient temperature upon the secretion of thyroxine in the young pig. J. Physiol. 264:511, 1977.

39. Ezrin, C., Kovacs, K., and Horvath, E.: A functional anatomy of the endocrine hypothalamus and hypophysis. Med. Clin. North Am. 62:229, 1978.

40. Falconer, I. R.: Studies of the congenitally goitrous sheep. The iodinated compounds of serum, and circulating thyroid-stimulating hormone. Biochem. J. 100:190, 1966.

41. Falconer, I. R.: Studies of the congenitally goitrous sheep. Composition and metabolism of goitrous thyroid tissue. Biochem. J. 100:197, 1966.

42. Ferguson, K. A., et al.: The influence of the thyroid on wool follicle development in the lamb. Aust. J. Biol. Sci. 9:575, 1956.

43. Ferguson, K. A., et al.: The hormonal regulation of wool growth. Acta Endocrinol. 51:1011, 1960.

44. Ferguson, K. A., et al.: Hormonal regulation of wool growth. *In*: Lyne, A. G., and Short, B. F. (eds.): *Biology of the Skin and Hair Growth.* New York, American Elsevier Publishing Co., Inc., 1965, p. 655.

45. Fitzpatrick, T. B., et al.: *Dermatology in General Medicine II.* New York, McGraw-Hill Book Company, 1979.

46. Friend, T. H., et al.: Adrenal glucocorticosteroid response to exogenous adrenocorticotropin mediated by density and social disruption in lactating cows. J. Dairy Sci. 60:1958, 1977.

47. Fulkerson, W. J.: Synchronous episodic release of cortisol in the sheep. J. Endocrinol. 79:131, 1978.

48. Fulkerson, W. J., and Tang, B. Y.: Ultradian and circadian rhythms in the plasma concentration of cortisol in sheep. J. Endocrinol. 81:135, 1979.

49. Ganjam, V.: Episodic nature of the -ENE and -ENE steroidogenic pathways and their relationship to the adrenogonadal axis in stallions. J. Reprod. Fertil. 27:67, 1979.

50. Glicksman, A. S., et al.: Modification of late radiation injury with L-triiodothyronine. Radiology 73:178, 1959.

51. Goolamali, S. K., et al.: Thyroid disease and sebaceous function. Br. Med. J. 1:432, 1976.

52. Green, D., and Moor, R. M.: The influence of anesthesia

on the concentrations of progesterone and cortisol in peripheral blood plasma of sheep. Res. Vet. Sci. 22:122, 1977.

53. Gribble, D. H.: The endocrine system. *In*: Mansmann, R. A., et al. (eds.): *Equine Medicine and Surgery II*. Santa Barbara, CA, American Veterinary Publications, Inc., 1972, p. 433.

54. Hart, I. C., et al.: Plasma thyroxine and free thyroxine index in high- and low-yielding cattle and calves of different breeds. J. Endocrinol. 80:52P, 1979.

55. Heitzman, R. J., et al.: Effect of anabolic steroids on plasma thyroid hormones in steers and heifers. Br. Vet. J. 136:168, 1980.

56. Held, J. P., and Oliver, J. W.: A sampling protocol for the thyrotropin-stimulation test in the horse. JAVMA 184:326, 1984.

57. Henneman, H. A., et al.: A determination of thyroid secretion rate in intact individual sheep. J. Anim. Sci. 11:794, 1952.

58. Hightower, D., and Miller, L. F.: Thyroid function tests in veterinary medicine. I. A review. Southwest. Vet. 22:200, 1969.

59. Hightower, D., et al.: Thyroid function tests in veterinary medicine. II. Results and applications. Southwest. Vet. 22:15, 1969.

60. Hightower, D., et al.: Comparison of serum and plasma thyroxine determinations in horses. JAVMA 159:449, 1971.

61. Hoffsis, G. F., et al.: Plasma concentration of cortisol and corticosterone in the normal horse. Am. J. Vet. Res. 31:1379, 1970.

62. Hoffsis, G. F., and Murdick, P. W.: The plasma concentrations of corticosteroids in normal and diseased horses. JAVMA 157:1590, 1970.

63. Holscher, M. A., et al.: Adenoma of the pars intermedia and hirsutism in a pony. Vet. Med. Small Anim. Clin. 73:1197, 1978.

64. Holt, P. J. A., et al.: The epidermis in thyroid disease. Br. J. Dermatol. 95:513, 1976.

65. Hudson, S., et al.: Diurnal variations in blood cortisol in the dairy cow. J. Dairy Sci. 58:30, 1975.

66. Ingraham, R. H., et al.: Seasonal effects of tropical climate on shaded and nonshaded cows as measured by rectal temperature, adrenal cortex hormones, thyroid hormone, and milk production. Am. J. Vet. Res. 40:1792, 1979.

67. Irvine, C. H. G., and Evans, M. J.: Post-natal changes in total and free thyroxine and triiodothyronine in foal serum. J. Reprod. Fertil. 23:709, 1975.

68. Irvine, C. H. G., and Evans, M. J.: Hypothyroidism in foals. N.Z. Vet. J. 25:354, 1977.

69. Irvine, C. H. G.: Protein bound iodine in the horse. Am. J. Vet. Res. 28:1687, 1967.

70. Irvine, C. H. G.: Thyroxine secretion rate in the horse in various physiological states. J. Endocrinol. 39:313, 1967.

71. Jaarsveld, P., et al.: Afrikander cattle congenital goiter: Purification and partial identification of the complex iodoprotein pattern. Endocrinology 91:470, 1972.

72. James, V. H. T., et al.: Adrenocortical function in the horse. J. Endocrinol. 48:319, 1970.

73. Jarrett, A.: *The Physiology and Pathophysiology of the Skin I*. New York, Academic Press, 1973.

74. Jarrett, A.: *The Physiology and Pathophysiology of the Skin IV*. New York, Academic Press, 1977.

75. Jensen, R., and Swift, B. L.: *Diseases of the Sheep II*. Philadelphia, Lea & Febiger, 1982.

76. Jones, C. T.: Normal fluctuations in the concentration of corticosteroids and ACTH in the plasma of foetal and pregnant sheep. Horm. Metab. Res. 11:237, 1979.

77. Jubb, K. V. F., and Kennedy, P. C.: *Pathology of Domestic Animals II*. New York, Academic Press, 1970.

78. Kahl, S., et al.: Plasma triiodothyronine and thyroxine in young growing calves. J. Endocrinol. 73:397, 1977.

79. Kahl, S., et al.: Effect of Synovex-S on growth rate and plasma thyroid hormone concentrations in beef cattle. J. Anim. Sci. 46:232, 1978.

80. Kallfelz, F. A., and Lowe, J. E.: Some normal values of thyroid function in horses. JAVMA 156:1888, 1970.

81. Kallfelz, F. A., and Erali, R. P.: Thyroid tests in domesti-

cated animals: Free thyroxine index. Am. J. Vet. Res. 34:1449, 1973.

82. Kallfelz, F. A.: The thyroid gland. *In*: Mansmann, R. A., et al. (eds.): *Equine Medicine and Surgery II*. Santa Barbara, CA, American Veterinary Publications, Inc., 1982, p. 891.

83. Kaneko, J. J.: Thyroid function. *In*: Cornelius, C. E., and Kaneko, J. J.: *Clinical Biochemistry of Domestic Animals II*. New York, Academic Press, 1970, p. 293.

84. Kelley, S. T., et al.: Measurement of thyroid gland function during the estrous cycle of nine mares. Am. J. Vet. Res. 35:657, 1974.

84a. Khurana, M. L., and Madan, M. L.: Effect of thyrotropin-releasing hormone on plasma tri-iodothyronine and thyroxine in bovine. Indian J. Anim. Sci. 55:647, 1985.

85. King, J. M., et al.: Diabetes mellitus with pituitary neoplasms in a horse and a dog. Cornell Vet. 52:133, 1962.

86. Kok, K., et al.: Prenatal diagnosis of a thyroglobulin synthesis defect in goats. Acta Endocrinol. 110:83, 1985.

87. Kumar, M. S. A., et al.: Diurnal variation in serum cortisol in ponies. J. Anim. Sci. 42:1360, 1976.

88. Lang, P. G.: Cutaneous manifestations of thyroid disease. Cutis 21:862, 1978.

89. Larsson, M., et al.: Plasma cortisol in the horse, diurnal rhythm and effects of exogenous ACTH. Acta Vet. Scand. 20:16, 1979.

90. Leiver, R., et al.: Pathophysiologische Untersuchungen zur Schilddrusenfunktion des Kalbes. 3. Mitteilung: Schilddrusenfunktion beim klinisch Kranken Kalb. Arch. Exp. Vet. Med. 38:234, 1984.

91. Leish, Z., and Panaretto, B. A.: Effect of intravenously infused dexamethasone on collagen metabolism in skin of Merino sheep. Aust. J. Biol. Sci. 32:561, 1979.

92. Leman, A. D., et al.: *Diseases of Swine V*. Ames, Iowa State University Press, 1981.

93. Lindner, H. R., and Ferguson, K. A.: Influence of the adrenal cortex on wool growth and its relation to "break" and "tenderness" of the fleece. Nature 177:188, 1956.

94. Liptrap, R. M., and Raeside, J. I.: A relationship between plasma concentrations of testosterone and corticosteroids during sexual and aggressive behavior in the boar. J. Endocrinol. 76:75, 1978.

95. Loeb, W. F., et al.: Adenoma of the pars intermedia associated with hyperglycemia and glycosuria in two horses. Cornell Vet. 56:623, 1966.

96. Long, J. F., et al.: The bovine protein bound iodine as related to age, sex, and breed. J. Anim. Sci. 10:1027, 1951.

97. Lothrop, C. D., and Nolan, H. L.: Equine thyroid function assessment with the thyrotropin-releasing hormone response test. Am. J. Vet. Res. 47:942, 1986.

98. Lowe, J. E.: Thyroid diseases. *In*: Robinson, N. E. (ed.): *Current Therapy in Equine Medicine*. Philadelphia, W. B. Saunders Co., 1983, p. 159.

99. Lowe, J. E., et al.: Equine hypothyroidism: The long-term effects of thyroidectomy on metabolism and growth in mares and stallions. Cornell Vet. 64:276, 1974.

100. Lundstrom, K., et al.: Peripheral plasma levels of corticosteroids in Swedish Landrace and Yorkshire boars. Swed. J. Agric. Res. 5:81, 1975.

101. MacHarg, M. A., et al.: Effects of multiple intramuscular injections and doses of dexamethasone on plasma cortisol concentrations and adrenal responses to ACTH in horses. Am. J. Vet. Res. 46:2285, 1985.

102. Maddocks, S., et al.: Effect on wool growth of thyroxine replacement in thyroidectomized Merino rams. Aust. J. Biol. Sci. 38:405, 1985.

103. Macadam, W. B., and Ebehart, R. J.: Diurnal variation in plasma corticoid concentration in dairy cattle. J. Dairy Sci. 55:1792, 1972.

104. Mansmann, R. A., et al.: *Equine Medicine and Surgery III*. Santa Barbara, CA, American Veterinary Publications, Inc., 1982.

105. Marston, H. R., and Pierce, A. W.: The effects of thyroidectomy in a Merino sheep. Aust. J. Exp. Biol. Med. Sci. 10:203, 1932.

106. McLaughlin, B. G., and Doige, C. E.: A study of ossification of carpal and tarsal bones in normal and hypothyroid foals. Can. Vet. J. 23:164, 1982.

107. McMullen, W. C.: The skin. *In* Mansmann, R. A., et al.

(eds.): *Equine Medicine and Surgery II.* Santa Barbara, CA, American Veterinary Publications, Inc., 1982, p. 783.

108. McNatty, K. P., et al.: Diurnal variation in plasma cortisol levels in sheep. J. Endocrinol. 54:361, 1972.

109. Mehregan, A. H., and Zamick, P.: The effect of triiodothyronine in healing of deep dermal burns and marginal scars of skin grafts. J. Cutan. Pathol. 1:113, 1974.

110. Melmed, S., et al.: A comparison of methods for assessing thyroid function in nonthyroidal illness. J. Clin. Endocrinol. 54:300, 1982.

111. Merritt, A. M.: Diabetes mellitus. *In*: Robinson, N. E. (ed.): *Current Therapy in Equine Medicine.* Philadelphia, W. B. Saunders Co., 1983, p. 169.

112. Moore, J., et al.: A case of pituitary adrenocorticotropin-dependent Cushing's syndrome in the horse. Endocrinology 104:576, 1979.

113. Morris, D. D., and Garcia, M.: Thyroid-stimulating hormone: Response test in healthy horses, and effect of phenylbutazone on equine thyroid hormones. Am. J. Vet. Res. 44:503, 1983.

114. Morris, D. D., and Garcia, M.: Effects of phenylbutazone and anabolic steroids on adrenal and thyroid gland function tests in healthy horses. Am. J. Vet. Res. 46:359, 1985.

115. Motley, J. S.: Use of radioactive triiodothyronine in the study of thyroid function in normal horses. Vet. Med. Small Anim. Clin. 67:1225, 1972.

116. Muller, G. H., et al.: *Small Animal Dermatology III.* Philadelphia, W. B. Saunders Co., 1983.

117. Nachreiner, R. F.: Radioimmunoassay and therapeutic monitoring. Proc. Am. Anim. Hosp. Assoc. 45:55, 1978.

118. Nathanielsz, P. W.: Plasma thyroxine levels in the young lamb from birth to 61 days. J. Endocrinol. 45:475, 1969.

119. Nicholson, W. E., et al.: Tissue and plasma levels of proopiolipomelanocortin (POLMC) peptides in the normal and Cushing's horse. Abstr. 62nd Annu. Meet. Endocrinol. Soc. 403:183, 1981.

120. Oliver, J. W., and Held, J. P.: Thyrotropin stimulation test—new perspective in value of monitoring triiodothyronine. JAVMA 187:931, 1985.

121. Oppenheimer, J. H., and Surks, M. I.: The peripheral action of the thyroid hormones. Med. Clin. North Am. 59:1055, 1975.

122. Orth, D. N., et al.: Equine Cushing's disease: Plasma immunoreactive proopiolipomelanocortin peptide and cortisol levels basally and response to diagnostic tests. Endocrinology 110:1430, 1982.

123. Orth, D. N., and Nicholson, W. E.: Bioactive and immunoreactive adrenocorticotropin in normal equine pituitary and in pituitary tumors of horses with Cushing's disease. Endocrinology 111:559, 1982.

124. Osanthanondh, R., et al.: Effects of dexamethasone on fetal and maternal thyroxine, triiodothyronine, reverse triiodothyronine, and thyrotropin levels. J. Clin. Endocrinol. Metab. 47:1236, 1978.

125. Paape, M. J., et al.: Response of plasma corticosteroids and circulating leukocytes in cattle following intravenous injection of different doses of adrenocorticotropin. Am. J. Vet. Res. 38:1345, 1977.

126. Palmer, J. E., et al.: The adrenal gland. *In*: Mansmann, R. A., et al. (eds.): *Equine Medicine and Surgery II.* Santa Barbara, CA, American Veterinary Publications, Inc., 1982, p. 900.

127. Panaretto, B. A.: Comparison of the plasma steroid concentration profiles and wool growth responses after administration of two forms of dexamethasone to sheep. Aust. J. Biol. Sci. 32:343, 1979.

128. Panaretto, B. A., et al.: Some effects of dexamethasone on nucleic acid metabolism in skin of Merino sheep. Aust. J. Biol. Sci. 35:579, 1982.

129. Paring, H. H., et al.: Mechanisms of edema formation in myxedema-increased protein extravasation and relatively slow lymphatic drainage. N. Engl. J. Med. 301:460, 1979.

130. Parker, R. O., et al.: Postnatal changes in concentrations of serum and urinary thyroxine and 3,3'-5-triiodothyronine in the pig. J. Anim. Sci. 51:132, 1980.

131. Pascoe, R. R.: *Equine Dermatoses.* Sydney, University of Sydney Post-Graduate Foundation in Veterinary Science, Veterinary Review No. 22, 1981.

132. Pauli, B. U., et al.: Swischenzelladenom der Hypophyse mit "Cushing-ahnlicher": Symptomatologie beim Pferd. Vet. Pathol. 11:417, 1974.

133. Pierzchala, K., et al.: The effect of shearing on the concentration of cortisol and thyroid hormones in the blood plasma of sheep. Zbl. Vet. Med. A 30:749, 1983.

134. Pipes, G. W., et al.: The biological half-life of L-thyroxine and L-triiodothyronine in the blood of the dairy cow. J. Dairy Sci. 42:1606, 1959.

135. Pochi, P. E., and Strauss, J. S.: Endocrinologic control of the development and activity of the human sebaceous gland. J. Invest. Dermatol. 62:191, 1974.

136. Premachandra, B. N., et al.: Variation in the thyroxine secretion rate of cattle. J. Dairy Sci. 41-1609, 1958.

137. Przekop, F., et al.: Changes in circadian rhythm and suppression of the plasma cortisol level after prolonged stress in sheep. Acta Endocrinol. 110:540, 1985.

138. Quaife, M. A., and Mason, S.: Triiodothyronine sponge resin uptake values in man and sheep. J. Nucl. Med. 6:192, 1965.

139. Rac, R., et al.: Congenital goitre in Merino sheep due to inherited defect in the biosynthesis of thyroid hormone. Res. Vet. Sci. 9:209, 1968.

140. Reap, M., et al.: Thyroxine and triiodothyronine levels in 10 species of animals. Southwest. Vet. 31:31, 1978.

140a. Redekopp, C., et al.: Spontaneous and stimulated adrenocorticotropin and vasopressin pulsatile secretion in the pituitary venous effluent of the horse. Endocrinology 118:1410, 1986.

141. Reece, R. P., and Man, E. B.: Serum precipitable and butanol extractable iodine of bovine sera. Proc. Soc. Exp. Biol. Med. 79:208, 1952.

142. Refetoff, S., et al.: Parameters of thyroid function in the serum of 16 selected vertebrate species: A study of PBI, serum T_4, free T_4, and the pattern of T_4 and T_3 binding to serum proteins. Endocrinology 86:793, 1970.

143. Reichlin, S.: Regulation of the endocrine hypothalamus. Med. Clin. North Am. 62:235, 1978.

144. Reichlin, S.: Regulation of the hypothalamic-pituitary-thyroid axis. Med. Clin. North Am. 52:305, 1978.

145. Reimers, T. J., et al.: Validation of radioimmunoassays for triiodothyronine, thyroxine, and hydrocortisone (cortisol) in canine, feline, and equine sera. Am. J. Vet. Res. 42:2016, 1981.

146. Ricketts, M. H., et al.: Autosomal recessive inheritance of congenital goiter in Afrikander cattle. J. Hered. 76:1, 1985.

147. Rinjberk, A., et al.: Congenital defect in iodothyronine synthesis. Clinical aspects of iodine metabolism in goats with congenital goitre and hypothyroidism. Br. Vet. J. 133:495, 1977.

148. Robbins, J., et al.: Abnormal thyroglobulin in congenital goiter of cattle. Endocrinology 78:1213, 1966.

149. Rook, A., et al.: *Textbook of Dermatology III.* Oxford, Blackwell Scientific Publications, Inc., 1979.

150. Ross, D. A., and Lewis, K. H. C.: The effect of thyroxine on the Romney two-tooth. Proc. N.Z. Soc. Anim. Prod. 18:141, 1958.

151. Rossdale, P. D., et al.: Changes in blood neutrophil/lymphocyte ratio related to adrenocortical function in the horse. Equine Vet. J. 14:293, 1982.

152. Rougeot, J.: The effect of thyroid hormones on the morphology of the wool cuticle. *In*: Lyne, A. G., and Short, B. F. (eds.): *Biology of the Skin and Hair Growth.* New York, American Elsevier Publishing Co., Inc., 1965, p. 625.

153. Rubenfeld, S., et al.: Euthyroid sick syndrome: Incidence and thyrotropin-releasing hormone (TRH) testing. Endocrinology 102:487, 1978.

154. Ryder, M. L.: Thyroxine and wool follicle activity. Anim. Prod. 28:109, 1974.

155. Satterlee, D. G., et al.: Effect of exogenous corticotropin and climatic conditions on bovine adrenal cortical function. J. Dairy Sci. 60:1612, 1977.

156. Schlotthauer, C. F.: The incidence and types of disease of the thyroid gland of adult horses. JAVMA 78:211, 1931.

157. Schulz, K. C. A., and Groenewald, J. W.: The familial incidence of "grey" Afrikander calves with and without goitre. J. S. Afr. Vet. Assoc. 54:147, 1983.

158. Scott, D. W.: Unpublished observations.
159. Shaver, J. R., et al.: Skeletal manifestations of suspected hypothyroidism in two foals. J. Equine Med. Surg. 3:269, 1979.
160. Shaw, K. E., et al.: Quantities of 17-hydroxycorticosteroids in the plasma of healthy cattle during various physiologic states. Am. J. Vet. Res. 21:52, 1960.
161. Slebodzinski, A.: Interaction between thyroid hormone and thyroxine-binding proteins in the early neonatal period. J. Endocrinol. 32:45, 1965.
162. Spielman, A. A., et al.: General appearance, growth, and reproduction of thyroidectomized bovine. J. Dairy Sci. 28:329, 1945.
163. Spurlock, G. M., and Clegg, M. T.: Wool characteristics of weaned lambs as influenced by the adrenals and gonads. J. Anim. Sci. 19:1336, 1960.
164. Spurlock, G. M., and Clegg, M. T.: Effect of cortisone acetate on carcass composition and wool characteristics of weaned lambs. J. Anim. Sci. 21:494, 1962.
165. Sreekumaran, T., and Rajan, A.: Pathology of the skin in experimental hypothyroidism in goats. Kerala J. Vet. Sci. 8:227, 1977.
166. Sreekumaran, T., and Rajan, A.: Clinicopathological studies in experimental hypothyroidism in goats. Vet. Pathol. 15:549, 1978.
167. Sreekumaran, T., and Rajan, A.: Pathology of gonads in experimental hypothyroidism in goats. Kerala J. Vet. Sci. 9:92, 1978.
168. Sreekumaran, T., and Rajan, A.: Thyroid pathology of experimental hypothyroidism in goats. Indian J. Vet. Res. 2:14, 1977.
169. Stanley, O., and Hillidge, C. J.: Alopecia associated with hypothyroidism in a horse. Equine Vet. J. 14:165, 1982.
170. Sterline, K.: Thyroid hormone action at the cell level. N. Engl. J. Med. 300:173, 1979.
171. Stith, R. D., and Bottoms, G. D.: Effects of metyrapone on concentrations of cortisol and corticosterone in plasma of pigs. Am. J. Vet. Res. 33:963, 1972.
172. Suda, A. K., et al.: The production and metabolism of 3,5,3'-triiodothyronine in normal and fasting subjects. J. Clin. Endocrinol. Metab. 47:1311, 1978.
173. Sutherland, R. L., and Irvine, C. H. G.: Total plasma thyroxine concentrations in horses, pigs, cattle, and sheep: Anion exchange resin chromatography and ceriarsenite colorimetry. Am. J. Vet. Res. 34:1261, 1973.
174. Swanson, E. W., et al.: Factors affecting the thyroid uptake of I^{131} in dairy cows. J. Anim. Sci. 16:318, 1957.
175. Swenson, M. J. (ed.): *Duke's Physiology of Domestic Animals IX*. Ithaca, Comstock Publishing Associates, 1978.
176. Talwar, K. K., et al.: Serum levels of thyrotropin, thyroid hormones, and their response to thyrotropin-releasing hormone in infective febrile illnesses. J. Clin. Endocrinol. Metab. 44:398, 1977.
177. Tasker, J. B., et al.: Diabetes mellitus in the horse. JAVMA 149:393, 1966.
178. Thomas, C. L., and Adams, J. C.: Radioimmunoassay of equine serum for thyroxine: Reference values. Am. J. Vet. Res. 39:1239, 1978.
179. Trum, B. F., and Wasserman, R. H.: Studies on the depression of radioiodine uptake by the thyroid after phenothiazine administration II. Effect of phenothiazine on the horse thyroid. Am. J. Vet. Res. 17:271, 1956.
180. Tveit, B., and Almlid, T.: T_4 degradation rate and plasma levels of TSH and thyroid hormones in 10 young bulls during feeding conditions and 48h of starvation. Acta Endocrinol. 93:435, 1980.
181. Urman, H. K., et al.: Pituitary neoplasms in two horses. Zbl. Vet. Med. 10:257, 1963.
182. van Zyl, A., et al.: Thyroidal iodine and enzymatic defects in cattle with congenital goiter. Endocrinology 76:353, 1965.
183. Vivrette, S. L., et al.: Skeletal disease in a hypothyroid foal. Cornell Vet. 74:373, 1984.
184. Wagner, W. C., and Oxenreider, S. L.: Adrenal function in the cow. J. Anim. Sci. 34:630, 1972.
185. Waldron-Mease, E.: Hypothyroidism and myopathy in racing thoroughbreds and standardbreds. J. Equine Med. Surg. 3:124, 1979.
186. Walton, E. A., and Humphrey, J. D.: Endemic goitre of sheep in the highlands of Papua, New Guinea. Aust. Vet. J. 55:43, 1979.
187. Wartofsky, L., and Burman, K. D.: Alterations in thyroid function in patients with systemic illness: The "euthyroid sick syndrome." Endocrin. Rev. 3:164, 1982.
188. Wilson, M. G., et al.: Proopiolipomelanocortin peptides in normal pituitary, pituitary tumor, and plasma of normal and Cushing's horses. Endocrinology 110:941, 1982.
189. Wilson, R. B., et al.: A procedure for assay of thyroid status in animals. Vet. Med. 56:285, 1961.
190. Zdelar, F., et al.: Istrazivanja o funkciji stitnjace junadi u tovu, s posebnim osvrtom na hipotireozu. I. Eksperimentalna hipotireoza: Klinicka slika, histopatoloske i histokemijske promjene. Veterinarski Arhiv. 51:243, 1981.
191. Zokolovick, A., et al.: Diurnal variation in plasma glucocorticosteroid levels in the horse (*Equus caballus*). J. Endocrinol. 35:249, 1966.

CHAPTER 14

DISORDERS OF PIGMENTATION AND EPIDERMAL APPENDAGES

DISORDERS OF PIGMENTATION

The melanosome, the specialized epidermal melanin-bearing organelle, is responsible for the color variation of skin and hair[22, 81] (see Chapter 1). Melanosomes are synthesized in the melanocytes, acquired by keratinocytes, and transported to the epidermal surface. The focal point of control of melanin synthesis is the epidermal melanin unit, which is a multicellular functional unit composed of a melanocyte and an associated cluster of keratinocytes.

The first step in melanin synthesis is the oxidation of tyrosine by the copper-containing enzyme tyrosinase, to dopa and dopaquinone. Subsequent intermediates polymerize to form melanin. Melanin deposition occurs in membrane-limited vesicles, which progress from spherical and clear (Stage I melanosomes) to oval and dark (Stage IV melanosomes).

Hyperpigmentation

Hyperpigmentation (melanosis) is frequently encountered as an acquired condition, usually associated with chronic inflammation and irritation (Fig. 14–1).[81] Hyperpigmentation may affect only the skin (melanoderma), only the hair (melanotrichia), or both.

Lentigo is an idiopathic macular melanosis of horses and swine (see Chapter 17, discussion on melanoma).

Hypopigmentation

Hypopigmentation (hypomelanosis), amelanosis (achromoderma, achromotrichia), and depigmentation are not synonymous.[22] Hypomelanosis refers to a decrease in normal melanin pigmentation. Amelanosis indicates a total lack of melanin. Depigmentation means a loss of pre-existing melanin. Leukoderma and leukotrichia are clinical terms used to indicate acquired depigmentation of skin and hair, respectively. Two other terms, rarely used in veterinary medicine, are poliosis (localized whitening of the hair) and canities (a more generalized whitening of the hair).

Theoretically, hypopigmentation and depigmentation may arise from any of the following:[22] (1) failure of migration of melanoblasts to the skin, (2) failure of differentiation of melanoblasts into melanocytes, (3) failure of mitotic division of melanocytes, (4) a defect in the synthesis of functional tyrosinase (e.g., copper deficiency), (5) failure of the synthesis of the melanosome matrix, (6) a defect in tyrosinase transport, (7) failure of melanosome formation, (8) failure of melanosome melanization, (9) a defect in melanosome transfer, (10) an alteration in the degradation of melanosomes, and (11) destruction of melanocytes (e.g., infections or physical or chemical trauma or intoxication).

ALBINISM

Albinism is an autosomal recessive disorder of melanin synthesis that affects the skin, hair, and eyes.[22] Affected animals have white skin and hair, pink eyes, and photophobia. The term albino is thought to be derived from the latin word for white, *albus*.

Albinism has rarely been documented in domestic animals.[10, 33, 81] It has been most completely documented in Icelandic sheep.[1, 2] In albinism, electron microscopy shows that melanocytes are present, but melanin synthesis is defective.

CHÉDIAK-HIGASHI SYNDROME

The Chédiak-Higashi syndrome is an autosomal recessive partial oculocutaneous albinism of Hereford cattle.[10, 14, 51, 53, 55, 61, 80] Affected

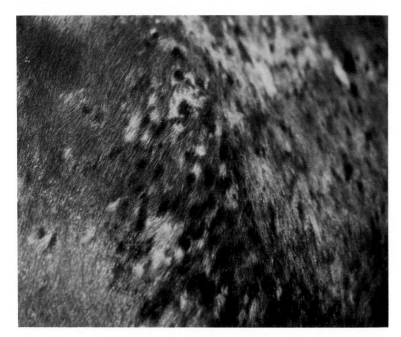

FIGURE 14–1. Melanotrichia over the neck of a horse, associated with insect hypersensitivity.

cattle also have photophobia, increased susceptibility to infections, hemorrhagic tendencies, and an average life span of about one year.

Light and electron microscopic examinations reveal abnormally large and clumped melanosomes, which are delivered with difficulty to keratinocytes. Enlarged cytoplasmic granules are also found in leukocytes.[10, 11, 53, 55] These granules are enlarged lysosomes, and the syndrome is thought to represent a lysosomal storage disease characterized by abnormal membrane fusion.[22, 29]

Other cellular abnormalities associated with the Chédiak-Higashi syndrome include (1) decreased bactericidal activity of leukocytes[17, 52, 54, 63] and (2) abnormal platelet function.[9, 47, 60]

LETHAL WHITE FOAL DISEASE

There are two forms of lethal white disease in foals. One is an autosomal dominant trait characterized by nonviable embryos in the homozygous state.[62] The other is an autosomal recessive disorder resulting from the breeding of two overo paints.[27, 30, 31, 66] Foals from such breedings may be characterized by albinism and congenital defects of the intestinal tract, especially colonic atresia.

LEUKODERMA

Leukoderma is an acquired depigmentation of the skin that follows various traumatic and inflammatory injuries to the skin.[33, 39, 49, 56, 58, 70, 75] Leukoderma is especially common in horses, may be localized or multifocal, and may be temporary or permanent. Leukoderma is often seen as a complication of onchocerciasis, dourine, herpes coital exanthema, lupus erythematosus, pressure sores, ventral midline dermatitis, regressing viral papillomatosis (Fig. 14–2), or freezing and burns (chemical, thermal, or radiation). Leukoderma has also been reported to follow contact with phenols and rubber bit guards, crupper straps, and feed buckets (Fig. 14–3).[33, 39, 49, 70, 75] Many rubbers contain monobenzyl ether of hydroquinone (antioxidant), which inhibits melanogenesis.[22]

VITILIGO

Vitiligo is an idiopathic acquired depigmentation.[22, 70] There are no preceding or concurrent signs of cutaneous inflammation or injury. The term vitiligo comes from the Latin word for blemish, *vitium*.

Etiologically, human vitiligo is divided into hereditary (autosomal dominant with variable expressivity and incomplete penetrance), autoimmune, dermatomal (neurologic?), and idiopathic types.[22] In large animals, vitiligo has been reported in horses and cattle* (in which the condition may be hereditary) and in horses and swine in conjunction with cutaneous melanomas[35, 48, 50] (in which the condition may

---

*References 39–46, 49, 56–58, 64, 68, 70

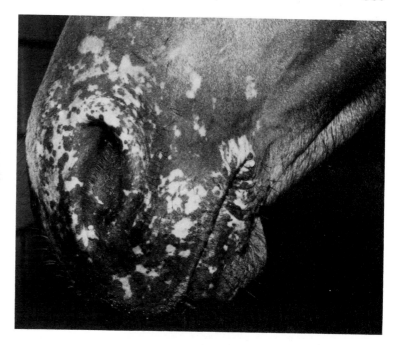

FIGURE 14–2. *Macular depigmentation on the muzzle of a horse after spontaneous regression of viral papillomatosis.*

be immune-mediated). Recently, vitiligo was reported in Japanese black cattle in conjunction with hyperthyroidism[64] and in Arabian horses in conjunction with circulating antibodies against the surface antigen of melanocytes.[50]

In horses, vitiligo is most commonly seen in Arabians (Arabian fading syndrome, pinky syndrome).[39, 49, 50, 56–68, 70, 81] Affected animals vary in age from weanlings to 23 years old, but most are young (one to two years old). It has been reported that vitiligo is more common in mares that are pregnant or that have just given birth,[39] suggesting a hormonal influence. Annular areas of macular depigmentation develop symmetrically on the muzzle, lips, and periocular area (Fig. 14–4) and occasionally involve the anus, vulva, sheath, and hooves and general body areas. The depigmented macules usually reach 1 cm in diameter and occasionally become patch size. The depigmentation may wax and wane in intensity but is usually permanent. Occasional horses will repigment within one year. In cattle, vitiligo has been most commonly reported in the Holstein-Friesian breed[41, 45, 46] and clinically resembles the disease in Arabian horses.

Diagnosis of vitiligo is based on history, physical examination, and skin biopsy (Fig. 14–5). Electron microscopy and dopa tissue reactions show a complete absence of melanocytes.[22, 36] For treatment, some authors have reported that vitamin-mineral dietary supplements are often effective.[39, 49] However, other authors report *no* benefit from dietary or any other form of therapy.[57, 70] Because of the probable hereditary nature of this disease, affected animals should not be used for breeding.

LEUKOTRICHIA

Leukotrichia is an acquired depigmentation of the hair that follows various traumatic and

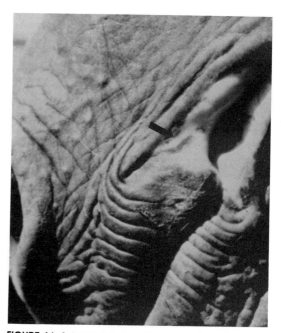

FIGURE 14–3. *Leukoderma of the lips (arrow) of a horse due to a rubber bit.*

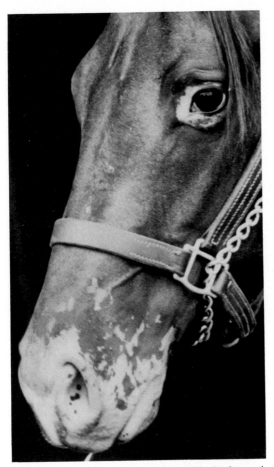

FIGURE 14—4. Macules and patches of leukoderma in a horse with vitiligo.

inflammatory injuries to the skin (see discussion on leukoderma).[33, 39, 49, 56, 58, 70] Leukotrichia has been reported in horses at the site of nerve blocks with epinephrine-containing local anesthetics.[39]

In the presence of the dominant allele W, a horse will, from birth, typically lack pigment in the skin and hair but have blue or brown eyes.[13, 62, 76] Such horses are often termed albino, blanco, or cremello. A similar appearance is produced by the C^{cr} allele of the C gene, which causes pigment dilution.[76]

A horse with the G allele is fully colored at birth but subsequently acquires an increasing number of white hairs with age.[3, 13, 23, 62, 74, 76] The earliest graying begins around the eyes, at two to four years of age, and by 10 years of age, such horses are practically all white. Skin and eyes remain pigmented. Examples include the Arabian, Camarque, Lippizaner, and Percheron breeds of horses. Recent studies[3] have

shown that the degree of coat pigmentation in white Camarque horses correlates directly with plasma α-MSH levels.

Precocious hereditary graying has been reported in Holstein-Friesian cattle in the Netherlands[44] and is called *blau*, or blue. Many black horses will sun-fade to brown, especially around the muzzle and flanks.[76]

RETICULATED LEUKOTRICHIA

Reticulated leukotrichia (variegated leukotrichia, tiger stripe) has been reported in quarter horses in the United States,[49, 71, 81] Thoroughbreds and Standardbreds in Australia,[49, 58] and rarely in other breeds.[71] The pathogenesis of the disorder is unclear, but it is believed to be hereditary.

There is no sex predilection, and animals usually develop clinical signs as yearlings. Linear crusts develop in a cross-hatched or netlike pattern symmetrically over the back, between the withers and tail. The eruption is asymptomatic. When the crusts are shed, a temporary alopecia is followed by the regrowth of white hair. The underlying skin is normal. The subsequent leukotrichia is permanent.

Diagnosis is based on history and physical examination. There is no effective therapy. Affected animals should not be used for breeding.

SPOTTED LEUKOTRICHIA

Spotted leukotrichia is an idiopathic disorder affecting mainly Arabian horses.[49, 81] Several white spots develop symmetrically or asymmetrically in the coat, especially over the rump and sides (Fig. 14–6). The condition is asymptomatic. Leukoderma is usually absent, although when present, the prognosis for recovery may be worse.

Diagnosis is based on history and physical examination. Individual lesions may come and go, and the condition may resolve spontaneously. There is no effective therapy.

HYPERESTHETIC LEUKOTRICHIA

Hyperesthetic leukotrichia is an idiopathic, rare, but highly characteristic equine dermatosis.[72] It has been described only in California. The disease affects mature horses, and there appear to be no breed or sex predilections.

The disorder is characterized by single or multiple extremely painful crusts, limited to

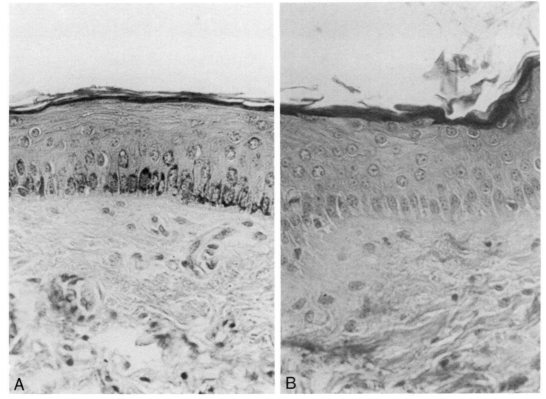

FIGURE 14–5. A, Equine vitiligo. Normal skin. Note heavy melanization of epidermal basal cells. B, Equine vitiligo. Depigmented skin. Absence of epidermal melanin.

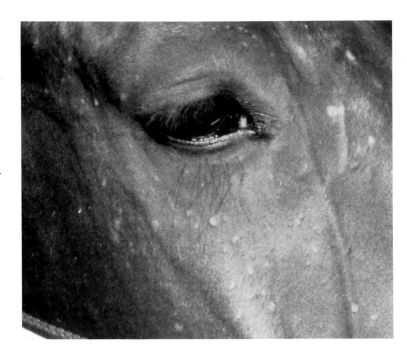

FIGURE 14–6. Spotted leukotrichia on the face of a horse.

the dorsal midline from the withers to the tail base. Affected horses react violently if the lesions are touched or even approached. Within a few weeks, white hairs appear in the area(s) of crusting. The disease runs a one- to three-month course, at which time the pain and crusts disappear. The leukotrichia persists.

Diagnosis is based on history and physical examination. Skin biopsy reveals marked subepidermal and intraepidermal edema. There is no known effective therapy. Even high doses of glucocorticoids are of no value. Occasional horses have recurrences.

Porcine Erythema and Cyanosis

Swine frequently develop noninflammatory erythema or cyanosis of the skin for a number of reasons.[10, 34, 73] Erythema may be seen with dermatosis erythematosa (especially on the ventrum, flanks, and ears), sunburn (especially the dorsum), transit erythema (especially the ventrum), carbon monoxide poisoning (all over), viral infections (especially the ears, tail, and extremities with hog cholera and African swine fever; see Chapter 5, discussion on hog cholera and African swine fever), and bacterial infections (streptococcosis; see Chapter 6, discussion on streptococcal infections). Cyanosis may be seen with benign peripartal cyanosis (sows at farrowing time, generalized), porcine stress syndrome (blotchy, then coalesced on dependent side), bacterial infections (especially on the ears, tail, and extremities with *Haemophilus parasuis* or *H. pleuropneumoniae* infections, *E. coli* enteritis, hemagglutinating encephalomyelitis, salmonellosis, pasteurellosis, erysipelas), thiamine deficiency, and organophosphate or carbamate poisoning (all over).

DISORDERS OF EPIDERMAL APPENDAGES

Hypotrichosis implies a less than normal amount of hair. The condition may be regional or multifocal but is usually generalized. It has been reported in all large animal species and is usually hereditary (see Chapter 11).

Curly Coat

Abnormal curliness of the hair coat has been reported as an inherited condition in cattle, horses, and swine (see Chapter 11).

Hypertrichosis

Hypertrichosis implies a greater than normal amount of hair. It has been reported as an inherited condition in cattle and swine (see Chapter 11) and as a result of maternal hyperthermia in sheep (see Chapter 11), *in utero* Border disease infection in lambs (see Chapter 11), and hyperadrenocorticism and chronic diseases in horses (see Chapter 13). Hypertrichosis may also be seen focally as a result of local injury or irritation, such as with wounds from ill-fitting tack.[33] The hair in these focal areas may become excessive, thicker, stiffer, and darker than normal.

Mane and Tail Dystrophy

Mane and tail dystrophy has been recognized in horses (see Chapter 11).[49]

Black and White Hair Follicle Dystrophies

Black and white hair follicle dystrophies have been recognized in horses (see Chapter 11).[49]

Abnormal Shedding

Normal shedding in large animals is basically controlled by photoperiod and, to a lesser extent, environmental temperature (see Chapter 1).[32, 33] Thus, most animals in temperate regions shed, to one degree or another, in spring and fall. In some animals, especially individual horses and cattle,[4, 32, 39, 49] abnormal spring shedding may result in excessive hair loss. Areas of marked hypotrichosis or alopecia may develop on the face, shoulders, and rump or may be fairly generalized and symmetric. The skin in affected areas is normal, and the animals are otherwise healthy. The pathogenesis of abnormal shedding is not understood.

Abnormal shedding may be mistaken for folliculitis (bacterial, fungal, or parasitic), anagen defluxion, alopecia areata, or endocrine skin disease. However, affected animals spontaneously and completely recover within one to three months.

Anagen Defluxion

So-called telogen defluxion (telogen effluvium, wool-break) has been reported in large animals.[10, 33, 39, 49] However, all such reports are most probably examples of anagen defluxion.

In telogen defluxion, a stressful circumstance (high fever, pregnancy, shock, severe illness, surgery, or anesthesia) causes the abrupt, premature cessation of growth in anagen hair follicles, and the sudden synchrony of many hair follicles in catagen, then telogen.[22] Two to three months later, a large number of telogen hairs are shed as a new wave of hair follicle cyclic activity begins.

In anagen defluxion, a circumstance (antimitotic drugs, infectious diseases, endocrine disorders, and metabolic disease) interferes with anagen, resulting in hair follicle and hair shaft abnormalities.[22] Hair loss occurs within days, as the growth phase continues. This is typical of the sudden hair loss that occurs within days of a very high fever, systemic illness, and malnutrition in large animals (Fig. 14–7).[10, 39, 49, 58, 70] In horses, the mane and tail are not affected.

Diagnosis is based on history, physical examination, and microscopic examination of affected hairs. Telogen hairs (club hairs) are characterized by a uniform shaft diameter and a slightly clubbed, nonpigmented root end that lacks root sheaths. Anagen defluxion hairs are characterized by irregularities and dysplastic changes. The diameter of the shaft may be irregularly narrowed and deformed, and breaking often occurs at such structurally weak sites, resulting in ragged points.

Both anagen and telogen defluxion spontaneously resolve when the constitutional stress is relieved.

Trichorrhexis Nodosa

Trichorrhexis nodosa (trichoclasis) is a hair shaft disorder recognized in horses and humans.[22, 33, 65] Most cases are associated with physical or chemical trauma, such as vigorous brushing or combing or harsh chemicals (e.g., insecticides, alcohol, solvents, and alkaline soaps and shampoos). In humans, hereditary and hair shaft structural defect forms exist.[22]

The characteristic lesions are small grayish white nodules along the hair shafts. These lesions may be visible with the naked eye. Breakage occurs through these nodules.

The differential diagnosis includes piedra (see Chapter 7, discussion on piedra). Diagnosis is based on history, physical examination, and microscopic examination of hairs. Microscopically, the hair shaft nodules have the appearance of two brooms pushed together end to end. The ends of broken hairs (split ends) have longitudinal splits and fracturing.

Therapy consists of stopping the external trauma.

Alopecia Areata

Alopecia areata is an idiopathic, clinically noninflammatory disorder characterized by

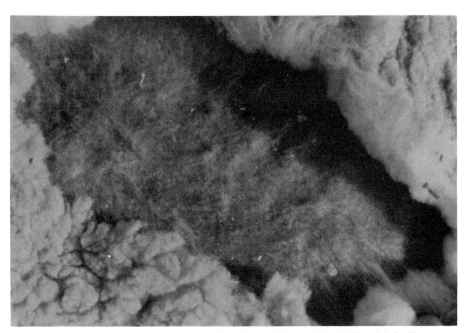

FIGURE 14–7. Ovine anagen defluxion ("wool break") associated with a febrile illness.

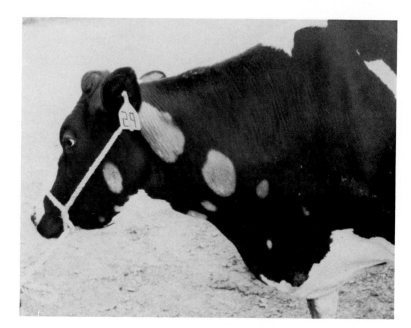

FIGURE 14–8. Alopecia areata in a cow. Multiple discrete areas of alopecia on the face and neck.

well-circumscribed patches of alopecia. It occurs in horses,[25, 33, 49] cattle,[67] and humans.[22] Although the exact pathogenesis of the disorder is unknown, genetic, endocrine, autoimmune, and psychologic factors have been thought to play a role.[22]

Clinically, alopecia areata is characterized by focal or multifocal, well-circumscribed, annular patches of noninflammatory alopecia (Figs. 14–8 and 14–9). In horses and cattle, lesions may be seen on the face, neck, and trunk. The dermatosis is asymptomatic, and affected animals are usually otherwise healthy. When hair grows back, it may be lighter than normal (leukotrichia).

The differential diagnosis includes folliculitis (bacterial, fungal, or parasitic), anagen defluxion, and occult sarcoid. Localized alopecia has also been reported to occur in horses fed excessive amounts of cane sugar and in certain infectious diseases.[26, 33] Diagnosis is based on history, physical examination, and skin biopsy. Histopathologic findings in early lesions are characterized by an accumulation of lymphoid cells ("swarm of bees") around the inferior segment of the anagen hair follicles (Figs. 14–10 and 14–11). However, this change may be difficult to demonstrate, requiring multiple biopsies from early lesions. Later histopathologic findings include a predominance of catogen and telogen hair follicles, follicular atrophy, orphaned sebaceous and apocrine glands, and no inflammation.

The prognosis for alopecia areata in humans is usually good, with the majority of patients making a complete recovery within three to five years, with or without therapy. The biologic behavior of alopecia areata in horses is unclear, although spontaneous recovery has occurred after several months to two years.[67]

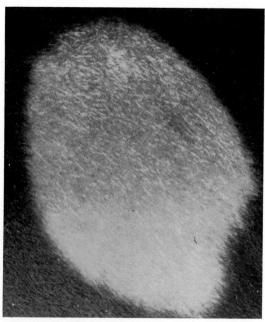

FIGURE 14–9. Alopecia areata in a cow. Hair regrowing within the lesion is white.

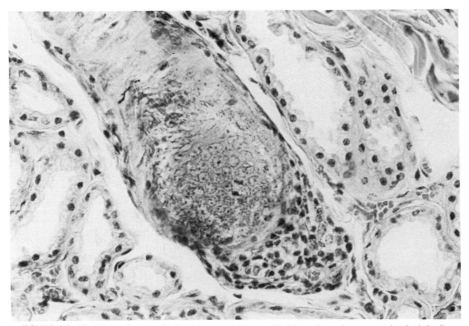

FIGURE 14–10. Alopecia areata in a horse. A "swarm" of lymphocytes around a hair bulb.

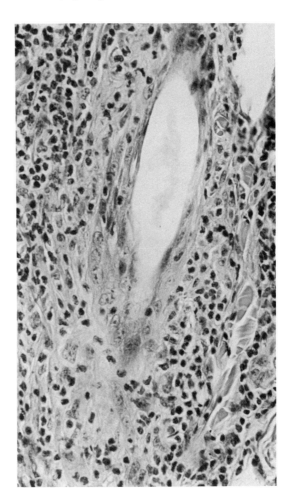

FIGURE 14–11. Equine alopecia areata. Transverse section through inferior segment of hair follicle with surrounding lymphoid infiltrate.

Anhidrosis

Anhidrosis is characterized by the inability to sweat in response to an adequate stimulus.[5, 10, 33, 49, 77-79, 79a] The condition is recognized commonly in horses and rarely in cattle. The etiology is uncertain, and no particular diet, vitamin-mineral supplement or lack thereof, or hereditary predilection can be identified.[79] The onset of the condition is not always associated with poor acclimatization but is precipitated by heat stress in a humid environment, whether previously experienced or not.[16, 77-79] Horses can lose up to 45 L of fluid per day via sweat in strenuous exercise, and the major electrolytes lost are chloride, potassium, and sodium.[12]

Pathogenetically, equine anhidrosis is believed to result from a conditioned insensitivity of sweat glands to epinephrine.[10, 39, 49, 70, 79] Blood epinephrine levels in horses in the tropics are higher than those in horses in temperate climates.[18-21, 70] Blood levels of epinephrine in normal and anhidrotic horses in the tropics are similar,[7, 18-21, 70] but anhidrotics have a very poor sweating response to intravenously or intradermally administered epinephrine. Recently, ultrastructural studies of the sweat glands of anhidrotic horses revealed a reduced number of cytoplasmic vesicles, compacted intercellular spaces, lack of evidence of myoepithelial cell contraction, and evidence of contracted ductal lumina, which often appeared to be completely occluded or obscured by cellular debris.[28] These investigators concluded that the findings suggested that a failure or impairment of sweat production had occurred.

Equine anhidrosis (dry-coat, nonsweating) has an incidence of up to 20 percent in some geographic areas and is an economically significant condition in horses in rigorous training for racing, endurance, polo, or show as well as in brood mares and idle pleasure horses.* In the United States, it is a particular problem in the Gulf Coast states. Horses of all ages, sexes, breeds, and colors may be affected. Native and imported horses are equally affected.

Acutely, equine anhidrosis is characterized by labored breathing, flared nostrils, fever (up to 42°C), and partial or complete lack of sweating. Collapse and death may occur. Chronically, a dry hair coat, excessive scaling (seborrhea sicca), and partial alopecia of the face

and neck may be seen. Pruritus, polydipsia, polyuria, poor appetite, and a loss of body condition may be present.

Diagnosis is based on history, physical examination, and intradermal skin testing.[10, 39, 49, 59, 70, 77-79] Epinephrine at concentrations of 1:1000, 1:10,000, 1:100,000, and 1:1,000,000 is injected intradermally at a dose of 0.5 ml each. In normal horses, sweating occurs over the injection sites within minutes, at all dilutions. Anhidrotic horses respond to *only* the 1:1000 dilution, and then only after a period of five hours or more.

Anhidrotic horses may have low blood levels of chloride and sodium,[10, 15, 24, 39, 49, 70] but hemograms, serum chemistry panels, and serum electrolyte levels are frequently normal.[77-79] Serum T_4 and T_3 levels may be low but return to normal as affected horses recover,[59] confirming the existence of the euthyroid sick syndrome (see Chapter 13, discussion on hypothyroidism). Light microscopic examination of the sweat glands in anhidrotic horses reveals no significant abnormalities.[6, 19] Ultrastructural examination reveals numerous abnormalities of unknown diagnostic significance.[28]

No form of medical treatment has any consistent benefit.[77-79] Medicaments reported to be effective include oral and intravenous electrolyte supplements,* 1000 to 3000 IU vitamin E/day orally,[10, 16, 38, 39, 49] 15 gm iodinated casein/day orally,[10, 16, 37, 39, 49] and injections of ACTH.[49] Reduction in dietary concentrates has been recommended[16, 49] but is of unknown benefit.

The most logical mode of therapy is to move the animal to a cooler, more arid climate.[39] If this is not feasible, affected animals should be kept in air-conditioned, low-humidity stalls and exercised during the cool periods of the day.[39, 49, 77-79]

Hyperhidrosis

Hyperhidrosis refers to excessive sweating and is most commonly seen in horses.[10, 22, 33, 39] Generalized hyperhidrosis in horses may be associated with high ambient temperatures, vigorous exercise, severe pain (e.g., colic), the administration of certain drugs (epinephrine, acetylcholine, promazine, colloidal silver, or prostaglandin $F_{2\alpha}$), hyperadrenocorticism, and pheochromocytoma.[10, 33, 39, 49] Localized hyperhidrosis in horses may be associated with local injections of epinephrine; dourine; and Hor-

---

*References 5, 10, 15, 16, 39, 49, 59, 70, 77-79

*References 5, 10, 15, 16, 24, 39, 49, 77-79

ner's syndrome (hypothalamic, brain stem, or spinal cord lesions; guttural pouch infections; careless intravenous injections).[33, 39, 49, 69]

Hematidrosis

Hematidrosis refers to the presence of blood in sweat and has been reported in horses with equine infectious anemia, purpura hemorrhagica, and various bleeding diatheses.[10, 33] In addition to blood-tinged or frankly bloody sweat, red to bluish-red vesicles and bullae may be seen.

REFERENCES

1. Adalsteinsson, S.: Depressed fertility in Icelandic sheep caused by a single colour gene. Ann. Genet. Select. Anim. 7:445, 1975.
2. Adalsteinsson, S.: Albinism in Icelandic sheep. J. Hered. 68:347, 1977.
3. Altmeyer, P., et al.: The relationship between α-MSH level and coat color in white Camarque horses. J. Invest. Dermatol. 82:199, 1984.
4. Amstutz, H. E.: Bovine skin conditions: A brief review. Mod. Vet. Pract. 60:821, 1979.
5. Arnold, T. F.: Panting in cattle and nonsweating horses. Vet. Rec. 62:463, 1950.
6. Barnes, J. E.: "Dry sweating" in horses. Vet. Rec. 50:977, 1938.
7. Beadle, R. E., et al.: Summertime plasma catecholamine concentrations in healthy and anhidrotic horses in Louisiana. Am. J. Vet. Res. 43:1446, 1982.
8. Bell, F. R., and Evans, C. L.: The relationship between sweating and the innervation of sweat glands in the horse. J. Physiol. 134:421, 1956.
9. Bell, T. G., et al.: Decreased nucleotide and serotonin storage associated with defective function in Chédiak-Higashi syndrome cattle and human platelets. Blood; 48:175, 1976.
10. Blood, D. C., et al.: *Veterinary Medicine VI.* Oxford, Baillière Tindall, 1983.
11. Blume, R. S., et al.: Grant neutrophil granules in the Chédiak-Higashi syndrome of man, mink, cattle and mice. Can. J. Comp. Med. 33:271, 1969.
12. Carlson, G., and Ocen, P.: Composition of equine sweat following exercise in high environmental temperatures and in response to intravenous epinephrine administration. J. Equine Med. Surg. 3:27, 1979.
13. Castle, W. E.: Coat color inheritance in horses and in other mammals. Genetics 49:35, 1954.
14. Collier, L. L., et al.: Ocular manifestations of the Chédiak-Higashi syndrome in four species of animals. JAVMA 175:587, 1979.
15. Correa, J. E., and Calderin, G. G.: Anhidrosis, dry coat syndrome in the Thoroughbred. JAVMA 149:1556, 1966.
16. Currie, A. K., and Seager, S. W. J.: Anhidrosis. Proc. Am. Assoc. Equine Pract. 22:249, 1976.
17. Davis, W. C., and Douglas, S. D.: Defective granule formation and function in the Chédiak-Higashi syndrome in man and animals. Semin. Hematol. 9:431, 1972.
18. Evans, C. L., and Smith, D. F. G.: The relationship between sweating and the catecholamine content of the blood in the horse. J. Physiol. 132:542, 1956.
19. Evans, C. L., et al.: A histological study of the sweat glands of normal and dry coated horses. J. Comp. Pathol. Ther. 67:397, 1957.
20. Evans, C. L., et al.: Physiologic factors on the condition of "dry-coat" in horses. Vet. Rec. 69:1, 1957.
21. Evans, C. L.: Physiological mechanisms that underlie sweating in the horse. Br. Vet. J. 122:117, 1966.
22. Fitzpatrick, T. B., et al.: *Dermatology in General Medicine II.* New York, McGraw-Hill Book Co., 1979.
23. Gebhart, W., and Niebauer, G. W.: Beziehungen Zwischen Pigment-Schwund und Melanomatose am Beispiel des Lipizzaner-schimmels. Arch. Dermatol. Res. 259:39, 1977.
24. Gilyard, R. T.: Chronic anhidrosis with lowered blood chlorides in race horses. Cornell Vet. 34:332, 1944.
25. Guilhon, J.: Alopecie psycho-somatique des animaux domestiques. Rec. Med. Vet. 138:839, 1962.
26. Hodgkins, J. R.: Alopecia toxica. Vet. Rec. 26:625, 1914.
27. Huston, R., et al.: Congenital defects in foals. J. Equine Med. Surg. 1:146, 1977.
28. Jenkinson, D. M., et al.: Ultrastructural variations in the sweat glands of anhidrotic horses. Equine Vet. J. 17:287, 1985.
29. Jolly, R. D., and Blakemore, W. F.: Inherited lysosomal storage diseases: An essay in comparative medicine. Vet. Rec. 92:391, 1973.
30. Jones, W. E., and Bogart, R.: *Genetics of the Horse.* Caballus Publ., East Lansing, 1971.
31. Jones, W. E.: The Overo white foal syndrome. J. Equine Med. Surg. 3:54, 1979.
32. Kilby, E.: How horses' hair reflects inner health. Equus 99, Jan. 1986, p. 41.
33. Kral, F., and Schwartzman, R. M.: *Veterinary and Comparative Dermatology.* Philadelphia, J. B. Lippincott Co., 1964.
34. Leman, A. D., et al.: *Diseases of Swine V.* Ames, Iowa State University Press, 1981.
35. Lerner, A. B., and Cate, G. W.: Melanoma in horses. Yale J. Biol. Med. 46:656, 1973.
36. Lever, W. F., and Schaumburg-Lever, G.: *Histopathology of the Skin VI.* Philadelphia, J. B. Lippincott Co., 1983.
37. Magsood, M.: Iodinated casein therapy for the "non-sweating" syndrome in horses. Vet. Rec. 68:475, 1956.
38. Marsh, J. H.: Treatment of "dry-coat" in Thoroughbreds with vitamin E. Vet. Rec. 73:1124, 1961.
39. McMullan, W. C.: The Skin. *In:* Mansmann, R. A., et al. (eds.): *Equine Medicine & Surgery III.* Santa Barbara, CA, American Veterinary Publications, Inc., 1982, p. 789.
40. Meijer, W. C. P.: Vitiligo. Tijdschr. Diergeneeskd. 85:592, 1960.
41. Meijer, W. C. P., and Eijk, W.: Vitiligo bijeen Zwartbante F. H. Stamboekvaars. Tijdschr. Diergeneeskd. 86:537, 1961.
42. Meijer, W. C. P.: Vitiligo bij het paard, de z.g. "neigeures." Tijdschr. Diergeneeskd. 86:1021, 1961.
43. Meijer, W. C. P., and Eijk, W.: Vitiligo bij paarden en runderen. Tijdschr. Diergeneeskd. 87:411, 1962.
44. Meijer, W. C. P.: Vekregen en aangeboren depigmentaties bij de huisdieren gezien in het licht van de recente stand der humane dermatologie. Tijdsch. Diergeneeskd. 87:1305, 1962.
45. Meijer, W. C. P.: Dermatological diagnosis in horse and cattle judging. Vet. Rec. 77:1046, 1965.
46. Meijer, W. C. P.: Pigment verlust des Integumentes und die dermatologische Diagnose bei der Beurteilung von Pferden und Rindern. Dtsch. Tierarztl. Wochenschr. 73:85, 1966.
47. Meyers, K. M., et al.: Storage pool deficiency in platelets from Chédiak-Higashi cattle. Am. J. Physiol. 237:R239, 1981.
48. Millikan, L. E., et al.: Gross and ultrastructural studies in a new melanoma model: The Sinclair swine. Yale J. Biol. Med. 46:631, 1973.
49. Mullowney, P. C.: Dermatologic diseases of horses part V. Allergic, immune-mediated, and miscellaneous skin diseases. Compend. Cont. Educ. 7:S217, 1985.
50. Naughton, G. K., et al.: Antibodies to surface antigens of pigmented cells in animals with vitiligo. Proc. Soc. Exp. Biol. Med. 181:423, 1986.
51. Padgett, G. A., et al.: The familial occurrence of the Chédiak-Higashi syndrome in mink and cattle. Genetics 49:505, 1964.
52. Padgett, G. A.: Neutrophil function in animals with the Chédiak-Higashi syndrome. Blood 29:906, 1967.
53. Padgett, G. A.: The Chédiak-Higashi syndrome. Adv. Vet. Sci. 12:239, 1968.
54. Padgett, G. A., et al.: Comparative studies of susceptibility to infection in the Chédiak-Higashi syndrome. J. Pathol. Bacteriol. 95:509, 1968.

55. Padgett, G. A., et al.: The Chédiak-Higashi syndrome: A comparative review. Curr. Top. Pathol. 51:1, 1969.
56. Page, E. H.: Common skin diseases of the horse. Proc. Am. Assoc. Equine Pract. 18:385, 1972.
57. Panel Report: Skin conditions in horses. Mod. Vet. Pract. 56:363, 1975.
58. Pascoe, R. R.: *Equine Dermatoses.* Sydney, University of Sydney Post-Graduate Foundation in Veterinary Science, Veterinary Review No. 22, 1981.
59. Peter, J. E., et al.: Anhidrosis in a Thoroughbred. Vet. Med. Small Anim. Clin. 76:730, 1981.
60. Prieur, D. J., et al.: Ultrastructural and morphogenetic studies of platelets from cattle with the Chédiak-Higashi syndrome. Lab. Invest. 35:197, 1976.
61. Prieur, D. J., and Collier, L. L.: Chédiak-Higashi syndrome. Am. J. Pathol. 90:533, 1978.
62. Pulos, W. L., and Hutt, F. B.: Lethal dominant white horses. J. Hered. 60:59, 1969.
63. Renshaw, H. W., et al.: Leukocyte dysfunction in the bovine homologue of the Chédiak-Higashi syndrome of humans. Infect. Immun. 10:928, 1974.
64. Sako, S.: Three cases of vitiligo vulgaris in Japanese black cattle. Jpn. J. Vet. Med. Assoc. 36:186, 1983.
65. Schindelka, H.: *Haut krankheiten bei Haustieren II.* Vienna, Braumuller, 1908.
66. Schneider, J. E., and Leipold, H. W.: Recessive lethal white in two foals. J. Equine Med. Surg. 2:479, 1978.
67. Scott, D. W.: Unpublished observations, 1986.
68. Sen, S., and Ansari, A. I.: Depigmentation (vitiligo) in animals and its treatment with "Meladinine." Indian J. Anim. Health 10:249, 1971.
69. Smith, T. S., and Mayhew, I. G.: Horner's syndrome in large animals. Cornell Vet. 67:529, 1977.
70. Stannard, A. A.: The skin. *In:* Mansmann, R. A., et al. (eds.): *Equine Medicine & Surgery II.* Santa Barbara, CA, American Veterinary Publications, Inc., 1972, p. 381.
71. Stannard, A. A.: Equine dermatology. Proc. Am. Assoc. Equine Pract. 22:273, 1976.
72. Stannard, A. A.: Hyperesthetic leukotrichia. *In:* Robinson, N. E. (ed.): *Current Therapy in Equine Medicine II.* Philadelphia, W. B. Saunders Co., 1987, p. 647.
73. Straw, B.: Diagnosis of skin disease in swine. Compend. Cont. Educ. 7:S650, 1985.
74. Sturtevant, A. H.: A critical examination of recent studies on colour inheritance in horses. J. Genet. 2:41, 1912.
75. Thomsett, L. R.: Noninfectious skin diseases of horses. Vet. Clin. North Am. Large Anim. Pract. 6:59, 1984.
76. Trommershausen-Smith, A.: Positive horse identification part 3: Coat color genetics. Equine Pract. 1:24, 1979.
77. Warner, A. E., and Mayhew, I. G.: Equine anhidrosis: A survey of affected horses in Florida. JAVMA 180:627, 1982.
78. Warner, A. E.: Equine anhidrosis. Compend. Cont. Educ. 4:S434, 1982.
79. Warner, A. E.: Anhidrosis. *In:* Robinson, N. E. (ed.): *Current Therapy in Equine Medicine.* Philadelphia, W. B. Saunders Co., 1983, p. 170.
79a. Warner, A. E.: Anhidrosis. *In:* Robinson, N. E. (ed.): *Current Therapy in Equine Medicine II.* Philadelphia, W. B. Saunders Co., 1987, p. 187.
80. Windhorst, D. B., and Padgett, G. A.: The Chédiak-Higashi syndrome and the homologous trait in animals. J. Invest. Dermatol. 60:529, 1973.
81. Yager, J. A., and Scott, D. W.: The skin and appendages. *In* Jubb, K. V., et al..: *Pathology of Domestic Animals.* Vol. 1. New York, Academic Press, 1985, p. 407.

CHAPTER 15

MISCELLANEOUS DERMATOSES

This chapter features a number of dermatoses for which the etiology and pathogenesis are unknown or multifactorial. Most important among these are syndromes that cause nodules on the skin of the horse. Single or multiple nodules are the most common equine skin lesion.[28] When the frequency of equine nodular skin disease is viewed in light of the plethora of potential causes (Table 15–1), the clinician's plight is readily appreciated. A complete discussion of the differential diagnosis of equine nodular skin disease is beyond the scope of this chapter, and the reader is referred to appropriate sections of this book for clinicopathologic details. Skin biopsy is a very useful and cost-effective diagnostic aid in equine dermatology. It is the only way to achieve a definitive diagnosis in most equine nodular skin diseases.

EQUINE EOSINOPHILIC GRANULOMA WITH COLLAGEN DEGENERATION

This disorder is probably the most common nodular skin disease of the horse.

Cause and Pathogenesis

The cause and pathogenesis of equine eosinophilic granuloma with collagen degeneration are unknown. Because the lesions often begin in warmer months, a hypersensitivity reaction to insect bites has been suspected.[16, 19–21, 23, 30, 32] However, in the northeastern United States, about one third of cases begin in winter. Thus, unless the insect hypersensitivity is a delayed immunologic reaction, there must be more than one etiology for a seemingly identical clinicopathologic entity. Because the lesions commonly occur in the saddle region, other authors have suggested that trauma may be an inciting cause.[4, 31, 33]

Clinical Features

Equine eosinophilic granuloma with collagen degeneration (nodular necrobiosis, nodular collagenolytic granuloma, acute collagen necrosis, eosinophilic granuloma) is seen most commonly in warmer months and has no apparent age, breed, or sex predilections.[8, 9, 19, 28, 30] Single or multiple lesions from 2 to 10 cm in diameter most commonly affect the neck, withers, and back (Figs. 15–1, 15–2, and 15–3). The lesions are usually rounded, well-circumscribed, firm, nonalopecic, nonulcerative, nonpainful, and nonpruritic. Cystic or plaquelike lesions are occasionally seen and may discharge a central, grayish-white caseous core. Affected horses are otherwise healthy.

Diagnosis

The differential diagnosis includes the conditions listed in Table 15–1. Definitive diagnosis is based on history, physical examination, exfoliative cytology (eosinophils, histiocytes, lymphocytes, and no microorganisms), skin biopsy, and culture (negative). Skin biopsy reveals multifocal areas of collagen degeneration followed by granulomatous inflammation containing eosinophils (Figs. 15–4 and 15–5). Older and larger lesions exhibit marked dystrophic mineralization (Fig. 15–6) and may be misdiagnosed as calcinosis circumscripta or tumoral calcinosis.

Clinical Management

Horses with solitary lesions, or a few lesions, may be treated by surgical excision or sublesional glucocorticoid injections.[8, 9, 16, 19, 28, 30] Triamcinolone acetonide (3 to 5 mg/lesion) or methylprednisolone acetate (5 to 10 mg/lesion) is effective. It has been recommended that no more than 20 mg of triamcinolone acetonide be administered sublesionally, at once, to any horse because of the potential of laminitis. Horses with multiple lesions may be treated with oral prednisone or prednisolone given orally at 1.1 mg/kg s.i.d. for two to three weeks.

Occasionally, horses may suffer relapses, and retreatment is successful. Some lesions

399

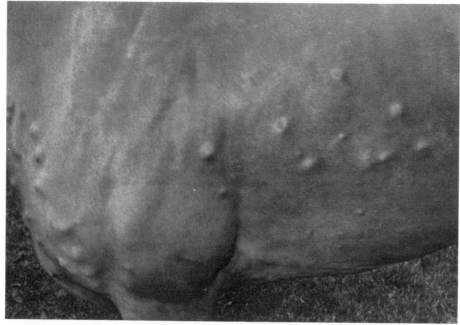

FIGURE 15–1. Equine eosinophilic granuloma. Multiple asymptomatic nodules on trunk.

undergo spontaneous remission. Older or larger lesions are often severely mineralized. Such lesions do not respond to glucocorticoid therapy, and surgical excision is required.

EQUINE AXILLARY NODULAR NECROSIS

Axillary nodular necrosis is a rare dermatosis of horses.[28] The cause and pathogenesis of this disorder are unknown.

There are no apparent age, breed, or sex predilections. One or two nodules are present near the girth and axillae (girth galls). The nodules are rounded, well-circumscribed, firm, nonalopecic, nonulcerative, nonpainful, and nonpruritic. Affected horses are otherwise healthy.

The differential diagnosis includes granulomatous disorders (infectious or sterile), neoplasia, and cysts. Definitive diagnosis is based on history, physical examination, exfoliative

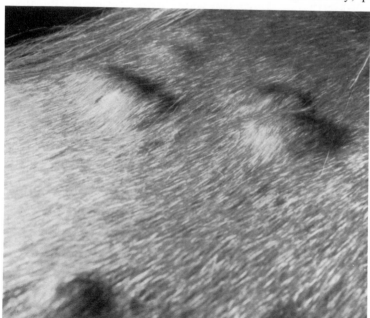

FIGURE 15–2. Equine eosinophilic granuloma. Cluster of nodules over withers.

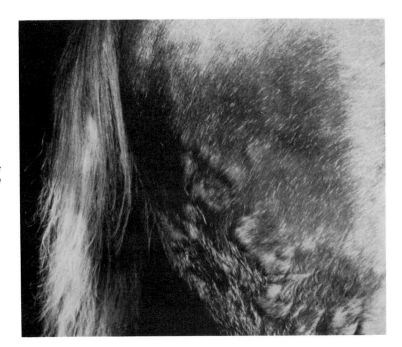

FIGURE 15–3. Equine eosinophilic granuloma. Cluster of nodules on thigh.

cytology (suppurative to pyogranulomatous inflammation, no microorganisms), skin biopsy (pyogranulomatous dermatitis with focal dermal necrosis, no microorganisms), and culture (negative).

If desired, treatment may include surgical excision or sublesional glucocorticoids. Triamcinolone acetonide (3 to 5 mg/lesion) or methylprednisolone acetate (5 to 10 mg/lesion) is effective.

EQUINE UNILATERAL PAPULAR DERMATOSIS

Unilateral papular dermatosis is an uncommon equine skin disorder.[16, 28, 30, 34, 37] The cause and pathogenesis of this disorder are unknown. Initial descriptions of this condition[16, 30] suggested that quarter horses had a genetic predilection. However, the disorder has been seen in several breeds of horses.[28, 34]

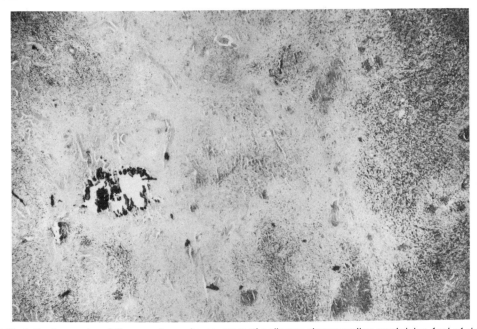

FIGURE 15–4. Equine eosinophilic granuloma. Large area of collagen degeneration containing foci of dystrophic mineralization.

TABLE 15–1. Differential Diagnosis of Nodular Skin Disease in the Horse

Disease	Common Site(s)
Bacterial	
Furunculosis (especially coagulase-positive staphylococci)	Saddle or tack areas
Ulcerative lymphangitis (especially *Corynebacterium pseudotuberculosis*)	Legs
Actinomycosis	Mandible and maxilla
Nocardiosis	?*
Abscess (especially *C. pseudotuberculosis*)	Chest and abdomen
Botryomycosis (especially coagulase-positive staphylococci)	Legs and scrotum
Tuberculosis	Ventral thorax and abdomen; medial thighs
Glanders	Medial hocks
Fungal	
Dermatophytosis	Saddle or tack areas
Mycetoma (*Curvularia geniculata*, black-grain; *Pseudoallescheria boydii*, white-grain)	?
Phaeohyphomycosis (*Drechslera specifera, Hormodendrum* sp.)	?
Sporotrichosis	Legs
Zygomycosis	
Basidiobolus haptosporus	Chest, trunk, neck, and head
Conidiobolus coronatus	Nostrils
Alternariosis (*Alternaria tenuis*)	?
Blastomycosis	?
Coccidioidomycosis	?
Cryptococcosis	?
Histoplasmosis farciminosi (*Histoplasma farciminosum*)	Face, neck, and legs
Pythiosis (*Pythium* sp.)	Legs, ventral chest, and abdomen
Parasitic	
Hypodermiasis (*Hypoderma bovis, H. lineatum*)	Withers
Habronemiasis (*Habronema muscae, H. majus, Draschia megastoma*)	Legs, ventrum, prepuce, and medial canthus
Parafilariasis (*Parafilaria multipapillosa*)	Neck, shoulders, and trunk
Viral	
Viral papular dermatitis (variola-like poxvirus)	Trunk
Immunologic	
Urticaria	Neck and trunk
Erythema multiforme	?
Amyloidosis	Head, neck, chest, and shoulders
Neoplastic	
Papilloma	Nose and lips
Aural plaques	Pinnae
Squamous cell carcinoma	Head and mucocutaneous junctions
Sarcoid	Head, ventrum, and legs
Apocrine gland adenoma	Pinnae, and vulva
Fibroma	Head, neck, saddle area, and legs
Hemangioma	Legs
Schwannoma	Eyelids and periorbital region
Mastocytoma	Head and legs
Melanoma	Perineum, perianal area, ventral tail, and base of ears
Lymphosarcoma	Trunk
Temporal teratoma	Base of ears
Miscellaneous	
Epidermoid or dermoid cysts	Dorsal midline
Eosinophilic granuloma	Neck, withers, and back
Axillary nodular necrosis	Near axilla and girth
Unilateral papular dermatosis	Trunk
Granulation tissue	Legs
Panniculitis	Trunk
Foreign body granuloma	Legs and ventrum
Pseudolymphoma	Lateral stifle
Calcinosis circumscripta†	Legs

*No apparent site(s) of predilection
†Calcinosis circumscripta (tumoral calcinosis) may, in some or all cases, be the end stage of eosinophilic granuloma or mastocytoma.

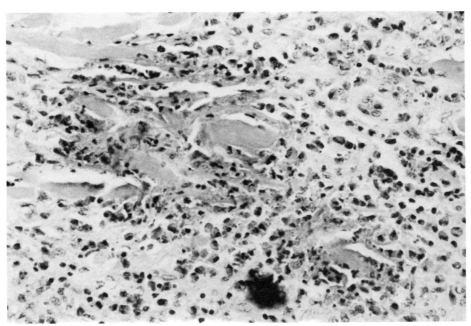

FIGURE 15–5. *Equine eosinophilic granuloma. Focus of early collagen degeneration and accumulation of eosinophils and histiocytes.*

Most horses develop lesions in spring and summer. There are no apparent age or sex predilections. The outstanding clinical feature of the disorder is the occurrence of multiple (30 to 300) papules and nodules limited to one side of the body (Fig. 15–7). The trunk is consistently affected. The lesions are usually rounded, well-circumscribed, firm, nonalope-cic, nonulcerative, nonpainful, and nonpruritic. Affected horses are otherwise healthy.

Diagnosis is based on history, physical examination, exfoliative cytology (predominantly eosinophils, no microorganisms), skin biopsy (eosinophilic folliculitis and furunculosis, no microorganisms) (Figs. 15–8 and 15–9) and culture (negative).

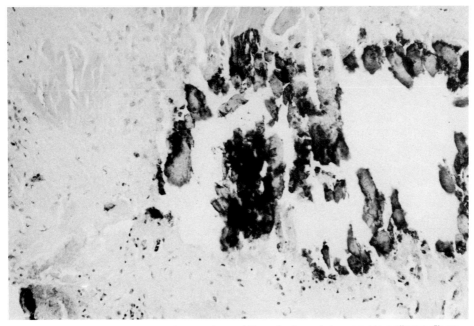

FIGURE 15–6. *Equine eosinophilic granuloma. Mineralization of degenerate collagen fibers.*

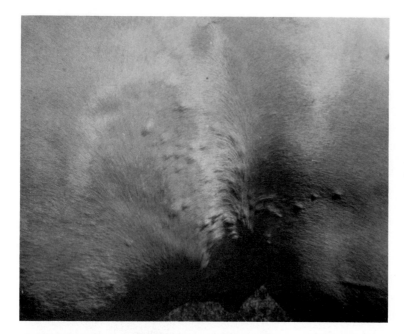

FIGURE 15–7. Equine unilateral papular dermatosis. Multiple papules in flank.

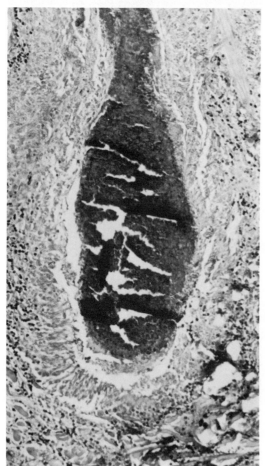

FIGURE 15–8. Equine unilateral papular dermatosis. Hair follicle filled with "eosinophilic mush" and surrounded by eosinophilic inflammation.

Equine unilateral papular dermatosis usually undergoes spontaneous remission within several weeks to months. Because of this and the asymptomatic nature of the disease, treatment is not usually attempted. Oral prednisone or prednisolone given orally at 1.1 mg/kg s.i.d. for two to three weeks is an effective treatment. Occasional horses suffer relapses (on the same side or the opposite side of the body) in subsequent years.

BOVINE STERILE EOSINOPHILIC FOLLICULITIS

Bovine sterile eosinophilic folliculitis is a recently reported, apparently rare disorder of cattle.[27] There are no apparent age, breed, or sex predilections. The cause and pathogenesis are unknown. The disorder is nonseasonal in occurrence and is characterized by a fairly symmetric papulocrustous eruption. Lesions progress to annular areas of alopecia, crusting, scaling, and plaques (Fig. 15–10). The head, neck, and trunk are commonly affected. There is no pain or pruritus, and affected cattle are otherwise healthy. Typically, only one animal of an entire herd is affected.

The differential diagnosis includes other causes of bovine folliculitis: dermatophytosis, dermatophilosis, demodicosis, staphylococcosis, stephanofilariasis, and *Pelodera* dermatitis. Definitive diagnosis is based on history, physical examination, exfoliative cytology

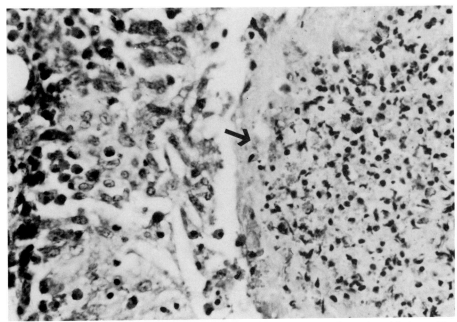

FIGURE 15–9. *Equine unilateral papular dermatosis. Pilary canal filled with necrotic eosinophils (arrow) bordered by inflamed outer root sheath.*

(predominantly eosinophils, no microorganisms), skin biopsy (eosinophilic folliculitis, no microorganisms) (Figs. 15–11 and 15–12), and culture (negative).

The natural course of the disease is unknown. Although the condition has been reported to clear with topical glucocorticoids,[27] relapses occurred when treatment was stopped.

PANNICULITIS

Panniculitis is a rare, multifactorial inflammatory condition of the subcutaneous fat in horses.

Cause and Pathogenesis

The lipocyte is particularly vulnerable to trauma, ischemia, and neighboring inflamma-

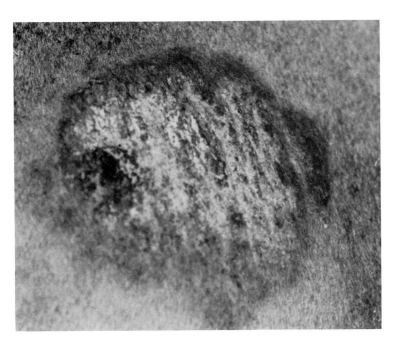

FIGURE 15–10. *Bovine sterile eosinophilic folliculitis. Annular alopecic, crusted plaque on thorax.*

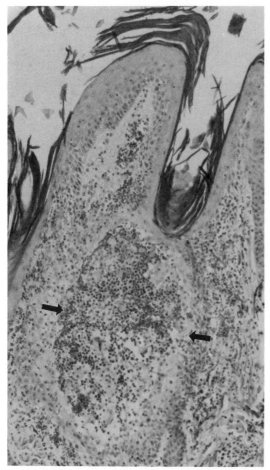

FIGURE 15–11. Bovine sterile eosinophilic folliculitis. Inferior segment of hair follicle filled with eosinophils (arrows).

tory disease. In addition, damage to lipocytes results in the liberation of lipid, which undergoes hydrolysis into glycerol and fatty acids. Fatty acids are potent inflammatory agents and incite further inflammatory reactions.

There are multiple etiologic factors involved in the genesis of panniculitis (Table 15–2). Nodular panniculitis refers to sterile subcutaneous inflammatory nodules and is not a specific disease. It is purely a descriptive term representing clinically the end result of several known and unknown etiologic factors.

Sterile panniculitis has been rarely reported in horses.[3, 5, 26, 28] The etiology was in all cases obscure but was suspected to be associated with vitamin E deficiency (yellow fat disease) in some animals.

Clinical Features

Panniculitis is manifested clinically as deep-seated cutaneous nodules and plaques (Fig. 15–13). The lesions may occur singly or in crops, either localized to specific areas or generalized, and may vary in size from a few millimeters to several centimeters in diameter. Nodules may be firm and well-circumscribed or soft and ill-defined. They are initially subcutaneous but may fix to the overlying skin as they progress. The lesions may become cystic, ulcerate, and develop draining tracts that discharge an oily, yellowish-brown to bloody substance. The lesions may or may not be painful and may heal with depressed scars. The nod-

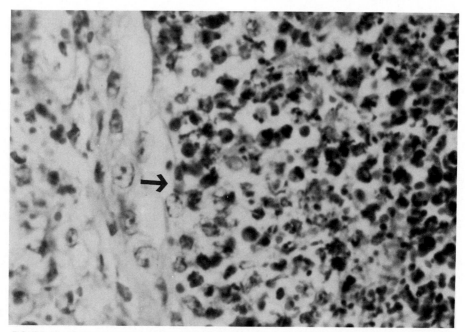

FIGURE 15–12. Bovine sterile eosinophilic folliculitis. Pilary canal filled with eosinophils (arrow).

TABLE 15–2. Differential Diagnosis of Panniculitis

Infections (bacterial, mycobacterial, actinomycetic, or fungal)
Immunologic (lupus erythematosus, drug eruption, or erythema nodosum)
Physicochemical (trauma, pressure, cold, foreign body, or result of subcutaneous injection of bulky, oily, or insoluble liquids)
Pancreatic disease
Result of glucocorticoid therapy
Vasculitis
Nutritional (vitamin E deficiency)
Enteropathies
Idiopathic

ules and plaques often have a predilection for the trunk.* Concurrent constitutional signs (anorexia, depression, lethargy, and pyrexia) may be present.

Diagnosis

The differential diagnosis includes granulomatous diseases (infectious or sterile), neoplasia, and cysts. Definitive diagnosis is based on history, physical examination, exfoliative cytology, skin biopsy, and culture. Direct smears reveal suppurative to pyogranuloma-

*References 1, 3, 133, 24–26, 28, 35, 36

tous inflammation with intra- and extracellular lipid droplets. Excisional biopsy is the *only* biopsy technique that is satisfactory for subcutaneous nodules, as punch biopsies fail to deliver sufficient tissue in about 75 percent of cases.[26] Skin biopsy reveals lobular to diffuse pyogranulomatous to granulomatous panniculitis (Figs. 15–14 and 15–15).

Clinical Management

Panniculitides with known causes (e.g., infectious) should be treated specifically (see appropriate sections of this book). Sterile panniculitides usually respond well to high doses of systemic glucocorticoids.[26, 28] Prednisone or prednisolone, given orally at 1.1 to 2.2 mg/kg/ day, as well as 20 to 30 mg dexamethasone/ day orally, has been used successfully. Lesions usually subside within 7 to 14 days. Relapses may occur and require long-term alternate-

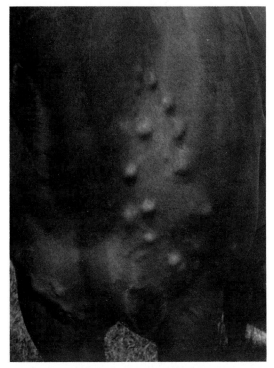

FIGURE 15–13. Equine sterile panniculitis. Multiple subcutaneous nodules on the chest.

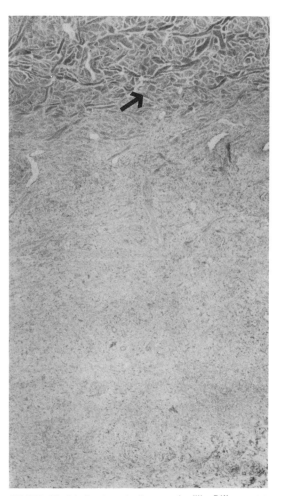

FIGURE 15–14. Equine sterile panniculitis. Diffuse panniculitis with overlying normal dermis (arrow).

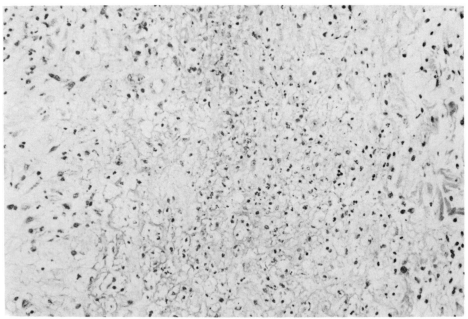

FIGURE 15–15. Equine sterile panniculitis. Diffuse, necrotizing, suppurative panniculitis.

morning prednisone or prednisolone maintenance therapy. In dogs, cats, and humans, sterile panniculitides have also been reported to respond to high doses of oral vitamin E or oral potassium iodide.[26]

PORCINE DERMATOSIS ERYTHEMATOSA

This is a poorly characterized dermatosis of swine.[6, 14] The etiology is unknown, and meaningful clinicopathologic studies have apparently not been conducted.

Porcine dermatosis erythematosa is reported to be quite common in white pigs and can occur in swine grazing new pasture or in fattening pigs and breeding stock housed entirely indoors. There is striking acute erythema over large areas of the body, including the ears, sides, and abdomen. There is no pruritus or pain, and affected swine are usually otherwise healthy.

Therapy is unnecessary, as complete, spontaneous recovery occurs within a few days.

EQUINE CALCINOSIS CIRCUMSCRIPTA

Equine calcinosis circumscripta (tumoral calcinosis) is characterized by firm nodules over the lateral stifle area that arise from a fibrosing granulomatous reaction to dystrophic mineralization.[2, 7, 11, 22] The cause and pathogenesis are

unknown. Although prolonged and chronic trauma to localized areas has been suggested, the condition frequently occurs in young horses, and usually in horses with no history of trauma. Calcium and phosphorus serum concentrations have been normal when measured.

Of 17 cases reported in the veterinary literature,[2, 11, 22] 10 (59 percent) have been Standardbreds, 15 (89 percent) have been males, and the majority have occurred in horses one and a half to four years of age. In 16 horses (94 percent), the lesions occurred over the lateral stifle region and were bilateral in five horses (30 percent). Rarely are any symptoms (e.g., lameness and local pain) attributable to the lesions. The lesions are hard, well-circumscribed, subcutaneous, and 3 to 12 cm in diameter and may be single or multiple. The overlying skin is usually normal.

The differential diagnosis includes granulomatous diseases (infectious or sterile) and neoplasia. Definitive diagnosis is based on history, physical examination, and skin biopsy.[7, 37] Skin biopsy reveals a multinodular deposition of mineral separated by variable degrees of fibrosis and granulomatous inflammation. The surrounding tissues should be carefully examined for evidence of mastocytoma or eosinophilic granuloma with collagen degeneration. The author[28] and others[30] have found some atypical occurrences (i.e., lesions at unusual sites) of equine calcinosis circumscripta to be chronic, heavily mineralized cases of the aforementioned disorders. Equine calcinosis circumscripta (and heavily mineralized lesions of equine mastocytoma and equine eosinophilic granuloma with collagen degeneration) appears radiographically as localized deposits of radiopaque material in soft tissues.

As equine calcinosis circumscripta (1) is rarely symptomatic, (2) is rarely progressive, and (3) is only treatable by surgical excision, which is fraught with complications, therapy is not usually recommended. When therapy is required for symptomatic relief or for cosmetic reasons, surgical excision is the only effective treatment.[7, 19] However, postoperative wound dehiscence and septic arthritis can be problems.

EQUINE PASTERN DERMATITIS

So-called grease-heel (scratches, mud fever) is *not* a specific disease: It is a cutaneous reaction pattern of the horse.[12, 16, 17, 19, 29] It is essential that the clinician realize that grease heel is a multifactorial dermatitis having many potential causes (Table 15–3).

This dermatitis typically involves the caudal aspect of the pasterns (Fig. 15–16). The hind limbs are most commonly affected, and the condition is almost always bilaterally symmetric. Initially, there is erythema and edema, which progresses to exudation and crusting. Secondary bacterial infection is a frequent

TABLE 15–3. Differential Diagnosis of Equine Pastern Dermatitis

Staphylococcal folliculitis
Dermatophilosis
Dermatophytosis
Horsepox
Chorioptic mange
Trombiculidiasis
Primary irritant contact dermatitis
Contact hypersensitivity
Photosensitization
Vasculitis
Pemphigus foliaceus

complication. The dermatitis can spread cranially and proximally on the limbs. Pain and pruritus are variable. In chronic cases, thickening of the skin, fissures, exuberant granulation tissue, and severe edema of the limbs may be seen. Lameness may be a problem.

The differential diagnosis of equine grease-heel is lengthy (Table 15–3). Successful management requires *early* specific diagnosis (see appropriate sections of this book) before severe chronic changes intervene. In such cases, the most uninformative term, grease heel, is abandoned for the precise etiologic diagnosis. In chronic cases, the etiology may be indeterminable. If so, the undesirable term grease heel should be cast off and replaced with "chronic, idiopathic equine pastern dermatitis," which is more precise and clinicopathologically correct.

Therapy is most successful when administered specifically and early. General sympto-

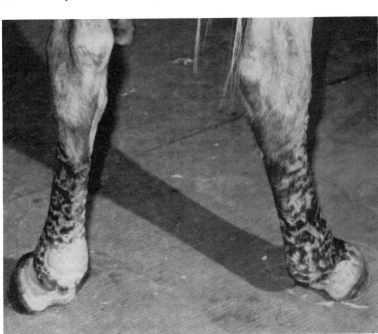

FIGURE 15–16. Equine pastern dermatitis. Alopecia and crusting of hind legs.

matic care includes (1) gentle clipping and cleansing, (2) topical application of astringent or antiseptic soaks (if moist) or emollient creams and ointments (if dry and thickened), (3) systemic antibiotics if needed, (4) systemic glucocorticoids or nonsteroidal anti-inflammatory agents, and (5) environmental hygiene. Chronic cases with exuberant granulation tissue may require surgical excision or cryosurgery.

EQUINE "BUMPS"

The veterinary literature is replete with unsatisfactory descriptions of horses with various papulonodular dermatoses that were variously termed heat bumps, feed bumps, grain bumps, fever bumps, protein bumps, and so on.[12, 15] Such terms attempt to relate an ill-defined dermatosis to some temporal occurrence. All such descriptions (1) fail to adequately characterize the skin disease clinically, (2) fail to characterize the skin disease pathologically, and (3) fail to establish any clear relationship between heat, protein, and anything else. In some cases, the dermatosis was probably equine eosinophilic granuloma with collagen degeneration or urticaria, and in others, it was probably unilateral papular dermatosis. We will never know!

I will, again, emphasize the differential diagnosis of equine nodular skin disease (Table 15–1). In most instances, a "bump is a bump," and a "lump is a lump," until it has been biopsied and examined histologically. The various "bumpish" terms referred to in this discussion are of no clinical or therapeutic benefit, are probably incorrect and misleading, and should be forever forgotten.

REFERENCES

1. Dodd, D. C.: Muscle degeneration and yellow fat disease in foals. N.Z. Vet. J. 8:45, 1960.
2. Dodd, D. C., and Raker, C. W.: Tumoral calcinosis (calcinosis circumscripta) in the horse. JAVMA 157:968, 1970.
3. Dyson, S., and Platt, H.: Panniculitis in an aged pony resembling Weber-Christian disease in man. Equine Vet. J. 17:145, 1985.
4. Finnochio, E. J.: Nodular necrobiosis. Mod. Vet. Pract. 62:76, 1981.
5. Foreman, J. H., et al.: Generalized steatitis associated with selenium deficiency and normal vitamin E status in a foal. JAVMA 189:83, 1986.
6. Gibbon, W. J.: Skin diseases. Mod. Vet. Pract. 43:76, 1962.
7. Goulden, B. E., and O'Callaghan, M. W.: Tumoral calcinosis in the horse. N.Z. Vet. J. 28:217, 1980.
8. Griffin, C. E.: Nodular collagenolytic granuloma (nodular necrobiosis). In: Robinson, N.E. (ed.): Current Therapy in Equine Medicine. Philadelphia, W. B. Saunders Co., 1983, p. 545.
9. Griffin, C. E.: Dermal nodules in horses. Mod. Vet. Pract. 66:704, 1985.
10. Hopes, R.: Skin diseases in horses. Vet. Dermatol. News. 1, August 1976.
11. Hutchins, D. R.: Tumoral calcinosis in the horse. Aust. Vet. J. 48:200, 1972.
12. Kral, F., and Schwartzman, R. M.: Veterinary and Comparative Dermatology. Philadelphia, J. B. Lippincott Co., 1964.
13. Kroneman, J., and Wensvoort, P.: Muscular dystrophy and yellow fat disease in Shetland pony foals. Neth. J. Vet. Sci. 1:42, 1968.
14. Leman, A. D., et al.: Diseases of Swine V. Ames, Iowa State University Press, 1981.
15. Lowe, J. E.: Heat bumps, sweet feed bumps, sweet itch. In Robinson, N. E. (ed.): Current Therapy in Equine Medicine. Philadelphia, W. B. Saunders Co., 1983, p. 110.
16. McMullen, W. C.: The skin. In Mansmann, R. A., et al. (eds.): Equine Medicine and Surgery III. Santa Barbara, CA, American Veterinary Publications, Inc., 1982, p. 789.
17. McMullen, W. C.: Scratches. In Robinson, N. E. (ed.): Current Therapy in Equine Medicine. Philadelphia, W. B. Saunders Co., 1983, p. 549.
18. Montes, L. F., and Vaughan, J. T.: Atlas of Skin Diseases of the Horse. Philadelphia, W. B. Saunders Co., 1983.
19. Mullowney, P. C.: Dermatologic diseases of horses part V. Allergic, immune-mediated, and miscellaneous skin diseases. Compend. Cont. Educ. 7:S217, 1985.
20. Murray, D. R., et al.: Granulomatous and neoplastic diseases of the skin of horses. Aust. Vet. J. 54:338, 1978.
21. Nicholls, T. J., et al.: Nodular necrobiosis in a horse. Aust. Vet. J. 60:148, 1983.
22. O'Connor, J. P., and Lucey, M. D.: Tumoral calcinosis (calcinosis circumscripta) in the horse. Irish Vet. J. 31:173, 1977.
23. Pascoe, R. R.: Equine Dermatoses. Sydney, University of Sydney Post-Graduate Foundation in Veterinary Science, Vet. Rev. No. 22, 1981.
24. Peyton, L. C., et al.: Fat necrosis in a foal. Equine Vet. J. 13:131, 1981.
25. Platt, H., and Whitewell, K. E.: Clinical and pathological observations on generalized steatitis in foals. J. Comp. Pathol. 81:499, 1971.
26. Scott, D. W.: Sterile nodular panniculitis in a horse. Equine Pract. 7:330, 1985.
27. Scott, D. W., et al.: Sterile eosinophilic folliculitis in cattle. Agri-Pract. 7:8, 1986.
28. Scott, D. W.: Nodular skin disease in the horse. In Robinson, N. E. (ed.): Current Therapy in Equine Medicine II. Philadelphia, W. B. Saunders Co., 1987, p. 634.
29. Stannard, A. A.: The skin. In Mansmann, R. A., et al. (eds.): Equine Medicine and Surgery II. Santa Barbara, CA, American Veterinary Publications, Inc., 1972, p. 381.
30. Stannard, A. A.: Equine dermatology. Proc. Am. Assoc. Equine Pract. 22:273, 1976.
31. Thomsett, L. R.: A nodular skin disease of horses. Vet. Dermatol. News. 3, March 1978.
32. Thomsett, L. R.: Skin diseases of the horse. In Pract. 1:15, 1979.
33. Thomsett, L. R.: Noninfectious skin diseases of horses. Vet. Clin. North Am. Large Anim. Pract. 6:57, 1984.
34. Walton, D. K., and Scott, D. W.: Unilateral papular dermatosis in the horse. Equine Pract. 4:15, 1982.
35. Wensvoort, P.: Age-linked features of generalized steatitis in equidae. Tijdschr. Diergeneeskd. 99:1067, 1974.
36. Wensvoort, P.: Morphogenesis of the altered adipose tissues in generalized steatitis in equidae. Tijdschr. Diergeneeskd. 99:1060, 1974.
37. Yager, J. A., and Scott, D. W.: The skin and appendages. In Jubb, K. V., et al.: Pathology of Domestic Animals III. Volume 1. New York, Academic Press, 1985, p. 407.

CHAPTER 16

DISORDERS OF KERATINIZATION

The epidermis normally undergoes an orderly pattern of differentiation and keratinization. The factors controlling these processes are incompletely understood (see Chapter 1, discussion on epidermopoiesis and keratogenesis). What is grossly recognized as altered keratinization may be due to a decreased epidermal turnover time, increased cohesiveness of the cells and layers of the stratum corneum, or possibly a combination of both.

SEBORRHEA

Seborrhea is an uncommon idiopathic dermatosis of the horse, characterized by increased scaling or greasiness, or both.

Cause and Pathogenesis

The term seborrhea is entrenched in veterinary literature as a broad classification for a variety of clinical syndromes ranging from simple dandruff to severe inflammation with scaling and crusting. Seborrhea literally means abnormal flow of sebum. However, the major clinical abnormality in seborrheic skin diseases is altered keratinization.

Most seborrheic skin diseases are secondary to such disorders as ectoparasitism, endoparasitism, dermatophytosis, dermatophilosis, staphylococcal folliculitis, abnormal lipid metabolism (malabsorption, liver disease), dietary deficiencies (fatty acids, protein, vitamin A, zinc, selenium), chronic catabolic states, and environmental factors (especially hot, dry conditions.)* Primary (idiopathic) seborrheic skin disease is uncommon in large animals.

In dogs and humans, the altered keratinization and lipid film that accompany seborrheic skin are associated with a marked increase in the number of surface bacteria per unit of skin.[1, 6, 19] In addition, the bacterial flora usually switches from the normally nonpathogenic resident micrococci to normally nonresident, pathogenic coagulase-positive staphylococci. Thus, seborrheic skin, regardless of the underlying cause, is often complicated by secondary bacterial infection.

Clinical Features

Whatever the underlying cause, seborrheic skin is characterized by altered keratinization, with or without altered glandular function. This is reflected grossly by varying degrees of scaling and crusting, with or without greasiness. Clinically, seborrhea is often separated into three morphologic types: (1) seborrhea sicca, characterized by dry skin with focal or diffuse flaking and accumulations of white to gray nonadherent scales; (2) seborrhea oleosa, characterized by focal or diffuse scaling associated with excessive lipid production, resulting in yellowish to brownish material that adheres to the skin and hair; and (3) seborrheic dermatitis, characterized by scaling and greasiness with gross evidence of local or diffuse inflammation. Pruritus or secondary bacterial infection, or both, are sometimes present with all three forms. This clinical categorization has little significance in terms of differential diagnosis.

In the horse, seborrhea is reported to be common[4, 10, 11] to rare.[5, 14, 18] Here, the confusion probably reflects failure to separate seborrhea into its primary and secondary forms. Whereas secondary seborrhea is common and has many causes (see later), primary (idiopathic) seborrhea is uncommon. The most common form of primary seborrhea in the horse is mane and tail seborrhea.[3, 4, 7, 19] No age, breed, or sex predilections have been noted. Moderate to severe scaling is seen in the mane or tail regions, or both (Fig. 16–1). Crusts may be present. Both dry and oily forms of the disease may be seen. There is little or no inflammation, pruritus, or alopecia.

Rarely, a generalized form of primary seborrhea is seen in horses.* The dermatosis is

---

*References 3, 5, 7, 14, 15, 18, 19

*References 2–5, 8, 9, 14, 15, 17, 18

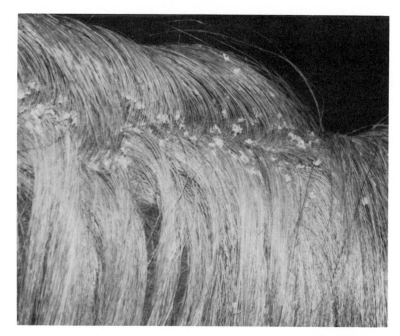

FIGURE 16–1. Equine mane seborrhea. Multiple flakes in mane.

usually symmetric (Figs. 16–2 and 16–3), tending to spare the extremities. Both dry and oily forms occur. With oily forms, a rancid odor is often present. Pruritus is rare.

Seborrhea has also been reported in cattle, sheep, and goats.[2, 4] However, because of the ancient and anecdotal nature of these reports, it is not known whether the animals described had primary or secondary seborrhea.

Diagnosis

The most important decision to be made is whether the seborrhea is primary (uncommon) or secondary (common). Primary (idiopathic) seborrhea is a diagnosis made by exclusion. Causes of secondary seborrhea include ectoparasitism (pediculosis, onchocerciasis); dermatophilosis; dermatophytosis; bacterial folliculitis; endoparasitism; abnormal lipid metabolism (malabsorption, liver disease); dietary deficiencies; chronic catabolic states; pemphigus foliaceus, in the horse and the goat; sarcoidosis, in the horse; environmental factors; and dermatosis responsive to vitamin E and selenium, in the goat.

Skin biopsy findings in primary seborrhea include superficial perivascular dermatitis with orthokeratotic and/or parakeratotic hyperkeratosis (Fig. 16–4).[4, 19] The parakeratotic hyperkeratosis is usually present multifocally (in "caps"), often overlying a squirting dermal papilla. The superficial dermal cellular infil-

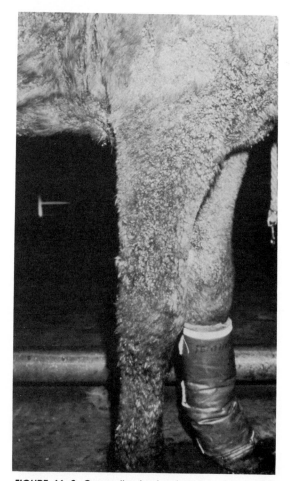

FIGURE 16–2. Generalized seborrhea in a horse associated with chronic cholangiohepatitis.

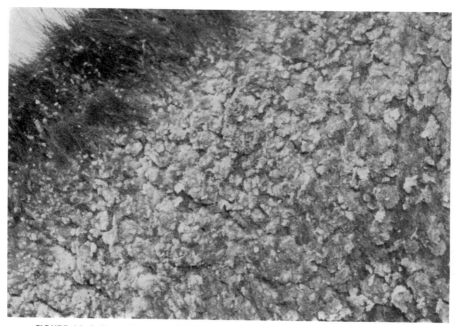

FIGURE 16–3. Same horse as in Figure 16–2. Severe scaling and crusting on neck.

FIGURE 16–4. Equine seborrheic dermatitis. Hyperplastic superficial perivascular dermatitis with papillary squirting (arrow) and focal parakeratotic hyperkeratosis.

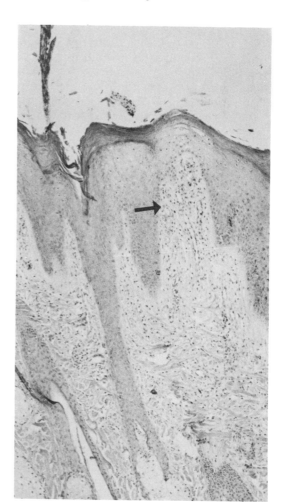

trate is composed of variable numbers of mononuclear cells and neutrophils.

Clinical Management

The successful management of seborrhea is dependent upon resolving the disorder into its primary and secondary forms. Secondary seborrhea is usually best managed by treating the underlying cause.

Primary seborrhea, being idiopathic, is usually incurable.[3, 7, 14, 15] It is important for the owner to understand that, similar to the case with dandruff in humans, control rather than cure is the goal of therapy. As equine seborrhea is essentially a cosmetic disease, many owners elect not to treat their horses.

Substantial benefit is usually seen with the regular use of antiseborrheic topical therapy.[3, 7, 14, 15] Therapeutic results are good when the effects of the antiseborrheic topicals are understood, and the correct topical applied to the morphologic variety of seborrhea at hand.[6] Sulfur (Sebbafon, Mycodex Tar and Sulfur, Lytar) is an excellent antiseborrheic agent and is often a good first-choice therapy. Dry seborrheas are frequently worsened by common medicated shampoos. When this occurs, emollient shampoos (Allergroom) and rinses (Humilac, Alpha-Keri Bath Oil) are indicated. Oily seborrheas often require a potent degreasing agent, such as benzoyl peroxide (Pyoben, OxyDex).

Whichever shampoo is chosen, it should be lathered well, allowed to stand for 10 to 15 minutes, and then rinsed thoroughly. Usually, shampooing is recommended twice weekly until control is achieved, followed by weekly or biweekly administration. Emollients (5 capfuls Humilac per liter of water; 1 capful Alpha-Keri per 4 liters of water) may be applied as rinses or sprays as needed.

EQUINE LINEAR KERATOSIS

Equine linear keratosis is an idiopathic, possibly inherited dermatosis of the horse, characterized by unilateral, linear, vertically oriented bands of hyperkeratosis over the neck and thorax.

Cause and Pathogenesis

The cause and pathogenesis of equine linear keratosis are unclear. Because of the early onset of lesions and the frequent occurrence of the disorder in related quarter horses, it has been suggested that the disorder may be hereditary.[3, 7, 16, 19] Clinicopathologically, equine linear keratosis closely resembles a linear epidermal nevus, a circumscribed developmental defect in the skin of humans.[1, 13]

Clinical Features

Equine linear keratosis has been reported most commonly in quarter horses, with most animals developing the condition between one and five years of age.[3, 5, 7, 13, 16] No sex predilection is apparent. The disorder appears to be uncommon.

Equine linear keratosis is characterized by the asymptomatic occurrence of one or more unilateral, linear, usually vertically oriented bands of alopecia and hyperkeratosis (Figs. 16–5 and 16–6), occurring most commonly over the neck and the lateral aspect of the thorax.[1, 13, 16] The lesions vary from 0.25 to 3.5 cm in width and from 5 to 70 cm in length. Often, the disorder is reported to begin as multiple hyperkeratotic papules, which coalesce into the vertical bands. Pruritus and pain are absent, and affected horses are otherwise healthy.

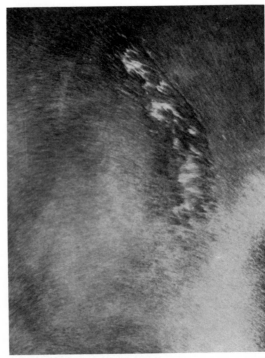

FIGURE 16–5. Equine linear keratosis. Linear, vertically oriented hyperkeratotic plaque on rump.

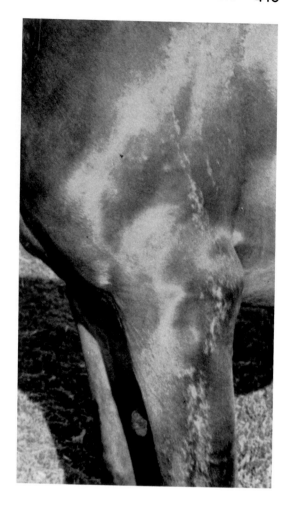

FIGURE 16–6. *Equine linear keratosis. Linear, vertically oriented hyperkeratotic papules and plaques on leg.*

Diagnosis

The diagnosis of equine linear keratosis rarely presents a problem. Scars resulting from linear trauma, such as scratches and whip marks, might be considered.[3, 7, 16]

Skin biopsy is characterized by regular to irregular to papillated epidermal hyperplasia with marked compact orthokeratotic hyperkeratosis (Fig. 16–7).[13, 16, 19] A mild superficial perivascular accumulation of mononuclear cells may or may not be present.

Clinical Management

Equine linear keratosis appears to have a chronic course, usually persisting for life.[3, 7, 13, 16] Topical antiseborrheic agents may be used, as needed, to minimize surface hyperkeratosis. However, because the disorder is asymptomatic, therapy may not be indicated.

Owners of affected horses should be advised of the potential problem of using them for breeding purposes.

EQUINE CANNON KERATOSIS

Equine cannon keratosis (stud crud) is an idiopathic dermatosis of horses, characterized by bilateral focal hyperkeratosis of the cranial surface of the rear cannon bone areas.

Cause and Pathogenesis

The cause and pathogenesis of equine cannon keratosis are unknown.

Clinical Features

Equine cannon keratosis has no reported age, breed, or sex predilections.[3, 7, 19] It appears to be uncommon. Moderately well-circumscribed plaques of scaling, crusting, and alo-

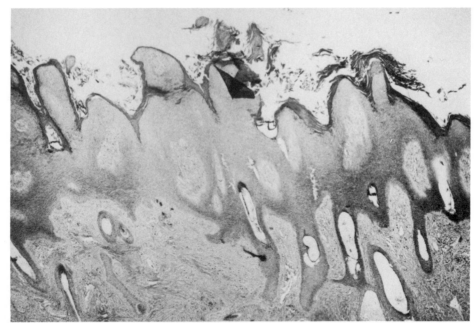

FIGURE 16–7. Equine linear keratosis. Papillated epidermal hyperplasia, papillomatosis, and hyperkeratosis.

pecia are seen bilaterally over the cranial surface of the rear cannon bone areas. Pruritus and pain are usually absent, and affected horses are otherwise healthy.

Diagnosis

Equine cannon keratosis is a readily recognizable dermatosis of the horse. The major differential diagnoses include dermatophilosis (see Chapter 6, discussion on dermatophilosis) and dermatophytosis (see Chapter 7, discussion on dermatophytosis).

Skin biopsy reveals irregular epidermal hyperplasia, marked orthokeratotic to parakeratotic hyperkeratosis, and a mild superficial perivascular accumulation of mononuclear cells and neutrophils.[19]

Clinical Management

Equine cannon keratosis usually persists for life.[3, 19] Topical antiseborrheic agents may be used, as needed, to minimize surface hyperkeratosis. In severe cases, topical glucocorticoid creams or ointments applied twice daily are beneficial.

PORCINE HYPERKERATOSIS

Porcine hyperkeratosis is a common, usually dorsally distributed dermatosis of intensively housed sows and boars.

Causes and Pathogenesis

The cause and pathogenesis of porcine hyperkeratosis are unknown.[12]

Clinical Features

Porcine hyperkeratosis is commonly seen in intensively housed sows and boars.[12] No age or breed predilections have been reported. In mild cases, brownish greasy scales accumulate over the dorsal neck and shoulders (Figs. 16–8 and 16–9). These accumulations can be rubbed off, revealing normal skin beneath. In severe cases, lesions extend over the entire dorsum and often down the flanks. Pruritus and pain are absent, and affected swine are otherwise healthy.

Diagnosis

The diagnosis of porcine hyperkeratosis is based on history, physical examination, and the ruling out of other disorders by laboratory tests (dermatophytosis, forage mites). Skin biopsy findings have not been reported.

Clinical Management

Because animals with this condition are usually asymptomatic, and its effects on production are insignificant, therapy is usually not undertaken. It has been reported that the feeding of 1 gallon of cod liver oil/50 sows/

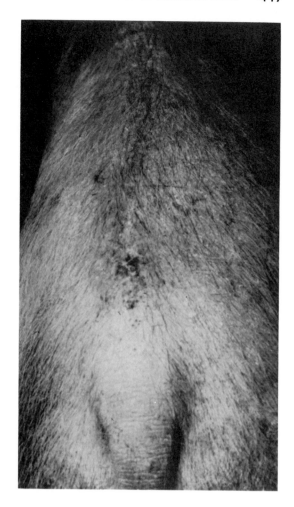

FIGURE 16–8. Porcine hyperkeratosis. Multiple waxy hyperkeratotic areas over the back.

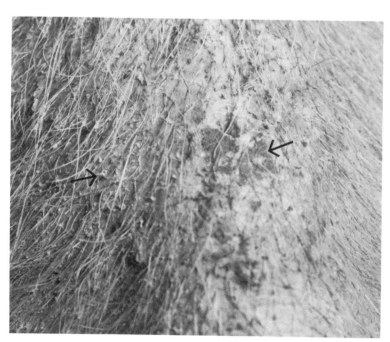

FIGURE 16–9. Porcine hyperkeratosis. Numerous small and large waxy hyperkeratotic areas (arrows) on the back.

week will markedly reduce the incidence of porcine hyperkeratosis.[12]

REFERENCES

1. Fitzpatrick, T. B., et al.: *Dermatology in General Medicine II.* New York, McGraw-Hill Book Co., 1979.
2. Hutyra, F., and Marek, J.: *Special Pathology and Therapeutics of the Diseases of Domestic Animals III.* Chicago, Alexander Eger Publisher, 1926.
3. Ihrke, P. J.: Diseases of abnormal keratinization (seborrhea). *In* Robinson, N. E. (ed.): *Current Therapy in Equine Medicine.* Philadelphia, W. B. Saunders Co., 1983, p. 546.
4. Kral, F., and Schwartzman, R. M.: *Veterinary and Comparative Dermatology.* Philadelphia, J. B. Lippincott Co., 1964.
5. McMullan, W. C.: The skin. *In:* Mansmann, R. A., et al. (eds.): *Equine Medicine and Surgery III.* Santa Barbara, CA, American Veterinary Publications, Inc., 1982, p. 789.
6. Muller, G. H., et al.: *Small Animal Dermatology III.* Philadelphia, W. B. Saunders Co., 1983.
7. Mullowney, P. C.: Dermatologic diseases of horses part V. Allergic, immune-mediated, and miscellaneous skin diseases. Comp. Cont. Educ. 7:S217, 1985.
8. Opperman, T.: Ueber das Eczema seborrhoicum siccum beim Pferde. Dtsch. Tierarztl. Wochenschr. 44:435, 1936.
9. Page, E. H.: Common skin diseases of the horse. Proc. Am. Assoc. Equine Pract. 18:385, 1972.
10. Panel Report: Skin conditions in horses. Mod. Vet. Pract. 56:363, 1975.
11. Panel Report: Dermatologic problems in horses. Mod. Vet. Pract. 62:75, 1981.
12. Penny, R. H. C., and Muirhead, M. R.: Skin. *In:* Leman, A. D., et al.: *Diseases of Swine V.* Ames, Iowa State University Press, 1981, p. 76.
13. Scott, D. W.: Equine linear keratosis. Equine Pract. 7:39, 1985.
14. Stannard, A. A.: The skin. *In:* Mansmann, R. A., et al. (eds.): *Equine Medicine and Surgery II.* Santa Barbara, CA, American Veterinary Publications, Inc., 1972, p. 381
15. Stannard, A. A.: Some important dermatoses in the horse. Mod. Vet. Pract. 53:31, 1972.
16. Stannard, A. A.: Equine dermatology. Proc. Am. Assoc. Equine Pract. 22:273, 1976.
17. Thomsett, L. R.: Skin diseases of the horse. In Pract. 1:15, 1979.
18. Thomsett, L. R.: Noninfectious skin diseases of horses. Vet. Clin. North Am. Large Anim. Pract. 6:59, 1984.
19. Yager, J. A., and Scott, D. W.: The skin and appendages. *In:* Jubb, K. V., et al.: *Pathology of Domestic Animals III. Volume I.* New York, Academic Press, 1985, p. 407.

CHAPTER 17

NEOPLASTIC DISEASES

CUTANEOUS ONCOLOGY

Veterinary oncology has come into its own as a specialty. Detailed information on the various aspects of the pathogenesis and immunology of neoplasia is available in other publications[323, 484] and will not be presented here. This chapter will serve as an overview of cutaneous neoplasia and selected non-neoplastic tumors in large animals.

In general, the risk of cutaneous neoplasia increases with age, except in horses.[397, 398, 484] Saddle horses (a composite of crossbreeds) are at increased risk for cutaneous neoplasia.[397, 398, 484] Specific sex predilections for cutaneous neoplasia are evident in female goats (udder papillomatosis; squamous cell carcinoma),[98, 94, 484, 486] female sheep (squamous cell carcinoma),[249, 498] male swine (scrotal hemangioma),[335, 346, 461] and male horses (mastocytoma).[5, 461] Breed predilections for cutaneous tumors are presented in Table 17–1.

Numerous surveys of skin tumors in large animals have been published.* In addition, surveys of skin tumors in cattle,† horses,‡ sheep,[31, 83, 94, 278, 296, 516] goats,[32, 94, 290, 535] and swine[32, 126] are numerous. The skin is the most common site of neoplasia in horses (mostly mesenchymal, mostly benign) and goats (mostly epithelial, mostly malignant), the second most common site in swine (mostly epithelial, mostly malignant), and the second or third most common site in cattle (mostly epithelial, mostly benign) and sheep (mostly epithelial, mostly malignant). The most common cutaneous neoplasms, by animal affected and in approximate descending order, are papilloma, squamous cell carcinoma, melanoma, and mast cell tumor (cattle); sarcoid, papilloma, squamous cell carcinoma, and mela-

noma (horses); melanoma, hemangioma, and squamous cell carcinoma (swine); squamous cell carcinoma and papilloma (sheep); and squamous cell carcinoma, papilloma, and melanoma (goats).

There are no completely satisfactory criteria for distinguishing benign neoplasms from certain proliferative inflammatory lesions and hyperplastic processes and for distinguishing benign from malignant neoplasms.[323, 484] In general, malignant neoplasms are usually characterized by sudden onset, rapid growth, infiltration, recurrence, and metastasis. The most important criterion for malignancy is metastasis.

The key to appropriate management and accurate prognosis of cutaneous neoplasms is *specific diagnosis*. This can be achieved only by biopsy and histologic evaluation. Exfoliative cytology (aspiration and impression smear) is easy and rapid and often gives valuable information on neoplastic cell type and differentiation. However, exfoliative cytology is inferior to, and no substitute for, biopsy and histopathology. Historical and clinical considerations often allow the experienced clinician to formulate an inclusive differential diagnosis on a cutaneous neoplasm, but variability renders such "odds playing" unreliable. In short, "a lump is a lump" until it is evaluated histologically.

A detailed histopathologic description of large animal cutaneous neoplasms is beyond the scope of this chapter. Only the histopathologic essence of individual neoplasms is presented here. For in-depth information and photomicrographic illustrations, the reader is referred to other publications on cutaneous neoplasia[323, 484, 518, 519, 534] and the individual references cited for each neoplasm.

Clinical management of cutaneous neoplasms may include surgery, cryosurgery, electrosurgery, hyperthermia, radiation therapy, chemotherapy, immunotherapy, and combinations of these. Detailed information on these various treatment modalities is available in a

---

*References 15, 50, 60, 85, 87, 98, 123, 178, 180, 214, 315, 318, 323, 326, 338, 348, 349, 393, 397, 429, 431–434, 442, 451, 484

†References 30, 108, 235, 327, 341, 445, 506

‡References 23, 33, 53, 84, 88, 95, 236, 337, 382, 422, 469

TABLE 17–1. Breed Predilections for Cutaneous Tumors

Breed	Tumor/Reference
Shorthorn cattle	Papillomatosis[397, 398, 484]
Saanen goats	Udder papillomatosis[324, 453, 486]
Hereford cattle	Squamous cell carcinoma[44, 134, 397, 484]
Angora goats	Squamous cell carcinoma[32, 93, 94, 214]; melanoma[32, 94, 214, 339, 488, 504]
Merino sheep	Squamous cell carcinoma[31, 83, 249, 278, 498]; follicular cysts[64, 81, 279]
Berkshire swine	Scrotal hemangioma[335, 346, 461]
Yorkshire swine	Scrotal hemangioma[335, 346, 461]
Angus cattle	Melanoma[9, 461, 484]
Suffolk sheep	Melanoma[180, 294]
Duroc-Jersey swine	Melanoma[187, 198]
Sinclair miniature swine	Melanoma[312]
Arabian horses	Melanoma[270, 312]
Percheron horses	Melanoma[270, 312]
Nubian goats	Wattle cysts[140, 453, 523]
Thoroughbred horses	Dermoid cysts[382]

number of excellent references.* Brief comments on treatment are included under clinical management sections for each tumor type.

EPITHELIAL NEOPLASMS

Papillomatosis

Papillomatosis (warts, verrucae) is common in cattle and horses, uncommon in goats and sheep, and apparently rare in swine.† In most instances, papillomatosis is known to be caused by DNA papovaviruses.

CAUSE AND PATHOGENESIS

In the last ten years, great advances have been made concerning the understanding and classification of papovaviruses in animals and humans.‡ Differentiation of papovavirus types by cleavage patterns produced by treating viral DNA with restriction endonucleases and the in vitro hybridization of viral DNA have emphasized the heterogeneity of papovaviruses within animal genera. In cattle, there are at least six types of papovaviruses that tend to have site specificity on the animal and, to a lesser extent, histologic specificity (see later).§ In addition, there is good clinicopathologic evidence that at least two different types of papillomatosis occur in horses (typical papillomatosis and aural plaques) and goats (papillomatosis of the head, neck, and forelegs and papillomatosis of the udder) (see later). Papovavirus antigens have been demonstrated in papillomas of horses and cattle by peroxidase-antiperoxidase technology.[232, 471]

In general, papovaviruses are host-specific.* Bovine papovaviruses (Types 1 and 2) can cause various mesenchymal neoplasms when injected into hamsters and calves,[72, 156, 363, 417, 461] and can cause fibroblastic skin tumors in horses (see discussion on equine sarcoid) but are not pathogenic for goats and sheep.[1, 152] Ovine papovavirus was pathogenic for hamsters but not for cattle and goats.[152]

Papillomatoses are infectious diseases and are transmitted by direct and indirect (fomite) contact. In general, infection requires damaged skin (e.g., environmental trauma, ectoparasites, and ultraviolet light damage). The incubation period varies from two to six months, probably depending on the papovavirus involved, the dose of virus, the route of exposure, and the immunity of the host.

Papovavirus antigens and antibodies have been studied using a number of techniques, including hemagglutination,[122, 389] agar gel immunodiffusion,[241, 267] indirect immunofluorescence,[389, 454] enzyme-linked immunosorbent assay,[114] peroxidase-antiperoxidase methods,[220, 232, 471] and DNA technology.[63, 255, 389, 457] In cattle, studies with bovine papovavirus Types 1 and 2 have demonstrated that precipitin and neutralizing antibodies develop, and titers correlate with immunity to virus challenge but *not* with growth or regression of existing papillomas.†

---

*References 102, 118, 119, 129, 133, 185, 186, 191, 226, 234, 244, 309, 383, 394, 395, 414, 484, 532, 533
†References 46, 110, 201, 206, 255, 290, 461, 484, 486
‡References 63, 206, 220, 255, 303, 389, 457, 458
§References 63, 206, 253–255, 303, 389, 457, 458

*References 61, 82, 165, 240, 255, 389, 461, 484
†References 27, 29, 241, 260, 266–268, 359–362, 419, 441

CLINICAL FEATURES

In cattle, papillomatosis is common and is caused by at least six different types of DNA papovaviruses.* Bovine papovavirus Type 1 (BPV 1) causes typical fibropapillomas on the teats and penises of animals less than two years of age.[46, 201, 206, 253, 254, 458] These lesions often spontaneously regress within 1 to 12 months. BPV 2 causes typical fibropapillomas on the head, neck (Figs. 17–1 and 17–2), dewlap, and occasionally the legs and teats of animals less than two years of age.† These lesions are usually multiple, gray, firm, hyperkeratotic, pedunculated or broad-based, and 1 mm to several centimeters in diameter and often spontaneously regress within 1 to 12 months. Immunity is not complete, however, and reinfection can occur.[20, 461] BPV 3 causes so-called atypical warts in cattle of all ages.[28, 206, 364, 389, 458] These lesions are low, flat, circular, and nonpedunculated, have delicate frondlike projections on their surfaces, and may occur anywhere on the body, including the teats. BPV 3–induced papillomas do *not* regress spontaneously. BPV 4 causes papillomas in the gastrointestinal tract.[63, 206, 389] BPV 5 causes so-called rice grain warts on the teats of cattle of all ages.[63, 206, 302, 303, 364] These lesions are small,

---

*References 9, 30, 46, 54, 135, 180, 201, 202, 206, 221, 233, 350, 358, 461, 484

†References 46, 201, 206, 253, 254, 274, 364, 390, 458

white, and elongated and do not regress spontaneously.

Interdigital papillomatosis has been described as a chronic problem in housed dairy cattle and has no age or breed predilections.[206, 409] Typical fibropapillomas occur on the dorsal and ventral aspects of the interdigital spaces, especially on the hind legs, and are often associated with pain, lameness, weight loss, decreased milk production, and decreased estrus detection. These lesions do not regress spontaneously. Viral etiology is suspected but not proved.

Ocular papillomas occur in range cattle and may be precursors of squamous cell carcinoma (see discussion on squamous cell carcinoma).[131, 206] Lesions may be long and frondlike or round and broad-based and tend to be attached to the eyelid or corneoscleral junction. Spontaneous regression may occur in 25 to 50 percent of these lesions. BPV has not been recovered from these lesions, but virions resembling papovavirus have been detected by electron microscopy.[131, 206]

Concern has been expressed over the potential infection of humans with BPV.[48, 390, 391] In one study, antibodies against BPV were found in humans with warts,[162] but another study failed to corroborate these findings.[391] At present, there is no direct evidence to suggest a causal relationship.

In horses, papillomatosis is common, is caused by a DNA papovavirus, occurs most

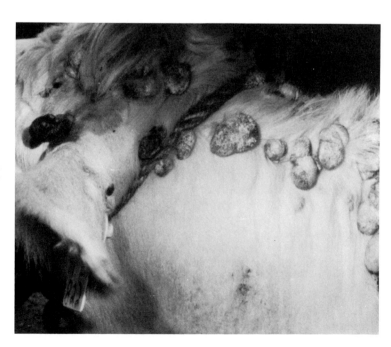

FIGURE 17–1. *Typical fibropapillomas (BPV 2) on the head and neck of a bovine.*

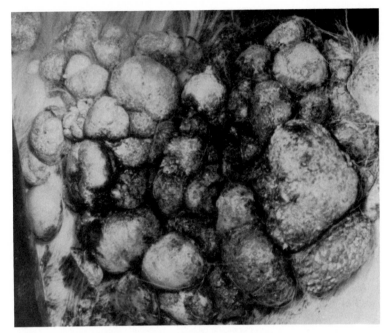

FIGURE 17–2. *Same animal as in Figure 17–1. Close-up of a cluster of fibropapillomas.*

frequently in animals younger than three years of age, and may be congenital.* There are no apparent sex or breed predilections. Lesions are usually multiple and verrucous and occur most commonly on the muzzle (Fig. 17–3), distal legs (Fig. 17–4), and genitalia. These lesions usually regress spontaneously within one to six months. Immunity is apparently complete. A clinically distinct variety of papillomatosis in horses is the so-called equine aural plaque (papillary acanthoma, hyperplastic dermatitis of the ear).[41, 80, 374, 460, 490] These lesions occur bilaterally on the lateral (inner) surface of the pinnae (Fig. 17–5), have no apparent age, breed, or sex predilections, and progress from small, smooth depigmented papules and plaques to larger, often coalescent hyperkeratotic plaques. Usually asymptomatic, the lesions may be more active in summer, in association with black fly bites. Similar plaques occasionally occur around the anus and vulva. These lesions do not regress spontaneously.

In sheep, papillomatosis is uncommon and has no apparent age, breed, or sex predilections.† The disease is caused by a DNA papovavirus.[152, 501, 502] Lesions are usually verrucous and multiple and occur most frequently on the hairy skin of the face and legs. Ovine papillomas have the potential of transforming into squamous cell carcinomas.[501, 502]

In goats, papillomatosis is uncommon and no age predilection is apparent.* Viral etiology is suspected but not proved. Caprine papillomatosis occurs in two clinical forms, and the lesions are usually verrucous. In one form, lesions occur commonly on the face, neck, shoulders, and forelegs and have no apparent sex or breed predilections.† These lesions usually regress spontaneously within 1 to 12 months. In the second form, lesions occur on the udder and teats, and white Saanens are predisposed.‡ In this second form, lesions do not usually regress spontaneously, and transformation into squamous cell carcinoma may occur.[125, 453, 486]

In swine, papillomatosis is rare, and no age, breed, or sex predilections are apparent.[110, 126, 243, 269, 378–380] Viral etiology is suspected but not proved. Lesions may be solitary or multiple and occur on the face (Fig. 17–6) and the genitalia.

HISTOPATHOLOGY

Histologically, papillomas are characterized by epithelial proliferation (squamous papilloma), with or without connective tissue proliferation (fibropapilloma). In cattle, papillomas caused by BPV 1 and BPV 2 show

---

*References 18, 33, 67, 82, 145, 180, 236, 255, 300, 347, 381, 383, 435, 461, 469, 484
†References 31, 94, 152, 180, 201, 216, 278, 281, 461

*References 32, 94, 97, 125, 201, 290, 324, 431, 451–453, 461, 486, 535
†References 94, 97, 278, 280, 332, 431, 453, 486
‡References 125, 290, 324, 332, 451–453, 486

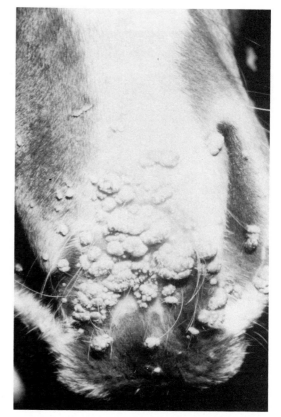

FIGURE 17–3. Typical squamous papillomas on the muzzle of a horse.

combined epithelial and fibrous proliferation (Fig. 17–7), whereas those caused by BPV 3, BPV 4, and BPV 5 show only epithelial proliferation.* In horses, typical papillomas and aural plaques show only epithelial proliferation (Figs. 17–8 and 17–9), with aural plaques ex-

*References 28, 54, 73, 141, 206, 409, 461, 477

hibiting concurrent epidermal hypomelanosis (Fig. 17–10).[142, 438, 460, 461] In goats, papillomas generally show only epithelial proliferation,[209, 324, 461, 486] whereas in sheep there is usually combined epithelial and fibrous proliferation.[152, 501]

Squamous papillomas are characterized by papillated epidermal hyperplasia and papillo-

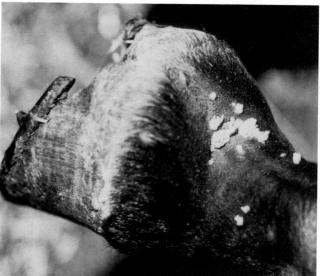

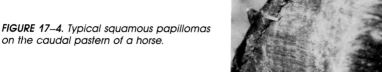

FIGURE 17–4. Typical squamous papillomas on the caudal pastern of a horse.

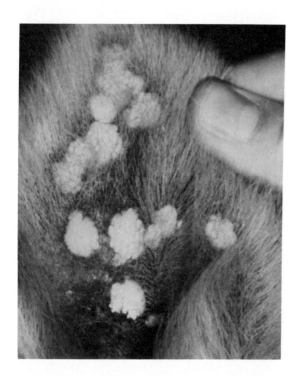

FIGURE 17–5. Aural plaques (squamous papillomas) on the pinna of a horse.

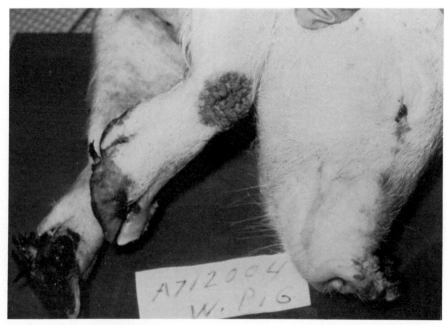

FIGURE 17–6. Multiple squamous papillomas on the snout and cranial carpus of a pig. (Courtesy J. M. King.)

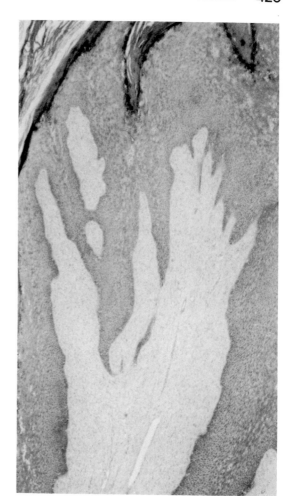

FIGURE 17–7. Bovine fibropapilloma (BPV2). Combined epithelial and connective tissue proliferation.

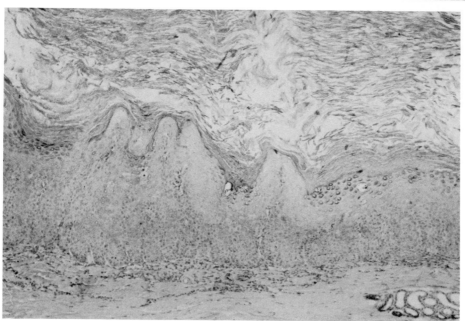

FIGURE 17–8. Equine aural plaque (squamous papilloma). Papillated epidermal hyperplasia and marked ortho-keratotic hyperkeratosis.

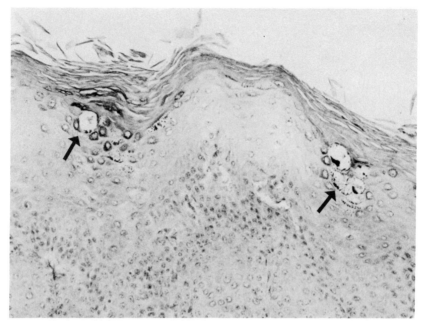

FIGURE 17–9. Equine aural plaque (squamous papilloma). Enlarged, vacuolated keratinocytes ("wart cells") in the stratum granulosum (arrows).

matosis. Ballooning degeneration, clumping of keratohyalin granules, and basophilic intranuclear inclusion bodies are variable findings (Figs. 17–11 and 17–12). Fibropapillomas are characterized by a fibroma-like proliferation of collagen with an overlying epidermis, as described earlier.

CLINICAL MANAGEMENT

The literature on the therapeutic management of papillomatosis is confusing and contradictory. Most of this confusion centers around two major points: (1) the failure to consider the self-limiting nature of many forms

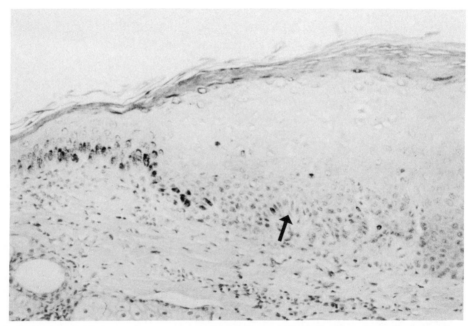

FIGURE 17–10. Equine aural plaque (squamous papilloma). Normal skin (left) with melanization of basilar epidermis and transition to papilloma with hypomelanosis (arrow).

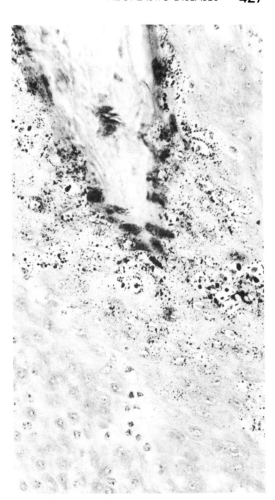

FIGURE 17–11. Caprine squamous papilloma. Vacuo-lated keratinocytes in stratum granulosum.

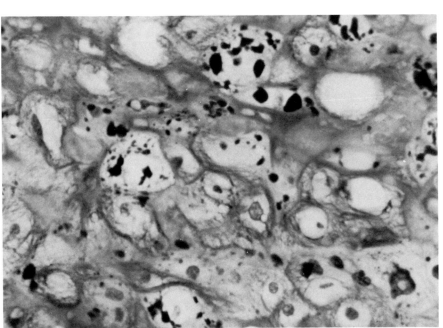

FIGURE 17–12. Caprine squamous papilloma. Ballooning degeneration of keratinocytes and clumping of kerato-hyalin granules.

of papillomatosis and (2) the recent discovery that there are many types of papovaviruses that produce papillomatosis in large animals.

In cattle, papillomatosis caused by BPV 1 and BPV 2 usually regresses spontaneously, as do typical papillomatosis in horses and sheep and papillomatosis of the head, neck, and forelegs in goats. Spontaneous regression usually occurs within 1 to 12 months, and animals that have persistent diseases should be suspected of having inappropriate immune responses.[109, 206, 484, 485] On the other hand, cattle with papillomatosis caused by BPV 3 or BPV 5, cattle with interdigital papillomatosis, horses with aural plaques, and goats with papillomatosis of the udder have persistent disease, with spontaneous regression occurring rarely.

For lesions that must be removed for aesthetic or health reasons, surgical excision or cryosurgery is effective.* It has been anecdotally stated that surgical excision of some larger lesions may encourage the others to regress.† There is no scientific support for such a statement. Controlled studies in horses[409] and cattle[357] designed to test this hypothesis showed that the duration of other lesions was *not* decreased and, in fact, may have been increased.

Many topical agents have been tried on individual lesions when surgery was impractical. The most commonly recommended agents include podophyllin (50 percent podophyllin; 20 percent podophyllin in 95 percent ethyl alcohol; 2 percent podophyllin in 25 percent salicylic acid) and dimethyl sulfoxide (undiluted medical grade DMSO).‡ These agents are usually applied once daily until remission occurs.

The subject of vaccination (autogenous or commercial) in the treatment and prevention of papillomatosis is very confusing, mostly because experimental and clinical trials were conducted prior to the recognition of the numerous types of papovaviruses involved in papillomatosis.[63, 206, 255, 303] As a result, vaccination has proponents and opponents.§

When one allows for the different types of papovaviruses, the following generalizations are possible: (1) autogenous vaccines and commercial bovine wart vaccines are ineffective for the treatment of caprine udder papillomatosis,[332, 452, 453, 486] (2) autogenous vaccines and commercial bovine wart vaccines are ineffective for the treatment or prevention of bovine papillomatosis caused by BPV 3 and BPV 5 and of bovine interdigital papillomatosis,[28, 303, 364, 409] and (3) autogenous vaccines and commercial bovine wart vaccines containing BPV 1 and BPV 2 are effective for the prevention but *not* the treatment of bovine papillomatosis caused by BPV 1 and BPV 2.[29, 266, 357, 359-361] At present, there is no scientific information on the benefits of vaccines in equine papillomatosis, ovine papillomatosis, and caprine papillomatosis of the head, neck, and forelegs.

Levamisole has been administered parenterally to goats with udder papillomatosis and to cattle with persistent papillomatosis caused by BPV 2.[332, 438, 452, 453] These attempts at immunostimulation have been unsuccessful.

There have been no reports of successful treatment of equine aural plaques.[333, 374, 460, 490]

General therapeutic adjuvants in all cases of papillomatosis, when feasible, include isolation of affected animals from noninfected animals, reduction of cutaneous injuries associated with the environment, and disinfection of the environment (e.g., formaldehyde and lye).*

Uncomplicated papillomatosis is usually of little concern, except in valuable animals in competitive shows or overseas sales.[46, 201, 206] Economic losses can occur through hide damage, secondary infection or myiasis, and carcass condemnation. In cattle, it has been stated that animals with papillomatosis affecting over 20 percent of their bodies have a poor prognosis.[46, 206, 221, 233, 350]

Basal Cell Tumor

Basal cell tumors are uncommon benign neoplasms of large animals arising from the basal cells of the epidermis, hair follicles, sebaceous glands, and sweat glands.† The cause of these neoplasms is unknown.

Basal cell tumors generally occur in adult to aged animals. Lesions are usually solitary, firm to cystic, rounded, elevated, well circumscribed, and dermoepidermal in position. They often become alopecic and ulcerated. In horses, the most common sites of occurrence are the neck, pectoral region, and trunk.[180, 382, 383, 438]

---

*References 9, 118, 226, 300, 309, 377, 383, 395, 409, 484, 485
†References 9, 46, 67, 206, 233, 329, 333, 374, 377, 383
‡References 9, 103, 104, 300, 329, 333, 383, 484, 503
§References 8, 9, 29, 104, 146, 201, 202, 206, 209, 273, 274, 329, 333, 357, 359–361, 374, 377, 387, 419, 461, 484, 485

---

*References 9, 46, 67, 206, 221, 233, 333, 377, 484, 485
†References 31, 49, 180, 334, 382, 383, 397, 461, 490, 518

Histologically, basal cell tumors are characterized by a proliferation of basaloid cells (Fig. 17–13). Frequent findings include uniform cell size, nuclear hyperchromasia, and mitotic figures. Several histologic patterns occur: solid, cystic, ribbon (garland), adenoid, and medusoid.

The therapy of choice is surgical excision or observation without treatment.

Squamous Cell Carcinoma

Squamous cell carcinomas are common malignant neoplasms of all large animals, except swine, and arise from squamous epithelial cells.* The etiology of squamous cell carcinoma is not clear in all cases but, in most instances, is related to the chronic exposure of poorly pigmented, poorly haired skin to ultraviolet light.† In some instances, squamous cell carcinomas may arise from papillomas or follicular cysts.[64, 125, 371, 484, 486] Squamous cell carcinoma has been reported to arise in burn wounds in a horse.[436a]

In horses, squamous cell carcinomas occur in animals with a mean age of 12 years, with no apparent breed or sex predilections.‡ The

*References 30–33, 87, 94, 178, 180, 214, 397, 451, 461, 484

†References 30–33, 83, 174, 181, 182, 249, 250, 278, 461, 484, 521

‡References 23, 33, 49, 84, 88, 95, 180, 214, 300, 383, 397, 461, 466, 469, 484

tumors occur most commonly on the head, mucocutaneous junctions (Fig. 17–14), and male and female genitalia (Fig. 17–15). Lesions are usually solitary, beginning as nonhealing, enlarging, granulating erosions or ulcers or as proliferative, often cauliflower-like masses. Necrosis and a foul odor are common. Generally, squamous cell carcinomas are locally invasive and slow to metastasize. Squamous cell carcinomas on the equine prepuce and penis are more aggressive, with frequent early metastases. The irritant and carcinogenic properties of equine smegma have been implicated in the etiology of squamous cell carcinoma of the penis and prepuce.[383, 392, 484] Papovavirus structural antigens were *not* detected in equine squamous cell carcinomas.[232, 471]

In goats, squamous cell carcinomas occur in adult to aged animals, with females and Angoras being predisposed.* The tumors are usually solitary and occur most commonly on the perineum, vulva, and udder of females and on the ears of both sexes. The lesions may be ulcerative or proliferative, and metastasis is not uncommon. Caprine squamous cell carcinomas are known to arise from papillomas of the udder, especially in Saanens.† The differential diagnosis of caprine vulvar squamous cell carcinoma includes ectopic mammary

*References 4, 32, 87, 93, 94, 111, 214, 405, 429, 432, 442, 451, 499, 535

†References 125, 290, 324, 452, 453, 484, 486

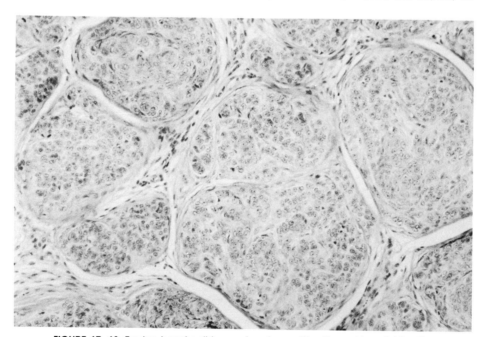

FIGURE 17–13. Equine basal cell tumor. Annular proliferations of basaloid cells.

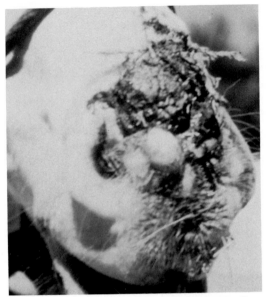

FIGURE 17–14. *Equine squamous cell carcinoma. Ulcerative, necrotizing tumor on muzzle of white horse.*

gland tissue,[140, 247, 452, 453] which presents as non-ulcerative bilateral enlargement of the vulvar lips. The ectopic tissue enlarges at parturition and spontaneously regresses over a two- to three-month period. Aspiration of the mass reveals milk, and biopsy reveals mammary gland tissue.

In sheep, squamous cell carcinomas occur in adult to aged animals with females and Merinos being predisposed.* The lesions may be solitary or multiple and commonly occur on the pinnae, eyelids, muzzle, lips, and perineal region. The lesions may be ulcerative or proliferative, and metastasis may occur. Ovine squamous cell carcinomas are thought to occasionally arise from viral papillomas,[501, 502] and vulvar squamous cell carcinomas occur most frequently in ewes that have had a radical Mule's operation to reduce susceptibility to fly-strike.[473, 498] Immunologic studies in naturally occurring ovine squamous cell carcinoma have revealed the following: (1) increasing tumor mass results in decreasing blastogenic responses of peripheral blood lymphocytes, which is associated with the presence of a serum suppressor factor,[6, 7, 229, 231] (2) surgical removal of the tumor results in normalization of blastogenic responses,[228, 230] and (3) immunotherapy results in tumor enhancement and increased metastasis.[227, 228]

*References 31, 83, 94, 214, 249, 250, 278, 281, 294, 318, 348, 349, 431, 473, 498, 516

In swine, squamous cell carcinomas are rarely reported.[32, 365, 436] Lesions occur in adult to aged animals and may be solitary or multiple, and metastasis may occur.

In cattle, squamous cell carcinomas occur in adult to aged animals, with no sex predilection.* Breed predilections include poorly pigmented animals, especially Herefords and Ayrshires. The lesions occur most commonly at mucocutaneous junctions, especially periocularly and on the vulva. So-called horn core cancer is a squamous cell carcinoma that arises from the frontal sinus mucosa and invades the horn core, causing the horn to become loose and eventually to drop off. The disease occurs in cattle, goats, and sheep.† Lesions may be ulcerative or proliferative. Metastasis is not uncommon but is rare in the horn core cancer form.[246, 340, 428] Papovavirus structural antigens were not detected in bovine squamous cell carcinomas in one study,[471] but papovavirus-like particles were seen with electron microscopy in cattle with periocular squamous cell carcinoma.[131]

*References 30, 158, 180–182, 211, 327, 330, 338, 341, 376, 393, 397, 461, 484, 521
†References 46, 59, 155, 184, 246, 251, 340, 372, 461, 484

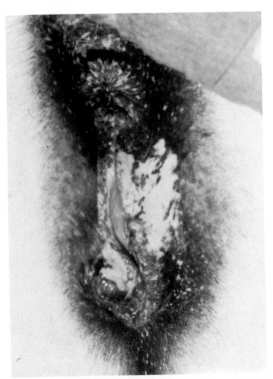

FIGURE 17–15. *Equine squamous cell carcinoma. Ulcerative tumor associated with leukoderma involving vulva.*

Bovine periocular squamous cell carcinoma (so-called cancer eye) is a common and economically important condition throughout North America.* It occurs most frequently in lower latitudes and under range conditions, and predilecting factors include ultraviolet light exposure, periocular lack of pigment, and possibly viral infection (papovavirus, herpesvirus) and heredity.† It typically arises from plaque (leukoplakia, solar keratosis) and papilloma precursors. Tumor-bearing cattle are immunocompromised[172, 181, 275] and can react to tumor-specific antigens.[219, 275, 456]

Histologically, squamous cell carcinomas are characterized by irregular masses or cords of epidermal cells that proliferate downward and invade the dermis (Fig. 17–16). Frequent findings include keratin formation, horn pearls, intercellular bridges, mitoses, and atypia. Lesions arising from precursors such as solar keratosis (see later) or papillomatosis (see earlier) may show features of these conditions as well.

The therapy of choice is wide surgical excision. Other treatment modalities that have been successful in squamous cell carcinoma include cryosurgery,[117–119, 185, 226, 383] radiofrequency hyperthermia,[163, 234, 528] and radiation therapy (including implants of gold-198, cobalt-60, cesium-157, iridium-192, and radon; and strontium-90 probes).*

Bovine horn core cancer usually recurs following surgery but may respond to immunotherapy (autogenous vaccine, *Corynebacterium parvum*).[46, 372, 428, 484, 505]

Bovine periocular squamous cell carcinoma may occasionally spontaneously regress[99, 134, 181] and has been found to respond to immunotherapy (autogenous vaccine and mycobacterial vaccine), radiofrequency hyperthermia, or cryosurgery.†

Immunotherapy with autogenous vaccine in ovine squamous cell carcinoma has been unsuccessful.[472]

Sebaceous Gland Tumors

Sebaceous gland tumors are rare epithelial growths in large animals, arising from sebaceous gland cells.‡ The cause of these tumors is unknown.

Sebaceous gland tumors usually occur in adult to aged animals. They are usually solitary and may occur anywhere on the body. The lesions vary from nodular and alopecic to lobulated (cauliflower-like), alopecic, shiny, and pinkish-yellow in color. The majority of seba-

---

*References 50, 108, 171, 181, 319, 459, 484

†References 11–14, 16, 44, 79, 116, 131, 134, 166, 181, 188, 190, 242, 421, 424, 425, 440, 459, 474, 481, 507, 530

---

*References 25, 101, 102, 133, 149, 272, 309, 447, 484, 532, 533

†References 119, 163, 189, 226, 234, 239, 408, 414, 456, 484, 500, 528

‡References 30, 33, 49, 299, 397, 438, 461, 490

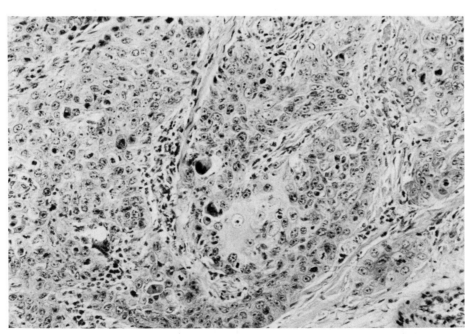

FIGURE 17–16. *Equine squamous cell carcinoma. Malignant proliferation of squamoid cells.*

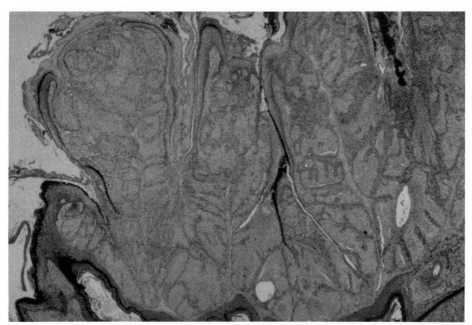

FIGURE 17–17. *Caprine nodular sebaceous hyperplasia. Exophytic, papillomatous, lobular proliferation of normal sebaceous gland cells.*

ceous gland tumors reported in large animals have been benign.

Histologically, sebaceous gland tumors are classified as *nodular sebaceous hyperplasia* (greatly enlarged sebaceous glands composed of numerous lobules grouped around centrally located sebaceous ducts) (Fig. 17–17); *sebaceous adenoma* (lobules of sebaceous cells of irregular shape and size, well demarcated from the surrounding tissue and containing mostly mature sebaceous cells and fewer undifferentiated germinative cells); *sebaceous epithelioma* (similar to basal cell tumor but containing mostly undifferentiated germinative cells and fewer mature sebaceous cells); and *sebaceous adenocarcinoma* (pleomorphism, atypia).

Clinical management of sebaceous gland tumors may include surgical excision, cryotherapy, and observation without treatment.

Sweat Gland Tumors

Apocrine sweat gland tumors are rare epithelial growths in large animals, arising from apocrine sweat gland cells.* The cause of these tumors is unknown.

Apocrine sweat gland tumors usually occur in adult to aged animals. Lesions are usually solitary, firm to cystic dermal nodules, which may be alopecic and ulcerated. In horses, apocrine adenomas occur most frequently on the pinnae and the vulva.[382, 383] Most apocrine sweat gland tumors reported in large animals have been benign.

Histologically, apocrine sweat gland tumors are characterized by benign or malignant proliferations of apocrine sweat gland epithelium, which may feature predominantly secretory or ductal epithelium, and may be solid or cystic in appearance.

The therapy of choice for apocrine sweat gland tumors is surgical excision.

MESENCHYMAL NEOPLASMS

Fibroma and Fibrosarcoma

Fibromas and fibrosarcomas are uncommon neoplasms in large animals and arise from dermal or subcutaneous fibroblasts.* The cause of these neoplasms is unknown. Fibrosarcoma has been reported to arise in burn wounds in a horse.[436a]

Fibromas and fibrosarcomas usually occur in adult to aged animals. Fibromas are usually solitary (Fig. 17–18) and may be firm (fibroma durum) or soft (fibroma molle), well-circum-

---

*References 110, 147, 334, 380, 382, 383, 461

*References 31–33, 49, 50, 60, 87, 94, 95, 180, 196, 235, 300, 301, 337, 338, 374, 381, 382, 393, 397, 402, 422, 461

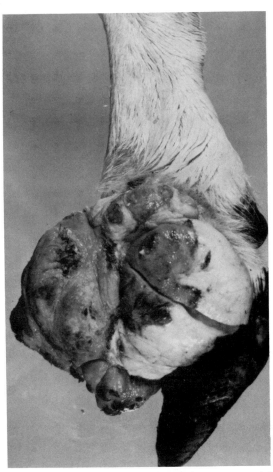

FIGURE 17–18. Bovine fibroma. Large tumor on cranial aspect of pastern. (Courtesy J. M. King.)

scribed dermal or subcutaneous nodules. Fibrosarcomas are usually solitary, poorly-demarcated, firm or fleshy, infiltrative subcutaneous masses that are frequently ulcerated and secondarily infected. In horses, fibromas and fibrosarcomas occur most commonly on the head (especially periocularly), neck, flanks, and legs.* Fibromatosis was reported in the pectoral region of an aged horse.[210] In swine, fibrous polyps occur most commonly in sows, on the pinnae, neck, and back.[62] Multiple subcutaneous fibrosarcomas with internal metastasis were reported in a two-month-old calf.[107] Fibromas are benign, but fibrosarcomas are locally invasive, with metastasis occurring in about 25 percent of reported cases.

Histologically, fibromas are characterized by whorls and interlacing bundles of fibroblasts

and collagen fibers. Tumor cells are usually fusiform, and mitotic figures are rare. Fibrosarcomas are characterized by interwoven bundles of immature, atypical fibroblasts and variable numbers of collagen fibers. Tumor cells are fusiform to stellate, and mitotic figures are common. Fibromatosis is characterized by a deep location, a relationship to muscular aponeuroses, diffuse growth of thick collagen bundles, and engulfment of muscle fibers.[210]

The therapy of choice for fibromas and fibrosarcomas is surgical excision. Radiation therapy is curative in only about 50 percent of the fibrosarcomas.* Chemotherapy is unlikely to be of benefit.[415, 447, 484] Cryosurgery may be useful.[395]

Exuberant Granulation Tissue

The horse is notorious for the formation of exuberant granulation tissue (proud flesh) in wounds, especially those on the distal extremities.† The cause of the condition is unknown. Exuberant granulation tissue differs from hypertrophic scar and keloid in that it lacks an epithelial covering and forms earlier in the healing process. Although there have been anecdotal reports of keloids in horses in the literature, none of these were corroborated by clinicopathologic data.

Equine exuberant granulation tissue is characterized clinically by a proliferation of hemorrhagic granulation tissue that fails to heal and epithelialize. The differential diagnosis includes equine sarcoid, squamous cell carcinoma, habronemiasis, and infectious granuloma (e.g., botryomycosis and pythiosis). Diagnosis is based on biopsy findings.

The management of equine exuberant granulation tissue is covered in other texts.[67, 138, 215, 300, 383, 387a]

Equine Sarcoid

Equine sarcoid is a unique, locally aggressive, fibroblastic skin tumor of horses.‡ It is the most common skin tumor of horses. There are no apparent breed, sex, or coat color predilections. Animals of any age may be affected, but over 70 percent of the cases occur in horses younger than four years of age.

---

*References 300, 337, 342, 381, 382, 412, 415

*References 101, 102, 153, 186, 447, 484, 532
†References 40, 67, 76, 138, 167, 215, 300, 383, 387a, 446
‡References 33, 84, 137, 175, 212, 214, 300, 381, 382, 402, 461, 467–469, 479, 510

CAUSE AND PATHOGENESIS

The etiology of equine sarcoids is not firmly established but is thought to be viral.[151, 159, 461, 468, 493] Lesions frequently occur in areas subjected to trauma, and there may be a history of a previous wound three to six months earlier.[214, 300, 354, 381, 402, 461] The lesions may be spread to other areas on the same horse or possibly to other horses through biting, rubbing, and fomites.[300, 383, 461] Epizootics of equine sarcoid have been described.[401, 461] Equine sarcoids have been autotransplanted[61, 321, 354, 403, 461, 508] but inconsistently with cell-free material.

Bovine papovavirus (probably types 1 and 2) was inoculated into horse skin and produced fibroblastic proliferations.[355, 400, 404, 441] Cultured fetal equine fibroblasts became transformed when exposed to BPV 2,[529] and common membrane neoantigens were found on BPV-induced tumor cells from cattle and horses.[26] However, (1) BPV-induced lesions in horses are distinguished by a short incubation period and rapid spontaneous regression uncharacteristic of equine sarcoid[400]; (2) the fibroblastic growths produced in horse skin with BPV differ histologically from equine sarcoids by lacking an epidermal component and active fibroblast proliferation interlaced at the dermoepidermal junction[400, 461, 479, 510]; (3) horses with naturally occurring sarcoids do not have serum-neutralizing antibodies against BPV,[399] whereas horses with BPV-induced lesions do[441]; and (4) attempts to produce papillomas in calves with equine sarcoid extracts are unsuccessful.[403] Papovavirus antigens were not detected in naturally occurring equine sarcoids by peroxidase-antiperoxidase technology.[471] Recent DNA hybridization studies have shown that equine sarcoids contain papovavirus sequences not directly derived from BPV 1 and BPV 2 but from a different, albeit closely related, papovavirus.[10, 159, 252, 256–258, 493]

Intracytoplasmic virus-like particles resembling retroviruses were observed in electron microscopic studies of equine sarcoid cell lines and tumors.[115, 461] Tumor-specific antigens were demonstrated in an equine sarcoid cell line,[514, 515] and cell-mediated immune responses against sarcoid antigens were demonstrated to occur in affected horses.[55] Recently, it has been shown that a retrovirus is released from cultured cells explanted from a naturally occurring equine sarcoid,[70] but this retrovirus does *not* exhibit in vitro transforming activity or replication when tested on equine fibro-

blasts.[71, 120, 121] It was concluded that this retrovirus was probably an endogenous virus, repressed in normal equine cells and expressed spontaneously by tumor cells.

Clinical studies have suggested that equine sarcoids may have familial tendencies.[217, 401, 461] Recently, the distributions of equine leukocyte antigens (ELA) in horses with equine sarcoid and in normal horses were determined and compared.[107a, 264] ELA haptotypes W5, W3, W13, and B1 occurred more frequently in horses with equine sarcoid, suggesting a predisposition to equine sarcoid associated with or linked to the major histocompatibility complex.

In summary, current information on the pathogenesis of equine sarcoid would suggest a papovavirus etiology (*not* BPV 1 and BPV 2, but another papovavirus of bovine, equine, or other origin) and a possible genetic predilection associated with the major histocompatibility complex.

CLINICAL FEATURES

Equine sarcoids may occur anywhere on the body, especially on the head (periocular, pinnae, and commissures of lips), legs, and ventral trunk.* About 30 to 50 percent of affected horses have multiple sarcoids. Equine sarcoids occur in four basic gross types: (1) verrucous (warty) (Fig. 17–19), (2) fibroblastic (proud flesh–like) (Figs. 17–20 and 17–21), (3) mixed verrucous and fibroblastic, and (4) occult (flat) (Fig. 17–22). The major differential diagnosis for verrucous sarcoids is papilloma and squamous cell carcinoma, and any "papilloma" in an atypical site in an adult horse must be considered to be a sarcoid until proved otherwise. The major differential diagnosis for fibroblastic sarcoids includes squamous cell carcinoma, exuberant granulation tissue, habronemiasis, and infectious granulomas (pythiosis, zygomycosis, botryomycosis, and mycetoma). Occult sarcoids present as one or a few annular areas of alopecia with variable scaling and crusting. Such lesions may remain static for long periods of time, before developing firm papules or nodules within the alopecic areas. The differential diagnosis includes dermatophytosis, dermatophilosis, demodicosis, staphylococcal folliculitis, onchocerciasis, and alopecia areata.

---

*References 33, 84, 88, 262, 381–383, 402, 461, 469

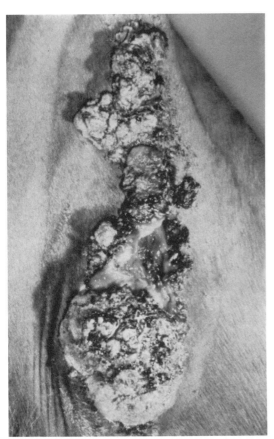

FIGURE 17-19. *Verrucous sarcoid on the neck of a horse.*

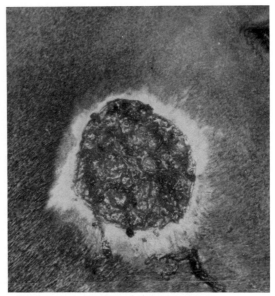

FIGURE 17-20. *Fibroblastic sarcoid on the face of a horse.*

found, but equine sarcoid cells exhibited an increased level of collagen synthesis.

CLINICAL MANAGEMENT

Equine sarcoids do not metastasize. Some lesions come and go, and many may undergo

HISTOPATHOLOGY

Equine sarcoids are characterized by fibroblastic proliferation with associated epidermal hyperplasia and dermoepidermal activity.[401, 461, 479, 510] The dermis shows variable amounts of collagen fibers and fibroblasts in a whorled, tangled, or occasionally herringbone pattern. Tumor cells are spindle-shaped or fusiform to stellate, often with hyperchromasia, atypia, and mitoses. Fibroblasts at the dermoepidermal junction frequently orient perpendicularly to the basement membrane zone in a picket-fence pattern. The overlying epidermis (if present) is hyperplastic and hyperkeratotic. Occult sarcoids are often overlooked histologically, as they are characterized by focal epidermal hyperplasia and hyperkeratosis with underlying junctional fibroblast proliferation (Fig. 17-23).

Recently, the connective tissue composition and organization of equine sarcoids were compared with those of normal adult equine skin.[524] No major qualitative differences were

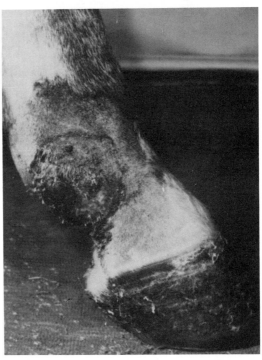

FIGURE 17-21. *Fibroblastic sarcoid on the fetlock of a horse.*

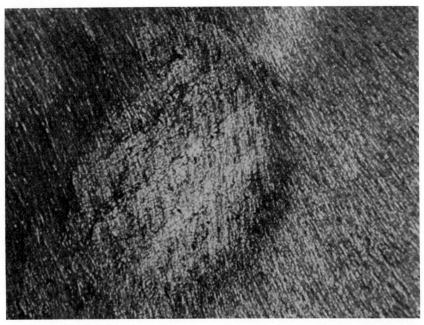

FIGURE 17–22. Occult or flat sarcoid on the neck of a horse. Annular area of alopecia and scaling. (Courtesy R. R. Pascoe.)

spontaneous remission, but this may take several years.[151, 214, 402, 461, 468] Static occult and verrucous sarcoids are perhaps best left alone, as the trauma of biopsy or surgical excision may cause a sudden increased growth and aggressive behavior.[151, 333, 402, 468]

In most instances, the therapy of choice for equine sarcoids is cryosurgery, with one-year cure rates varying from 80 to 90 percent.* Spontaneous regression of multiple nontreated sarcoids has been reported following cryosurgical treatment of one of the lesions.[300]

Immunotherapy with mycobacterial products (commercial bacillus Calmette-Guérin [BCG]; mycobacterial cell wall preparation in oil; mycobacterial cell wall skeleton–trehalose dimycolate combination) has been very effective for equine sarcoids, especially periocular lesions.[129, 263, 336, 410a, 437, 526, 531] These products are administered intralesionally, every two to three weeks, for an average of four treatments. Inflammatory reactions are common, especially three to ten days after injection and may lead to necrosis, ulceration, and discharge. Owners must be informed that the lesions usually look worse before healing occurs. Occasional horses show transient malaise or anorexia after injection. Fatal anaphylaxis has occurred following repeated injections of the

commercial BCG product, and medication with flunixin meglumine and prednisolone 30 minutes prior to treatment with this BCG product is recommended.[129, 526] Immunotherapy with autogenous vaccines, commercial bovine wart vaccine, and poxvirus vaccines has been unsuccessful.[300, 373, 374, 383, 416, 522]

Surgical excision of equine sarcoids is followed by recurrence in at least 50 percent of cases.[56, 151, 354, 383, 461, 468] Radiation therapy is also effective in only about 50 percent of cases.[153, 186, 447, 484, 532, 533] Radiofrequency hyperthermia has been effective in some cases of equine sarcoid.[191] Local treatment with 50 percent podophyllin in alcohol has been effective in some cases.[300, 304, 383] The podophyllin is applied topically, once daily, with care taken to remove the exudate each time and to protect surrounding normal skin with Vaseline. Remission usually occurs within about 30 days.

Myxoma and Myxosarcoma

Myxomas and myxosarcomas are rare neoplasms of large animals and arise from dermal or subcutaneous fibroblasts.[30, 33, 316, 395, 406, 461] The cause of these neoplasms is unknown.

Myxomas and myxosarcomas occur predominantly in adult or aged animals. The lesions are usually solitary infiltrative growths that are soft, slimy, poorly circumscribed, and without

---

*References 56, 117, 118, 137, 225, 226, 244, 259, 309, 383, 395, 410a

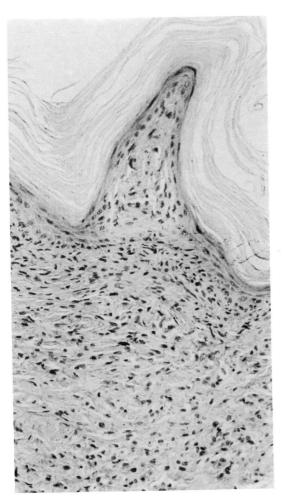

FIGURE 17–23. Flat equine sarcoid. Proliferation of fibroblasts at the dermoepidermal junction ("picket fence") and overlying orthokeratotic hyperkeratosis.

definite shape. They can occur anywhere on the body.

Histologically, these tumors are characterized by stellate to fusiform tumor cells distributed in a vacuolated, basophilic, mucinous stroma that may be partitioned by collagenous connective tissue septae.

Myxomas are benign. Myxosarcomas are malignant but apparently rarely metastasize. The therapy of choice is radical surgical excision. Both neoplasms frequently recur following surgery, because of their infiltrative growth patterns. Cryosurgery has been effective in some cases.[395]

Schwannoma

Schwannomas (neurofibromas, neurilemmomas, neurinomas, perineural fibroblastomas, and nerve sheath tumors) are uncommon in horses and cattle and rare in other large animals.[*] Malignant schwannomas (neurofibrosarcomas) are very rare in all species. These tumors arise from dermal or subcutaneous Schwann's cells (nerve sheath). The cause of schwannomas is unknown. Virus-like particles have been seen in tumor cells from cattle.[106]

Schwannomas are seen in horses three to six years of age, with no apparent breed or sex predilections.[†] Lesions begin as single or multiple, firm, 2 to 3 mm in diameter subcutaneous papules, especially on the upper or lower eyelids. Lesions may enlarge to 10 mm in diameter and may or may not become alopecic and ulcerated.

In cattle, schwannomas are usually seen in mature animals but may be seen in calves.[‡] Multiple schwannomas (neurofibromatosis) may have a genetic basis and have been likened to von Recklinghausen's disease in humans.[448, 450] Attempts to transmit the disorder to normal calves with cell suspensions and cell-free extracts were unsuccessful.[448, 450] Lesions are usually multiple, firm, round to flat, subcutaneous, and up to 8 cm in diameter and occur most commonly on the head and trunk. Most affected cattle have extracutaneous lesions as well, especially in the heart, brachial plexus, and intercostal nerves.

Histologically, schwannomas are characterized by areas of spindle-shaped cells exhibiting nuclear palisading and faintly eosinophilic, thin, wavy fibers (Antoni Type A tissue) alternating with areas of edematous stroma containing relatively few haphazardly arranged cells (Antoni Type B tissue) (Fig. 17–24).[151, 317, 323]

The therapy of choice is surgical excision. In horses, periocular schwannomas recur in about 50 percent of animals treated with surgical excision, usually within six months.[382, 383] Two or more operations may be necessary to effect a cure.

Lipoma and Liposarcoma

In large animals, lipomas are uncommon and liposarcomas are rare. Both neoplasms arise from subcutaneous lipocytes (adipocytes).[§] Their cause is unknown.

Usually, lipomas and liposarcomas occur in

*References 31, 49, 177, 224, 294, 317, 318, 323, 382, 383, 402, 448, 484, 490

†References 151, 224, 382, 383, 402, 469, 532

‡References 46, 177, 214, 317, 318, 323, 448, 450

§References 31, 32, 43, 49, 52, 180, 334, 382, 397, 461, 469

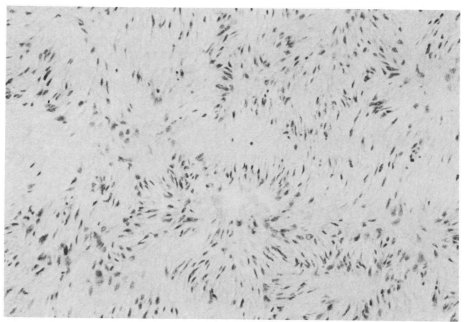

FIGURE 17–24. Equine schwannoma. Palisading of spindle-shaped cells (Antoni Type A) alternating with edematous stroma (Antoni Type B).

adult to aged animals. Lesions are usually solitary, rounded, well circumscribed, flabby to firm, variable in size, and subcutaneous. Lesions occur most commonly on the trunk and proximal limbs.[52, 180, 469]

Histologically, lipomas are characterized by a well-circumscribed proliferation of normal-appearing lipocytes. Liposarcomas are characterized by a cellular, infiltrative proliferation of atypical lipocytes with abundant, eosinophilic, finely vacuolated cytoplasm.

The therapy of choice is surgical excision.

Hemangioma and Hemangiosarcoma

Hemangiomas are uncommon in horses, swine, and cattle and rare in sheep and goats.* These benign tumors arise from the endothelial cells of blood vessels. The cause of hemangiomas is unknown, and some authors consider them to be hamartomas or nevi. Hemangiosarcomas (hemangioendotheliomas) are rare in all large animals.

In horses, hemangiomas are seen often in animals younger than one year, and some animals are born with the lesions.† Equine hemangiomas are usually solitary and most

commonly affect the distal limbs. The lesions may be (1) well circumscribed, nodular, firm to fluctuant, bluish to blackish, and dermal or subcutaneous or (2) dark, hyperkeratotic, and verrucous (verrucous hemangioma, angiomatosis, Fig. 17–25). They frequently ulcerate and bleed easily, occasionally to the point of causing anemia.

In cattle, hemangiomas usually occur in mature animals but may occur congenitally (Fig. 17–26).* Lesions may be single or multiple and may occur anywhere on the body. Angiomatosis has been described in European and United States dairy and beef cattle with an average age of five and a half years.[86, 283, 461, 509] One or several reddish-gray to pink, soft, sessile or pedunculated masses, 0.5 to 2.5 cm in diameter, are most commonly found over the back. These lesions are usually first detected because of recurrent hemorrhage, which can be profuse.

In swine, hemangiomas occur most commonly in the scrotum of Yorkshire and Berkshire boars.[204, 265, 335, 346, 461] The condition may be genetically determined. Lesions are usually multiple, beginning as tiny purple papules and progressing to hyperkeratotic, verrucous lesions. Other porcine hemangiomas may occur anywhere on the body and may be congenital.†

---

*References 33, 34, 65, 126, 173, 180, 335, 382, 397, 461, 475, 484, 511

†References 23, 65, 173, 207, 213, 236, 337, 382, 430, 469

*References 22, 180, 201, 237, 341, 393, 461

†References 15, 77, 98, 335, 380, 461, 520

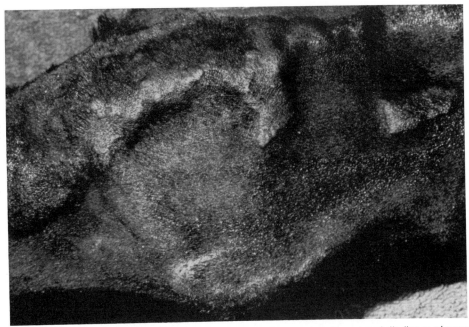

FIGURE 17–25. Verrucous hemangioma on the fetlock of an equine. Hyperkeratotic linear plaques.

Hemangiosarcomas usually occur in adult to aged animals.[173, 461] Lesions are usually solitary, rapidly growing, poorly circumscribed, firm to friable, and dermal to subcutaneous. The lesions often undergo necrosis, ulceration, and bleeding and have no site predilection.

Histologically, hemangiomas are characterized by the proliferation of blood-filled vascular spaces lined by single layers of well-differentiated endothelial cells (Fig. 17–27). Hemangiomas are often subclassified as capillary or cavernous, depending on the size of the vascular spaces. Equine verrucous hemangioma is characterized as a multinodular capillary hemangioma with hyperplasia and hyperkeratosis of the overlying epidermis (Figs. 17–28 and 17–29).[213, 334, 439] Bovine angiomatosis is characterized as a multinodular hemangioma with the frequent presence of intervening inflamed connective tissue stroma, a histopathologic picture similar to so-called pyogenic granuloma in humans.[86, 271, 461] Hemangiosarcomas are characterized by an invasive proliferation of atypical endothelial cells with areas of vascular space formation.

The therapy of choice for hemangiomas and hemangiosarcomas is surgical excision. Equine verrucous hemangioma of the leg is often difficult to excise, and cryosurgery may be beneficial. The prognosis for hemangiosarcoma is poor, with frequent local recurrence and metastasis.

Lymphangioma

Lymphangiomas are rare benign neoplasms of large animals, arising from the endothelial cells of lymphatic vessels.* The cause of lymphangiomas is unknown, and some authors consider them to be hamartomas.

---

*References 84, 110, 180, 331, 334, 380, 382, 461, 469, 494

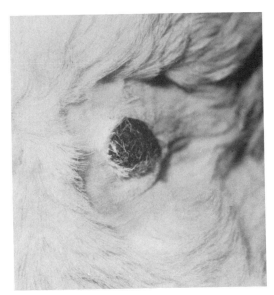

FIGURE 17–26. Congenital hemangioma in a calf. Alopecic, hyperpigmented nodule on lateral thorax.

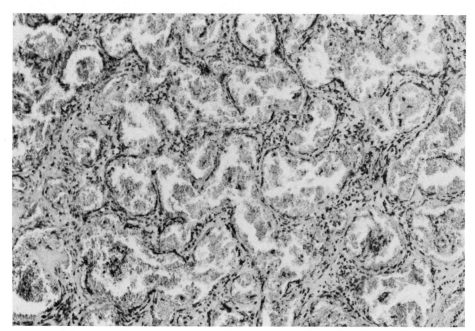

FIGURE 17–27. Bovine hemangioma. Proliferation of well-differentiated blood vessels.

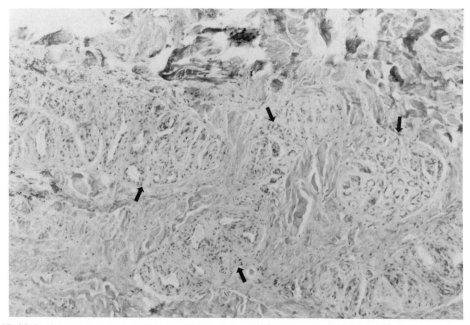

FIGURE 17–28. Equine verrucous hemangioma. Multinodular proliferation of well-differentiated blood vessels (arrows).

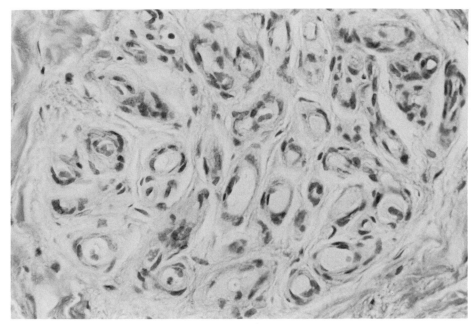

FIGURE 17–29. Equine verrucous hemangioma. Nodular proliferation of well-differentiated blood vessels.

Most reported lymphangiomas have occurred as congenital lesions or lesions recognized within the first few months of life. They have been multinodular or fluctuant masses in the inguinal and axillary regions.

Histologically, lymphangiomas are characterized by a proliferation of variably sized cystic spaces lined by a single layer of flattened endothelial cells within the dermis or subcutis, or both (Fig. 17–30). The vascular structures are irregularly shaped, the endothelial cells are widely spaced, the vessels do not contain blood, and there are no pericytes.

The therapy of choice for lymphangiomas is surgical excision.

Mast Cell Tumor

Mast cell tumors are uncommon in horses and cattle, rare in swine, and not reported in sheep and goats.* Mast cell tumors may be benign or malignant, and they arise from tissue mast cells. The cause of these tumors is unknown.

In horses, mast cell tumors occur in animals 1 to 15 years (average seven years) old, with no breed predilection but with a marked predilection for males (five times as many males

affected as females).* In addition, multiple mast cell tumors, resembling urticaria pigmentosa of humans, may occur in newborn foals.[74, 396, 438] Equine mast cell tumors are usually solitary and occur most commonly on the head and legs. Lesions are 2 to 20 cm in diameter, well to poorly circumscribed, firm to fluctuant, and dermal or subcutaneous and may or may not be alopecic, ulcerated, and hyperpigmented. Lesions on the legs tend to be very firm and immovable (Fig. 17–31). Equine mast cell tumors appear to be hyperplastic rather than neoplastic growths. Spontaneous remissions may occur in young animals and following incomplete surgical excision, and metastasis has never been reported.[74, 383, 396, 461]

In cattle, mast cell tumors occur in animals six months to seven years of age, with no breed or sex predilections.† Lesions are usually multiple, 1 to 40 cm in diameter, firm to fluctuant, and dermal or subcutaneous and may or may not be alopecic and ulcerated. They can occur anywhere, especially over the neck and trunk. The majority of bovine mast cell tumors are malignant and metastatic.

In swine, mast cell tumors have been reported in animals 6 to 18 months of age, with

---

*References 45, 180, 201, 289, 300, 331, 368, 461, 484, 517

*References 5, 105a, 136, 289, 300, 352, 383, 427, 460, 461, 463, 484, 490

†References 45, 164, 179, 180, 285, 289, 298, 305, 368a, 461, 464

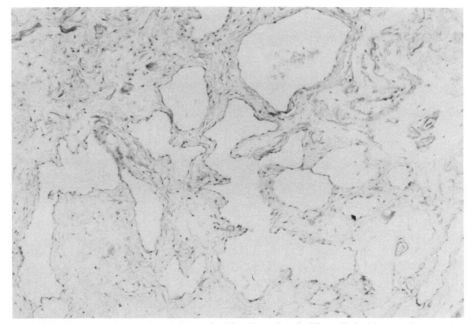

FIGURE 17–30. *Equine lymphangioma. Proliferation of well-differentiated lymphatic vessels.*

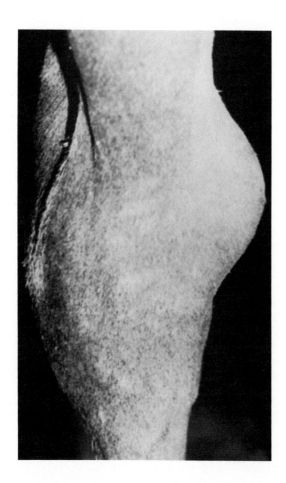

FIGURE 17–31. *Equine mastocytoma. Firm, poorly demarcated nodule on hock.*

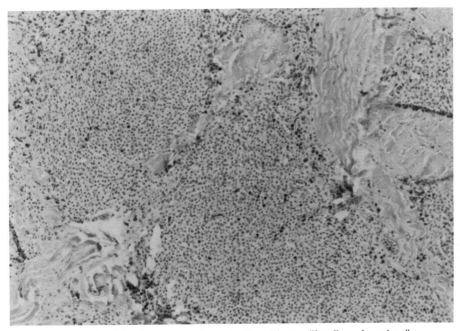

FIGURE 17–32. Equine mastocytoma. Multinodular proliferation of mast cells.

no breed or sex predilections.[57, 306, 461] Lesions may be single or multiple, 2 to 20 mm in diameter, firm to fluctuant, well circumscribed, and dermal to subcutaneous and may occur anywhere on the body. Porcine mast cell tumors may be limited to the skin or may involve internal organs.

Histologically, mast cell tumors are charac-terized by a diffuse to multinodular prolifera-tion of mast cells (Figs. 17–32 and 17–33). Tumor cells may be well differentiated (typical of equine mast cell tumors) or pleomorphic and atypical. Tissue eosinophilia and focal areas of collagen degeneration are usually present (Figs. 17–34 and 17–35). A variety of vascular lesions (hyalinization, fibrinoid degen-

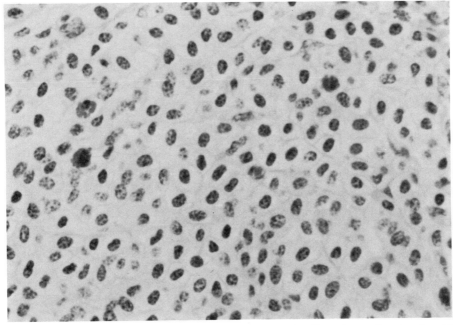

FIGURE 17–33. Equine mastocytoma. Well-differentiated mast cells and occasional eosinophils.

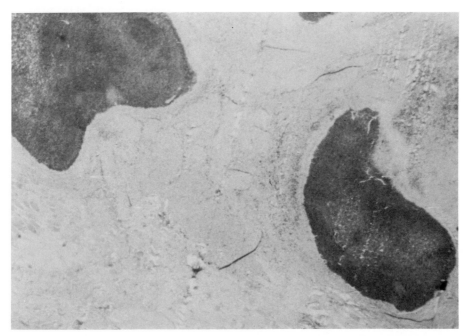

FIGURE 17–34. Equine mastocytoma. Multifocal areas of collagen degeneration and eosinophilic inflammation.

eration, eosinophilic vasculitis) may be seen. In horses, large areas of dystrophic mineralization are frequently seen (Fig. 17–36), which may lead to a misdiagnosis of calcinosis circumscripta (tumoral calcinosis).[438, 461, 463]

The therapy of choice is wide surgical excision when practical. In horses, solitary mast cell tumors have been successfully treated with sublesional injections of 5 to 10 mg of triamcinolone acetonide or 10 to 20 mg of methylprednisolone acetate. Cryosurgery and radiation therapy are treatment options.

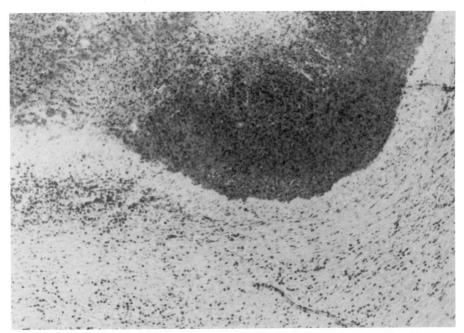

FIGURE 17–35. Equine mastocytoma. Area of collagen degeneration bordered by an infiltration of eosinophils and histiocytes.

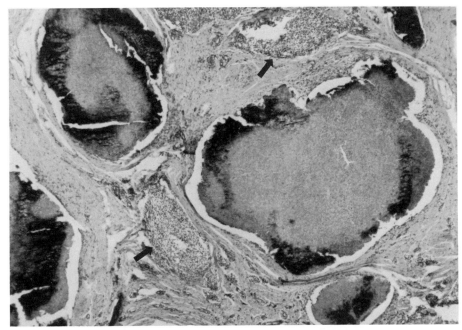

FIGURE 17–36. *Equine mastocytoma. Multifocal areas of dystrophic mineralization. Unless small residual clusters of mast cells are noted (arrows), this lesion could be misdiagnosed as calcinosis circumscripta.*

LYMPHORETICULAR NEOPLASMS

Histiocytoma

Histiocytomas are benign neoplasms arising from dermal histiocytes.[23, 328, 420] The cause of these tumors is unknown.

Histiocytomas appear to be very rare in large animals. Two cases have been reported in goats.[290, 420] Both animals were bucks with solitary, firm, well-demarcated scrotal nodules (Fig. 17–37). Congenital histiocytosis, resembling the Letterer-Siwe syndrome of humans,[271] was reported in a piglet.[482] The piglet had generalized purpuric macules and papules.

Histologically, histiocytomas are characterized by uniform sheets of pleomorphic histiocytes infiltrating the dermis and subcutis (Fig. 17–38). A characteristic feature of this neoplasm is a high mitotic index. Lymphocytic infiltration and areas of necrosis develop in regressing neoplasms.

The therapy of choice may include surgical excision or observation without treatment. In one goat,[420] the scrotal histiocytoma regressed completely six months after biopsy.

Malignant Fibrous Histiocytoma

Malignant fibrous histiocytoma (extraskeletal giant cell tumor, giant cell tumor of soft parts) is a rare neoplasm that is thought to arise from histiocytes.[271, 328, 413] The cause of this neoplasm is unknown.

Malignant fibrous histiocytoma has been reported only in horses.[96, 130, 413] Lesions are solitary, firm, poorly circumscribed, and variable in size and occur most frequently on the neck and proximal limbs. These neoplasms are locally invasive but apparently slow to metastasize.

Histologically, malignant fibrous histiocy-

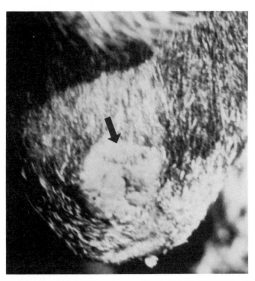

FIGURE 17–37. *Histiocytoma (arrow) on scrotum of a buck. (Courtesy J. M. King.)*

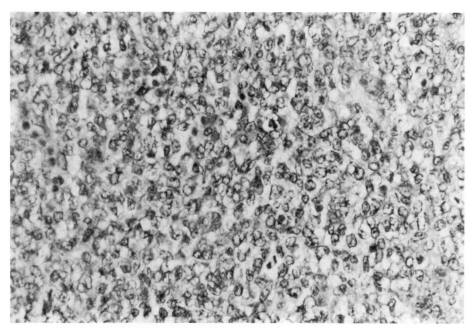

FIGURE 17–38. Caprine histiocytoma. Proliferation of pleomorphic histiocytes.

toma is characterized by an infiltrative mass composed of varying mixtures of pleomorphic histiocytes, fibroblasts, and multinucleated histiocytic giant cells. Mitotic figures and a storiform (cartwheel) arrangement of fibroblasts and histiocytes are common features.

The therapy of choice is radical surgical excision. However, recurrence following surgery is common because of the infiltrative growth pattern of the tumor.

Lymphosarcoma

Cutaneous lymphosarcoma is a rare malignancy of horses and cattle* and is extremely rare in sheep,[294, 323, 421a] goats,[21, 89] and swine.[75, 78, 148] In cattle, enzootic lymphosarcoma (bovine leukemia, lymphomatosis, enzootic bovine leukosis) is caused by a retrovirus (bovine leukemia virus, BLV), but most cases of bovine cutaneous lymphosarcoma are sporadic and not BLV-associated.† Enzootic bovine lymphosarcoma can be transmited to sheep, and the enzootic form of ovine lymphosarcoma is caused by a retrovirus (ovine leukemia virus, OLV).[181a, 222, 286, 294, 335, 386, 421a]

In horses, cutaneous lymphosarcoma usually occurs in adult to aged animals (but with a range of 4 months to 22 years old), with no sex or breed predilections.* Most horses have concurrent systemic illness, including depression, weight loss, anemia, and peripheral lymphadenopathy. Lesions are usually multiple and dermoepidermal to subcutaneous and may occur anywhere on the body, especially the trunk (Fig. 17–39). Lesions may be firm or soft (resembling urticaria), and the overlying skin is usually normal. Horses with lymphosarcoma may be immunosuppressed.[105] The disease is usually fatal. Histiocytic varieties of equine cutaneous lymphosarcoma may have a better prognosis, with less frequent involvement of internal organs.[426, 443]

In cattle, cutaneous lymphosarcoma usually occurs in young adult animals (usually one to four years of age), with no sex or breed predilections.† The lesions are usually multiple and dermoepidermal to subcutaneous and may occur anywhere on the body, especially the neck and trunk (Fig. 17–40). The overlying skin may be normal or alopecic, crusted, hyperkeratotic, and ulcerated. Initially, affected cattle are often otherwise healthy. Frequently, the cutaneous lesions spontaneously regress. However, remission is usually followed by relapse and internal involvement. The disease is usually fatal.

---

*References 33, 289, 308, 330, 410, 460, 484
†References 36, 124, 201, 289, 308, 366, 367

*References 33, 105, 154, 168, 180, 197, 300, 334, 343, 344, 397, 402, 410, 426, 443, 460, 483, 490, 512, 525
†References 35, 36, 46, 124, 180, 183, 199, 205, 277, 289, 293, 308, 323, 330, 399

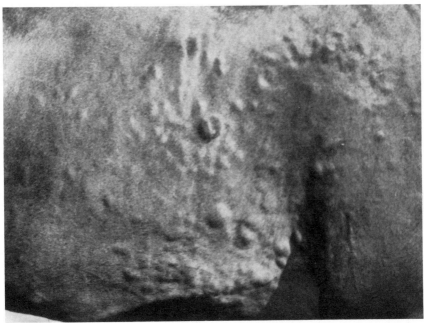

FIGURE 17–39. Equine lymphosarcoma. Multiple papules and nodules over the trunk. (Courtesy W. C. Rebhun.)

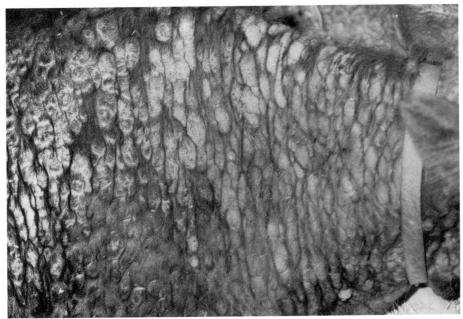

FIGURE 17–40. Bovine lymphosarcoma. Multiple alopecic, hyperkeratotic plaques and nodules over neck and shoulder.

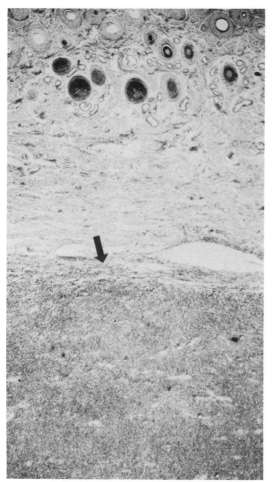

FIGURE 17–41. Equine lymphosarcoma. Diffuse infiltration of subcutis with malignant lymphocytes (arrow).

Histologically, lymphosarcoma is usually characterized by diffuse dermal and subcutaneous infiltration by malignant lymphocytes (nonepitheliotropic or B-cell pattern) (Figs. 17–41 through 17–44). Immunologic studies of bovine lymphosarcoma have suggested that the enzootic (BLV-associated) form is primarily a B-cell disease, whereas the sporadic (non–BLV-associated) form is a null-cell proliferation.[46, 124, 366, 367] Immunologic studies of ovine lymphosarcoma have demonstrated proliferations of T, B, and null cells.[100, 222] Therapy for lymphosarcoma is ineffective.

Pseudolymphoma

Pseudolymphomas are papular to nodular skin lesions arising from chronic antigenic stimulus, such as seen in response to arthropod and insect bites and drug reactions.[271] Pseudolymphomas have occasionally been recog-

nized in horses.[438] Lesions are commonly seen in late summer and fall, are normally solitary, and occur most frequently over the head and trunk. They are usually firm and asymptomatic, and the overlying skin is normal.

Diagnosis is based on history, physical examination, and skin biopsy. Histologic examination reveals dense dermal, and occasionally subcutaneous, inflammatory infiltrate consisting of lymphocytes, histiocytes, plasma cells, and eosinophils. Lymphoid nodules are present (Fig. 17–45).

Therapy has consisted of surgical excision, and recurrences have not been seen.

MELANOCYTIC NEOPLASMS

Melanoma

Melanomas are benign or malignant neoplasms arising from melanocytes or melanoblasts. Melanomas are common in horses and certain breeds of swine, uncommon in cattle and goats, and rare in sheep.[*] In general, the cause of these tumors is unknown. In Sinclair miniature and Duroc-Jersey swine, melanomas appear to have a genetic basis.[198, 312] In horses, melanomas usually occur in adult to aged animals (congenital to 20 years old), with no sex predilection.[†] They are especially common in Arabians, Percherons, and specifically bred subsets of these genetic stocks.[‡] There is a striking relationship between the incidence of melanoma and gray coat color. Equine melanotic disease occurs almost exclusively in horses that first turn dappled gray and then white as they age.[169, 270, 496, 497] The horses may originally be any color, and only the hair turns gray, the skin remaining pigmented. Concurrent with the coat depigmentation is the development of a widespread melanosis with the deposition of pigment and possibly tumor cells in systemic tissues. It has been estimated that about 80 percent of gray horses over 15 years of age have clinical melanomas.[297, 461] Equine melanomas may be solitary or multiple and dermoepidermal or subcutaneous and occur most commonly on the perineal region, undersurface of the tail (Fig. 17–46), pinnae, periocular region, and distal limbs. The tumors are usually firm and nodular and may or may not be alopecic, ulcerated,

---

*References 30, 87, 180, 289, 294, 312, 461
†References 33, 87, 170, 178, 180, 300, 382, 383, 461, 469
‡References 144, 270, 287, 297, 312, 322, 383, 422, 461

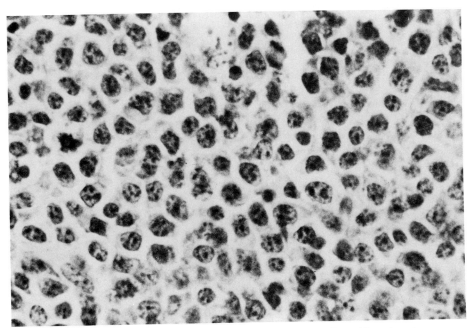

FIGURE 17–42. Equine lymphosarcoma. Proliferation of malignant lymphocytes.

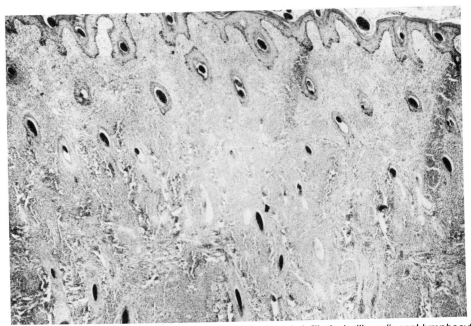

FIGURE 17–43. Bovine lymphosarcoma. Entire dermis is diffusely infiltrated with malignant lymphocytes.

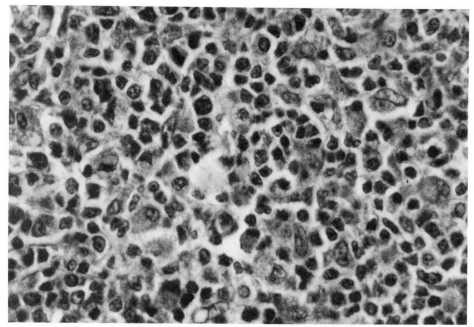

FIGURE 17–44. Bovine lymphosarcoma. Proliferation of malignant lymphocytes.

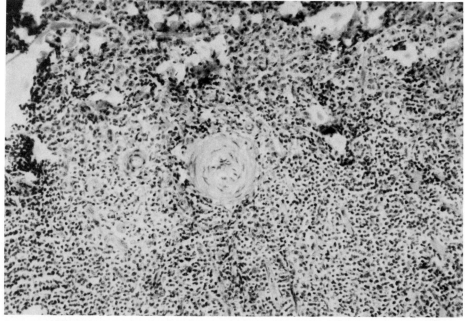

FIGURE 17–45. Equine pseudolymphoma (tick bite). Nodular proliferation of normal lymphocytes admixed with eosinophils and plasma cells.

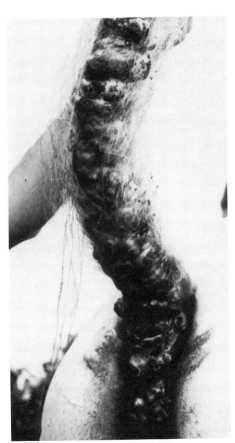

FIGURE 17–46. Equine melanoma. Multiple melanotic nodules on undersurface of tail and perianally.

and grossly hyperpigmented. The appearance of equine melanomas may be heralded by the appearance of vitiligo (see Chapter 14, discussion on vitiligo).[270, 496, 497] Three growth patterns have been described for equine cutaneous melanomas: (1) slow growth for years without metastasis, (2) slow growth for years with sudden rapid growth and malignancy, and (3) rapid growth and malignancy from the onset.[460, 461]

Approximately two thirds of all reported equine melanomas have been malignant and metastatic.*

In cattle, melanomas occur in animals of any age (newborn to aged), with no sex predilection.† Dark-haired breeds appear to be predisposed, especially Angus. Lesions may be solitary or multiple and dermoepidermal or subcutaneous and may occur anywhere on the

body, especially the legs (Fig. 17–47). Congenital melanomas resembling human melanotic progonoma were reported on the jaws of two calves.[527] Most bovine cutaneous melanomas are benign, although metastasis can occur.[87, 180, 261, 289, 291]

In goats, melanomas occur most commonly in adult to aged animals with no sex predilection.* Angora goats appear to be predisposed. Lesions may be solitary or multiple and dermoepidermal or subcutaneous and occur most commonly on the perineum, udder, pinnae, and coronets. Caprine cutaneous melanomas commonly metastasize.

In sheep, melanomas usually occur in adult to aged animals, with no sex predilection.[24, 180, 284, 294, 296, 461] Suffolk and Angora sheep appear to be predisposed. Lesions are often multiple and subcutaneous and tend to occur in pigmented skin. Metastases are frequent.

In swine, melanomas occur in animals of any age (newborn to adult), with no sex pre-

---

*References 50, 87, 94, 214, 322, 431, 455, 488, 504, 535

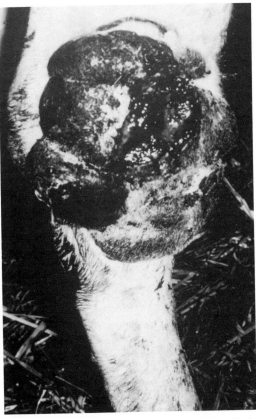

FIGURE 17–47. Bovine melanoma. Large melanotic tumor on lateral hock.

---

*References 33, 49, 150, 158, 160, 170, 180, 238, 248, 292, 320, 322, 444, 491, 492

†References 9, 30, 87, 92, 180, 214, 289, 318, 341, 341, 397, 449, 461, 527

dilection.* Duroc-Jersey and Sinclair miniature swine are genetically predisposed.† The incidence of melanomas in some swine herds can reach 20 percent,[312, 351, 461, 465] and litter mates may be affected. Lesions may be solitary or multiple and may occur anywhere on the body, especially the trunk. In general, they may be flat, well circumscribed, and evenly pigmented (lentigo, melanocytic nevus) or raised, black, and frequently ulcerated (melanoma).[312, 369] The smaller, flatter lesions often spontaneously regress, and regression may be associated with the development of vitiligo and halo nevi (see Chapter 14, discussion on vitiligo).[312, 313] Larger, raised lesions are frequently metastatic. Clinical, pathologic, and immunologic studies have demonstrated the usefulness of the Sinclair miniature swine melanoma as a model for melanoma in humans.[192, 195, 198, 223, 310–313] Leukocytes from Sinclair swine recognize and react in vitro with autologous and allogeneic swine melanoma extracts and cultured allogeneic swine melanoma cells; leukocyte reactivity has been found to correlate with tumor load and spontaneous regression of swine melanomas.[19, 37–39, 192, 194, 223]

*References 66, 68, 98, 110, 126, 161, 187, 208, 218, 314, 351, 388, 465, 476, 487

†References 62, 69, 126–128, 187, 198, 208, 218, 288, 312, 369, 461, 465

Histologically, cutaneous melanocytic lesions are divided into the following types:*
I. Benign melanomas
   A. Benign melanoma with junctional activity (melanocytic nevi: junctional and compound types)
   B. Benign dermal melanoma
     1. Cellular type
     2. Fibrous type
II. Malignant melanomas
   A. Epithelioid type (Figs. 17–48 and 17–49)
   B. Spindle-cell type
   C. Epithelioid and spindle-cell type
   D. Superficial spreading (intraepidermal) type

In addition, perifollicular (pilar neurocristic hamartoma)[496, 497] and melanotic progonoma (epithelioid melanocytes and lymphocytes in a fibrous stroma)[527] variants have been reported.

The treatment of choice is early radical surgical excision. Cryosurgery has been reported to be effective in some cases.[395]

MISCELLANEOUS NEOPLASMS

Other neoplasms that have been rarely reported in the skin of large animals include

*References 144, 271, 312, 313, 369, 461, 518

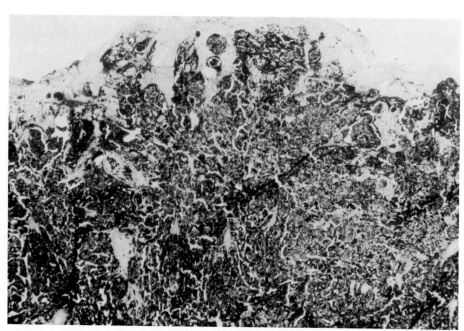

FIGURE 17–48. Equine malignant melanoma. Diffuse dermal proliferation of malignant melanocytes.

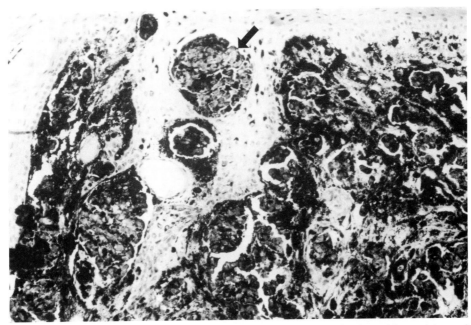

FIGURE 17–49. Equine malignant melanoma. Nests of malignant melanocytes (arrow) in overlying epidermis.

metastatic embryonal nephroma (swine),[269, 307, 378] rhabdomyoma (swine),[180, 378] hemangiopericytoma (horse),[397] osteoma (horse),[397] and organoid nevi (cow and swine).[438, 489]

KERATOSES

Keratoses are firm, elevated, circumscribed areas of excessive keratin production.[271, 328]

Solar keratoses (actinic keratoses) have been recognized in cattle, sheep, and horses.* They are caused by excessive exposure to ultraviolet light. Solar keratoses may be single or multiple, appear in lightly haired and lightly pigmented skin, and vary in appearance from ill-defined areas of erythema, hyperkeratosis, and crusting to indurated, crusted, hyperkeratotic plaques. Histologically, they are characterized by atypia and dysplasia of the epidermis, parakeratotic hyperkeratosis, and solar elastosis (basophilic degeneration) of the dermis. Solar keratoses are premalignant lesions capable of becoming invasive squamous cell carcinoma.

Cutaneous horns have been recognized in cattle, sheep, goats, and horses.† The cause of cutaneous horns is unclear; they may originate from epidermal lesions such as papillomas, squamous cell carcinomas, solar keratoses, and dermatophilosis (see Chapter 6, discussion on dermatophilosis). They may be single or multiple and are firm, hornlike projections up to 10 cm in length. Histologically, cutaneous horns are characterized by extensive, compact, laminated hyperkeratosis. The base of a cutaneous horn must always be inspected for the possible underlying cause.

The therapy of choice for most keratoses is surgical excision or cryosurgery. Solar keratoses are always premalignant lesions, and cutaneous horns may have a neoplastic process at their bases.

CYSTS

Cutaneous cysts are uncommon in horses, goats, and sheep and rare in cattle and swine.* These cysts are benign non-neoplastic lesions characterized by an epithelial wall, with keratinous to amorphous contents. Cutaneous cysts are subdivided into six types, based on clinicopathologic findings.

Epidermoid cysts (epidermal cysts, epidermal inclusion cysts) are thought to arise congenitally or to be acquired (traumatically?)

*References 174, 181, 182, 278, 281, 438, 480, 521
†References 31, 131, 181, 245, 278, 281, 411, 438, 473

*References 140, 157, 276, 279, 290, 334, 370, 371, 383, 518, 534

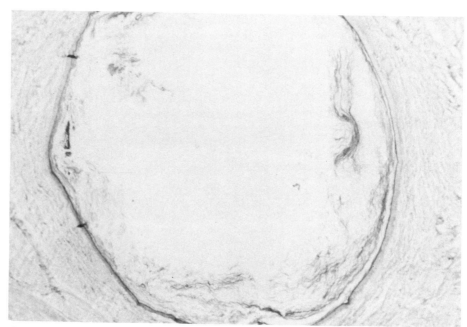

FIGURE 17–50. Equine epidermal cyst. Keratin-containing cyst lined by squamous epithelium.

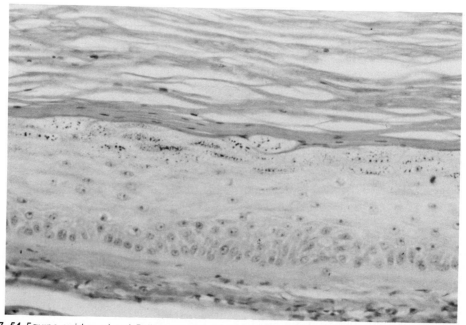

FIGURE 17–51. Equine epidermal cyst. Epithelium of cyst wall undergoes differentiation identical to that of epidermis.

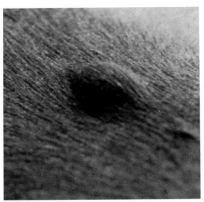

FIGURE 17-52. Equine dermoid cyst. Solitary nodule on dorsal midline in middle of back.

from displaced fragments of epithelium. The cysts may be solitary or multiple, firm to fluctuant, well circumscribed, smooth, and round, and usually, the overlying skin is normal. Epidermoid cysts occur most commonly in the horse, especially at the base of the ear, where they may discharge a mucoid material (dentigerous cyst), or unilaterally in the false nostril (atheroma, false nostril cyst).[157, 334, 383, 385] Epidermoid cysts in the false nostril may be present at birth but are usually not noticed until the animal is three to six months of age. They may attain a size of 8 cm and contain a gray porridge-like material. Epidermoid cysts also occur in cattle.[370] Histologically, epidermoid cysts are characterized by an epithelial lining that undergoes maturation and keratinization typical of epidermis and contains no adnexal structures (Figs. 17-50 and 17-51).

Dermoid cysts are usually congenital or hereditary lesions.[2, 328, 334, 345, 478] The cysts may be solitary or multiple, firm to fluctuant, well circumscribed, smooth, and round, and usually, the overlying skin is normal. Dermoid cysts occur most commonly in the horse, especially on the dorsal midline (Fig. 17-52), between the withers and the rump.[157, 334, 382, 383] Affected horses range from six months to nine years of age, and in one survey,[382] all 16 cases involved Thoroughbreds. Histologically, dermoid cysts are characterized by an epithelial lining that contains adnexa (Fig. 17-53).

Follicular cysts develop by retention of follicular or glandular products resulting from congenital or acquired loss or obliteration of follicular orifices.[371, 518] The cysts may be solitary or multiple, firm to fluctuant, well circumscribed, smooth, and round, and usually, the overlying skin is normal. Follicular cysts are most commonly seen in sheep,[81, 279, 371] and ovine lesions are often multiple, occur without apparent site or sex predilection, and may have an inherited basis in Merinos. Ovine follicular cysts cause esthetic damage, damage to hides and fleece, and increased difficulty in shearing. Secondary squamous cell carcinomas may develop in the cyst walls.[64] Histologically, follic-

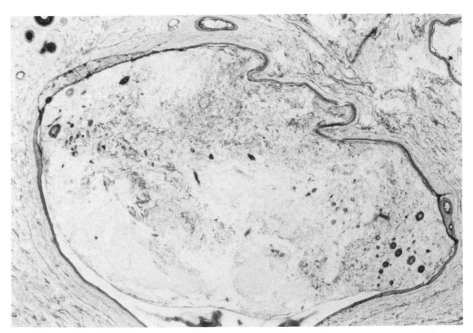

FIGURE 17-53. Equine dermoid cyst is filled with keratin and hair shafts. Epithelial lining of cyst contains appendages.

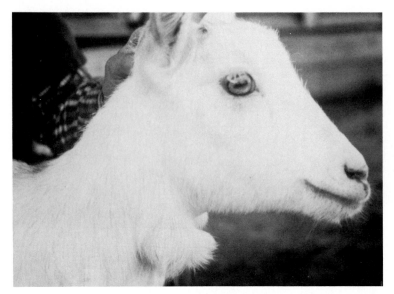

FIGURE 17–54. Wattle cyst in a goat.

ular cysts are characterized by marked dilatation and hyperkeratosis of hair follicles.

Periauricular cysts (conchal fistula, cyst, or sinus; dentigerous cyst, temporal teratoma or odontoma; ear fistula or ear tooth) are reported infrequently in the horse.* These cysts are thought to represent developmental defects. There are no apparent breed or sex predilections, and lesions may be present at birth or may not be recognized until the animal

*References 34, 49, 84, 88, 113, 132, 207, 276, 295, 345, 353, 383, 384, 513

is seven years of age. Lesions are solitary and occur at or near the base of the ear or in relationship to the zygomatic process. They may appear as typical cysts or as sinuses that discharge a grayish, mucoid material. Histologically, periauricular cysts may be epidermoid, dermoid, or dentigerous (containing a tooth or teeth).

Wattle cysts have been reported in goats.[140, 143, 290, 452, 453, 523] These cysts are believed to be developmental abnormalities, possibly arising from the branchial cleft. Nubian goats and Nubian crossbreeds are most commonly af-

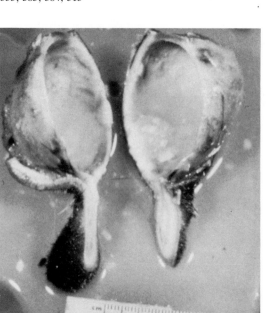

FIGURE 17–55. Excised and hemisected wattle cyst from a goat.

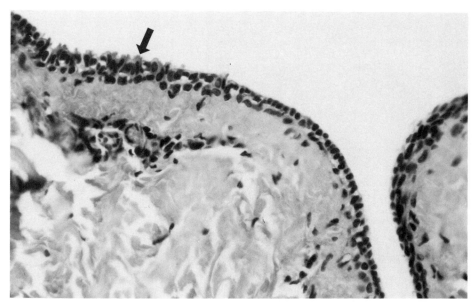

FIGURE 17–56. Caprine wattle cyst. Cyst wall composed of cuboidal to columnar epithelium exhibiting apical "budding" (arrow).

fected, and the lesions may have a hereditary basis. The cysts are present at the base of the wattle at birth but may not be noticed until the animal is two to three months of age. They are usually rounded, smooth, soft, and fluctuant, and the overlying skin is normal (Fig. 17–54). Wattle cysts contain a clear fluid (Fig. 17–55) and, if aspirated, will re-form. Histologically, wattle cysts are characterized by a cyst wall composed of a single to double layer of cuboidal to columnar epithelial cells that often exhibit the apical budding (decapitation secretion) typical of apocrine sweat gland secretory epithelium (Fig. 17–56).

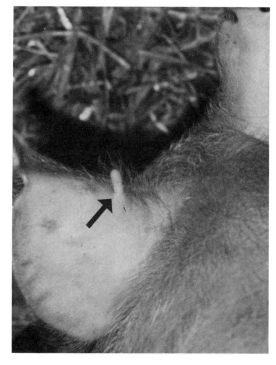

FIGURE 17–57. Organoid nevus (arrow) on the pinna of a pig.

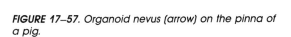

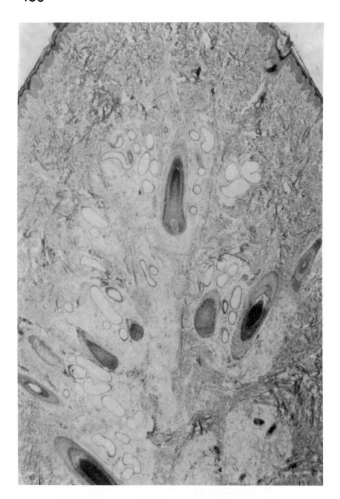

FIGURE 17–58. Porcine organoid nevus. Hyperplasia of hair follicles and apocrine glands.

Udder cysts are reported in sheep, especially older ewes.[140] The lesions are frequently multiple, 1 to 5 cm in diameter, soft, reducible, and filled with milk in the lactating mammary gland. Aspiration yields milk. The cause of udder cysts is unknown, and no treatment is required.

The treatment of choice for most cutaneous cysts is surgical excision or observation without therapy. It has been recommended that equine epidermoid cysts of the false nostril be incised on the inner aspect of the nostril, drained, and packed with iodine. However, recurrence is a problem, and surgical excision is preferable when practical.[383, 384]

NEVI

A nevus (hamartoma) is a circumscribed developmental (hyperplastic) defect of the skin.[271, 328] Nevi may arise from any skin component or combination thereof. They may or may not be congenital. Nevi are apparently rare in large animals. Melanocytic (see earlier), vascular (see earlier), and organoid nevi (Figs. 17–57 and 17–58)[438] have been recognized in large animals. These lesions are benign, and surgical excision is the treatment of choice when necessary or practical.

REFERENCES

1. Abu-Samra, M. T., et al.: Clinical observations on bovine papillomatosis (warts). Br. Vet. J. 138:139, 1982.
2. Adams, S. B., et al.: Periocular dermoid cyst in a calf. JAVMA 184:1255, 1983.
3. Akerejola, O. O., et al.: Equine squamous cell carcinoma in Northern Nigeria. Vet. Rec. 103:336, 1978.
4. Al-Saleem, T. I.: Cancer in Iraq. Iraqi Med. J. 22:12, 1974.
5. Altera, K., and Clark, L.: Equine cutaneous mastocytoma. Pathol. Vet. 7:43, 1970.
6. Al-Yaman, F., and Willenborg, D. O.: Successful isolation, cultivation, and partial characterization of naturally occurring ovine squamous cell carcinomata. Vet. Immunol. Immunopathol. 5:273, 1983.
7. Al-Yaman, F., and Willenborg, D. O.: Immune reactivity to autochthonous ovine squamous cell carcinomata. Vet. Immunol. Immunopathol. 7:153, 1984.

8. Amstutz, H. E.: Bovine skin conditions: A brief review. Mod. Vet. Pract. 60:821, 1979.

9. Amstutz, H. E.: *Bovine Medicine and Surgery II.* Santa Barbara, CA, American Veterinary Publications, 1980.

10. Amtmann, E., et al.: Equine connective tissue tumors contain unintegrated bovine papillomavirus DNA. J. Virol. 35:962, 1980.

11. Anderson, D. E., et al.: Nutrition and eye cancer in cattle. J. Natl. Cancer Inst. 45:697, 1979.

12. Anderson, D. E.: Effects of pigment on bovine ocular squamous cell carcinoma. Ann. N.Y. Acad. Sci. 100:436, 1963.

13. Anderson, D. E., et al.: Studies on bovine ocular squamous cell carcinoma ("cancer eye"). II. Relationship between eyelid pigment and occurrence of cancer eye lesions. J. Anim. Sci. 45:739, 1977.

14. Anderson, D. E., and Skinner, P. E.: Studies on bovine ocular squamous cell carcinoma ("cancer eye"). XI. Effects of sunlight. J. Anim. Sci. 20:474, 1961.

15. Anderson, L. J., et al.: A British abattoir survey of tumours in cattle, sheep, and pigs. Vet. Rec. 84:547, 1969.

16. Anson, M. A., et al.: Bovine herpesvirus-5 (DN-599) antigen in cells derived from bovine ocular squamous cell carcinoma. Can. J. Comp. Med. 46:334, 1982.

17. Abu-Samra, M. T.: *Dermatophilus* infection: The clinical disease and diagnosis. Zbl. Vet. Med. B 25:641, 1978.

18. Atwell, R. B., and Summers, P. M.: Congenital papilloma in a foal. Aust. Vet. J. 53:229, 1977.

19. Aultman, M. D., and Hook, R. R.: In vitro lymphocyte reactivity to soluble tumor extracts in Sinclair melanoma swine. Intl. J. Cancer 24:673, 1979.

20. Bagdonas, V., and Olson, C.: Observations on the epizootiology of cutaneous papillomatosis (warts) of cattle. JAVMA 122:393, 1953.

21. Baker, J. C., and Sherman, D. M.: Lymphosarcoma in a Nubian goat. Vet. Med. Small Anim. Clin. 77:557, 1982.

22. Baker, J. C., et al.: Disseminated cavernous hemangioma in a calf. JAVMA 181:172, 1982.

23. Baker, J. R., and Leyland, A.: Histological survey of tumours of the horse, with particular reference to those of the skin. Vet. Rec. 96:419, 1975.

24. Baker, J. R.: A case of an invasive melanoma in a new-born lamb. Vet. Rec. 97:496, 1975.

25. Banks, W. C., and England, R. B.: Radioactive gold in the treatment of ocular squamous cell carcinoma of cattle. JAVMA 163:745, 1973.

26. Barthold, S. W., and Olson, C.: Common membrane neoantigens on bovine papillomavirus-induced fibroma cells from cattle and horses. Am. J. Vet. Res. 39:1643, 1978.

27. Barthold, S. W., and Olson, C.: Fibroma regression in relationship to antibody and challenge immunity to bovine papillomavirus. Cancer Res. 34:2436, 1974.

28. Barthold, S. W., et al.: Atypical warts in cattle. JAVMA 165:276, 1974.

29. Barthold, S. W., et al.: Precipitin response of cattle to commercial wart vaccine. Am. J. Vet. Res. 37:449, 1976.

30. Bastianello, S. S.: A survey of neoplasia in domestic species over a 40-year period from 1935 to 1974 in the Republic of South Africa. I. Tumours occurring in cattle. Onderstepoort J. Vet. Res. 49:195, 1982.

31. Bastianello, S. S.: A survey of neoplasia in domestic species over a 40-year period from 1935 to 1974 in the Republic of South Africa. II. Tumours occurring in sheep. Onderstepoort J. Vet. Res. 49:205, 1982.

32. Bastianello, S. S.: A survey of neoplasia in domestic species over a 40-year period from 1935 to 1974 in the Republic of South Africa. III. Tumours occurring in pigs and goats. Onderstepoort J. Vet. Res. 50:25, 1983.

33. Bastianello, S. S.: A survey of neoplasia in domestic species over a 40-year period from 1935 to 1974 in the Republic of South Africa. IV. Tumours occurring in Equidae. Onderstepoort J. Vet. Res. 50:91, 1983.

34. Bello, T. R.: Surgical removal of a dentigerous cyst from a horse. Southwest. Vet. 21:152, 1962.

35. Bendixen, H. J., and Friis, N. F.: Die haut leukose bei rindern in danemark. Wien. Tierarztl. Monatschr. 52:496, 1965.

36. Bendixen, H. J.: Bovine enzootic leukosis. Adv. Vet. Sci. 10:129, 1965.

37. Berkelhammer, J., et al.: Growth and spontaneous regression of swine melanoma: Relation of in vitro leukocyte reactivity. J. Natl. Cancer Inst. 68:461, 1982.

38. Berkelhammer, J., et al.: Adaptation of Sinclair swine melanoma cells to long-term growth in vitro. Cancer Res. 39:2960, 1979.

39. Berkelhammer, J., et al.: Correlation of in vitro lymphocyte reactivity with in vivo swine melanoma growth and regression. Am. Assoc. Cancer Res. Abst. 318, 1981.

40. Bertone, A. L., et al.: Effect of wound location and the use of topical collagen gel on exuberant granulation tissue formation and wound healing in the horse and pony. Am. J. Vet. Res. 46:1438, 1985.

41. Binninger, C. E., and Piper, R. C.: Hyperplastic dermatitis of the equine ear. JAVMA 153:69, 1968.

42. Black, P. H., et al.: Transformation of bovine tissue–culture cells by bovine papilloma virus. Nature 199:1016, 1963.

43. Blackwell, J. G.: Unusual adipose tissue growth in a colt. JAVMA 161:1141, 1972.

44. Blackwell, R. L., et al.: Age incidence and heritability of cancer eye in Hereford cattle. J. Anim. Sci. 15:943, 1956.

45. Bliss, E. L., and Iverson, W. D.: Mastocytoma in the dairy cow: Two case reports. Vet. Med. Small Anim. Clin. 76:79, 1981.

46. Blood, D. C., et al.: *Veterinary Medicine VI.* Philadelphia, Lea & Febiger, 1983.

47. Boiron, M., et al.: Some properties of bovine papilloma virus. Nature 201:423, 1964.

48. Bosse, K., and Christophers, B.: Beitrag zur epidemiologie der warzen. Hautarzt 15:80, 1964.

49. Bostock, D. E., and Owen, L. H. N.: *A Color Atlas of Neoplasia in the Cat, Dog and Horse.* Chicago, Year Book Medical Publishers, Inc., 1975.

50. Brandly, P. J., and Migaki, G.: Types of tumours found by federal meat inspectors in an eight-year survey. Ann. N.Y. Acad. Sci. 108:872, 1963.

51. Bridges, C. H.: Dermatological conditions in equidae. Proc. Am. Assoc. Equine Pract. 9:147, 1963.

52. Bristol, D. G., and Fubini, S. L.: External lipomas in three horses. JAVMA 185:791, 1984.

53. British Equine Veterinary Association Survey of Equine Diseases. Vet. Rec. 77:528, 1965.

54. Brobst, D., and Hinsman, E. J.: Electron microscopy of bovine cutaneous papilloma. Pathol. Vet. 3:196, 1966.

55. Brostrum, H., et al.: Cell-mediated immunity in horses with sarcoid cells in vitro. Am. J. Vet. Res. 40:1701, 1979.

56. Brown, M. P.: Surgical treatment of equine sarcoid. *In:* Robinson, N. E. (ed.): *Current Therapy in Equine Medicine.* Philadelphia, W. B. Saunders Co., 1983, p. 537.

57. Bundza, A., and Dukes, T. W.: Porcine cutaneous and systemic mastocytosis. Vet. Pathol. 19:453, 1982.

58. Burdin, M. L.: Squamous-cell carcinoma of the vulva of cattle in Kenya. Res. Vet. Sci. 5:497, 1964.

59. Burggraaf, H.: Kanker aan de basis van de hoorns bij zebus. Tijdschr. Diergeneeskd. 62:1121, 1935.

60. Bwangamoi, O.: Tumors of domestic animals in Uganda. Vet. Rec. 81:525, 1967.

61. Cadeac, C.: Sur la transmission expérimentales des papillomas des diverses espèces. Bull. Soc. Sci. Vet. Lyon 4:333, 1901.

62. Cameron, R. D. A.: *Skin Diseases of the Pig.* Sydney, University of Sydney Post-Graduate Foundation in Veterinary Science, Veterinary Review No. 23, 1984.

63. Campo, M. S., et al.: Molecular heterogeneity and lesion site specificity of cutaneous bovine papillomaviruses. Virology 113:323, 1981.

64. Carne, H. R., et al.: Squamous cell carcinoma associated with cysts in the skin in Merino sheep. J. Pathol. Bacteriol. 86:305, 1963.

65. Cannon, S. R. L., and Loh, H.: Treatment of a cavernous haemangioma-like lesion in a polo pony. Equine Vet. J. 14:254, 1982.

66. Case, M. T.: Malignant melanoma in a pig. JAVMA 144:1129, 1964.

67. Catcott, E. J., et al.: *Equine Medicine and Surgery II.* Santa Barbara, CA, American Veterinary Publications, 1972.

68. Caylor, H. D., and Schlotthauer, C. F.: Melano-epitheliomas of swine: Transplantation and culture experiments. Arch. Pathol. 2:343, 1926.

69. Cameron, R. D. A.: Skin diseases of the pig. Proc. Univ. Sydney Post-Grad. Comm. Vet. Sci. 56:445, 1981.
70. Cheevers, W. P., et al.: Isolation of a retrovirus from cultured equine sarcoid tumor cells. Am. J. Vet. Res. 43:804, 1982.
71. Cheevers, W. P., et al.: Spontaneous expression of an endogenous retrovirus by the equine sarcoid-derived MC-1 cell line. Am. J. Vet. Res. 47:50, 1986.
72. Cheville, N. F.: Studies on connective tissue tumors in the hamster produced by bovine papilloma virus. Cancer Res. 26:2334, 1966.
73. Cheville, N. F., and Olson, C.: Epithelial and fibroblastic proliferation in bovine papillomatosis. Pathol. Vet. 1:248, 1964.
74. Cheville, N. F., et al.: Generalized equine cutaneous mastocytosis. Vet. Pathol. 9:394, 1972.
75. Chevrel, M. L., et al.: Le lymphosarcomeporcin. Rec. Med. Vet. 145:135, 1969.
76. Chvapil, M., et al.: Dynamics of the healing of skin wounds on the horse as compared with the rat. Exp. Mol. Pathol. 30:349, 1979.
77. Clarenburg, A.: Haemangioma cavernosum (cysticum) in der subkutis bei einem schwein. Dtsch. Tierärztl. Wochenschr. 40:814, 1932.
78. Claussen, C.: Multiple Sarkome in der haut einen schweines. Dtsch. Tierärztl. Wochenschr. 48:401, 1940.
79. Cleaver, J. E., et al.: Ocular squamous cell carcinoma (cancer eye) in Hereford cattle: Radiation repair processes and a comparison of cultured cells with xeroderma pigmentosum in man. Am. J. Vet. Res. 33:1131, 1979.
80. Cohrs, P.: Lehrbuch der speziellea pathologischen Anatomie der Haustiere IV. Stuttgart, Gustav Fischer Verlag, 1962.
81. Communal, R.: Anomalies folliculaires cutanées chez le mouton. Bull. Acad. Vet. Fr. 26:471, 1953.
82. Cook, R. H., and Olson, C.: Experimental transmission of cutaneous papillomas of the horse. Am. J. Pathol. 27:1087, 1951.
83. Cordes, D. O., and Shortridge, E. H.: Neoplasms of sheep. N.Z. Vet. J. 19:55, 1971.
84. Cotchin, E.: A general survey of tumours in the horse. Equine Vet. J. 9:16, 1977.
85. Cotchin, E.: Neoplasms of the Domesticated Mammals. England, Commonwealth Agricultural Bureaux, 1956.
86. Cotchin, E., and Swarbrick, O.: Bovine cutaneous angiomatosis: A lesion resembling human "pyogenic granuloma." Vet. Rec. 75:437, 1963.
87. Cotchin, E.: Tumours of farm animals. Vet. Rec. 72:816, 1960.
88. Cotchin, E., and Baker-Smith, J.: Tumours in horses encountered in an abattoir survey. Vet. Rec. 97:339, 1975.
89. Craig, D. R., et al.: Lymphosarcoma in goats. Compend. Cont. Educ. 8:S190, 198.
90. Crawshaw, H. A.: Further observations upon the use of "anthiomaline" in the treatment of multiple papillomata in the bovine. Vet. Rec. 64:596, 1952.
91. Creech, G. T.: Experimental studies of the etiology of common warts of cattle. J. Agric. Res. 39:723, 1929.
92. Crowell, W. A., et al.: Melanoma in cattle: Fine structure and a report of two cases. Am. J. Vet. Res. 34:1591, 1975.
93. Curasson, M. G.: Le cancer cutané de la chèvre Angora. Bull. Acad. Vet. Fr. 6:346, 1933.
94. Damodaran, S., and Parthasarathy, K. R.: Neoplasms of goats and sheep. Indian Vet. J. 49:649, 1972.
95. Damaradaran, S., and Ramachandran, P. V.: A survey of neoplasms of Equidae. Indian Vet. J. 52:531, 1975.
96. Danks, A. G., and Olafson, P.: Giant-cell sarcoma. Cornell Vet. 29:68, 1939.
97. Davis, C. L., and Kemper, H. E.: Common warts (papillomata) in goats. JAVMA 88:175, 1936.
98. Davis, C. L., et al.: Neoplasms encountered in federally inspected establishments in Denver, Colorado. JAVMA 83:229, 1933.
99. Dennis, M. W., et al.: Autotransplantation of bovine ocular squamous cell carcinoma and effects on primary tumor growth. Am. J. Vet. Res. 45:1225, 1984.
100. Dixon, R. J., et al.: An immunological classification of ovine lymphomas. J. Comp. Pathol. 94:107, 1984.
101. Dixon, R. T.: Radiation therapy in horses. Aust. Vet. J. 43:508, 1967.
102. Dixon, R. T.: Results of Radon[222] gamma radiation therapy in an equine practice. Aust. Vet. J. 48:279, 1972.
103. Donovan, C. A.: DMSO and bovine warts: A practitioner's experience. Vet. Med. Small Anim. Clin. 78:1278, 1983.
104. Donovan, C. A.: Bovine warts: Treatment with DMSO is justified. Vet. Med. Small Anim. Clin. 78:1813, 1983.
105. Dopson, L. C., et al.: Immunosuppression associated with lymphosarcoma in two horses. JAVMA 182:1239, 1983.
105a. Doran, R. E., et al.: Mastocytoma in a horse. Equine Vet. J. 18:500, 1986.
106. Doughty, F. R.: Virus particles in a bovine neurofibroma. Aust. Vet. J. 48:365, 1972.
107. Dozsa, L., and Weiss, R.: Multiple fibroblastic tumor in a two-month-old calf. Cornell Vet. 61:705, 1971.
107a. Dubath, M. L.: Recherche d'association entre le systeme ELA et une predisposition aux sarcoides equins. Schweiz. Arch. Tierheilkd. 129:41, 1987.
108. Dukes, T. W., et al.: Bovine neoplasms encountered in Canadian slaughterhouses: A summary. Can. Vet. J. 23:28, 1982.
109. Duncan, J. R., et al.: Persistent papillomatosis associated with immunodeficiency. Cornell Vet. 65:205, 1975.
110. Dunne, H. W., et al.: Diseases of Swine IV. Ames, Iowa State University Press, 1975.
111. Dutt, B., et al.: Note on the occurrence of squamous cell carcinoma in a goat. Indian Vet. J. 49:433, 1972.
112. Dwiredy, J. N.: Squamous cell carcinoma in a goat. Indian Vet. J. 46:124, 1969.
113. Elkins, A. D., and Walter, P. A.: Managing a dentigerous cyst in a Hackney pony. Vet. Med. 79:1294, 1984.
114. El Shazly, M. O., et al.: Enzyme-linked immunosorbent assay for the detection of bovine papillomavirus. Am. J. Vet. Res. 46:1737, 1985.
115. England, J. J., et al.: Virus-like particles in an equine sarcoid cell line. Am. J. Vet. Res. 34:1601, 1973.
116. Epstein, B.: Isolation of bovine rhinotracheitis virus from ocular squamous cell carcinoma of cattle. Rev. Med. Vet. 53:105, 1972.
117. Farris, H., et al.: Cryosurgery of equine cutaneous neoplastic and non-neoplastic lesions. Proc. Am. Assoc. Equine Pract. 21:177, 1975.
118. Farris, H., et al.: Cryotherapy of equine sarcoid and other lesions. Vet. Med. Small Anim. Clin. 71:325, 1976.
119. Farris, H., and Fraunfelder, F. T.: Cryosurgical treatment of ocular squamous cell carcinoma of cattle. JAVMA 168:213, 1976.
120. Fatemi-Nainie, S., et al.: Identification of a transforming retrovirus from cultured equine dermal fibrosarcoma. Virology 120:490, 1982.
121. Fatemi-Nainie, S., et al.: Cultural characteristics and tumorigenicity of the equine sarcoid-derived MC-1 cell line. Am. J. Vet. Res. 45:1105, 1984.
122. Favre, M., et al.: Hemagglutinating activity of bovine papillomavirus. Virology 60:572, 1974.
123. Feldman, W. H.: Neoplasms of Domesticated Animals. Philadelphia, W. B. Saunders Co., 1932.
124. Ferner, J. F.: Bovine lymphosarcoma. Adv. Vet. Sci. Comp. Med. 24:1, 1980.
125. Ficken, M. D., et al.: Papilloma–squamous cell carcinoma of the udder of a Saanen goat. JAVMA 183:467, 1983.
126. Fisher, L. F., and Olander, H. J.: Spontaneous neoplasms of pigs. A study of 31 cases. J. Comp. Pathol. 88:505, 1978.
127. Flatt, R. E., et al.: Pathogenesis of benign cutaneous melanomas in miniature swine. JAVMA 153:936, 1968.
128. Flatt, R. E., et al.: Melanotic lesions in the internal organs of miniature swine. Arch. Pathol. 93:71, 1972.
129. Fleming, D. D.: BDG therapy for equine sarcoid. In: Robinson, N. E. (ed.): Current Therapy in Equine Medicine. Philadelphia, W. B. Saunders Co., 1983, p. 539.
130. Ford, G. H., et al.: Giant cell tumor of soft parts: A report of an equine and a feline case. Vet. Pathol. 12:428, 1975.
131. Ford, J. N., et al.: Evidence for papillomaviruses in ocular lesions in cattle. Rev. Vet. Sci. 32:257, 1982.

132. Frank, E. R.: *Veterinary Surgery Notes*. Minneapolis, Burgess Publishing Co., 1947.
133. Fraunfelder, H. C., et al.: ^{90}Sr for treatment of periocular squamous cell carcinoma in the horse. JAVMA 180:307, 1982.
134. French, G. T.: A clinical and genetic study of eye cancer in Hereford cattle. J. Anim. Sci. 9:578, 1959.
135. Frenz, K.: Ausgedehnte Papillomatose in einem Jungrinderbestand. Dtsch. Tierarztl. Wochenschr. 49:158, 1941.
136. Frese, K.: Mastzelkutumoren beim Pferd. Berl. Munch. Tierarztl. Wochenschr. 18:342, 1969.
137. Fretz, P. B., and Barber, S. M.: Prospective analysis of cryosurgery as the sole treatment for equine sarcoids. Vet. Clin. North Am. Small Anim. Clin. 10:847, 1980.
138. Fretz, P. B., et al.: Treatment of exuberant granulation tissue in the horse: Evaluation of four methods. Vet. Surg. 12:137, 1983.
139. Frost, J. N., and Danks, A. G.: Papillomas in a heifer. Cornell Vet. 29:73, 1939.
140. Fubini, S. L., and Campbell, S. G.: External lumps on sheep and goats. Vet. Clin. North Am. Large Anim. Pract. 5:457, 1983.
141. Fujimoto, Y., and Olson, C.: The fine structure of the bovine wart. Pathol. Vet. 3:659, 1966.
142. Fulton, R. E., et al.: The fine structure of equine papillomas and equine papilloma virus. J. Ultrastruct. Res. 30:328, 1970.
143. Gamlem, T., and Crawford, T. B.: Dermoid cysts in identical locations in a doe goat and her kid. Vet. Med. Small Anim. Clin. 72:616, 1977.
144. Garma-Avina, A., et al.: Cutaneous melanomas in domestic animals. J. Cutan. Pathol. 8:3, 1981.
145. Garma-Avina, A., et al.: Equine congenital papillomatosis: A report of five cases. Equine Vet. J. 13:59, 1981.
146. Garma-Avina, A., and Rendon-Fernandez, H.: Giant papilloma on a heifer. Vet. Med. Small Anim. Clin. 77:1530, 1982.
147. Garma-Avina, A., and Valli, V. E.: Mixed sweat gland tumor in a bull (a case report). Vet. Med. Small Anim. Clin. 76:557, 1981.
148. Gaus, O.: Leukose des Gesauges beim Schwein. Dtsch. Tierarztl. Wochenschr. 47:340, 1939.
149. Gavin, P. R., and Gillette, E. L.: Interstitial radiation therapy of equine squamous cell carcinoma. Am. Vet. Radiol. Soc. J. 19:138, 1978.
150. Gebhart, W., and Neibauer, G. W.: Beziehungen Zwischen Pigmenschward und Melanomatose am Beispeil des Lippiozanerschimmels. Arch. Dermatol. Forsch. 259:29, 1977.
151. Genetzky, R. M., et al.: Equine sarcoids: Causes, diagnosis, and treatment. Compend. Cont. Educ. 5:S416, 1983.
152. Gibbs, E. P. J., et al.: Identification of a papilloma virus and transmission of infection to sheep. J. Comp. Pathol. 85:327, 1975.
153. Gillette, E. L., and Carlson, W. D.: An evaluation of radiation therapy in veterinary medicine. Am. Vet. Radiol. Soc. J. 5:58, 1964.
154. Gillis, M. F.: Lymphosarcoma in a mare. Vet. Med. Small Anim. Clin. 60:609, 1966.
155. Gimbo, A.: [Horn base tumours in a cow and a goat]. Nuova Vet. 39:105, 1963.
156. Gordon, D. E., and Olson, C.: Meningiomas and fibroblastic neoplasia in calves induced with the bovine papillomavirus. Cancer Res. 28:2423, 1968.
157. Gordon, L. R.: The cytology and histology of epidermal inclusion cysts in the horse. J. Equine Med. Surg. 2:371, 1978.
158. Gorham, S., and Robl, M.: Melanoma in the gray horse: The darker side of equine aging. Vet. Med. 81:446, 1986.
159. Gorman, N. T.: Equine sarcoid—time for optimism. Equine Vet. J. 17:412, 1985.
160. Grant, B., and Lincoln, S.: Melanosarcoma as a cause of lameness in a horse. Vet. Med. Small Anim. Clin. 67:995, 1972.
161. Greene, J. J., et al.: Melanosarcoma of the spinal cord in a piglet. Irish Vet. J. 27:108, 1973.
162. Grenier, R., et al.: Les verrues animales sont-elles vraiment inoffensives pour l'homme? Vie Med. Can. Fr. 5:263, 1976.
163. Grier, R. L., et al.: Treatment of bovine and equine ocular squamous cell carcinoma by radiofrequency hyperthermia. JAVMA 177:55, 1980.
164. Groth, A. H., et al.: Bovine mastocytoma—a case report. JAVMA 137:241, 1960.
165. Grunder, H. D.: Sammelreferat: Die Tierpapillomatosen. Dtsch. Tierarztl. Wochenschr. 66:159, 1959.
166. Guilbert, H. R., et al.: Observations on pigmentation of eyelids of Hereford cattle in relation to occurrence of ocular epitheliomas. J. Anim. Sci. 7:426, 1948.
167. Gunson, D. E.: Collagen in normal and abnormal tissues. Equine Vet. J. 11:97, 1979.
168. Gupta, B. N., et al.: Cutaneous involvement of malignant lymphoma in a horse. Cornell Vet. 62:205, 1972.
169. Hadwen, S.: The melanomata of grey and white horses. Can. Med. Assoc. J. 25:519, 1931.
170. Hamilton, D. P., and Byerly, C. S.: Congenital malignant melanoma in a foal. JAVMA 164:1040, 1974.
171. Hamir, A. N., and Parry, O. B.: An abattoir study of bovine neoplasms with particular reference to ocular squamous cell carcinoma in Canada. Vet. Rec. 106:551, 1980.
172. Hamir, A. N., et al.: An immunopathological study of bovine ocular squamous cell carcinoma. J. Comp. Pathol. 90:535, 1980.
173. Hargis, A. M., and McElwain, T. F.: Vascular neoplasia in the skin of horses. JAVMA 184:1121, 1984.
174. Hargis, A. M.: A review of solar-induced lesions in domestic animals. Compend. Cont. Educ. 4:287, 1981.
175. Harmon, K. S.: A case of equine sarcoid. Cornell Vet. 39:432, 1949.
176. Hawkins, C. D., et al.: Attempted immunotherapy and auto transplantation of bovine vulvar squamous cell carcinoma. Aust. Vet. J. 55:604, 1979.
177. Hayes, H. M., et al.: Occurrence of nerve tissue tumors in cattle, horses, cats, and dogs. Intl. J. Cancer 15:39, 1975.
178. Head, K. W.: Skin diseases: Neoplastic disease. Vet. Rec. 65:926, 1953.
179. Head, K. W.: Cutaneous mast-cell tumours in the dog, cat and ox. Br. J. Dermatol. 70:389, 1958.
180. Head, K. W.: Some data concerning the distribution of skin tumours in domestic animals. *In*: Rook, A. J., and Walton, G. S.: *Comparative Pathology and Physiology of the Skin.* Oxford, Blackwell Scientific Publications, 1965, p. 615.
181. Heeney, J. L., and Valli, V. E. O.: Bovine ocular squamous cell carcinoma: An epidemiological perspective. Can. J. Comp. Med. 49:21, 1985.
181a. Henry, E. T., et al.: Rectal transmission of bovine leukemia virus in cattle and sheep. Am. J. Vet. Res. 48:634, 1987.
182. Herrmann, H. J., and Prietz, G.: Zur karzinomatosen entdifferenzievung der dermatitis solaris chronica des rindes. Monat. Vet. Med. 21:826, 1966.
183. Herzog, A., and Hoffmann, W.: Hautleukose beim einem jungbullen vom typ des reticulosarkoms. Dtsch. Tierarztl. Wochenschr. 74:491, 1967.
184. Hewlett, K.: Cancer of the horn-core of cattle. J. Comp. Pathol. Ther. 18:161, 1905.
185. Hilbert, B. J., et al.: Cryotherapy of periocular squamous cell carcinoma in the horse. JAVMA 170:1305, 1977.
186. Hilmas, D. E., and Gillette, E. L.: Radiotherapy of spontaneous fibrous connective-tissue sarcomas in animals. J. Natl. Cancer Inst. 56:365, 1976.
187. Hjerpe, C. A., and Theilen, G. H.: Malignant melanomas in porcine littermates. JAVMA 144:1129, 1964.
188. Hod, I., and Perk, K.: Intranuclear microspherules in bovine ocular squamous cell carcinoma. Refuah Vet. 30:41, 1973.
189. Hoffman, D., et al.: Immunotherapy of bovine ocular squamous cell carcinoma with phenol-saline extracts with allogeneic carcinomas. Aust. Vet. J. 57:159, 1981.
190. Hoffman, D., et al.: Autografting and allografting of bovine ocular squamous cell carcinoma. Res. Vet. Sci. 31:48, 1981.
191. Hoffman, K. D., et al.: Radio-frequency current induced hyperthermia for the treatment of equine sarcoid. Equine Pract. 5:24, 1983.
192. Hook, R. R., et al.: Melanoma: Sinclair swine melanoma. Am. J. Pathol. 108:130, 1982.
193. Hook, R. R., et al.: The biopsy of cutaneous exophytic

melanomas in Sinclair miniature swine. Am. Assoc. Cancer Res. 18:46, 1977.

194. Hook, R. R., et al.: Cell-mediated immune reactivity of Sinclair melanoma-bearing swine to 3 mm KCl extracts of swine and human melanoma. Intl. J. Cancer 31:633, 1983.

195. Hook, R. R., et al.: Influence of selective breeding in the incidence of melanomas in Sinclair miniature swine. Intl. J. Cancer 24:668, 1979.

196. Hopes, R.: Skin diseases in horses. Vet. Dermatol. News. 1:4, 1976.

197. Horbright, M. B., et al.: Equine lymphosarcoma. Compend. Cont. Educ. 5:53, 1983.

198. Hordinsky, M. K., et al.: Inheritance of melanocytic tumors in Duroc swine. J. Hered. 76:385, 1985.

199. Horvath, Z., et al.: A case of cutaneous leukosis in Hungary. Acta Vet. Acad. Sci. Hung. 26:131, 1976.

200. Howard, J. L. (ed.): *Current Veterinary Therapy. Food Animal Practice.* Philadelphia, W. B. Saunders Co., 1986.

201. Howard, J. L. (ed.): *Current Veterinary Therapy. Food Animal Practice II.* Philadelphia, W. B. Saunders Co., 1986.

202. Houck, R. A.: Bovine papillomatosis. Vet. Bull. 35:475, 1965.

203. House, P. D., et al.: Cryogenic and immunotherapeutic treatment of myxoma in the horse. Can. Vet. J. 17:216, 1976.

204. Hua, L. C.: Haemangioendotheliomata in a herd of pure-bred middle white swine. J. Malay. Vet. Med. Assoc. 2:164, 1957.

205. Hugoson, G.: A case of congenital skin leukosis in a calf. Zbl. Vet. Med. B 13:748, 1966.

206. Hunt, E.: Infectious skin diseases of cattle. Vet. Clin. North Am. Large Anim. Pract. 6:155, 1984.

207. Huston, R., et al.: Congenital defects in foals. J. Equine Med. Surg. 1:146, 1977.

208. Huston, R., et al.: Congenital defects in pigs. Vet. Bull. 48:645, 1978.

209. Hutchins, D. R.: Skin diseases of cattle and horses in New South Wales. N.Z. Vet. J. 8:85, 1960.

210. Ihrke, P. J., et al.: Fibromatosis in a horse. JAVMA 183:1100, 1983.

211. Ingmire, C. U.: Carcinoma in the vulva of a cow. Vet. Med. 42:427, 1947.

212. Ivascu, I., et al.: Clinical and pathological observations on five cases of equine sarcoidosis identified in Romania. Zbl. Vet. Med. A 21:815, 1974.

213. Jabara, A. G., et al.: A congenital vascular naevus in a foal. Aust. Vet. J. 61:286, 1984.

214. Jackson, C.: The incidence and pathology of tumours of domesticated animals in South Africa. Onderstepoort J. Vet. Res. Anim. Sci. Ind. 6:3, 1936.

215. Jacobs, K. A., et al.: Comparative aspects of the healing of excisional wounds on the leg and body of horses. Vet. Surg. 13:83, 1984.

216. James, C. K., et al.: Report on five ovine neoplasms. Ceylon Vet. 15:138, 1967.

217. James, V. S.: A family tendency to equine sarcoids. Southwest. Vet. 21:235, 1968.

218. Jayasekara, U., and Leipold, H. W.: Congenital melanomas in swine. Bovine Pract. 2:25, 1981.

219. Jennings, P. A., et al.: Tumor-associated immunity in bovine ocular squamous cell carcinoma detected by leukocyte adherence inhibition microassay. J. Natl. Cancer Inst. 63:775, 1979.

220. Jensen, A. B., et al.: Immunologic relatedness of papillomaviruses from different species. J. Natl. Cancer Inst. 64:495, 1980.

221. Jensen, R., and Mackey, D. R.: *Diseases of Feedlot Cattle III.* Philadelphia, Lea & Febiger, 1979.

222. Johnstone, A. C., and Manktelow, B. W.: The pathology of spontaneously occurring malignant lymphoma in sheep. Vet. Pathol. 15:301, 1978.

223. Jones, D. H., and Amoss, M. S.: Cell-mediated immunity response in miniature Sinclair swine bearing cutaneous melanomas. Can. J. Comp. Med. 46:209, 1982.

224. Jones, S. A., and Strafuss, A. C.: Scanning electron microscopy of nerve sheath neoplasms. Am. J. Vet. Res. 39:1069, 1978.

225. Joyce, J. R.: Cryosurgery for removal of equine sarcoids. Vet. Med. Small Anim. Clin. 70:200, 1975.

226. Joyce, J. R.: Cryosurgical treatment of tumors of horses and cattle. JAVMA 168:226, 1976.

227. Jun, M. H., et al.: Enhancement and metastasis after immunotherapy of ovine squamous-cell carcinoma. Br. J. Cancer 38:382, 1978.

228. Jun, M. H., and Johnson, R. H.: Effect of cyclophosphamide on tumour growth and cell-mediated immunity in sheep and ovine squamous cell carcinoma. Res. Vet. Sci. 27:155, 1979.

229. Jun, M. H., et al.: In vitro response of lymphocytes of normal and ovine squamous cell carcinoma–bearing sheep to phytomitogens and tumour extracts. Res. Vet. Sci. 27:144, 1979.

230. Jun, M. H., and Johnson, R. H.: Effect of removal of ovine squamous cell carcinoma on peripheral lymphocyte stimulation by tumour extracts and phyto-hemagglutinin. Res. Vet. Sci. 27:149, 1979.

231. Jun, M. H., and Johnson, R. H.: Suppression of blastogenic response of peripheral lymphocytes by serum from ovine squamous cell carcinoma–bearing sheep. Res. Vet. Sci. 27:161, 1979.

232. Junge, R. E., et al.: Papillomas and squamous cell carcinomas of horses. JAVMA 185:656, 1984.

233. Kahrs, R. F.: *Viral Diseases of Cattle.* Ames, Iowa State University Press, 1981.

234. Kainer, R. A., et al.: Hyperthermia for treatment of ocular squamous cell tumors in cattle. JAVMA 176:356, 1980.

235. Kenney, J. E.: Some observations on bovine neoplasia. Vet. Rec. 56:149, 1944.

236. Kerr, K. M., and Alden, C. L.: Equine neoplasia—a ten-year survey. Proc. Am. Assoc. Vet. Lab. Diagn. 17:183, 1974.

237. Kirkbride, C. A., et al.: Hemangioma of a bovine fetus with a chorioangioma of the placenta. Vet. Pathol. 10:238, 1973.

238. Kirker-Head, C. A., et al.: Pelvic limb lameness due to malignant melanoma in a horse. JAVMA 186:1215, 1985.

239. Kleinschuster, S. J., et al.: Regression of bovine ocular carcinoma by treatment with a mycobacterial vaccine. J. Natl. Cancer Inst. 58:1807, 1977.

240. Koller, L. D., and Olson, C.: Attempted transmission of warts from man, cattle, and horse and of deer fibroma to selected hosts. J. Invest. Dermatol. 58:366, 1972.

241. Koller, L. D., et al.: Quantitation of bovine papilloma virus and serum antibody by immunodiffusion. Am. J. Vet. Res. 35:121, 1974.

242. Kopecky, K. E., et al.: Biological effects of ultraviolet radiation on cattle: Bovine ocular squamous cell carcinoma. Am. J. Vet. Res. 40:1783, 1979.

243. Krafft, H.: Ein seltener fall von diffuses hautpapillomatose beim schwein. Monat. Vet. Med. 12:415, 1957.

244. Krahwinkel, D. J., et al.: Cryosurgical treatment of cancerous and noncancerous diseases of dogs, horses, and cats. JAVMA 169:201, 1976.

245. Kral, F., and Schwartzman, R. M.: *Veterinary and Comparative Dermatology.* Philadelphia, Lea & Febiger, 1964.

246. Kulkarni, H. V.: Carcinoma of the horn in bovines of the old Baroda state. Indian Vet. J. 29:415, 1953.

247. Kulkarni, P. E., and Marudwar, S. S.: Unusual location of mammary glands in the vulva lips of she-goats. Vet. Rec. 90:385, 1972.

248. Kunze, D. J., et al.: Malignant melanoma of the coronary band in a horse. JAVMA 188:297, 1986.

249. Ladds, P. W., and Entwistle, K. W.: Observations on squamous cell carcinoma of sheep in Queensland, Australia. Br. J. Cancer 35:410, 1977.

250. Ladds, P. W., and Daniels, P. W.: Ovine squamous cell carcinoma. Am. J. Pathol. 107:122, 1982.

251. Lall, H. K.: Incidence of horn cancer in Meerat Circle, Uttar Pradesh. Indian Vet. J. 30:205, 1953.

252. Lancaster, W. D., et al.: Bovine papilloma virus: Presence of virus-specific DNA sequences in naturally occurring equine tumors. Proc. Natl. Acad. Sci. 74:524, 1977.

253. Lancaster, W. D.: Physical maps of bovine papillomavirus type 1 and type 2 genomes. J. Virol. 32:684, 1979.

254. Lancaster, W. D., and Olson, C.: Demonstration of two

distinct classes of bovine papillomavirus. Virology 89:372, 1978.

255. Lancaster, W. D., and Olson, C.: Animal papillomaviruses. Microbiol. Rev. 46:191, 1982.

256. Lancaster, W. D., et al.: Hybridisation of bovine papillomavirus type 1 and type 2 DNA from virus-induced hamster tumours and naturally occurring equine tumours. Intervirology 11:227, 1979.

257. Lancaster, W. D., and Olson, C.: State of bovine papillomavirus DNA in connective-tissue tumours. *In* Essex, M., et al. (eds.): *Viruses in Naturally Occurring Cancers.* Cold Spring Harbor, Cold Spring Harbor Lab., 1980, p. 223.

258. Lancaster, W. D.: Apparent lack of integration of bovine papillomavirus DNA in virus-induced equine and bovine tumour cells and virus-transformed mouse cells. Virology 180:251, 1981.

259. Lane, J. G.: The treatment of equine sarcoids by cryosurgery. Equine Vet. J. 9:127, 1977.

260. Lanfranchi, A., and Seren, E.: Ricerche su la trasmissione sperimentale e su la immunizzazione nella papillomatosi cutanea dei bovini. Nuova Vet. 16:32, 1938.

261. Lapin, D. R., et al.: Malignant melanoma in a steer. Vet. Med. Small Anim. Clin. 78:587, 1983.

262. Lavach, J. D., and Severin, G. A.: Neoplasia of the equine eye, adnexa, and orbit: A review of 68 cases. JAVMA 170:202, 1977.

263. Lavach, J. D., et al.: BCG treatment of periocular sarcoid. Equine Vet. J. 17:445, 1985.

264. Lazary, S., et al.: Equine leukocyte antigens in sarcoid-affected horses. Equine Vet. J. 17:283, 1985.

265. Lee, C. H.: Haemangioendotheliomata in a herd of pure-bred middle white swine. J. Malay. Vet. Med. Assoc. 1:164, 1957.

266. Lee, K. P., and Olson, C.: Response of calves to intravenous and repeated intradermal inoculation of bovine papillomavirus. Am. J. Vet. Res. 29:2103, 1968.

267. Lee, K. P., and Olson, C.: A gel diffusion precipitin test for bovine papillomavirus. Am. J. Vet. Res. 30:725, 1969.

268. Lee, K. P., and Olson, C.: Precipitin response of cattle to bovine papillomavirus. Cancer Res. 29:1393, 1969.

269. Leman, A. D., et al.: *Diseases of Swine IV.* Ames, Iowa State University Press, 1981.

270. Lerner, A. B., and Case, G. W.: Melanomas in horses. Yale J. Biol. Med. 46:646, 1973.

271. Lever, W. F., and Schaumburg-Lever, G.: *Histopathology of the Skin VI.* Philadelphia, J. B. Lippincott, 1983.

272. Lewis, R. E.: Radon implant therapy of squamous cell carcinoma and equine sarcoid. Proc. Am. Assoc. Equine Pract. 10:217, 1964.

273. Liess, J.: Zur Genese und Behandlung der Papillomatose des Rindes. Dtsch. Tierarztl. Wochenschr. 42:521, 1934.

274. Lindley, W. H.: Malignant verrucae of bulls. Vet. Med. Small Anim. Clin. 69:1548, 1974.

275. Lindsay, G. C., et al.: Ocular squamous cell carcinoma: Immunological responses to tumor tissue and phytomitogens. Res. Vet. Sci. 24:113, 1978.

276. Lindsay, W. A., and Beck, K. A.: Temporal teratoma in a horse. Compend. Cont. Educ. 8:S168, 1986.

277. Linzell, J. L.: Diffuse lymphoid leukosis of the skin in a dairy cow. Vet. Rec. 55:19, 1943.

278. Lloyd, L. C.: Epithelial tumors of the skin of sheep. Br. J. Cancer 15:780, 1961.

279. Lloyd, L. C.: The etiology of cysts in the skin of some families of Merino sheep in Australia. J. Pathol. Bacteriol. 88:219, 1964.

280. Lloyd, S.: Goat medicine and surgery. Br. Vet. J. 138:70, 1982.

281. Lofstedt, J.: Dermatologic diseases of sheep. Vet. Clin. North Am. Large Anim. Pract. 5:427, 1983.

282. Lombard, C., et al.: Adenopapillome de la muqueuse pituitaire chez la chèvre. Bull. Acad. Vet. Fr. 39:199, 1966.

283. Lombard, L., and Levesque, L.: Une affection nouvelle en France: Hemangiomatose cutanée et de la muqueuse pituitaire des vaches normandes. C. R. Acad. Sci. Paris 258:3137, 1964.

284. Lund, L.: Generalisierte Melanosarkomatose beim Schaf. Dtsch. Tierarztl. Wochenschr. 31:561, 1923.

285. Madewell, B. R., et al.: Ultrastructure of canine, feline, and bovine mast cell neoplasms. Am. J. Vet. Res. 45:2066, 1984.

286. Mammerickx, M., et al.: Study on the oral transmission of bovine leukosis to sheep. Vet. Microbiol. 1:347, 1976.

287. Mangrulkar, M. Y.: Melanomata in domesticated animals. Indian J. Vet. Sci. 14:178, 1944.

288. Manning, P. J., et al.: Congenital cutaneous and visceral melanomas of Sinclair miniature swine: Three case reports. J. Natl. Cancer Inst. 52:1559, 1974.

289. Manning, T. O.: Noninfectious skin diseases of cattle. Vet. Clin. North Am. Large Anim. Pract. 6:175, 1984.

290. Manning, T. O., et al.: Caprine dermatology. Part III. Parasitic, allergic, hormonal, and neoplastic disorders. Compend. Cont. Educ. 7:S437, 1985.

291. Maraduar, S. S., et al.: Melanomas in bullocks. Indian Vet. J. 55:667, 1978.

292. Markel, M. D., and Dorr, T. E.: Multiple myeloma in a horse. JAVMA 188:621, 1986.

293. Marshak, R. R., et al.: Observations on a heifer with cutaneous lymphosarcoma. Cancer 19:724, 1966.

294. Martin, W. B.: *Diseases of Sheep.* Oxford, Blackwell Scientific Publications, 1983.

295. Mason, B. J. E.: Temporal teratoma in the horse. Vet. Rec. 95:226, 1974.

296. McCrea, C. T., and Head, K. W.: Sheep tumours in northeast Yorkshire. I. Prevalence on seven moorland farms. Br. Vet. J. 134:456, 1978.

297. McFadyean, J.: Equine melanomatosis. J. Comp. Pathol. Ther. 38:186, 1933.

298. McGavin, M. D., and Leis, T. J.: Multiple cutaneous mastocytomas in a bull. Aust. Vet. J. 44:20, 1968.

299. McMartin, D. N., and Gruhn, R. F.: Sebaceous carcinoma in a horse. Vet. Pathol. 14:532, 1977.

300. McMullan, W. C.: The skin. *In:* Mansmann, R. A., et al. (eds.): *Equine Medicine & Surgery III.* Santa Barbara, CA, American Veterinary Publications, 1982, p. 789.

301. Medreck, B.: [Malignant fibrosarcoma in the mammary gland of a mare]. Med. Weter. 34:23, 1978.

302. Meischke, H. R. C.: A study of bovine teat papillomatosis. Vet. Rec. 104:28, 1979.

303. Meischke, H. R. C.: Experimental transmission of bovine papillomavirus (BPV) extracted from morphologically distinct teat and cutaneous lesions and the effects of inoculation of BPV-transformed fetal bovine cells. Vet. Rec. 104:360, 1979.

304. Metcalf, J. W.: Improved technique in sarcoid removal. Proc. Am. Assoc. Equine Pract. 17:45, 1971.

305. Migaki, G., and Carey, A. M.: Malignant mastocytoma in a cow. Am. J. Vet. Res. 33:253, 1972.

306. Migaki, G., and Langheinrich, K. A.: Mastocytoma in a pig. Pathol. Vet. 7:353, 1970.

307. Migaki, G., et al.: Prevalence of embryonal nephroma in slaughtered swine. JAVMA 159:441, 1971.

308. Miller, J. M.: Bovine lymphosarcoma. Mod. Vet. Pract. 61:588, 1980.

309. Miller, R.: Treatment of some equine cutaneous neoplasms: A review. Aust. Vet. Pract. 10:119, 1980.

310. Millikan, L. E., et al.: Gross and ultrastructural studies in a new melanoma model: The Sinclair swine. Yale J. Biol. Med. 46:631, 1973.

311. Millikan, L. E., et al.: Melanoma in Sinclair swine: A new animal model. J. Invest. Dermatol. 62:20, 1974.

312. Millikan, L. E., et al.: Animal models in melanoma. *In* Maibach, H. I., and Lowe, N. J. (eds.): *Models in Dermatology.* Vol. 1. Basel, Kanger, 1985, p. 23.

313. Millikan, L. E., et al.: Vitiligo and halo nevus in the Sinclair swine. J. Invest. Dermatol. 70:219, 1978.

314. Misdorp, W.: Tumors in newborn animals. Pathol. Vet. 2:328, 1965.

315. Misdorp, W.: Tumours in large domestic animals in the Netherlands. J. Comp. Pathol. 77:211, 1967.

316. Misra, S. S., et al.: Interdigital myxoma in a Hariana cow. Vet. Med. Small Anim. Clin. 76:381, 1981.

317. Monlux, A. W., and Davis, C. L.: Multiple schwannomas of cattle (nerve sheath tumors; multiple neurilemmomas; neurofibromatosis). Am. J. Vet. Res. 14:499, 1953.

318. Monlux, A. W., et al.: A survey of tumors occurring in cattle, sheep, and swine. Am. J. Vet. Res. 17:646, 1956.

319. Monlux, A. W., et al.: The diagnosis of squamous cell carcinoma of the eye (cancer eye) in cattle. Am. J. Vet. Res. 18:5, 1957.

320. Montes, L. F., et al.: Equine melanoma. J. Cutan. Pathol. 6:234, 1979.

321. Montpellier, J. R., et al.: Greffe d'une tumeur schwannienne chez le mulet. Bull. Acad. Vet. Fr. 12:91, 1939.

322. Mostafa, M. S. E.: A case of malignant melanoma in a bay horse. Br. Vet. J. 109:201, 1953.

323. Moulton, J. E.: *Tumors in Domestic Animals.* Berkeley, University of California Press, 1978.

324. Moulton, J. E.: Cutaneous papillomas on the udder of milk goats. North Am. Vet. 35:29, 1954.

325. Moulton, J. E., et al.: Morphological changes in cells transformed in vitro by bovine papilloma virus. Cornell Vet. 56:427, 1966.

326. Moulton, J. E.: Occurrence and types of tumours in large domestic animals. Ann. N.Y. Acad. Sci. 108:620, 1963.

327. Mugara, G. M.: Study of bovine neoplasms in Kenya. Bull. Epizoot. Dis. Afr. 16:513, 1958.

328. Muller, G. H., et al.: *Small Animal Dermatology III.* Philadelphia, W. B. Saunders Co., 1983.

329. Mullowney, P. C.: Dermatologic diseases of cattle. Part II. Infectious diseases. Compend. Cont. Educ. 4:S3, 1982.

330. Mullowney, P. C.: Dermatologic diseases of cattle. Part III. Environmental, congenital, neoplastic, and allergic diseases. Compend. Cont. Educ. 4:S138, 1982.

331. Mullowney, P. C., and Hall, R. F.: Skin diseases of swine. Vet. Clin. North Am. Large Anim. Pract. 6:107, 1984.

332. Mullowney, P. C., and Baldwin, E. W.: Skin diseases of goats. Vet. Clin. North Am. Large Anim. Pract. 6:143, 1984.

333. Mullowney, P. C., and Fadok, V. A.: Dermatologic diseases of horses. Part II. Bacterial and viral skin diseases. Compend. Cont. Educ. 6:S16, 1984.

334. Mullowney, P. C.: Dermatologic diseases of horses. Part IV. Environmental, congenital, and neoplasia diseases. Compend. Cont. Educ. 7:S22, 1985.

335. Munro, R., et al.: Scrotal haemangiomas in boars. J. Comp. Pathol. 92:109, 1984.

336. Murphy, J. M., et al.: Immunotherapy in ocular equine sarcoid. JAVMA 174:269, 1979.

337. Murray, D. R., et al.: Granulomatous and neoplastic diseases of the skin of horses. Aust. Vet. J. 54:338, 1978.

338. Murray, M.: Neoplasms of domestic animals in East Africa. Br. Vet. J. 124:514, 1968.

339. Mustafa, I. F., et al.: Melanoma in goats. Sudan Med. J. 4:113, 1966.

340. Naik, S. N., et al.: Epidemiology of horn cancer in Indian Zebu cattle: Breed incidence. Br. Vet. J. 125:222, 1969.

341. Nair, K. P. C., and Sastry, G. A.: A survey of neoplasia in the Madras State (bovine). Indian Vet. J. 30:325, 1954.

342. Nakamura, Y., et al.: Tumor of the neck of a Thoroughbred. J. Vet. Med. Tokyo 608:138, 1974.

343. Neufeld, T. L.: Lymphosarcoma in the horse: A review. Can. Vet. J. 14:129, 1973.

344. Neufeld, T. L.: Lymphosarcoma in a mare and review of cases at Ontario Veterinary College. Can. Vet. J. 14:149, 1973.

345. Nieberle, C. P.: *Textbook of Special Pathological Anatomy of Domestic Animals.* New York, Pergamon Press, 1967.

346. Niimi, D.: Patho-histological studies on the characteristic haemangiomata in the scrotum of swine. J. Jpn. Soc. Vet. Sci. 10:31, 1931.

347. Njoku, C. O., and Burwash, W. A.: Congenital cutaneous papilloma in a foal. Cornell Vet. 62:54, 1972.

348. Nobel, T. A., et al.: Neoplasms in domestic mammals in Israel (1959–1969). Refuah Vet. 27:115, 1970.

349. Nobel, T. A., et al.: Neoplasms in domestic mammals in Israel (1969–1979). Refuah Vet. 36:23, 1979.

350. Nooruddin, M., and Das, J. G.: Bovine cutaneous papillomatosis. Agri-Pract. 5:33, 1984.

351. Nordby, J. E.: Congenital melanotic skin tumors in swine. J. Hered. 24:361, 1933.

352. Nyrop, K. A., et al.: Equine cutaneous mastocytoma. Compend. Cont. Educ. 8:757, 1986.

353. O'Connor, J. J.: *Dollar's Veterinary Surgery IV.* London, Baillière, Tindall and Cox, 1950.

354. Olson, C.: Equine sarcoid, a cutaneous neoplasm. Am. J. Vet. Res. 9:333, 1948.

355. Olson, C., and Cook, R. H.: Cutaneous sarcoma-like lesions of the horse caused by the agent of bovine papilloma. Proc. Soc. Exp. Biol. Med. 77:281, 1951.

356. Olson, C., et al.: Transmission of lymphosarcoma from cattle to sheep. J. Natl. Cancer Inst. 45:1463, 1972.

357. Olson, C., and Skidmore, L. V.: Therapy of experimentally produced bovine cutaneous papillomatosis with vaccines and excision. JAVMA 135:339, 1959.

358. Olson, C.: Cutaneous papillomatosis in cattle and other animals. Ann. N.Y. Acad. Sci. 108:1042, 1963.

359. Olson, C., et al.: Induced immunity of skin, vagina and urinary bladder to bovine papillomatosis. Cancer Res. 22:463, 1962.

360. Olson, C., et al.: Cutaneous and penile bovine fibropapillomatosis and its control. JAVMA 153:1189, 1968.

361. Olson, C., et al.: Immunity to bovine cutaneous papillomatosis produced by vaccine homologous to the challenge agent. JAVMA 135:499, 1959.

362. Olson, C., et al.: Further observations on immunity to bovine cutaneous papillomatosis. Am. J. Vet. Res. 21:233, 1960.

363. Olson, C., et al.: Oncogenicity of bovine papilloma virus. Arch. Environ. Health 19:827, 1969.

364. Olson, R. O., et al.: Papillomatosis of the bovine teat (mammary papilla). Am. J. Vet. Res. 43:2250, 1982.

365. Omar, A. R., and Chong, S. N.: Multiple squamous cell carcinoma in the skin of a pig associated with cutaneous microfilariasis. Kajian Vet. 2:202, 1970.

366. Onuma, M., et al.: Tumor-associated antigen and cell surface markers in cells of bovine lymphosarcoma. Ann. Rech. Vet. 9:825, 1978.

367. Onuma, M., et al.: Studies on the sporadic and enzootic forms of bovine leukosis. J. Comp. Pathol. 89:159, 1979.

368. Orkin, M.: Mastocytosis in animals. Arch. Dermatol. 96:381, 1967.

368a. Osame, S., et al.: [Mastocytoma in a cow]. J. Jpn. V.M.A. 39:247, 1986.

369. Oxenhandler, R. W., et al.: Malignant melanoma in the Sinclair miniature swine. Am. J. Pathol. 96:707, 1979.

370. Oz, H. H., et al.: Epidermal inclusion cysts in a cow. JAVMA 187:504, 1985.

371. Oz, H. H., et al.: Follicular cysts in sheep. JAVMA 187:502, 1985.

372. Pachauri, S. P., and Pathak, R. C.: Bovine horn cancer: Therapeutic experiments with autogenous vaccine. Am. J. Vet. Res. 30:475, 1969.

373. Page, E. H., and Tiffany, L. W.: Use of an autogenous equine fibrosarcoma vaccine. JAVMA 150:177, 1967.

374. Page, E. H.: Common skin diseases of the horse. Proc. Am. Assoc. Equine Pract. 18:385, 1972.

375. Pascoe, R. R.: *Equine Dermatoses.* Sydney, University of Sydney Post-Graduate Foundation in Veterinary Science, Veterinary Review No. 14, 1974.

376. Paine, R.: Two cases of carcinoma of the vulva in cows. J. Comp. Pathol. Ther. 22:349, 1899.

377. Panel Report: Dermatologic problems in cattle. Mod. Vet. Pract. 60:172, 1979.

378. Parish, W. E.: A transmissible genital papilloma of the pig resembling condyloma accuminatum of man. J. Pathol. Bacteriol. 81:331, 1961.

379. Parish, W. E.: An immunological study of the transmissible genital papilloma of the pig. J. Pathol. Bacteriol. 83:429, 1962.

380. Parish, W. E., and Done, J. T.: Seven apparently congenital non-infectious conditions of the skin of pigs resembling congenital defects in man. J. Comp. Pathol. 72:286, 1962.

381. Pascoe, R. R.: Infectious skin diseases of horses. Vet. Clin. North Am. Large Anim. Pract. 6:27, 1984.

382. Pascoe, R. R., and Summers, P. M.: Clinical survey of tumors and tumor-like lesions in horses in southeast Queensland. Equine Vet. J. 13:235, 1981.

383. Pascoe, R. R.: *Equine Dermatoses.* Sydney, University of Sydney Post-Graduate Foundation in Veterinary Science, Veterinary Review No. 22, 1981.

384. Pascoe, R. R.: The nature and treatment of skin conditions of horses in Queensland. Aust. Vet. J. 49:35, 1973.

385. Pascoe, R. R.: Conchal fistula in two horses. Aust. Vet. Pract. 11:109, 1981.
386. Paulsen, J., et al.: Comparative studies on ovine and bovine C-type particles. Biblio. Haematol. 43:190, 1976.
387. Pearson, J. K. L., et al.: Tissue vaccines in the treatment of bovine papillomas. Vet. Rec. 70:971, 1958.
387a. Peyton, L. C., and Pattio, N.: Wound care and excessive granulation tissue. *In* Robinson, N. E. (ed.): Current Therapy in Equine Medicine II. Philadelphia, W. B. Saunders Co., 1987, p. 642.
388. Pickens, E. M.: Generalized melanosis in a pig. JAVMA 52:707, 1918.
389. Pfister, H.: Biology and biochemistry of papillomaviruses. Rev. Physiol. Biochem. Pharmacol. 99:111, 1984.
390. Pfister, H., et al.: Partial characterization of a new type of bovine papillomavirus. Virology 96:1, 1979.
391. Pfister, H., et al.: Seroepidemiological studies of bovine papillomavirus infections. J. Natl. Cancer Inst. 62:1423, 1979.
392. Plaut, A., and Kohn-Speyer, A. C.: The carcinogenic action of smegma. Science 105:391, 1947.
393. Plummer, P. J. G.: A survey of six hundred and thirty-six tumours from domesticated animals. Can. J. Comp. Med. 20:239, 1956.
394. Podkonjak, K. R.: Veterinary cryotherapy-1. Vet. Med. Small Anim. Clin. 77:51, 1982.
395. Podkonjak, K. R.: Veterinary cryosurgery-2. Vet. Med. Small Anim. Clin. 77:183, 1982.
396. Prasse, K. W., et al.: Generalized mastocytosis in a foal, resembling urticaria pigmentosa of man. JAVMA 166:68, 1975.
397. Priester, W. A.: Skin tumors in domestic animals. Data from 12 United States and Canadian Colleges of Veterinary Medicine. J. Natl. Cancer Inst. 50:457, 1973.
398. Priester, W. A., and Mantel, N.: Occurrence of tumors in domestic animals. Data from 12 United States and Canadian Colleges of Veterinary Medicine. J. Natl. Cancer Inst. 47:1333, 1971.
399. Ragland, W. L., and Spencer, G. R.: Attempts to relate bovine papilloma virus to the cause of equine sarcoid: Immunity to bovine papilloma virus. Am. J. Vet. Res. 29:1363, 1968.
400. Ragland, W. L.: Attempts to relate bovine papilloma virus to the cause of equine sarcoid. Equidae inoculated intradermally with bovine papilloma virus. Am. J. Vet. Res. 30:743, 1969.
401. Ragland, W. L., et al.: An epizootic of equine sarcoid. Nature 210:1399, 1966.
402. Ragland, W. L., et al.: Equine sarcoid. Equine Vet. J. 2:2, 1970.
403. Ragland, W. L., et al.: Attempts to relate bovine papilloma virus to the cause of equine sarcoid: Horses, donkeys, and calves inoculated with equine sarcoid extracts. Equine Vet. J. 2:168, 1970.
404. Ragland, W. L., et al.: Experimental viral fibromatosis of the equine dermis. Lab. Invest. 14:598, 1965.
405. Ramadan, R. O.: Squamous cell carcinoma in the perineum of the goat. Br. Vet. J. 113:347, 1975.
406. Ramakumar, V., et al.: Resection of the anterior nares in a bullock. Indian Vet. J. 55:583, 1978.
407. Rama Rao, P., et al.: Neurofibrosarcoma in bovines. Indian Vet. J. 47:208, 1970.
408. Rapp, H., et al.: Immunotherapy of experimental cancer as a guide to the treatment of human cancer. Ann. N.Y. Acad. Sci. 276:550, 1976.
409. Rebhun, W. C., et al.: Interdigital papillomatosis in dairy cattle. JAVMA 177:437, 1980.
410. Rebhun, W. C., and Bertone, A.: Equine lymphosarcoma. JAVMA 184:720, 1984.
410a. Rebhun, W. C.: Immunotherapy for sarcoids. *In:* Robinson, N. E. (ed.): Current Therapy in Equine Medicine II. Philadelphia, W. B. Saunders Co., 1987, p. 637.
411. Reed, M. G.: Cutaneous horn on a Hereford cow. Vet. Med. Small Anim. Clin. 70:37, 1975.
412. Reinertson, E. L.: Fibrosarcoma in a horse. Cornell Vet. 64:617, 1974.
413. Render, J. A., et al.: Grant cell tumor of soft parts in six horses. JAVMA 183:790, 1983.
414. Ribi, E., et al.: Immunotherapy of ocular squamous-cell carcinoma in cattle using a mycobacterial biologic. Mod. Vet. Pract. 67:451, 1986.
415. Riggott, J. M., and Quarmby, W. B.: Treatment of fibrosarcoma in a horse. Equine Vet. J. 12:193, 1980.
416. Roberts, D.: Experimental treatment of equine sarcoid. Vet. Med. Small Anim. Clin. 65:67, 1970.
417. Robl, M. G., and Olson, C.: Oncogenic action of bovine papilloma virus in hamsters. Cancer Res. 28:1596, 1968.
418. Rosenberger, G.: Ursache und behandlung der papillomatose des rinds. Dtsch. Tierarztl. Wochenschr. 49:177, 1941.
419. Rosenberger, G., and Grunder, H. D.: Untersuchungen uber die Immunitats bildung und Immunotherapie bei der Papillomatose des Rindes. Dtsch. Tierarztl. Wochenschr. 66:661, 1959.
420. Roth, L., and Perdrizet, J.: Cutaneous histiocytoma in a goat. Cornell Vet. 75:303, 1984.
421. Roudicek, C. E., et al.: Genetics of cancer eye in beef cattle. J. Ariz. Acad. Sci. 10:31, 1975.
421a. Roussel, A. J., et al.: Lymphosarcoma in sheep. Compend. Cont. Educ. 9:F182, 1987.
422. Runnells, R. A., and Benbrook, E. A.: Connective tissue tumors of horses and mules. Am. J. Vet. Res. 2:427, 1941.
423. Runnells, R. A., and Benbrook, E. A.: Epithelial tumors of horses. Am. J. Vet. Res. 3:176, 1942.
424. Russell, W. C., et al.: Incidence and heritability of ocular squamous cell tumors in Hereford cattle. J. Anim. Sci. 43:1156, 1976.
425. Russell, W. C., et al.: Studies on bovine ocular squamous cell carcinoma ("cancer eye"). I. Pathological anatomy and historical review. Cancer 9:1, 1956.
426. Rutgers, H. C., et al.: Huidleukose bij een paard. Tijdschr. Diergeneeskd. 104:511, 1979.
427. Sabrazes, J., and Lafon, C. H.: Granulome de la lèvre a mastzellen et a eosinophiles chez un cheval. Folia Haematol. 6:3, 1908.
428. Sahu, S.: The effectiveness of the advocated methods of treatment of horn cancer in bovine—a report of 27 cases. Indian Vet. J. 45:965, 1968.
429. Sandersleben, J.: [Epithelial tumors of the skin in domestic animals, particularly benign epithelioma]. Berl. Munch. Tierarztl. Wochenschr. 80:285, 1967.
430. Sartin, E. A., and Hodge, T. G.: Congenital hemangioendothelioma in two foals. Vet. Pathol. 19:569, 1982.
431. Sastry, G. A.: Neoplasms of animals in India. Indian Vet. J. 42:332, 1957.
432. Sastry, G. A.: Neoplasms in animals in India. An account of neoplasms collected in 12 years. Vet. Med. 54:428, 1959.
433. Sastry, G. A., and Tweihaus, H. J.: A study of the animal neoplasms in Kansas State. Indian Vet. J. 41:454, 1964.
434. Sastry, G. A., and Tweihaus, H. J.: A study of the animal neoplasms in Kansas State. IV. Others. Indian Vet. J. 42:332, 1965.
435. Scheuler, R. L.: Congenital equine papillomatosis. JAVMA 162:640, 1973.
436. Schulz, K. C. A., and Schutte, J. A.: Multiple acanthoma in the skin of swine. J. S. Afr. Vet. Med. Assoc. 31:437, 1960.
436a. Schumacher, J., et al.: Burn-induced neoplasia in two horses. Equine Vet. J. 18:410, 1986.
437. Schwartzman, S. M., et al.: Immunotherapy of equine sarcoid with cell wall skeleton (CWS)–trehalose dimycolate (TDM) biologic. Equine Pract. 6:13, 1984.
438. Scott, D. W.: Unpublished observations.
439. Scott, D. W., and Hackett, R. P.: Cutaneous hemangioma in a mule. Equine Pract. 5:8, 1983.
440. Scottish Veterinary Inspection Service Report: Eye lesions associated with infectious bovine rhinotracheitis virus infection. Vet. Rec. 104:398, 1983.
441. Segne, D., et al.: Neutralization of bovine papillomavirus with serums from cattle and horses with experimental papillomas. Am. J. Vet. Res. 16:517, 1955.
442. Seiler, R. J., and Punita, I.: Neoplasia of domestic mammals: Review of cases diagnosed at Universiti Pertanian, Malaysia. Kajian Vet. 11:80, 1979.
443. Sheahan, B. J., et al.: Histiolymphocytic lymphosarcoma in the subcutis of two horses. Vet. Pathol. 17:123, 1980.

444. Shokry, M., and Lotfi, M. M.: Malignant perianal melanoma in a horse. Mod. Vet. Pract. 65:226, 1984.

445. Shortridge, E. H., and Cordes, D. O.: Neoplasms in cattle: A survey of 372 neoplasms examined at the Ruakura Veterinary Diagnostic Station. N.Z. Vet. J. 19:5, 1971.

446. Silver, I. A.: Basic physiology of wound healing in the horse. Equine Vet. J. 14:7, 1982.

447. Silver, I. A., and Cater, D. B.: Radiotherapy and chemotherapy for domestic animals. I. Treatment of malignant tumors and benign conditions in the horse. Acta Radiol. 2:226, 1964.

448. Simon, J., and Brewer, R. L.: Multiple neurofibromas in a cow and calf. JAVMA 142:1102, 1963.

449. Sividas, C. G., et al.: Congenital melanoma in a calf: A review and case report. Br. Vet. J. 127:289, 1971.

450. Slanina, L., et al.: Kongenital Neurofibromatose der Haut bei Kalbern. Dtsch. Tierarztl. Wochenschr. 85:41, 1978.

451. Smit, J. D.: Skin lesions in South African domestic animals with specific reference to the incidence and prognosis of various skin tumors. J. S. Afr. Vet. Med. Assoc. 33:363, 1962.

452. Smith, M. C.: Caprine dermatologic problems: A review. JAVMA 178:724, 1981.

453. Smith, M. C.: Dermatologic diseases of goats. Vet. Clin. North Am. Large Anim. Pract. 5:449, 1983.

454. Smithies, L. K., and Olson, C.: Antigen of bovine cutaneous papilloma detected by fluorescent antibodies. Cancer Res. 21:1557, 1961.

455. Sockett, D. C., et al.: Malignant melanoma in a goat. JAVMA 185:907, 1984.

456. Spradbrow, P. B., et al.: Immunotherapy of bovine ocular squamous cell carcinoma. Vet. Rec. 100:376, 1977.

457. Spradbrow, P. B., et al.: Papillomaviruses with unusual restriction endonuclease profiles from bovine skin warts. Aust. Vet. J. 60:259, 1983.

458. Spradbrow, P. B., and Ford, J.: Bovine papillomavirus type 2 from bovine cutaneous papillomas in Australia. Aust. Vet. J. 60:78, 1983.

459. Spradbrow, P. B., and Hoffman, D.: Bovine ocular squamous cell carcinoma. Vet. Bull. 50:449, 1980.

460. Stannard, A. A.: The skin. In: Mansmann, R. A., et al. (eds.): Equine Medicine and Surgery II. Santa Barbara, CA, American Veterinary Publications, 1972, p. 381.

461. Stannard, A. A., and Pulley, L. T.: Tumors of the skin and soft tissues. In: Moulton, J. E.: Tumors in Domestic Animals II. Berkeley, University of California Press, 1978, p. 16.

462. Stannard, A. A.: Some important dermatoses in the horse. Mod. Vet. Pract. 53:31, 1972.

463. Stannard, A. A.: Equine dermatology. Proc. Am. Assoc. Equine Pract. 22:273, 1976.

464. Stephens, K. A., and Mullowney, P. C.: Disseminated mastocytoma in an Angus bull. Compend. Cont. Educ. 8:S307, 1986.

465. Strafuss, A. C., et al.: Cutaneous melanoma in miniature swine. Lab. Anim. Care 18:165, 1968.

466. Strafuss, A. C.: Squamous cell carcinoma in horses. JAVMA 168:61, 1976.

467. Strafuss, A. C., et al.: Sarcoid in horses. Vet. Med. Small Anim. Clin. 68:1246, 1973.

468. Sullins, K. E., et al.: Equine sarcoid. Equine Pract. 8:21, 1986.

469. Sundberg, J. P., et al.: Neoplasms of Equidae. JAVMA 170:150, 1977.

470. Sundberg, J. P., et al.: Equine papillomatosis: Is partial resection of lesions an effective treatment? Vet. Med. 80:71, 1985.

471. Sundberg, J. P., et al.: Immunoperoxidase localization of papilloma viruses in hyperplastic and neoplastic epithelial lesions of animals. Am. J. Vet. Res. 45:1441, 1984.

472. Swan, R. A., et al.: Attempted transmission and immunotherapy of squamous cell carcinoma of the vulva of ewes. Aust. Vet. J. 60:314, 1983.

473. Swan, R. A., et al.: The epidemiology of squamous cell carcinoma of the perineal region of sheep: Abattoir and flock studies. Aust. Vet. J. 61:146, 1984.

474. Sykes, J. A., et al.: Bovine ocular squamous cell carcinoma. IV. Tissue culture studies of bovine ocular squamous cell carcinoma and its benign precursor lesions. J. Natl. Cancer Inst. 26:445, 1961.

475. Szezech, G. M., et al.: Hemangioma of the scrotum in a Chester White boar. Can. Vet. J. 14:16, 1973.

476. Tacal, J. V., et al.: Melanoma in a piglet. Indian Vet. J. 38:622, 1961.

477. Tajima, M., et al.: Electron microscopy of bovine papilloma and deer fibroma. Am. J. Vet. Res. 29:1185, 1968.

478. Tanwar, R. K., et al.: Congenital dermoid-like cyst in a neonatal calf. Vet. Med.79:706, 1984.

479. Tarwid, J. N., et al.: Equine sarcoids: A study with emphasis on pathologic diagnosis. Compend. Cont. Educ. 7:S293, 1985.

480. Taylor, R. L., and Kunks, M. A.: Developmental changes in precursor lesions of bovine ocular carcinoma. Vet. Med. Small Anim. Clin. 67:669, 1972.

481. Taylor, R. L., and Hanks, M. A.: Viral isolations from bovine eye tumors. Am. J. Vet. Res. 30:1885, 1969.

482. Teredesai, A.: Kongenitale Histiozytose der Haut beim Ferkel. Berl. Munch. Tierarztl. Wochenschr. 87:253, 1974.

483. Theilen, G. H., and Fowler, M. E.: Lymphosarcoma (lymphocytic leukemia) in the horse. JAVMA 140:923, 1962.

484. Theilen, G. H., and Madewell, B. R.: Veterinary Cancer Medicine. Philadelphia, W. B. Saunders Co., 1979.

485. Theilen, G. H.: Papillomatosis (warts). In: Robinson, N. E. (ed.): Current Therapy in Equine Medicine. Philadelphia, W. B. Saunders Co., 1983, p. 536.

486. Theilen, G. H., et al.: Goat papillomatosis. Am. J. Vet. Res. 46:2519, 1985.

487. Thirloway, L., et al.: Malignant melanomas in a Duroc boar. JAVMA 170:345, 1977.

488. Thomas, A. D.: Skin cancer of the Angora goat in South Africa. Rep. Dir. Vet. Serv. S. Afr. 15:659, 1929.

489. Thomsett, L. R.: Hamartoma in the calf. Vet. Dermatol. News. 3:56, 1978.

490. Thomsett, L. R.: Noninfectious skin diseases of horses. Vet. Clin. North Am. Large Anim. Pract. 6:59, 1984.

491. Traub, J. L., and Schroeder, W. G.: Malignant melanoma in a horse. Vet. Med. Small Anim. Clin. 75:261, 1980.

492. Traver, D. S., et al.: Epidural melanoma causing posterior paresis in a horse. JAVMA 170:1400, 1977.

493. Treufield, K., et al.: Sequences of papillomavirus DNA in equine sarcoids. Equine Vet. J. 17:449, 1985.

494. Turk, J. R., et al.: Cystic lymphangioma in a colt. JAVMA 174:1228, 1979.

495. Turner, C. B.: An oral papilloma in a young calf. Vet. Rec. 95:367, 1974.

496. Tuthill, R. J., et al.: Equine melanotic disease: A unique animal model for human dermal melanocytic disease. Lab. Invest. 46:85A, 1982.

497. Tuthill, R. J., et al.: Pilar neurocristic hamartoma: Its relationship to blue nevus and equine melanotic disease. Arch. Dermatol. 118:592, 1982.

498. Vandergraff, R.: Squamous cell carcinoma of the vulva in Merino sheep. Aust. Vet. J. 52:21, 1976.

499. Van der Heide, L.: Some cases of cutaneous carcinoma in goat and cow in Curacao. Tijdschr. Diergeneeskd. 88:510, 1963.

500. Van Kampen, K. R., et al.: The immunologic therapy of squamous cell carcinoma. Am. J. Obstet. Gynecol. 116:569, 1975.

501. Vanselow, B. A., et al.: Papilloma viruses, papillomas, and squamous cell carcinomas in sheep. Vet. Rec. 110:561, 1982.

502. Vanselow, B. A., and Spradbrow, P. B.: Squamous cell carcinoma of the vulva, hyperkeratosis and papillomas in a ewe. Aust. Vet. J. 60:194, 1983.

503. Vaughan, J. T., et al.: Condyloma acuminata. J. Cutan. Pathol. 3:244, 1976.

504. Venkatesan, R. A., et al.: A note on the incidence of melanoma on goat skin. Indian J. Anim. Sci. 49:154, 1979.

505. Vijaykumar, D. S., et al.: Corynebacterium parvum–induced regression of horn cancer in a bullock. Vet. Med. Small Anim. Clin. 78:1905, 1983.

506. Vitovec, J.: Statistical data on 370 cattle tumours collected over the years 1964–1973 in South Bohemia. Zbl. Vet. Med. A 23:445, 1976.

507. Vogt, D. W., and Anderson, D. E.: Studies on bovine ocular

squamous cell carcinoma "cancer eye." XV. Heritability of susceptibility. J. Hered. 55:133, 1964.

508. Voss, J. L.: Transmission of equine sarcoid. Am. J. Vet. Res. 30:183, 1969.

509. Waldvogel, A., and Hauser, B.: Bovine kutane angiomatose in der Schweiz. Schweiz. Arch. Tierheilkd. 125:329, 1983.

510. Walker, D.: Defining the equine sarcoid. Vet. Rec. 96:494, 1975.

511. Waller, T., and Rubarth, S.: Hemangioendothelioma in domestic animals. Acta Vet. Scand. 8:234, 1967.

512. Ward, J. M., and Whitlock, R. H.: Chemotherapy of equine leukemia with amethopterin. Vet. Med. Small Anim. Clin. 62:1003, 1967.

513. Watrous, B. J., and Rendano, V. T.: Radiographic interpretation—a case report. Mod. Vet. Pract. 61:188, 1980.

514. Watson, R. E., et al.: Cultural characteristics of a cell line derived from an equine sarcoid. Appl. Microbiol. 24:727, 1972.

515. Watson, R. E., and Larson, K. A.: Detection of tumor-specific antigens in an equine cell line. J. Immunol. 9:714, 1974.

516. Webster, W. M.: Neoplasia in food animals with special reference to the high incidence in sheep. N.Z. Vet. J. 14:203, 1966.

517. Weiss, E.: The pathology of the tissue mast cell in domestic animals. *In*: Rook, A. J., and Walton, G. S.: *Comparative Physiology and Pathology of the Skin.* Oxford, Blackwell Scientific Publications, 1965, p. 413.

518. Weiss, E., and Frese, K.: Tumours of the skin. Bull. WHO 50:79, 1974.

519. Weiss, E.: Tumours of the soft (mesenchymal) tissues. Bull. WHO 50:101, 1974.

520. Wells, G. A. H., and Morgan, G.: Multifocal haemangioma in a pig. J. Comp. Pathol. 90:483, 1980.

521. Wettimuny, S. G.: Das Vulvakarzinom bei Rindern auf Ceylon. Zbl. Vet. Med. A 21:834, 1974.

522. Wheat, J. D.: Therapy for equine sarcoids. Mod. Vet. Pract. 45:62, 1964.

523. Williams, C. S. F.: Differential diagnosis of caseous lymphadenitis in the goat. Vet. Med. Small Anim. Clin. 75:1165, 1980.

524. Williams, I. F., et al.: Connective tissue composition of the equine sarcoid. Equine Vet. J. 14:305, 1982.

525. Wilson, R. G., et al.: Alimentary lymphosarcoma in a horse with cutaneous manifestations. Equine Vet. J. 17:148, 1985.

526. Winston, M., et al.: Treatment of equine sarcoids. JAVMA 175:775, 1979.

527. Wiseman, A., et al.: Melanotic neuro-ectodermal tumour of infancy (melanotic progonoma) in two calves. Vet. Rec. 101:264, 1977.

528. Witt, R. P.: Treating ocular carcinoma in cattle. Vet. Med. 80:1087, 1984.

529. Wood, A. L., and Spradbrow, P. B.: Transformation of cultured equine fibroblasts with a bovine papillomavirus. Res. Vet. Sci. 38:241, 1985.

530. Woodward, R. R., and Knapp, B.: The hereditary aspects of cancer eye in Hereford cattle. J. Anim. Sci. 9:578, 1950.

531. Wyman, M., et al.: Immunotherapy in equine sarcoid: A report of two cases. JAVMA 171:449, 1977.

532. Wyn-Jones, G.: Treatment of periocular tumours of horses using radioactive gold[198] grains. Equine Vet. J. 11:3, 1979.

533. Wyn-Jones, G.: Treatment of equine cutaneous neoplasia by radiotherapy using iridium[192] linear sources. Equine Vet. J. 15:361, 1983.

534. Yager, J. A., and Scott, D. W.: The skin and appendages. *In*: Jubb, K. V., et al.: *Pathology of Domestic Animals III.* Vol. I. New York, Academic Press, 1985, p. 407.

535. Zubaidy, A. J.: Caprine neoplasms in Iraq: Case reports and review of the literature. Vet. Pathol. 13:460, 1976.

INDEX

Note: Numbers in *italics* refer to illustrations; numbers followed
by t refer to tables.